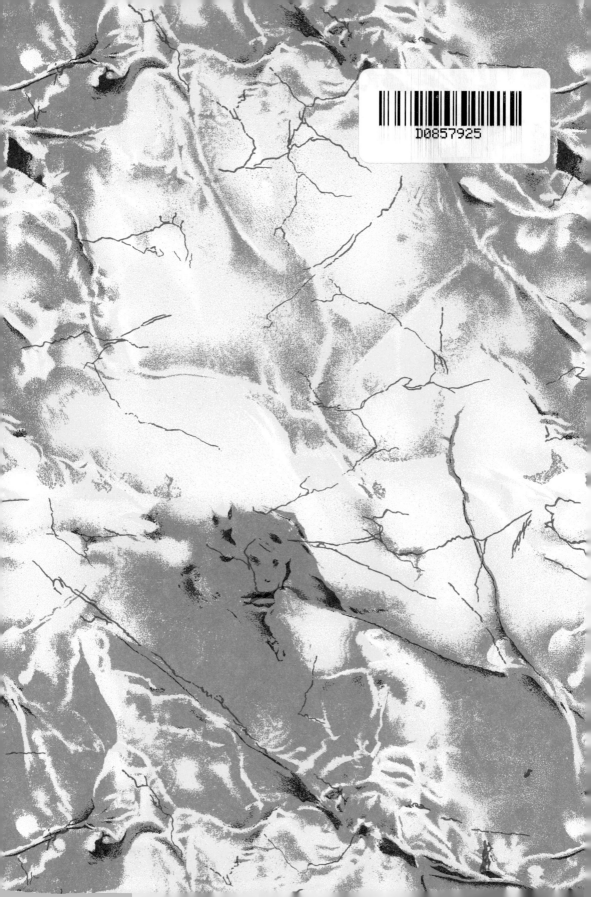

ACCOMMODATION
AND
REFRACTION OF THE EYE

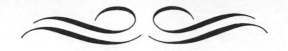

ACCOMMODATION
AND
REFRACTION OF THE EYE

by

F. C. DONDERS

(Fascimile of 1864 Edition)

ROBERT E. KRIEGER PUBLISHING COMPANY
1979

ORIGINAL EDITION 1864
REPRINT WITH NEW INTRODUCTION
1979

PRINTED AND PUBLISHED BY
ROBERT E. KRIEGER PUBLISHING COMPANY INC.
645 NEW YORK AVENUE, HUNTINGTON, NEW YORK 11743

Library of Congress Cataloging in Publication Data

Donders, Franciscus Cornelis, 1818-1889.
    On the anomalies of accommodation and refraction of the
eye.

    (Classics in opthalmology)
    Reprint of the 1864 ed. published by the New Sydenham
Society, London, as v. 22 of its Publications.
    Includes index.
    1. Eye—Accommodation and refraction. I. Title.
    II. Title:Accommodation and refraction of the eye.
    III. Series. IV. Series:
New Sydenham Society. Publications; v. 22.
[DNLM: WW D679o 1864a]
RE925.D68   1979   617.7'55   78-27045
ISBN 0-88275-839-X

INTRODUCTION

by

PAUL HENKIND, M.D., Ph.D.

Frans Cornelius Donders (1818-1889) a physiologist and ophthalmologist, was one of three men who lifted ophthalmology into the stream of modern medicine. This trio, von Graefe, a German; Bowman, an Englishman; and Donders, a Dutchman; met as young men and maintained a close association as long as they lived. They are immortalized by the three most important prizes in ophthalmology, the von Graefe, Bowman and Donders medals.

In 1862, Dr. Donders published a monograph on astigmatism and cylindrical lenses at a time when ophthalmologists knew little about the subject and trial cases contained only spherical lenses. He was working on a more definitive manuscript dealing with refractive errors and accommodation when this work became known to Jonathan Hutchinson, Secretary of the New Sydenham Society who arranged for it to be translated and published. Thus, this great work by a Dutchman appeared in print for the first time in English and was later translated into French, German, and Italian. A revised summary was eventually prepared for Dutch readers by Donders in 1969.

There can be no doubt that this was the most influential book on refraction that appeared in the nineteenth century. The work is laced with practical points and illustrative cases and it is surprising how relevant it seems today. The reader will certainly smile when he comes across information that is the source of the modern day practice of refraction. This is a book which has stood the test of time and which glows more brightly as the years pass.

THE NEW SYDENHAM SOCIETY.

INSTITUTED MDCCCLVIII.

VOLUME XXII.

ON THE ANOMALIES OF

ACCOMMODATION

AND

REFRACTION OF THE EYE.

WITH A PRELIMINARY ESSAY ON

PHYSIOLOGICAL DIOPTRICS.

BY

F. C. DONDERS, M.D.,

PROFESSOR OF PHYSIOLOGY AND OPHTHALMOLOGY IN THE UNIVERSITY OF UTRECHT.

TRANSLATED FROM THE AUTHOR'S MANUSCRIPT BY

WILLIAM DANIEL MOORE, M.D., Dub., M.R.I.A.,

HONORARY FELLOW OF THE SWEDISH SOCIETY OF PHYSICIANS, OF THE NORWEGIAN MEDICAL SOCIETY, AND OF
THE ROYAL MEDICAL SOCIETY OF COPENHAGEN.

THE NEW SYDENHAM SOCIETY,
LONDON.

MDCCCLXIV.

LONDON :
Printed by J. W. ROCHE, 5, Kirby Street,
Hatton Garden.

TO

WILLIAM BOWMAN, F.R.S.,

WHOSE MERITS IN THE

ADVANCEMENT OF PHYSIOLOGY AND OPHTHALMOLOGY

ARE EQUALLY RECOGNISED AND HONOURED

IN EVERY COUNTRY,

THIS WORK ON THE ANOMALIES OF REFRACTION AND

ACCOMMODATION IS,

IN TESTIMONY OF THE WARMEST FRIENDSHIP

AND OF THE HIGHEST ESTEEM,

INSCRIBED BY

THE AUTHOR.

PREFACE.

My essay upon *Ametropie en hare gevolgen* ("Ametropia and its Results"), published in 1860, was confined to the anomalies of refraction, and treated of these exclusively from the dioptric point of view.

In the preface, however, I announced my intention of producing, subsequently to the appearance of that essay, a complete system of the anomalies of refraction and accommodation: the anomalies of refraction, including the subject of astigmatism, were to be treated of also from an anatomical and practical point of view, and the anomalies of accommodation were to be developed both in their opposition to, and their connexion with, the anomalies of refraction.

When, later, I was honoured with a request, on the part of the New Sydenham Society, to prepare my essay for an English edition, I felt bound to endeavour to complete my work on the plan alluded to. This I have done to the best of my ability. The experience of many years, the examination of many thousands of eyes, in which I have been zealously assisted by several of my pupils, have been made available. I believe that my work has gained by its enlargement. I cannot, however, fail to regret that its bulk has increased beyond my expectation, and I feel bound to apologise to the Council both for the delay in its appearance, and for the inconsiderate manner in which I have used the liberty allowed me for its extension. May the intrinsic value of the additions made plead successfully in my behalf.

One object I have kept constantly in view,—to make the book, notwithstanding its great size, useful and, in all its parts, easily accessible to the practical physician. To this end, in the first place, each subject is fully treated of in the body of the text;

consequently, only those who wish to penetrate more deeply into the subject, need attend to the details of the investigation, to the mathematical demonstration, and to the history, added as an appendix, in smaller type. And, in the second place, to facilitate reference to the several parts, each chapter is so drawn up, that the reader's knowledge of what has gone before, is not taken for granted. The work forms, in a certain sense, a series of lesser monographs, united in a single volume, which is the emblem of their mutual connexion.

For the oculist it is perhaps an additional advantage that I am no mathematician. I freely admit that I am not competent to follow the investigations of Gauss and of Bessel in this department, and even the study of the physiological dioptrics of Helmholtz required an effort on my part. I have, therefore, sought a way of my own, and, as I believe, I have found it. The whole theory of the cardinal points of compound dioptric systems, as it is here put forward, is quite explicit and elementary, depending almost exclusively upon the mutual comparison of similar triangles. If the road has thus become somewhat longer, it presents this advantage, that it lies open to all. To guard against the possibility of its leading on any point to error, I have requested my friend Hoek, our Professor of Astronomy, to look over it, and to his kindness I am indebted for many improvements in the form of the demonstration.

In the doctrine of the anomalies of refraction and accommodation, the connexion between science and practice is more closely drawn together than in any part of medicine.

Science here celebrates her triumph; for it is at her hand that this branch has acquired the exact character, which makes it also worthy of the attention of natural philosophers and physiologists. It is, indeed, satisfactory to see, how in the accurate distinction between anomalies of refraction and accommodation, with exclusion of every condition foreign to these anomalies, the system assumed, as if spontaneously, an elegant simplicity, and how the cause and mode of origin of many an obscure type of disease emerged into the clearest light.

Practice, in connexion with science, here enjoys the rare, but splendid satisfaction, of not only being able to give infallible precepts based upon fixed rules, but also of being guided by a clear insight into the principles of her actions—advantages the more highly to be estimated as the anomalies in question are of more frequent occurrence, and as they more deeply affect the use and functions of the eyes.

Is it then strange that the study and treatment of my subject have been to me a labour of love? the more so, as I felt proud in having been called upon to elaborate it for a country in which Young, Wells, Ware, Brewster, and Airy have pointed out to us the track which we had only to follow, and happy in being able to offer my work in this form to my highly esteemed friends and colleagues, whose proofs of kindness and affection have left with me the most agreeable recollection of my visits to England.

Among the privileges, which my task has procured me, dear friend Moore, is the agreeable relation into which it has brought me with you. If I have admired your talent, and highly appreciated your unwearied care, I have, above all, to thank you heartily for the interest and the love, with which the difficult task of the translation of my work has been accomplished by you. I feel that we have become friends, and friends we shall continue. You will, I am certain, gladly join me in thanking the Rev. Professor Haughton, for the solution of many doubtful points, and for his kind revision of certain portions of the work.

F. C. DONDERS.

UTRECHT, 27th February, 1864.

NOTICE BY THE TRANSLATOR.

THE author having mentioned in his preface the circumstances which have led to the appearance of the present volume, it now remains only to state, in addition, that every page of the book has received his careful correction and revision. I should wish also to observe, that the chapter on Astigmatism is not a mere translation of his essay on that subject, published in the year 1862, but that it has received so many amendments and additions, as to represent a second edition of the work in question, brought down to the present day, and enriched with the results of the latest researches bearing upon that remarkable phenomenon.

While I have to congratulate myself, that the free and unrestricted correspondence with Professor Donders, which it has been my privilege to enjoy during the translation of his work, his courtesy and readiness to solve the difficulties arising from the complicated nature of the subject-matter of the book, and his accurate knowledge of the English language, have enabled me to avoid any serious misconceptions of his meaning; I am only too painfully conscious of many defects in the manner of the translation, some of which my present experience would have enabled me to avoid. These, as the wiser course, I would here have passed over in silence, were it not that I think it absolutely necessary to explain one or two points connected with some of them.

For example, when I first met with the words *zenuwvlak* and *gezigtszenuwvlak*, I translated them too literally (pp. 354 *et seq.*) by the terms "nerve-surface," "surface of the optic nerve," "plane of the optic nerve," instead of by the shorter phrase "optic disc," by which this part is now designated by several modern ophthalmological writers, and which I have in the later sheets of the volume exclusively employed.

In like manner I have to apologise for having followed the Dutch orthography of the term "kyklitis" (p. 370), instead of that of English, French, and German writers, in accordance with which the word should have been written "cyclitis."

But I may, in reference to this point, mention, that the word in question is not to be found in any Medical Dictionary (Mayne, Dunglison, Palmer, &c.) which I have had an opportunity of consulting. For this reason, I sometime since requested Professor Donders to supply me with a footnote, giving the meaning and derivation of the term. But as the note did not reach me in time for insertion in its proper place, I venture to introduce it here, giving a reference in the index, by which it may at once be found.

" Kyklitis, the cyclitis of English and German ophthalmological writers, the *cyclíte* of the French, is a term recently introduced to signify inflammation of the ciliary muscle (or ligament) and the neighbouring parts of the sclerotic, and ciliary processes. It is derived from the Greek word κύκλος, the circle or orbiculus ciliaris."

Having mentioned these, as it seems to me, necessary matters, I shall not dwell longer upon my own deficiencies, nor find fault with the kindness of the author, which has led him to take a far too favourable view of the manner in which I have discharged the humble part assigned to me in the production of the English (and in point of priority of publication, original) version of his important work; I shall content myself with thanking him heartily for his courtesy and readiness on all occasions to solve every difficulty submitted to him, and for the care with which he has revised at least two proofs of every sheet of the translation. Nor can I sufficiently express my thanks to the Rev. Samuel Haughton, M.D., F.R.S., Fellow of Trinity College, and Professor of Geology in the University of Dublin, for the trouble he has taken in correcting for the press the mathematical portions of the work. Professor Haughton has also been good enough to furnish me with a few footnotes, to which he has, at my request, attached his initials. To Mr. Bowman, F.R.S., I am deeply indebted for many valuable suggestions, and for much important help, freely and kindly offered, and most willingly afforded.

7, South Anne Street, Dublin,
March 4th, 1864.

CONTENTS.

GENERAL PART.

CHAPTER IV.

SPECIAL PART.

CHAPTER V.

CHAPTER VI.

CHAPTER VII.

CHAPTER VIII.

CHAPTER IX.

SIGNS AND ABBREVIATIONS USED IN THIS WORK.

ρ, radius.

ρ^0, radius of the cornea in the visual line.

n, coefficient of refraction.

k, nodal point.

h, principal point.

k' and k'', anterior and posterior nodal points of the same system.

h' and h'',   ,,   ,,   principal   ,,   ,,

ϕ' and ϕ'',   ,,   ,,   focal   ,,   ,,

k_1 and k_2, two nodal points of two different systems.

h_1 and h_2, ,,   principal   ,,   ,,

ϕ_1 and ϕ_2, ,,   focal   ,,   ,,

o, optical centre.

F′ and F″, anterior and posterior principal focal distances.

G′ and G″, the principal focal distances calculated from k' and k''.

F, principal focal distance where F′ and F″ are equal.

G, the same, calculated from k, where G′ and G″ are equal.

f' and f'', conjugate focal distances calculated from h' and h''.

g' and g'',   ,,   ,,   ,, k' and k''.

B, an object; β, its image.

i, a point in the axis; j, its image.

i', a point outside the axis; j', its image.

p, (proximum) absolute nearest point of distinct vision.

p_1, (,,   ) relative   ,,   ,,   ,,

p_2, (,,   ) binocular   ,, .   ,,   ,,

r, (remotissimum) absolute farthest point of distinct vision.

r_1,   relative   ,,   ,,   ,,

r_2,   binocular   ,,   ,,   ,,

P, P$_1$, and P$_2$, distances from p, p_1, and p_2 to k'.

R, R$_1$, and R$_2$,   ,, r, r_1, and r_2 ,,

P′ P″, and R′ R″,   ,, p, and from r to a lens or another given point.

1 : A, absolute range of accommodation.

1 : A$_1$, relative   ,,   ,,

1 : A$_2$, binocular   ,,   ,,

O, the eye; D or R, right; S or L, left.

C, the cornea.

L, crystalline lens.

l, a lens.

N, the retina.

V, the vitreous humour.

D, the thickness of a lens.

x, distance of a lens from a point.

a, angle between visual line and axis of the cornea.

S, Acuteness of vision.

E, Emmetropia.

H, Hypermetropia.

Hm, manifest H.

Hl, latent H.

Ht, total H.

M, Myopia.

Pr, Presbyopia.

As, Astigmatism.

Ah, Hypermetropic astigmatism.

Am, Myopic   ,,

Amh and Ahm, mixed ,,

In H, in the horizontal principal meridian.

In V, in the vertical   ,,   ,,

M_o, principal meridian of maximum of curvature of the eye.

M_c,   ,,   ,,   ,,   ,,   ,, cornea.

M_l,   ,,   ,,   ,,   ,,   ,, crystalline lens.

A_s, Astigmatism of the whole eye.

A_{sc},   ,,   ,, cornea.

A_{sl},   ,,   ,, crystalline lens.

<, less than.

>, greater than.

$^0/_0$, per cent.

′ (after a numeral) foot or feet, as 2′, 2 feet.

″ (,,   ,,) inch or inches, as 2″, 2 inches.

‴ (,,   ,.) line or lines, as 2‴, 2 lines.

ERRATA.

Page 23, line 17 from above—*For* "`Moreover," *read* " We admit that."

  "   40, "   6 from below—*Dele* "to."

  "   67, "   7 from below—*For* "19·875," *read* "14·858."

  "   75, " 21 from above—The words, "the correctness," &c., and the following lines, 22 to 32, are incorrect, and may be entirely omitted.

  "   75, "   4 from below—*For* " $\phi'\,h' = \phi''\,h''$," *read* " $\phi'\,h' = \phi'\,k''$."

  "   "   "   4 from below—*For* " $\phi''\,h''$," *read* " $\phi''\,k''$."

  "   "   "   3, 4, and 5—*For* " ij," *read* " y."

  "   81, line 17 from below—*For* "measure," *read* "mean."

  "   83, " 15 from above—*For* "adjoining," *read* "nearer."

  "   91, "   7 to 15 from below, " : 18 " should throughout be " 12."

  " 143—*For* " § 12," *read* " § 13."

  " 169—*For* " Note to § 12," *read* " Note to § 13."

  " 170, line 10 from above—*For* "should," *read* "would."

  " 173, " 13 from above—*For* " can," *read* " cannot."

  " 173, " 13 from above—*For* " and," *read* "but."

  " 173, " 16 from above—*For* " § 13," *read* " § 14."

  " 174, "   8 from below—*For* " taxation," *read* "determination."

  " 178, " 19 from below—*For* " ϕ'," *read* " ζ."

  " 178, " 19 from below—*For* " ζ," *read* " $\phi_{,}$."

  " 204—*For* " § 16," *read* " § 17."

  " 212, line 4 from below—*After* " care," *read* "not."

  " 256, " 20 from below—*For* " another," *read* " excessive."

  " 273, "   5 from below—New line should not begin until after " free."

  " 358, "   3 from below—*For* " Artl," *read* " Arlt."

  " 389, "   3 from above—"Among" should begin a new line.

  " 396, "   7 from below—*For* "limitations," *read* "interruptions."

  " 398, " 14 from below—*For* " limitations," *read* " limitations and interruptions."

  " 400, " 19 from above—*For* " disproportionate," *read* " irregular."

  " 533, "   9 from below—"II. Acquired regular astigmatism" should be in italics, to correspond to " 1. Congenital astigmatism," p. 512.

GENERAL PART.

INTRODUCTION.

§ 1.—On the conditions of accurate vision.—Function of
the retina.

In order to see an object distinctly and accurately, two conditions
must be fulfilled. In the first place, an inverted, but well-defined,
image of the object must be formed on the surface of the membrana
Jacobi or layer of rods and bulbs of the retina.* In the second place,
the local change here excited must be conveyed to the fibres of the
optic nerve, communicated to the brain, and again, in an inverted
direction, projected outwards.

Through this double inversion the projected image corresponds to
the object, and we therefore say that we see the object, although,
properly speaking, only the projected retinal image stands, as it were,
before our eyes.

Every disturbance of vision depends on a disturbance in one of
these two conditions, or in both together. If the projection outwards be disturbed, by anomalies in the retina, in the optic nerve,
or in the brain, the affection belongs to the domain of amblyopia or
amaurosis. If no image be formed, or if the image be clouded
through diffusion of light in the eye, obscurities in the way of the
radiation of light through the organ are the foundation of the mis-
chief. Lastly, if the image of objects placed at the ordinary distances
of distinct vision, be not formed on the layer of rods and bulbs, or
even if, through abnormity in the curving of the surfaces, no defined
image is on the whole produced, anomalies of refraction or of
accommodation are developed.

The lesions of vision, for each eye separately, may therefore all
be referred to *three* principal classes: amblyopia, obscurities, anomalies of refraction and of accommodation. If the power of vision of

* See note to § 1.

1

an eye be impaired, one of these three species of disturbance must necessarily exist.

A glance with the ophthalmoscope into such an eye will show whether obscurity of the light-refracting media be present or not. If such be not found, we may infer the existence of either amblyopia or of disturbance of refraction or of accommodation. If now, even with the aid of convex glasses, perfectly-defined vision can at no distance be obtained, the case is one of amblyopia. If, on the contrary, the power of vision be, at one distance or other, accurately defined; or if, at least, by the employment of a convex glass, a perfect definition be attainable, we have to deal with an anomaly of refraction or accommodation, opacity and amblyopia are excluded.

The difference between lesions of refraction and of accommodation is deducible from the words themselves. The lesions of refraction are to be sought in the structure of the eye, in the condition of rest, without attendant action of accommodation. The disturbances of accommodation, on the other hand, have their foundation in abnormal action of the internal muscular system of the eye. This will be more fully explained in Chapter II.

NOTE ON § 1.

At the termination of the nerves of sense, especially of the optic and acoustic nerves, peripheric apparatus are found, which are of great importance in the reception of the stimulus. This, anatomy has taught us. Anatomy has shown that the retina is not a simple expansion of the optic nerve, but that behind the fibres of the latter several layers are developed. To investigate the signification of these is the task of the physiologist.

In order to see and to distinguish these layers, it is merely necessary to macerate in a watery fluid, thin sections of the fresh, but slightly dried, connected membranes of the eye.

To study them accurately, the methods proposed by H. Mueller are made use of. Reckoning from without, we find the following layers (Fig. 1., taken from the drawing by Mueller and Kölliker, in Ecker's *Icones*).

    I. The layer of rods, or staff-like bodies, and bulbs.

    II. The external granular layer.

    III. The middle granular layer.

    IV. The internal granular layer.

    V. The finely granular layer.

    VI. The layer of nerve-cells.

    VII. The layer of the optic-fibres.

These layers are thickest close to the optic nerve, where the figure is taken, and all become attenuated towards the ora serrata, particularly VII. which here terminates.

In the yellow spot the structure is peculiar. The nerve-cells VI. here form a very thick layer, not covered by a layer of optic fibres, but merely interwoven with a small number of these fibres ; the layers V., IV., III., and II. are in this situation particularly thin, and layer I. possesses no staff-like bodies, or rods, but consists exclusively of bulbs. In proportion as we withdraw from the yellow spot, the several bulbs become surrounded by more and more numerous rods.

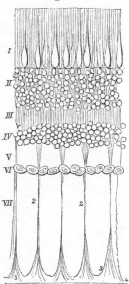

Fig. 1.

The central portion of the yellow spot, the fovea centralis, the most important part of the retina, is now particularly to be distinguished : the expansion in this situation becomes exceedingly thin ; layer I., consisting exclusively of slender bulbs, is here covered only by scarcely perceptible traces of the other layers.

The elements of the several layers are united and enveloped by a proper connective tissue, wherein, after the action of chromic acid, bundles of radiating fibres (2) are separately distinguished ; these extend from (1) the boundaries between I. and II. to an innermost investing vitreous membrane (membrana limitans (4), into which they are divergingly (3) inserted (radiating fibres of Mueller). Omitting the connective tissue, we may in a physiological point of view provisionally reduce the layers of the retina to three :—1. the fibrous layer, belonging to the optic nerve ; 2. the layer of rods and bulbs, the perceptive layer ; 3. the intervening layers, effecting the connexion between the two first-named.

1. The fibrous layer, distinguished above as VII :—It is the immediate continuation of the optic nerve, whose fibres, even before they have entered the eye, lose the medullary sheath, and in their membranous expansion, as the innermost layer of the retina, continue quite unchanged. The fibres of the optic nerve themselves are insensible to the stimulus of the vibrations of light. Its entrance into the eye may be demonstrated as the blind spot of Mariotte ; and if we allow the little image of a distant flame to move to and fro on the papilla nervi optici, it is, as we can observe in ourselves, and in others with the ophthalmoscope, imperceptible ; it is not until the little image passes the boundary of the papilla, where the other layers of the retina are also present, that the feeble glimmering of light through the whole eye gives way to a completely circumscribed image.

As the membranous expansion is precisely similar to the fibres of the papilla, we cannot expect to find in that expansion more sensibility to the vibrations of light than exists in the nerve itself. And if we consider, that everywhere many layers of these transparent fibres

2

lie over one another, and that the same fibre runs from the ora serrata to the papilla of the optic nerve, it is evident that rays, derived from the same point of an object pass, and necessarily irritate the fibres of different layers, and that the same fibre is struck by rays derived from different points of an object. Therefore, if the fibres were sensitive to the oscillations of light, the localized projection from the retina, or vision, as actually takes place, would be excluded.*

2. The layer of rods and bulbs, which is at least pretty generally considered as the perceptive layer :—The supposition is, that the bulbs and rods, while they are traversed by the undulations of light, undergo a molecular change, and that this change, whatever it may be, excites a secondary modification in the fibres, which were incapable of directly experiencing the stimulus of the light itself.

3. The intervening layers II., III., IV., V., and VI., formed of fibres, nuclear bodies and nerve-cells, whose mutual connection is not yet completely ascertained :—It appears that rods and bulbs are connected with the granules, are continued, as thin nerve-filaments, into the intervening granular and finely-granular layers, enter into connexion with the nerve-cells, which are also mutually connected, and are finally united with the proper nerve-fibres. The meaning of these several layers is as yet quite obscure. For the present we can only say, that they represent the connexion between the perceptive layer of bulbs and rods, and the fibrous layer.

The reasons why the layer of rods and bulbs is considered to be the immediately perceptive lamina, have been designedly passed over in silence under 2, in order to admit of their being here more fully examined. In the first place, the fibrous lamina, as has been shown, does not perceive. One of the other layers must therefore be the directly perceptive layer. The nerve-cells lie in the yellow spot, where perception is more accurate, over one another in numerous laminæ, and therefore appear not to be adapted to the purpose. The same is true of the two granular layers over the whole retina. Thus we come by exclusion to the layer of rods and bulbs. This view is further supported by the following positive reasons :—

1. Precisely in the fovea centralis, where acute, accurately localized, direct vision takes place, the layer of bulbs is present in perfection, and consists of smaller bulbs, from which more defined distinction is to be expected. Almost all the other elements are here wanting. They are pushed aside in the yellow spot, and therefore do not receive the light which excites the images in the fovea centralis, but effect only the transition of the modification to the nerve-fibres. Consequently, the bulbs here lie almost naked, and are immediately accessible to the light. Even the adjoining parts of the yellow spot, which by the accumulation of the elements, particularly of the nerve-cells, are placed in a relatively unfavourable condition, perceive much less acutely and accurately than the fovea centralis itself. That direct vision actually takes place in the latter, I satisfied myself by examination with the ophthalmoscope.

---

* Bowman, *Lectures on the parts concerned in the operations on the Eye.*— London, 1849, p. 82.

2. PURKINJE's experiment proves that the perceptive layer is situated tolerably far behind the fibrous layer. This experiment consists in making the vessels of the retina visible to ourselves. In it, properly speaking, we perceive the shadows of these vessels. The characteristic ramifications are made to appear, by moving a candle to and fro beside the eye, opened and directed towards an uniformly dark chamber ; and still more easily are they rendered visible to any one, by turning the cornea as much as possible towards the nose, and moving the dioptric image of a flame, formed by a convex lens of one or two Parisian inches' focus, to and fro, or up and down on the exposed sclerotic. In either case an image of light is formed on a circumscribed part of the membranes of the eye, which sends out light through the whole eye, but must necessarily in the deeper layers cast shadows of the great vessels of the fibrous layer. The shadows now change their place with the movements of the image of light, and the object (in this case the blood-vessels), which produces the shadows, can therefore not be situated in the layer which perceives the shadows. From the amount of this displacement H. Mueller has inferred, that the perceptive curtain actually lies about where the surface of the layer of bulbs and rods is to be found. (*Verh. der physik.-med. Gesellschaft zu Würzburg*, V. p. 411.)

3. In the eye of the Cephalopodes the layer of rods and bulbs is directed forwards, and immediately receives the incident light, while the other layers situated more posteriorly, are cut off by a dark layer of pigment from the access of the light.

4. The rods and bulbs are traversed over their whole length by the same waves of light, and are therefore in a position to be strongly affected by the latter. Bruecke was the first to point out this. His idea of the layer of rods as a catoptric system is so far perfectly correct, that the rays of light which have entered a rod or bulb, cannot again leave it. In the first place, the most of the rays coming directly from without fall in the direction of these radiatingly-placed elements, and therefore do not reach to the lateral surfaces of boundary ; but, so far as they might reach them, total reflexion must take place in consequence of the obtuse angle of incidence and the so-much-less light-refracting power of the intervening matter. In comparison to this quantity of light, which is limited to the same rods, the quantity of diffuse light reflected by the choroid and sclerotic behind the rods, which is dispersed through various rods in all directions, is very small, and does not interfere with the accuracy of perception. In connexion with the isolated condition of the bundle of rays falling upon each bulb or rod, the most perfect accommodation is obtained, if the accurate image be formed precisely on the surface of the layer of rods and bulbs, consequently in the fovea centralis, exactly at the surface. If it fell first in the middle of the bulbs, there would be at the surface a distribution of light starting from a point and extending over more than a bulb : the accommodation would not be perfect. Therefore, too, the so-called line of accommodation, of which we shall hereafter speak, cannot depend upon the length of the rods, as has been stated. The traversing of the rods in their whole longitudinal direction by the waves of light must produce a very powerful influence, in like manner as a nerve is more strongly affected by a galvanic action, when the latter

passes through a portion in the longitudinal direction of the nerve, than when it permeates the nerve only in a transverse course.

5. Many phenomena respecting the limits of the smallest angles of perception, and the change of form of fine lines, &c., thence arising, agree only with the idea that the layer of bulbs and rods is affected by light.

The question has been started, whether perhaps the bulbs alone, and not the rods, receive the impressions of the light. This suggestion has arisen from the anatomical fact, that in the yellow spot, where perception is most acute, bulbs exclusively occur, immediately touching one another, and that between the bulbs a progressively greater number of rods appear, in proportion as we remove from the yellow spot. The latter circumstance seems, indeed, to indicate, that the acuteness of perception is connected with the number of bulbs; and the same view is corroborated by the great number of nerve-cells occurring here, and the numerous nerve-fibres which are directed towards the yellow spot, and have their peripheric termination in this locality. But we are not thereby justified in denying the capacity of the rods for the impression of light. It is a fact, that every rod cannot have its nerve-fibre; to that end (the place occupied by a rod and nerve-fibre on section being assumed to be equal) the nerve must have a section equal to the surface of the whole retina. There does not even appear to be a nerve-fibre for each bulb. But this by no means proves that each rod may not convey its action to a nerve-fibre, which should then equally receive the stimulus of several adjoining rods, thus precisely furnishing a very intelligible reason why the acuteness of perception of the retina, should constantly diminish from the yellow spot to the ora serrata. The very recent anatomical investigations carried on independently of one another by W. Krause[*] and Braun,[†] have revealed morphological peculiarities in the rods, which still more strongly bring to light their analogy to the bulbs, and thus prove much in favour of the harmony, if not of the similarity of their functions.

---

[*] *Sitzungsberichte der kaiserl. Akademie der Wissenschaften.* Wien, 1860. Bd. XLII., p. 15.

[†] *Nachrichten von der G. A. Universität u. d. königl. Gesellsch. der Wissensch. zu Göttingen.* 1861.

w of the rays proceeding from them being brought, if
, at least into a converging direction.

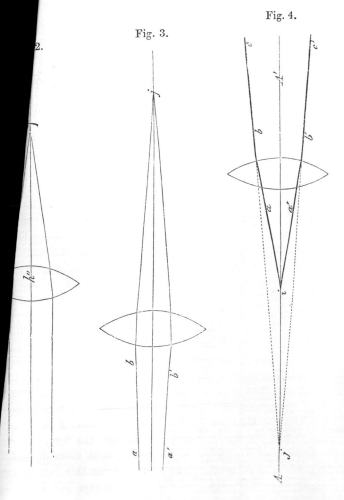

Fig. 4.

Fig. 3.

2.

the normal eye, the retina is placed precisely at the focal dis-
e of the dioptric system. Parallel rays, derived from infinitely
ant objects, are therefore brought into union exactly in the retina.
 objects are accurately perceived. From near objects, as we have
erved, the rays proceed in a diverging direction, and their point
 union in the normal eye, consequently, lies behind the retina,
 yet the organ is capable of perceiving near objects also accurately.

the eye to all
not into unio

Fig.

S″

§ 2.—Proofs o

The media of th
we can accurately
by being acquainte
number of question
as a single lens, wit
is then sufficient to

It is well known
convex lens (Fig. 2), t
nearly into a point,
between a particular
termed the *focal distan*
nitely distant objects.
finite distance, proceed r
such rays fall on the len
almost into a point *j*, but
the principal focus. Such
principal focus is the focus
rays may fall on the lens in
a degree of divergence behin
(Fig. 4 *i*), whence the rays
from the lens than amounts t
rays then acquire after refrac
a direction as if they had com
lens. In the explanation of o
no importance, inasmuch as ob

* This point is called the centre
on the curvatures of the two surface
† Or focus *conjugate* to the point
writers use the word focus, in genera
the focus of parallel rays is by them
rays are not parallel, the points of di
called *conjugate foci.*—S. H.

I
tan
dist
The
obs
of
an

It therefore has the further power of bringing divergent rays into union on the retina. Now, this power of bringing at will rays of different directions into union on the retina is the *power of accommodation of the eye*.

We can easily convince ourselves that the normal eye possesses such a power. That we are able clearly and accurately to distinguish objects at different distances, everyone knows by experience. We need, therefore, only assure ourselves that we *cannot at the same time* plainly distinguish remote and proximate objects, to obtain a proof that an accommodating power exists; in other words, that in the eye a change is produced in connexion with the distance at which we can see accurately. It is almost superfluous to adduce a direct proof in support of this statement. Ordinary observation will abundantly demonstrate it. It is well illustrated by holding a veil at some inches from the eye, and a book at a greater distance; we can then at will see accurately either the texture of the veil, or the letters of the book, but never both together. If we see the texture of the veil, we cannot distinguish the letters of the book; if we read, the veil produces only a feeble, almost uniform obscuration of the field of vision; of the separate threads we see scarcely anything. The circle of diffusion in imperfect accommodation can be most distinctly seen at an illuminated point, or at a darker spot on a piece of ordinary window-glass. The latter is held close to one eye (while the other eye is shut), but so that the point can still be accurately perceived—the objects situated at a certain distance on the other side of the glass are then observed without defined contours. We can now, however, at will, immediately see, in the direction of the point, the objects at the remote side of the glass distinctly, whereupon the point appears as a larger, diffused spot. A change has consequently taken place in the eye. Of this we are ourselves distinctly conscious. When we looked at distant objects through the glass, the eye was adjusted for almost parallel rays; the diverging rays proceeding from the point had therefore their point of union behind the retina. When the point was accurately seen, the eye was accommodated to the diverging rays proceeding from it, and the almost parallel rays derived from the distant objects, had already united in front of the retina, and had decussated in a focus. In uniting, whether before or behind the retina, the rays proceeding from each separate point formed a *round* spot on the retina, instead of a point. The section of these rays has, in fact, nearly the *form of the pupil*, and, if the rays of the cone have not yet been brought into union, or if they have already decussated, they form on the retina a little spot of the form of the pupil. All the little spots, which represent the several points of the object in the retinal picture, are now like so many blotted points of an accurate image covering one another, and it is evident, that the former must, therefore, lose its sharp contour and be diffused on the surface. But as the retinal, so is the projected picture, and we therefore say, that we see the object diffused. In such a state do all objects appear, for which the eye is not accommodated.

§ 3. — CHANGE OF THE DIOPTRIC SYSTEM OF THE EYE IN ACCOMMODATION.

That in the eye, in accommodation, a change is produced, has in the preceding section been placed beyond a doubt. The question now is, in what that change consists? Since Kepler first attempted to answer it, the inquiry has been the constant source of much difference of opinion among natural philosophers and physiologists. All imaginable hypotheses have been advanced. Alteration of situation of the lens, elongation of the axis of vision, contraction of the pupil, change of form of the lens, have all in turns been made use of in the explanation, and those who were satisfied with none of these theories, were sometimes bold enough altogether to deny the existence of an accommodating power. The ophthalmoscope, which enables us to see, in the fundus of the eye, the diffused images of objects for which the eye is not accommodated, effectually silences these last.

It is not my intention to subject anew to criticism the long series of incorrect views upon the subject. I am not writing a history of errors. We now know what change the dioptric system undergoes in accommodation, and the source of this knowledge alone can here be sketched in its leading features. *The change consists in an alteration of form of the lens: above all, its anterior surface becomes more convex and approaches to the cornea.*

It is now nearly sixty years since Thomas Young* had satisfied himself that the power of accommodation depends upon a change of form in the lens. Nor was he led to this conviction merely by the exclusion of other hypotheses; he adduced reasons which, properly

* *Philosophical Transactions*, 1801, vol. xcii. p. 23. Conf. *Miscellaneous Works* of the late TH. YOUNG, edited by GEORGE PEACOCK, Vol. I. p. 12. London, 1855.

understood, should be taken as positive proofs. As an hypothesis the idea had already existed ; but previously to the time of Young it could be considered as little more than a loose assertion, to which no value was to be attached. The force of Young's experiments was, however, not understood, and his doctrine scarcely found a place in the long list of incorrect opinions and hazardous suggestions, which were constantly anew brought forward. Perhaps the necessary attention was not paid to Young's demonstration, because physiologists, not being acquainted with any muscular elements in the eye, could scarcely imagine by what mechanism the crystalline lens should change its form, and they were little inclined to believe with Young [*] in the contractility of the fibres of the lens. It was not until after direct proofs (within the reach of every one's observation and comprehension) of the change of form of the lens had been brought forward by others, that Helmholtz[†] placed the able investigation of Thomas Young in its proper light. The direct proofs were given a few years ago, and to our fellow-countryman Cramer,[‡] too early snatched from science, belongs the highest honour in the matter.

For many years the reflected images of the anterior and posterior surfaces of the lens were generally known. Purkinje had discovered them in 1823, and Sanson had made them available in the diagnosis of cataract (1837). If some doubt still remained respecting the origin of the two reflected images, observed in the eye behind that of the cornea, the doubt was removed by the experiments of Meyer.[§] For the recognition of cataract they lost their value, when more decisive means of attaining it were discovered. But it was they which could give an infallible answer to the question, whether the lens in the accommodation of the eye undergoes a change, either in form or in situation.

Maximilian Langenbeck [‖] was the first to whom it occurred to investigate the reflected images of the lens with reference to this important question. He examined them, however, only with the naked eye, moreover at a very unfavourable angle, almost solely with respect to the depth of their situation in the eye, and we can, therefore, scarcely assume that this investigation was sufficiently

---

[*] *Miscellaneous Works*, Vol. I. pp. 1 *et seq.*

[†] *Allgemeine Encyclopædie der Physik*, herausgegeben von G. Karsten. Erste Lieferung, B. I. pp. 112 *et seq.*

[‡] *Het accommodatie-vermogen, physiologisch toegelicht.* Haarlem, 1853.

[§] *Zeitschrift f. ration. Medizin*, Band V. p. 262. 1846.

[‖] *Klinische Beiträge aus dem Gebiete der Chirurgie u. Ophthalmologie.* Göttingen, 1849.

decisive to produce conviction. Nevertheless, he announced the most important fact : namely, that *in accommodation for near objects the anterior surface of the lens becomes more convex.* This statement lay hidden in a work, whose title was little adapted to attract the attention of physiologists. Accidentally the book fell into my hands. Struck with Langenbeck's fortunate idea, I immediately endeavoured to satisfy myself of the correctness of his assertion ; but owing to defects in the means I employed, no satisfactory result was obtained. That on examination with a magnifier the reflected images should show with certainty, whether in accommodation a change of the crystalline lens arises, I did not hesitate to predict.* I soon heard that Cramer, led by this prediction, had taken up the question.† He comprehended its full importance, solved it in the manner pointed out by me, and so put forward his result, that its correctness was in a very short time universally admitted.

I have above observed, that from the reflected images of the lens we may learn both the *curvature* and the *situation* of its surfaces. Cramer had already deduced both from his investigations.

In the first place, as relates to the curvature, we know that convex mirrors produce a diminished image behind, concave mirrors before the reflecting surface, and that the images are smaller in proportion as the radius of curvature is less. This is easily seen by comparing the reflected image of a flame formed by biconvex spectacles ground with different radii. We see an erect reflected image behind the anterior surface of the glass, and an inverted image before the glass, and both are smaller in proportion to the convexity of the surfaces of the glass employed. The posterior erect image is formed by reflexion on the anterior surface of the glass ; the anterior inverted image is formed by reflexion on the posterior surface, or, to speak more correctly, on the concave surface of the air contiguous with the posterior convex surface. Now, the anterior surface of the crystalline lens is a convex mirror ; the posterior surface, or rather the anterior surface of the vitreous humour corresponding thereto, represents a concave mirror. The reflected images are feebly illuminated, because the difference in refraction between the fluids of the eye and the lens being small, the reflexion is not considerable. They are, how-ever, clearly discernible, when we hold a bright flame at one side of the eye, and look into the organ at the other side. If a line, drawn from the flame to the eye, forms an angle of about 30° with the axis of vision, and if we look at the other side, likewise at an

    * *Nederl. Lancet*, 2ᵉ Sér., D. V., pp. 135 and 147.   † *loc. cit.*

angle of about 30° with the axis of vision, into the eye, the three little images appear flat, close to one another, in the pupil (Fig. 5).

Fig. 5.

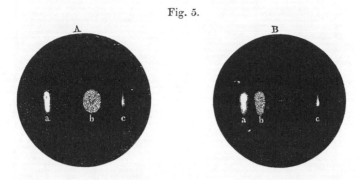

A represents their situation in the eye accommodated for distance; B in the eye accommodated for near objects. In both *a* is the reflected image of the cornea; *b* that of the anterior surface, and *c* that of the posterior surface of the lens. Cramer viewed them magnified 10 or 20 times. He thus convinced himself that the image *b* reflected by the anterior surface of the lens is, in accommodation for near objects, considerably smaller, and he thence correctly inferred that the anterior surface of the lens increases in convexity, that the radius of curvature diminishes. Subsequently Helmholtz,* who, independently of Cramer, had discovered the true principle of accommodation,† has stated that also of the little inverted image *c* formed by reflexion on the surface of the vitreous humour, not only the apparent, but the actual size diminishes a little in accommodation for near objects, and that, consequently, the posterior surface of the lens, too, increases in convexity, although this increase is very slight.

As to the change in situation of the curved surfaces of the lens, this can be determined from the alteration of place of the reflected images. If we compare Fig. 5, A and B, we shall see that in B the image *b* reflected by the anterior surface of the lens, is approximated much more to the reflected image of the cornea *a*, than in A; and Cramer hence inferred that the anterior surface of the lens, which had become more convex, now comes also to lie closer to the cornea.

* *Arch. f. Ophthalmologie*, herausgegeben von Artl, Donders und von Graefe, Bd. I. Abth. 2, p. 1.

† *Monatsberichte der Akademie zu Berlin*, Febr. 1853, p. 137.

The next figure (6) clearly decides this.   A A′ is the axis of the

Fig. 6.

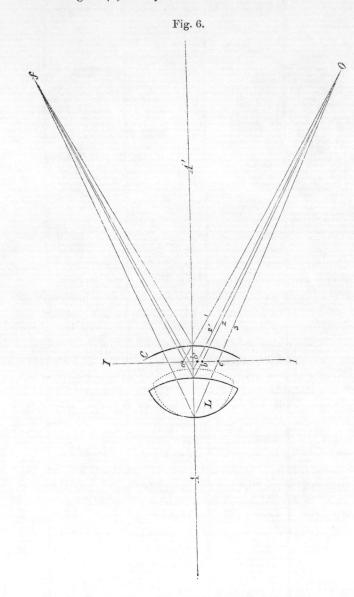

cornea, with which we here assume that the axis of the lens L coincides. The lens is drawn in a double form, namely, with continuous lines in the form of accommodation for distant, and with dotted lines in the form of accommodation for near objects. At f is a flame; at o the eye of the observer. These two are so placed that lines proceeding from them cut each point of the axis at similar angles. Therefore, the rays thrown back by the reflecting surfaces of the observed eye, where these surfaces are cut by the axis, reach the eye of the observer.

The reflected image of the cornea is consequently seen in the direction $O\,1$, and (disregarding refraction on surfaces situated in front) that of the anterior surface of the lens in the direction $O\,2$, that of the posterior surface in the direction $O\,3$. Projected on the surface $I\,I'$, they appear close to one another as a, b, and c (compare also Fig. 5, A). If now the anterior surface of the lens advances to the dotted line, the second image is seen in the direction $O\,2'$, and is therefore projected in the surface $I\,I'$, as b'; it has consequently approached the reflex image a of the cornea (compare the preceding Fig. 5 B). From this change of place, which is easily observed, we therefore infer that, in accommodation for near objects the anterior surface of the lens approaches the cornea. It is, indeed, true that we do not see the images b and b' exactly in the direction of the point where the axis cuts the surface of the lens, because both the incident and the reflected ray is refracted by the cornea in front. But in consequence of the symmetry of the cornea, which, moreover, does not change its form, and the symmetrical position of the eye O, and the flame f, with respect to the axis, the deviations so produced are equally great on both sides, and the above inference, therefore, remains quite correct. If we determine the direction of the radius of the cornea in this place, where the ray reflected on the anterior surface of the lens enters and leaves the latter, we can, from the distance between the images a and b and a and b', calculate the distance from the anterior surface of the lens to the cornea.

Cramer did not observe any displacement of the posterior image. He thence inferred that the situation of the surface did not alter. This inference was hazardous, so long as it was not ascertained how far the change of form of the lens in accommodation might have influence on the place where the image c was seen. Now, however, since the mathematical investigation of Helmholtz has shown, that in consequence of an incidental compensation, such an influence does not at all, or scarcely exist, we are really justified in concluding, from the unaltered situation of the image *c*, that the posterior surface of the crystalline lens in accommodation does not change its situation.

The changes in the dioptric system, observed in accommodation for near objects, therefore, consist in: 1. That the anterior surface of the lens becomes more convex and approaches the cornea, both these alterations taking place to a considerable degree; 2. That the posterior surface of the lens becomes a little more convex, but, notwithstanding, remains at a nearly equal distance from the cornea.—Besides the changes here described, none others occur in the dioptric system in accommodation.   In the first place, Dr. Knapp has proved that the changes occurring in particular persons in the crystalline lens, are, in general, sufficient to account for their range of accommodation; and, in the second place, I have satisfied myself that where the crystalline lens is absent, even in young people, not the slightest trace of accommodating power remains.   Knapp's results are spoken of at the end of the first Chapter; mine shall be subsequently more fully communicated.

NOTE TO § 3.

In order to observe the reflected images, Cramer made use of an instrument, by him called the *ophthalmoscope*, a term which is now generally and more correctly applied to the eye-speculum.   This instrument I have so modified that it can be used for measurements, and I have given to it in this form the name of *phacoidoscope*, which word fully expresses its object.   The most essential elements of this instrument are—(Fig. 7) 1. A horizontal quadrant, divided into degrees; 2. A flame *f* reflected in the observed eye O′; 3. A microscope *m*, through which the observer's eye O sees the observed eye O′ magnified from 15 to 30 times, and in which the slit between two movable vertical surfaces present in the eye-piece, serves as a micrometer; 4. A sight *v*, capable of being placed at different distances from the eye.   The flame impinges unchanged upon 0°, the sight and the microscope can turn horizontally around the middle point from which the quadrant is described; the observed eye O′ is so placed, that its crystalline lens coincides with the middle point of this quadrant.   We can thus alternately fix the sight, placed near the eye, and a distant point situated in the direction of the sight, after having first given a proper position to the microscope and to the sight.   The flame remains, as has been said, in the direction of 0°.   If the microscope be now placed at 60° and the sight close to 30°, we shall usually, on altering the accommodation, see very distinctly the displacement and change of size of the middle image. Properly speaking, the sight ought not to stand at 30°, but at about 5° or 6° from it, as the observed eye must

Fig. 7.

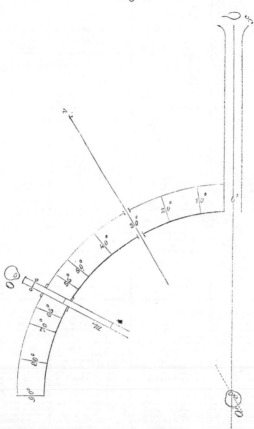

look 5° or 6° more inwards. The axis of vision lies, viz., in general, to the outside of the line of vision (that is the line extending from the yellow spot to the fixed point), and the line of vision must therefore be turned inwards, in order to direct the axis of vision to 30°. If we wish to determine the position of the surface of reflexion of the lens from the distance between the reflected images *a* and *b*, the direction of the axis of the cornea must first be sought in order to place the sight correctly with respect to it.

Helmholtz constructed a peculiar instrument, called by him the *ophthalmometer*, for the purpose of determining the magnitude of the reflected images. This instrument is one of the great treasures for which we are indebted to his genius. Kohlrausch, and also Senff, had already measured the reflected

images, at least that of the cornea, with a magnifying glass. But the ophthalmometer possesses a great advantage over an ordinary magnifier, inasmuch as the trouble and inaccuracy, which in the successive measurements
of the borders of the image must necessarily result from slight movements of
the head and eyes, are avoided in this instrument. The mode of measurement with the heliometer, which enables astronomers accurately to determine
minute dimensions of the planets in constant motion, suggested its construction to Helmholtz. These measurements are accomplished by doubling the
images; the same is true of the ophthalmometer. Objects which are seen
through a plate of glass, bounded by perfectly flat and parallel surfaces,
held obliquely to the line of vision, appear to be in some measure laterally
displaced, and this displacement increases with the magnitude of the angle
of incidence of the rays of light upon the plate. On this simple fact depends the action of the ophthalmometer.

In Fig. 8, let A be a Galilean telescope, before whose object-glass two plano-

Fig. 8.

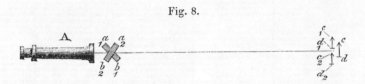

parallel glass-plates, seen in profile in $a_1 b_1$ and $a_2 b_2$, are so placed obliquely
to its axis, that the right half of the object-glass receives its light through
the plate $a_2 b_2$, the left half through the plate $a_1 b_1$, then the image $c d$, to
which the telescope is directed, appears not at $c d$, but through the plate
$a_1 b_1$ at $c_1 d_1$ and through the plate $a_2 b_2$ at $c_2 d_2$. The two images stand at the
same time close to one another in the field of vision of the telescope. If now
the glass-plates be turned so far, that the extremity d_1 of the first coincides
with the extremity c_2 of the second image, and if we know the angle through
which the glass-plates have revolved, with their thickness and the coefficient
of the refracting power of the glass, we can calculate the length $c d$, even
without knowing the distance from A to $c d$. The ophthalmometer is
further so arranged that, on turning round the glass plates, both traverse
equal angles, and it can be read with great accuracy at what angle they are.
Those who desire to learn the details of the construction of the instrument
should consult Helmholtz (*Archiv für Ophthalmologie*, herausgegeben
von Artl, Donders und von Graefe, Bd. 1, Abth. 2, p. 1). At the option
of the observer, $c d$ need not be calculated. If we have a finely divided
measuring-rod, we can empirically determine by what number of degrees
of the ophthalmometer known magnitudes are measured, and prepare a table
of the results. For reasons elsewhere detailed (*Verslagen en Mededeelingen
van de Koninklijke Akademie van Wetenschappen*, Amsterdam, 1861. D.
XI., p. 159), I have even given the preference to this method. From the
degrees on the ophthalmometer, by which a reflected image is measured, we
then immediately find its magnitude in the table; and if we know at the

same time the distance and magnitude of the object, whose image we measure on a curved surface, we can, by a tolerably simple formula, calculate the radius of the curve. If we always use the same object (represented, for example, by the distance between two flames), and if this is always at the same distance from the observed eye, we can in the tables easily add, after the magnitudes of the images, the corresponding radii of curvature, and so immediately read from each observed number of degrees on the ophthalmometer the radius of curvature of the reflecting surface. Such an arrangement exists in the Netherlands Hospital for Diseases of the Eye at Utrecht.

The application of the ophthalmometer to the measurement of the clear reflected images of the cornea is very easy. We observe that in accommodation for each distance the magnitudes of the images, and consequently the radius, remain unalterably the same.

On the anterior surface of the lens the image is too weak and too ill-defined, to allow of the measurement of double images thereof with the ophthalmometer. Helmholtz therefore produced, close to the reflected image of the lens, a changeable reflected image on the cornea, and made this last equal in magnitude to the first, of which he could accurately judge with the naked eye. The magnitude of that of the cornea can then in every case be calculated or measured. The magnitude is estimated most precisely when each reflected image consists of two little tapers, whose mutual distance then represents the size. We obtain the doubling by two candles, or by the reflexion of one candle in a mirror held under the observed eye. The accuracy of the method, however, according to Knapp, who somewhat modified it (*Archiv für Ophthalmol.*, Bd. VI., Abth., 2, p. 1), still left much to be desired. For easy as it is to satisfy one's self of the *alteration* in magnitude of the reflected image *b*, it is difficult, on account of its faintness and want of sharp contours, to determine the *absolute* size of it with the desirable accuracy. The little inverted image of the posterior surface of the lens is well defined. In this instance the ophthalmometer was again applicable, and Helmholtz satisfied himself that the radius of curvature in accommodation for near objects here becomes a little smaller. More accurate determinations, obtained by a modified method,* have led to the same result.

In order to ascertain the place of the anterior surface of the lens, Helmholtz determined that of the margin of the pupil which lies against the lens. The position of the posterior surface, in the determination of which the ophthalmometer again rendered good service, was deduced in a rather complex manner, from that of the reflected image. These determinations of the places of the surfaces of refraction might, as has been already observed, also be obtained with the phacoidoscope.

So far respecting the methods, with reference to which Helmholtz and Knapp may further be compared. As to the results obtained, the necessary statements will be made at the end of this Chapter.

---

* Conf. Knapp, *l. c.* p. 34.

§ 4. On the Mechanism of Accommodation.

So soon as the changes which the dioptric system undergoes in accommodation had become known, physiologists were in a position to investigate, with some hope of success, the mechanism whereby those changes are produced. Many modes of solving this question have been tried. By some, experiment has been resorted to; others have instituted an accurate examination of the anatomy of the parts which appear to be concerned in the mechanism referred to; pathology, finally, has been made use of in prosecuting the inquiry. But, notwithstanding all these efforts, it cannot be said that any theory brought forward has as yet been fully proved: the utmost we have attained to is, that by exclusion, the limits wherein our views may range have been much restricted.

It has been in general tacitly assumed that the accommodation for distance, and even for the farthest point of distinct vision, is purely passive,—that in it only relaxation of the parts which actively produce accommodation for near objects takes place. I believe that this idea was in all respects fully justified. But, if we endeavour to explain the mechanism of accommodation, it is, as a preliminary question, so important, that it may well be specially treated of, the more so, because some advocate an active accommodation also for distant objects. The grounds on which it may, in my opinion, be maintained that accommodation for near objects only is active, while that for distant objects is passive, are the following:—

1. The subjective sensation;—for myself this is conclusive.

2. The phenomena produced by mydriatics. If we drop into the eye, a solution of one part of sulphate of atropia in 120 of water, the pupil, after ten or fifteen minutes, begins to dilate, and soon afterwards the nearest point of distinct vision removes farther and farther from the eye. At the end of forty minutes all action is destroyed, and the eye remains accommodated to its farthest point. The muscular system for accommodation is now paralysed, and paralysis, that is, the highest degree of relaxation, is thus proved to be equivalent to accommodation for the farthest point. Now, did we assume the existence of a distinct system, working actively in accommodation to the farthest point, we ought to maintain—1st, That this system is not paralysed by atropia; 2nd, That it is by this agent brought into a condition in which it

is incapable of relaxation. This supposition would not be quite absurd. Something of the kind is said to occur in the action of atropia upon the iris : the circular fibres of the latter are thereby paralysed, but at the same time its radiating (?) fibres are said to be brought into the condition of spasm, so that the pupil becomes much wider than in cases of paralysis of the sphincter, and is also not at all or scarcely capable of further dilatation by irritation of the sympathetic nerve in the neck.*   But though the supposition is not absurd, it is nevertheless far-fetched and little admissible. That it is incorrect appears further :—

3. From the phenomena attending paralysis of the oculo-motor nerve. In this affection the power of accommodation is not unfrequently wholly lost. This condition may occur with paralysis of some or of all the muscles governed by the oculo-motor nerve ; but it may also exist quite independently. In it the refraction corresponds to the original *farthest point*, as cases of recovery have satisfactorily proved to me. The pupil is immovable and dilated, although not highly so. On instillation of atropia, the diameter becomes much greater, but the refraction of the eye remains unaltered. Accommodation for the farthest point corresponds, therefore, to total paralysis. In imperfect paralysis (paresis of accommodation) the nearest point is always removed further from the eye, the farthest remaining unaltered. Cases of paralysis, where the farthest point should be approximated to the eye, do not occur : they should necessarily occur, did a muscular system exist, actively producing accommodation for remote objects.

4. The lens, enclosed in its capsule, has an important property, which must here be expressly pointed out. It possesses a high degree of elasticity. On gentle pressure its form is easily altered, but it immediately regains its original form when the pressure ceases.

Hence, too, it appears, that only the mechanism of accommodation for near objects is explicable by muscular action, and that the return to accommodation for distant objects occurs spontaneously (with the co-operation of elastic parts) when the active muscular operation ceases. The efforts of myopic individuals to see distinctly at a greater distance, are confined, as we shall subsequently observe, to diminishing

* See de Ruyter, *De actione Atropæ Belladonnæ in iridem*, Trajeni ad Rhenum, 1856. Kuyper, *Onderzoekingen betrekkelijk de kunstmatige verwijding van den oogappel.* Utrecht, 1860.

the circles of diffusion, by excluding a part of the pupil: they produce no true accommodation—no change of the dioptric system.

Now the accommodation for near objects must take place through the intervention of muscular action. The accommodation is produced voluntarily, and we know no voluntary movement without the intervention of contractile—of muscular elements.

Before physiologists were acquainted with the changes of the dioptric system, they often attached importance to the *external* muscles in the production of accommodation. Now that we know that the accommodation depends on a change of form in the lens, this opinion seems scarcely to need refutation. That with converging lines of vision, through the action of the musculi recti interni, we are capable of producing a higher degree of accommodation than is attainable by parallel lines, proves only that the muscular action of accommodation and the contraction of the musculi recti interni are associated: we can by no means thence infer that the musculi recti interni have a direct influence upon the accommodation. That they do not possess this, I learned from cases where the musculus rectus internus was completely paralysed, and the accommodation nevertheless had its normal range. The same might already have been inferred from the fact, that when the near object fixed upon lies to the side, the rectus internus in one eye is not active, and, nevertheless, accommodation for near objects in this case equally takes place. Many instances further occur, where the accommodation is wholly destroyed by paralysis, without the external muscles of the eye being in the least impeded in their action; and, finally, some cases are on record of paralysis of all, or of nearly all, the muscles of the eye, and of deficiency of the same, without diminution of the power of accommodation. We hence conclude that the external muscles of the eye exercise no direct influence on accommodation.

The contractile elements, which produce the accommodation, must consequently be situated exclusively *in* the eye. Now we are acquainted, in the eye of the mammalia, solely with unstriped muscular fibres or fibre-cells: there are no striped muscular fibres or fasciculi. These last, however, replace the former in the eye of birds, and therefore we may attribute to the unstriped muscular fibres the same signification and the same voluntary action. Indeed it is as little strange that fibre-cells should here be subject to the will as that the striped fibres of the heart should be withdrawn from it. Furthermore, if we consider that Cramer saw accommodation for near objects supervene on galvanic irritation of the eye of various animals, deprived of its external muscles, and that paralysis of the iris and paralysis of accommodation almost always go hand in hand, there can be no doubt that internal muscular elements, under the control of the ciliary nerves, by their contraction produce the accommodation.

Now the muscular elements known to exist in the eye of the mammalia are (Fig. 9) :—

1. The muscular fibres of the iris. The circular fibres (sphincter pupillæ [1]) are easily seen and isolated, most easily in white rabbits or rats.

Independent radiating fasciculi of fibres are less easily demonstrated. The vascular trunks [2], which likewise have a radiating direction, possess a distinct muscular layer; and it is generally difficult to prove that the fibrous bundles found do not belong to the vessels. However, most anatomists think that they have satisfied themselves as to their presence. In this I never completely succeeded. Moreover, it is difficult to explain dilatation of the pupil from atropia, in cases of paralysis of the sphincter pupillæ (whether the result of disease or of division of the oculo-motor nerve), without assuming the existence of radiating fibres. But even admitting the presence of radiating muscular fibres, I consider the explanation to be unsatisfactory, as it makes it necessary to assume that the same substance which stimulates them should paralyse the circular fibres.—I have shown with certainty from experiments on white rabbits,* that the blood-vessels of the iris, on irritation of the sympathetic nerve in the neck, become narrower while the pupil dilates. As to the connexion between these two phenomena, I do not venture to give an opinion.

2. The ciliary muscle.

That the organ formerly known under the name of ciliary ligament is of a muscular nature, has been proved, independently of one another, by my esteemed friends Bowman and Bruecke. The fibres arise in great part from the outer layers [3] of vitreous fibres, in which the membrana Descemetii (D) subdivides, while the innermost layers of these fibres spread as ligamentum pectinatum on the iris. The muscular fibres form fasciculi, of which the most external, connected in long extended networks, run backwards parallel to the upper surface of the sclerotic (S) and pass into the several laminæ of the choroid (C). Internally [6] the meshes of the nets become gradually shorter, and

* Compare Kuyper, *l. c.* p. 19.

finally, mostly spread out in a circular direction, so that the fasciculi here acquire rather a circular than an antero-posterior direction.

Fig. 9.

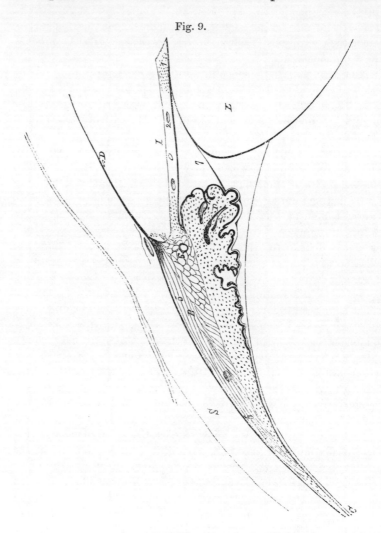

This innermost portion of the ciliary muscle is connected with the choroidal tissue in the place where the corpus ciliare (P) passes from without inwards. If we cut out a piece of the conjoined membranes, and with a pincers seize the whole breadth of the portion of the iris near its insertion and tear it off, the innermost part [6] of the ciliary muscle remains attached to the outer surface of the ciliary process, while the most external portion [5] continues lying on the sclerotic and connected with the extreme outer layers of the choroid, which are not torn off. We can thus divide the muscle into two parts, as is described in von Reeken's dissertation.* The networks of the fasciculi of the innermost portion possess, as is there also represented, a more circular direction. H. Müller[†] has subsequently described these as a separate muscle. He has the merit of having thereby directed attention to this innermost part. That it does not, however, deserve to be considered as a separate muscle, is clearly shown by the above-described gradual transition from the one direction to the other.

3. In other elements also of the eye of the mammalia, contractility has been suspected, though not demonstrated. Max. Langenbeck has assumed the existence of a musculus compressor lentis immediately around the lens. Others, however, have not succeeded in finding this. After the action of acetate of lead and acetic acid, the Zonula Zinnii (Fig. 9, 7) acquires, as Nuhn has shown, a most deceptive appearance, as if it possessed transversely striped primitive bundles; but the attempt to establish the existence of contractility, or of other reasons for assuming the presence of muscular elements in that membrane, has not been successful. In the choroid, Schweigger has found cells presenting quite the appearance of ganglionic cells, and it seems that they must really be considered as such; and Heinrich Müller appears inclined to attribute contractility to the choroid. Each of these views is, however, still problematical.

From this sketch it seems most probable, that no contractile elements, except those of the iris and of the ciliary muscle, can come into play in accommodation. Accordingly Cramer thought that the change of form of the lens might be explained by the action of the iris: simultaneous contraction of the circular and radiating fibres producing pressure on the lens, and thus giving to the part of the crystalline corresponding to the pupil greater convexity, and causing it to protrude through the pupil. Pathology has, however, shown that the iris takes no direct part in the accommodation of the lens. It may

---

* *Ontleedkundig onderzoek van den toestel voor accommodatie van het oog.* Utrecht, 1855.

† *Archiv für Ophthalmologie*, B. iv. p. 1.

be adherent to the cornea, leaving a space between the iris and the lens; it may float without tension in the aqueous humour (iridodenosis); it may be in part removed by iridectomy; it may even be wholly absent, without the power of accommodation being perceptibly disturbed. In an extremely important case, where the whole iris was removed by operation, von Graefe* recently instituted an accurate investigation, and established the existence of the range of accommodation normally corresponding to the patient's age, while the change of the anterior reflected image of the lens, too, in accommodation was admirably seen. We are therefore justified in denying to the iris any, or almost any, influence on the change of form of the crystalline lens in accommodation, and in estimating the contraction of the pupil, in accommodation for near objects, as a simply associated movement.

It therefore remains only to attribute to the musculus ciliaris the important quality of accommodation-muscle. Thus far we have arrived by exclusion. But the mechanism whereby the contraction of this little muscle alters the form of the lens is—to however small a compass the question may now seem to be reduced—not yet satisfactorily and convincingly brought to light. The accompanying changes of the eye have been studied with great accuracy : the advance of the surface of the pupil and the retrocession of the periphery of the iris, in the accommodation for near objects; the light-phenomenon (phosphène) at the termination of this accommodation (Czermak), etc.; but to a perfect solution we have not attained. I shall here confine myself to a short statement of the views of Helmholtz, who numbers the most adherents, and of H. Müller. Helmholtz, by measurement during life, found the lens, in accommodation for distance, thinner than it occurs in the dead body. It is said that this may depend on elongation of the lens (Fig. 9 L), through tension of the Zonula Zinnii [7], which is stated to be present during life, certainly as a result of the pressure of the vitreous humour. It is further stated that after death, when the pressure ceases, the tension may diminish and the lens consequently become thicker. But during life the action of the ciliary muscle may effect the same. It is evident that the outermost layers of the ciliary muscle, in contracting, must cause the origin at the fibrous layers [3] of the membrana Descemetii and the termination at the choroid (C), both of which are elastic, to approach one another. According to this, the iris (I), which is mediately connected with the anterior part of the ciliary muscle, recedes in ac-

* Archiv für Ophthalmologie, B. vii.

commodation for near objects; and, on the contrary, the place of insertion in the choroid will advance a little forwards. Now with this the origin of the Zonula Zinnii is connected; and as, therefore, the latter at the same time advances, its tension ceases, and the equator of the lens becomes smaller, the lens itself becomes thicker in the middle, and its two surfaces are rendered more convex. Helmholtz supposes that to this may be added a pressure of the iris, which may make the equatorial surface of the lens arched anteriorly, and thus increase the convexity of the anterior surface and diminish that of the posterior.

H. Müller's theory is based upon his anatomical investigations of the ciliary muscle. He distinguishes, as we have seen, a circular muscle capable of exercising pressure on the margin of the lens, and thus of rendering the lens thicker, while it would at the same time draw the periphery of the iris backwards. Moreover, he attaches, with Helmholtz, importance to the relaxation of the Zonula Zinnii. Lastly, he sees in the action of the most external layers of the ciliary muscle a means of augmenting the pressure of the vitreous humour, of pushing the lens forwards, of diminishing the increased convexity of the posterior surface, and, by the resistance of the simultaneous contraction of the iris, of increasing that of the anterior surface.

Against these two theories I have difficulties which I shall not further develop. It would, moreover, be easy to bring forward other hypotheses, but from this too I shall refrain. I am afraid of depriving this work of the character I desire, above all, to see attached to it,—the character of exact science.

NOTE TO § 4.

One point I shall take leave to remark upon is, that in the case of acquired aniridesis with normal range of accommodation, described by von Graefe, in accommodation for near objects, no displacement of the then visible ciliary process was observed; that, moreover, nothing is mentioned of the possibility of a direct pressure of the ciliary muscle on the margin of the lens; and, finally, that nothing is said of any diminution of the circumference of the lens, although the increased convexity of its anterior surface is proved from the reflected images. On former occasions I have also in vain endeavoured, after iridectomy, in which the margin of the lens became visible, to satisfy myself of the diminution of the circumference of the lens in accommodation for near objects. Thus far it has not been directly observed. It is evident that, if it be wanting, with the increase in thickness in the middle, which has certainly been witnessed, attenuation of the parts situated near the equator must be combined, and thus the curved surfaces would obtain such an irregular form, that it becomes difficult to explain the tolerably accurate power of vision in the case of aniridesis described by von Graefe, in accommodation also for near objects. What we must, in the first place, therefore, endeavour to clear up is the question, whether the circumference of the lens, in accommodation for near objects, becomes perceptibly smaller? The answer will have great influence on our further considerations.

---

§ 5. Range of accommodation.

In all the investigations respecting the cause and mechanism of accommodation, observers appear not to have thought of defining the range of accommodation under various circumstances, and of seeking a simple numerical expression for the same. And yet the necessity for such existed almost still more for the oculist than for the physiologist. If it be desired to investigate the accommodation, whether in reference to the changes observed in the eye, either at different periods of life, or with respect to myopia, hypermetropia, asthenopia, strabismus, paresis, etc., it is evidently necessary to have an easily comparable standard of its magnitude or range.

Had the necessity been felt, it would not have been difficult to have provided for it. The knowledge alone of the distance R from the farthest point of distinct vision, and of the distance P from the nearest, is sufficient. With the knowledge of these distances the range of accommodation $\frac{1}{A}$ may be found by a very simple formula.

The formula is *

$$\frac{1}{A} = \frac{1}{P} - \frac{1}{R}.$$

The distances P and R may be calculated from the nearest point p, and from the farthest point r of distinct vision to a point situated about 3″ behind the anterior surface of the cornea in the eye, called

---

* English writers on optics would say—

$$\frac{1}{A} = \frac{1}{R} - \frac{1}{P},$$

the negative sign of A denoting that the lens is convex.—S. H.

the anterior nodal point k'. The latter coincides in the eye nearly with the second nodal point k'', both of which may therefore here be considered as one point. This point corresponding nearly to what is termed the optical centre, has a very important signification; the rays, which in front of the cornea are directed to the node, in the vitreous humour continue parallel to their primitive direction, and also nearly exactly directed to the same point; these rays may therefore be considered not to have been refracted. This is represented in the subjoined figure 10.

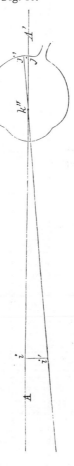

Fig. 10.

The ray $i'\,k''$, proceeding from the point i', continues as $k''\,j'$, and since all the rays, which proceed from the point i', unite in one point, this must occur where they meet conjointly the ray $k''\,j'$. Now if the eye be accommodated, the union takes place in the retina, and then the image of the point i' lies in j'. In like manner the image of the point i lies in j, both being situated in the axis A A′. Therefore, $j\,j'$ is the image of $i\,i'$, and it immediately appears that their reciprocal magnitudes are as their distances from the point k'' where the rays $i\,j$ and $i'\,j'$ cross one another. If we express the distance $i\,k''$ by g', and the distance $j\,k''$ by g'', the magnitudes of the object B and the image β are to one another, in the accurately accommodated eye, as g' to g''.

$$\mathrm{B} : \beta = g' : g''.$$

In the normal eye g'' is about 15 millimètres. Therefore, if an object be accurately seen at 15 mètres distance, the retinal image is 1000 times smaller than the object; if the object lies at 1.5 mètres (= 1500 mm.) the retinal image is $\dfrac{1500}{15} = 100$ times smaller. Hence it clearly appears, how important the posterior nodal point (Knotenpunkt) k'' is. If we connect the corresponding points of the object and image by right lines with one another, these all, just as $i'\,j'$, pass through the point k'', and they are therefore called lines of direction; *the posterior nodal point k'' is consequently the point of decussation of the lines of direction.*

The meaning of the formula for the range of accommodation—

$$\frac{1}{A} = \frac{1}{P} - \frac{1}{R}$$

is easily understood. In this formula, A is the focal length of a lens, which gives a direction to the rays from the nearest point of distinct vision p, as if they came from the farthest point r. The subjoined figure (11) illustrates this. The eye in the condition of rest is accommodated for the distance $r\ k' = R$; in the strongest tension of accommodation for the distance $p\ k' = P$. In the former case the rays diverging from r are united on the retina, in the latter those diverging from p. In accommodation the eye must therefore be so altered that the rays proceeding from p, in the vitreous humour acquire a direction equal to that of the rays proceeding from r in the non-accommodated eye. This can be effected by placing an auxiliary lens in k', and we may thus imagine the eye away, and suppose that the auxiliary lens in k' is in the air. The lens now represents the accommodation of the eye, and its power the range of accommodation. Its focal distance A is found by the formula mentioned:

$$\frac{1}{P} - \frac{1}{R} = \frac{1}{A}.$$

Consequently A is the focal distance of the auxiliary lens, of which the eye avails itself in accommodation, and as the power of a lens is inversely proportional to its focal distance, $\frac{1}{A}$ or

1 : A expresses the range of accommodation. It is convenient to represent the value of A in Parisian inches, especially as the focal distance of lenses is usually stated in the same, and this applies also more particularly to spectacles.*

I may be allowed to illustrate the calculation of the range of accommodation by a couple of examples.

Fig. 11.

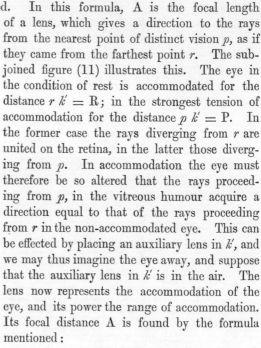

* In the boxes of Glasses, prepared by Paetz and Flohr, of Berlin, for

Let the distance P of the nearest point $= 4''$, that of the farthest point of distinct vision $R = 12''$, then the range of accommodation will be—

$$\frac{1}{4} - \frac{1}{12} = \frac{1}{6}$$

If the farthest point lies at an infinite distance, $R = \infty$, the nearest point at $5''$, the range of accommodation will be—

$$\frac{1}{5} - \frac{1}{\infty} = \frac{1}{5}.$$

In the first case, the range of accommodation is represented by an auxiliary lens of six, in the latter by one of five Parisian inches. The same form of expression I now apply to all lenses. The power may always be regarded as inversely proportional to the focal distance F, and therefore find its expression in $1 : F$. If the focal distance be negative, it becomes $-1 : F$. Glasses of $\frac{1}{10}$, of $-\frac{1}{8}$, &c., therefore mean glasses of ten Parisian inches positive, eight Parisian inches negative focal distance, &c. We shall subsequently see that the degrees of anomalies of refraction may be expressed in a similar mode, and that it is thereby at the same time shown, by what glasses they may be neutralized.

We have above seen that the range of accommodation is contained in the formula

$$\frac{1}{A} = \frac{1}{P} - \frac{1}{R}.$$

Therefore it is necessary to possess a simple method of determining the points p and r with sufficient accuracy for practical purposes. The determination of r is accomplished with a nearly parallel state of the lines of vision, that is, by fixing with both eyes an object at least 5 mètres distant. We know, namely, that when the lines of vision converge, accommodation necessarily takes place, and that consequently the true farthest point in total relaxation of accommodation cannot thus be found. As an object we may use groups of vertical black lines, each line $2\frac{1}{2}$ millimètres thick and 10 millimètres from one another, and examine whether they can at the distance of five mètres be seen with perfect accuracy with the naked eye, or whether the sharpness of the object can be increased by glasses. If no improve-

oculists, they are defined in Prussian inches, which are less than Parisian inches. In England, English inches are employed, one English inch being equal to about 0·94 Parisian inch, and differing but little from the Prussian. In practice a reduction will rarely be necessary.

ment is attainable by glasses, r lies at least 5 mètres distant, which may here be equally represented by an infinite distance ∞. Where nearsightedness exists, concave glasses, with negative focal distance, are required to obtain perfect accuracy : in this case we determine what is the weakest glass of this nature with which the sharpest possible vision is obtained. In the determination the distance of the farthest point is ascertained ; thus when parallel rays (Fig. 12), $a\,b$ and $a'\,b'$, derived from a distant object, fall on a concave lens l, they are, after refraction, divergent, as $c\,d$ and $c'\,d'$, and appear now to be derived from the point ϕ'. The distance $\phi'\,l$ is the negative focal distance F of the lens l. If we now designate the distance $l\,k'$ by x, it is clear that the point ϕ', for which the nearsighted eye is accommodated with parallel lines of vision, is at the distance $F + x$ from the point k'. Consequently, $R = F + x$. Let us illustrate this by an example. A nearsighted eye, to see accurately at a distance, needs a glass of 15 Parisian inches negative focal distance ($F = 15$), placed at a quarter of an inch in front of the cornea, that is, half an inch before the nodal point k' in the eye ($x = \frac{1}{2}$), then $R = F + x = 15\frac{1}{2}$ Parisian inches.

In place of the above-mentioned black lines we may, in the determination, make use of definite letters or numbers, whereby, by causing them to be named, we may obtain still more objective certainty with what glass they are accurately seen. A sharp-sighted eye recognises letters such as the subjoined in good light — (Fig. 13) — at a distance of about 20 feet. In Dr. Snellen's system of test-types, each number corresponds to the number of feet at which a sharp-sighted eye distinguishes them. The following letters (Fig. 13) correspond, therefore, to No. XX. of Snellen. They are the lowest in the Table appended to this work, in which

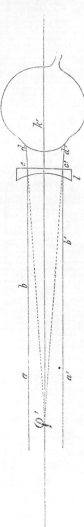

Fig. 12.

also XXX, XL, LX, LXXX, C, and CC occur. For practical purposes, these experiments with vertical lines and letters afford

Fig. 13.

quale non
si dia una

a sufficiently accurate result. If a very exact determination be required, we must employ a little point of light, which changes form on the slightest alteration of accommodation. This shall be more fully explained in treating of astigmatism.

The determination of the nearest point is effected by means of a wire optometer. This consists of a little frame (Fig. 14 A), of the size represented in the figure, in which some fine black wires are vertically extended, and wherewith a measure, B, capable of being rolled up, is connected, the scale commencing at the frame, and the bobbin c being applied to the temple, on a line with the anterior surface of the cornea. This bobbin is, by moving the frame out from the eye, unwound until the vertical wires are seen with perfect accuracy. It is, indeed, possible to determine by means of such wires with sufficient accuracy whether they are exactly seen, as by a slight deviation the margins lose their sharp outlines, and more of these lines appear. The persons examined for the most part state this very easily. The reading of print, capable of being distinguished at given distances in due accommodation and by a sharp eye, may be used to control the result.

Most optometers are based upon the principle of the well-known experiment of Scheiner: through two openings or slits, placed closer to one another than the diameter of the pupil, the object, for example a wire, is seen, and this appears double if the eye is not accurately adjusted to this distance. If we now cause any one to

3

look into such an optometer and to determine when he sees the wire

Fig. 14.

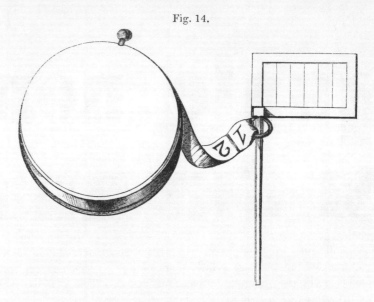

single, we shall in general obtain a distance to which the person easily accommodates his vision, but this distance will not correspond to either the nearest or the farthest point. This is looked upon as *the mean distance of distinct vision*. But to this we must not attach too much importance, for such a mean distance does not exist, or at least it has a very wide range; this appears when a number of determinations are made, for example with Stampfer's optometer: the same person never obtains, even under the same circumstances, similar results, and where circumstances differ, the results vary very much. Only when a person has learned to control his power of accommodation, and can voluntarily bring it into the condition of the highest action and of perfect relaxation, can we with such optometers successively determine his farthest and his nearest point of distinct vision. But such voluntary control of the power of accommodation is acquired only by great practice. Ordinary individuals accommodate for their farthest point only when they actually look at a distant object, and for their nearest only when they very distinctly see an object approaching, whose diminishing distance they meanwhile observe and follow in their imagination. Then, by the effort actually to

see the object distinctly as long as possible, the greatest possible tension
of the power of accommodation is excited. Such
an approaching object is the frame above described, while in the optometer, the distance of
the object not being known, no stimulus to
tension is created.

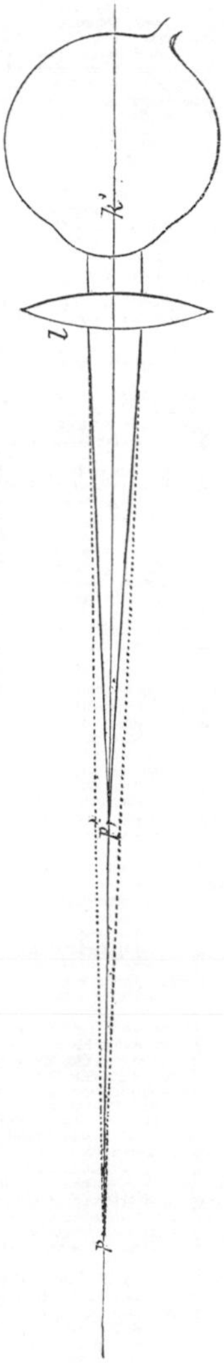

If greater accuracy be desired, as in observations intended for the solution of scientific
questions, it is advisable to employ another instrument, which shall be described in treating of
the relative range of accommodation.

The partial dependence of accommodation on
the convergence of the lines of vision has already
been alluded to. In the determination of the
nearest point this should be borne in mind.
Theoretically we should, in order to be able to
institute a comparison, always determine the nearest point at the same angle of convergence, as the
farthest point is examined with parallel lines of
vision. This would, however, be attended with
great practical difficulties, and, as I shall hereafter
show, would moreover lead to wholly incorrect results. The only thing required in this respect is,
that in all the cases where the nearest point lies
farther from the eye than 8″, the determination
should be made with the use of such convex
glasses, that the nearest point should be brought
to about 8″ from the eye. It will then be necessary to calculate at what distance the eye should
have been brought into this state of accommodation without the use of the convex glasses.
The calculation is not attended with any difficulty :—Let x be the distance of the convex
lens l (Fig. 15) from k' : F the focal distance of
the convex lens, P″ the distance from p' to l.
The rays proceeding from p' when refracted
through the lens $l\,l$, assume a direction as if
they came from p. The eye is therefore accommodated not for p' but
for p. The distance P′ from the point p to the lens is now found
by the simple formula :—

Fig. 15.

2

$$\frac{1}{P'} = \frac{1}{P''} - \frac{1}{F}.$$

The distance P of the nearest point is $= P' + x$.—An example will illustrate this. With a lens of $12''$ focal distance ($F = 12$), removed $\frac{1}{2}'$ from k' ($x = \frac{1}{2}$) the point p', situated $7\frac{1}{2}''$ from the lens, is accurately seen. We therefore find the distance P' from

$$\frac{1}{7\frac{1}{2}} - \frac{1}{12} = \frac{1}{20}$$

to be $20'$ from the eye, and P is therefore $= 20\cdot5$ inches.

Lastly, I would here state a method of expressing the *ranges of accommodation* by the *lengths of lines*, which exhibits at the same time the commencement and termination of the range of accommodation, that is the nearest and farthest points of distinct vision. Above parallel lines, situated at equal distances from each other (Fig. 16), let numbers be placed, expressing the distances of distinct

Fig. 16.

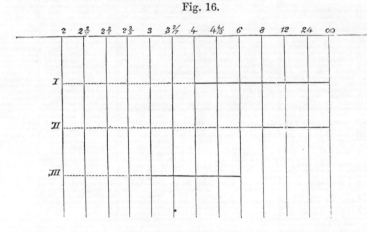

vision, and in such an order, that the distance between two lines may everywhere represent an equal range of accommodation, for example, $\frac{1}{24}$. It is evident that in Fig. 16 the differences of the distances from line to line always amounts to $\frac{1}{24}$ of the range of accommodation: this is true from ∞ to 24, from 24 to 12, from 12 to 8, &c.; for

$$\frac{1}{24} - \frac{1}{\infty} = \frac{1}{24}$$

$$\frac{1}{12} - \frac{1}{24} = \frac{1}{24}$$

$$\frac{1}{8} - \frac{1}{12} = \frac{1}{24}.$$

etc.

A single horizontal line now immediately shows the extent and range of accommodation. In Fig. 16 three such lines occur.

I. represents a person whose farthest point of distinct vision lies at an infinite distance, his nearest point at 4″. His range of accommodation is

$$\frac{1}{4} - \frac{1}{\infty} = \frac{1}{4}$$

and is expressed by six lines distance, each of $\frac{1}{24}$ of this range of accommodation, consequently $\frac{6}{24} = \frac{1}{4}$.

II. has likewise his farthest point at an infinite distance, his nearest at 6 inches. His range of accommodation is

$$\frac{1}{6} - \frac{1}{\infty} = \frac{1}{6}, \text{ expressed by } \frac{4}{24}.$$

III. has his farthest point at 6 inches (he is therefore near-sighted) his nearest at 3 inches. His range of accommodation is

$$\frac{1}{3} - \frac{1}{6} = \frac{1}{6};$$

corresponding to four lines distance

$$= \frac{4}{24} = \frac{1}{6}.$$

It need not be demonstrated how easily observations may in this manner be registered. We shall hereafter have much occasion to employ this method in exhibiting in print the several anomalies of refraction and accommodation.

NOTE TO THE FIRST CHAPTER.

FIRST PART.

DIOPTRICS OF THE EYE.

I. *Literature.*

In order to give an idea of the necessity of accommodation, the eye has hitherto been regarded as a simple lens, with a positive focus. This has been, so far, sufficient for our purpose. But if we wish to go more deeply into many questions relating to the refraction and accommodation of the eye, we shall require more accurate knowledge of the dioptric system of the organ. This knowledge is a necessity, to enable us to form an idea what range of accommodation is obtained by definite changes of the crystalline lens, and how each range of accommodation may be expressed by an imaginary lens, applied to the eye. It will hereafter be serviceable to us in the right understanding of many other questions.

I shall therefore endeavour, in a simple manner, to give a satisfactory description of the dioptric system of the eye. Those who are not deterred by the higher mathematics, may consult Moser (Dove's *Repertorium der Physik*), who has applied to the eye the theoretical investigations of Bessel (*Astronomische Nachrichten*, xviii., No. 415), and Listing, who, in his *Dioptrik des Auges* (Wagner's *Handwörterbuch der Physiologie*, Bd. IV., p. 451) has followed the mode adopted by Gauss (*Dioptrische Untersuchungen*, Göttingen, 1841); lastly, Helmholtz, who in his *Physiologische Optik* (Karsten's *Allgemeine Encylopædie der Physik*, 1ste Lief. Leipzig, 1858), has, together with thorough explanation, made the whole theory more generally accessible.

II. *Refracting surfaces in the Eye.*

In the eye three refracting surfaces are to be distinguished, whose curvatures may be assumed to be spherical.

1. *The anterior surface of the cornea*, approaching to an ellipsoid, with the apex in the middle of the cornea. The radius at the apex, which defines the focal distance, amounts on an average to something less than 8 millimètres. The slight thickness of the cornea, and the almost perfect parallelism of the outer and inner surfaces, together with the slight difference in refracting power of the cornea and aqueous humour, justify us in considering the system as if the aqueous humour extended to the anterior surface of the cornea. For the cornea and aqueous humour we have therefore to assume only one refracting surface of nearly 8 millimètres radius of curvature, and with a refracting proportion of 1·3366, found by Sir David Brewster for the aqueous humour.

2. *The anterior surface of the lens*, 3·6 millimètres from the anterior surface of the cornea, with a radius of about 10 millimètres. In accommodation for near objects, this surface approaches to about 3·2 millimètres from

the anterior surface of the cornea, and diminishes in radius to about 6 millimètres.

3. *The posterior surface of the lens* (or the anterior surface of the vitreous humour), 7·2 millimètres from the anterior surface of the cornea, and with a radius of 6 millimètres during accommodation for distance, of 5·5 millimètres when looking at near objects.

The lens is, however, no homogeneous mass, but consists of layers of refractive power, increasing towards the centre. In the lens itself, therefore, innumerable refractions take place from layer to layer, which cannot, nevertheless, be separately traced. Consequently, we cannot regard the lens otherwise than as formed of a homogeneous substance, and the question then is, what index of refraction we ought to ascribe to this substance. For a long time physiologists assumed an index, the mean of that of the nucleus and that of the periphery, notwithstanding that Young (*On the Mechanism of the Eye*, in the *Philosophical Transactions* for 1801, vol. xcii., and in the *Miscellaneous Works of the late Thomas Young*, edited by G. Peacock; London, 1855, vol. i., pp. 28 and 29) had already shown that, in consequence of the laminated structure of the lens, with refractive power increasing towards the centre, an index must be adopted, greater even than that of the nucleus. Subsequently, the same was observed by Senff (*see* Volkmann's article *Sehen* in Wagner's *Handwörterbuch für Physiologie*, Bd. III., Abth. 1), to whom the honour of having first made the observation is in general incorrectly ascribed. The subject is one of importance; for it is only by taking this higher index of refraction into account that we get rid of the paradoxical result, that in a well-formed eye parallel incident rays should be brought to a focus behind the retina. The coefficient of refraction is now fixed by Listing at 1·455.

As a conclusion from these considerations, we may repeat, that in the dioptric system of the eye three refracting surfaces are to be distinguished.

1. The anterior surface of the cornea.
2. The anterior surface of the lens.
3. The anterior surface of the vitreous humour.

The index of refraction of the vitreous humour differs so little from that of the aqueous humour that we may consider it as equal to it.

III. *Cardinal Points.—Their Object.*

In a compound dioptric system we can successively follow the refraction in the different surfaces, each time determining from or towards what point originally parallel rays converge. Thus we find, lastly, the situation of the focal point after the last refraction. But in order also to determine the point of union of rays falling upon the first surface under different degrees of convergence or divergence, and to find the magnitude of the dioptric images, a separate calculation would be necessary for each case.

For this purpose a particular method has been adopted. Optical mathematicians seek, namely, for a given system of refracting surfaces, certain fixed points, called *cardinal points;* and the knowledge of these is sufficient to enable us to construct and calculate the situation and size of the images of given objects. The conditions are :—1st, that the system be centred, that is, that the centres of curvature of all the refracting surfaces lie in a right line, the axis of the system : 2ndly, that the rays intersect the axis at only small angles. The first condition appears to be amply fulfilled by the structure of the eye, as the second is by direct vision, that is by looking nearly in the direction of the line of vision.

The situation and signification of the cardinal points are best understood by studying them :—*A* in the case of only a single refracting surface; *B* for a biconvex lens, with two refracting surfaces; *C* for a combination of these two into a compound system, such as the eye is.

Fig. 17.

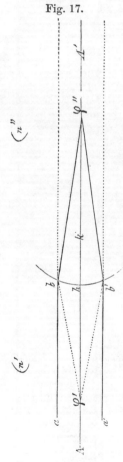

A.—Refraction by a Spherical Surface.

IV.—*Cardinal Points.*

In Fig. 17, let *k* be the central point of the spherical surface *h*, on which, parallel to the axis *A A'*, rays of light fall, *a b* and *a' b'*, coming from the medium with index *n'*, and passing into the medium with index *n''*. If *n''* is $>$ *n'*, the parallel rays unite in the axis nearly in a point, the posterior focal point ϕ''. The distance $h\ \phi''$ $= F''$, that is, the posterior focal distance is found by the known formula $F'' = \dfrac{n''\ \rho,}{n'' - n'} \dots 1\ a$, wherein ρ the radius of the surface of curvature is $= h\ k$.

If on the same refracting surface, but in the direction from *A'* to *A*, rays fall, which in the medium with index *n''* run parallel to the axis (they are in the figure represented by dots), these also unite nearly in a point in the axis, the anterior focal point ϕ'. The distance $h\ \phi' = F'$, called the anterior focal distance, is found by the formula,

$$F' = \frac{n'\ \rho}{n'' - n'} \dots \dots 1\ b.$$

The formulas 1 *a* and 1 *b* obtain only for rays which run close to the axis. As such they are deducible in a simple mode.

In Fig. 18, *a b* is the incident ray; *b* the point of incidence ;

k b v the normal on the spherical surface at the point of incidence;

b ϕ'' the refracted ray, bent towards to the normal *b k ;*

a b v is the angle of incidence, $\alpha = b\ k\ h$, and thus corresponding to arc *h b;*

$\phi''\ b\ k$ is the angle of refraction β, and if we draw *d k* parallel to *b* ϕ'', we have the angle *b k d*, corresponding to the arc *d b :*

$h\,k\,d$ is the angle of deviation, $\gamma = \alpha - \beta$.

The relation of each of the focal distances $h\,\phi'' = F''$ and $h\,\phi' = F'$, to the radius $h\,k = \rho$ is now to be found.

For small segments $h\,k\,d$ and $h\,\phi''\,b$ may be regarded as rectilineal triangles. They are in this case uniform and rectangular in h. Consequently

$$k\,h : \phi''\,h = \text{arc}\; h\,d : \text{arc}\; h\,b.$$

$$\rho : F'' = \alpha - \beta : \alpha.$$

For small arcs we may substitute the sines, and thus alter the above formula into

$$F'' : \rho = \sin\alpha : \sin\alpha - \sin\beta.$$

Then the law of refraction is, as experience teaches, the following :—

$$n'\,\sin\alpha = n''\,\sin\beta.$$

Consequently, if we substitute the value of $\sin\alpha$ in our proportion,

$$F'' : \rho = n'' : n'' - n'$$

$$F'' = \frac{\rho\,n''}{n'' - n'}.$$

The relation of F' to F'' is, moreover, easily found. The ray $a'\,b$, running parallel to the axis in $n,''$ is bent from the normal $b\,v$, and proceeds as $b\,\phi^1$. By this deflection the angle of refraction $v\,b\,\phi' = \beta'$ becomes greater than the angle of incidence $\alpha' = \alpha$. However, the law of refraction must here also find its application, and thus the proportions remain the same, as immediately appears by considering $\phi'\,b$ as the incident, and $b\,a'$ as the refracted ray. There is a general law, of which we shall hereafter often make use; it is this: if a ray, proceeding from a point, passes through an optical system, in order to come to a second point, a ray from this second point will, *vice versâ*, be able to reach the first point, only by following precisely the same route in an opposite direction. As the angles of deviation are proportional[*] to the angles of refraction, we here obtain

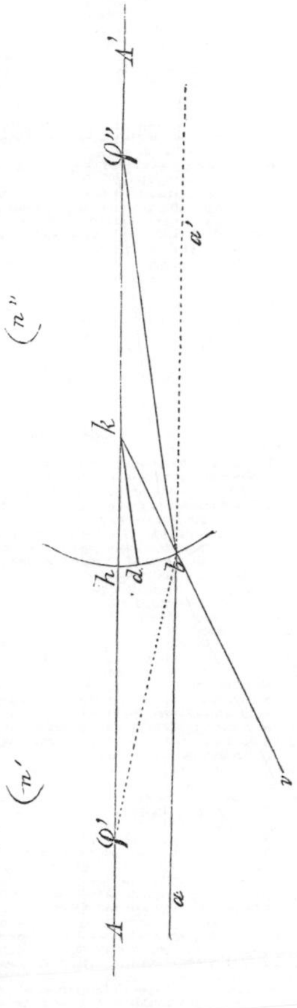

$$b\,\phi'\,h : b\,\phi''\,h = v\,b\,a : \phi''\,b\,k,$$

that is, for small angles,

$$\gamma' : \gamma = \alpha : \beta = n'' : n'.$$

Now as

$$F' : F'' = \gamma : \gamma',$$

we have

$$F' = F''\,\frac{n'}{n''} \;\ldots\ldots\; 1\,c.$$

But,

$$F'' = \frac{\rho\,n''}{n'' - n'},$$

---

[*] Because they are very small, and therefore proportional to their sines.
—S. H.

Fig. 18.

therefore,

$$F' = \frac{\rho\; n'}{n'' - n'}.$$

Moreover,

$$F'' - F' = \rho\, \frac{n'' - n'}{n'' - n'} = \rho$$

$$F'' = F' + \rho \;\ldots\ldots\ldots 1\; d.$$

If we regard n' as unity, we obtain n'', the symbol of the relative index of refraction with respect to the air, and we obtain

$$F' \quad \frac{\rho}{n'' - 1}$$

$$F'' \quad \frac{\rho\; n''}{n'' - 1}.$$

Thus we recognise *four cardinal points* in the axis:—

ϕ', the anterior focus.

h, the point of section of the spherical surface with the axis.

k, the centre of curvature.

ϕ'', the posterior focus.

From the distances between these points flow the following values:—

$h\; \phi'$, the anterior focal distance F'.

$h\; \phi''$, the posterior focal distance F''.

We further distinguish—

$k\; \phi'$ as G', $k\; \phi''$ as G'',

then :

$$G' = F' + \rho = F'' \ldots.\; 2\; b$$
$$G'' = F'' - \rho = F' \ldots.\; 2\; a$$
$$G' = G'' + \rho \;\ldots\ldots.\; 2\; d$$
$$\frac{G''}{G'} = \frac{F'}{F''} = \frac{n'}{n''} \;\ldots.\; 2\; c$$

V.—*Conjugate foci and relation between magnitude B of the object, and magnitude β of the image.*

Having ascertained these values, we can, by a simple construction, find both the conjugate *foci* and the relation between the magnitude of the object and that of the image $B : \beta$.

Let i' (Fig. 19) be a given point of light; if we wish to find its image:

From i' proceeds: 1. The ray $i'\; k\; j'$, which being directed to k coincides with the normal of the refracting surface, and passes through unrefracted; 2. the ray $i'\; b$, which, as being parallel to the axis, after refraction passes through ϕ''. *All* the rays proceeding from i' unite in one point. Consequently, where two rays, proceeding from i', cut one another, is its conjugate focus. This point is j', and j' is therefore the image of the point of light i'.

The points of an object, which lie in a line perpendicular to the axis, are also in the image situated in a line perpendicular to the axis. Consequently, the image of the point of light i is in j. The object $i\; i' = B$ will therefore have an image β, the magnitude of which is $j\; j'$.

It is of importance to prove this last proposition. From the point of light i' (Fig. 19), proceed, as we saw, two rays, the direction of which we know; the ray $i'\; j'$, and the ray $i'\; b\; \phi''$, in whose point of intersection lies j' the image of i'. To find this, we draw the perpendicular $s\,d$ at a point of the axis arbitrarily taken, provided only that the perpendicular cut the two rays $i'\,j'$ and $b\,j'$. We thus obtain two pairs of similar triangles, $\phi''\,h\,b$ and $\phi''\,s\,c$, and $k\,i\,i'$ and $k\,s\,d$; moreover, $h\,b$ is $= i\,i'$. The said triangles give us now the subjoined proportions :—

$$\phi''\,h : h\,b = \phi''\,s : s\,c \text{ and}$$
$$k\,i : h\,b = k\,s : s\,d,$$

consequently,

$$s\,c = \frac{h\,b \times \phi''\,s}{\phi''\,h} \text{ and } s\,d = \frac{h\,b \times k\,s}{k\,i}$$

we see that $s\,c$ will be $= s\,d$, if

$$\frac{\phi''\,s}{\phi''\,h} = \frac{k\,s}{k\,i}.$$

This is evidently the case, if the point s is removed towards j. The situation of the point j is therefore determined by

$$\phi''\,j : \phi''\,h = k\,j : k\,i.$$

On the perpendicular from j, we have $s\,c = s\,d$, and here, therefore, the ray passing through k crosses that passing through ϕ''. This is the case for every value of $h\,b$ or $i\,i'$, which term does not occur in the proportion. Every point of the perpendicular $j\,j'$, therefore, has its image on the perpendicular $i\,i'$. Q. E. D.

In the above figure,

$$h\,\phi'' = F'' = G'$$
$$k\,\phi'' = G'' = F'.$$

If we now call the conjugate focal distances, measured from h, $h\,i = f'$ and $h\,j = f''$, and, measured from k, $k\,i = g'$ and $k\,j = g''$, we obtain, in place of,

$$\phi''\,j : \phi''\,h = k\,j : k\,i, \dots A$$

the proportion

$$g'' - G'' : G' = g'' : g',$$

and hence directly

$$g' = \frac{G'\,g''}{g'' - G''} \quad \dots (3\,a$$

or,
$$g'\,g'' - g'\,G'' = G'\,g''$$
$$g'\,g'' - G'\,g'' = g'\,G''$$
$$g''\,(g' - G') = g'\,G''$$
$$g'' = \frac{G''\,g'}{g' - G'} \quad \dots 3)\,b$$

In place of the proportion A we may equally write

$$f'' - F'' : F'' = F' + f'' - F'' : f' + F'' - F'.$$

Fig. 19.

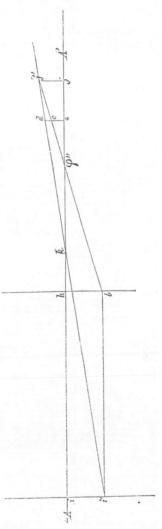

Hence follows,

$$f'f'' - f'\,F'' + f''F'' - F''\,F'' - f''\,F' + F'\,F'' = f''\,F'' - F''\,F'' + F'\,F''$$

$$f'f'' - f'\,F'' - f''\,F' = 0$$

$$f'\,(f'' - F''') = f''\,F' \quad f''\,(f' - F') = f'\,F''$$

$$f' = \frac{f''\,F'}{f'' - F''} \ \cdots \ 3\,c) \qquad\qquad f' = \frac{f'\,F''}{f' - F'} \ 3\,d.)$$

In the same figure we find still two pairs of similar triangles,

$$i\,i'\,k \text{ and } k\,j'\,j.$$

and

$$h\,b\,\phi'' \text{ and } \phi''\,j\,j'.$$

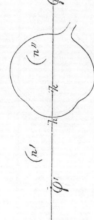

Fig. 20.

Hence we have two proportions, expressing the relation between the magnitudes of object and image, namely,

$$j'j : i\,i' = k\,j : k\,i \text{ or } \beta : B = g'' : g' \ \cdots \ (4\,a$$

and

$$j'j : i\,i' = \phi''\,j : \phi''\,h \text{ or } \beta : B = f'' - F'' : F'' \ \cdots \ (4\,b.$$

The first is applied above, in Figure 10. Of the second we shall hereafter make much use.

VI.—*Application to the Eye.*

All that has been brought forward is applicable to the refraction of the rays through the cornea. If, therefore, the crystalline lens be absent (aphakia), no other formulas than those above given need be used.

The principal point lies on the anterior surface of the cornea, the nodal point 8 mm. behind its apex. The radius of the cornea being 8 mm. (compare 1 *a* and 1 *b*) we find

$$F'' = \frac{8 \times 1\cdot3366}{1\cdot3366 - 1} = \frac{10\cdot6928}{0\cdot3366} = 31\cdot692 \text{ millimètres.}$$

$$F' = \frac{8}{1\cdot3366 - 1} = \frac{8}{0\cdot3366} = 23\cdot692 \text{ millimètres.}$$

Herewith are also given $G' = F''$ and $G'' = F'$ (Compare 2 *a* and 2 *d*).

The above Figure (20) shows the situation of the cardinal points in such an eye.

In the normal eye, refraction through a biconvex lens is combined herewith. We shall now investigate the cardinal points of such a lens.

B.—REFRACTION THROUGH A BICONVEX LENS.

VII.—*With the exception of the axis-ray, all rays are refracted in a lens.*

It has above been shown how, by the determination of four cardinal points, the position, as well as the magnitude of the dioptric images, formed by a single refracting surface, may be constructed and calculated. The question is, whether we can also, for a system composed of various refracting surfaces, find such points, and whether we can likewise make use of the same in the determination of the size and position of the dioptric images.

In the eye there is a biconvex lens, which, just as every lens, has two refracting surfaces. We shall therefore examine the question specially with respect to a biconvex lens.

Does a lens possess a nodal point in this sense, that all rays directed thereto pass through unrefracted?

A lens possesses such a point only when the nodal points (the central points of curvature) of both surfaces coincide. This takes place only in a lens having the form of Fig. 21; the two surfaces of curvature are at h_1 and h_2, described for this lens from the point k, and every ray directed to this point, as $a\,b$ and $a'\,b'$, therefore coincides on both the anterior and the posterior surface with the radius. Such a lens is not biconvex, but convex-concave,* and with a negative focal distance.

In every other form of lens every ray is refracted, except that which coincides with the axis. This is easily demonstrated. In Fig. 22 k_1 is the centre of curvature of the anterior surface h_1, and k_2, that of the posterior surface h_2. Now if the ray $a\,b$ be directed to k_1, it is not refracted on the surface h_1; but arrived at c, it is bent from the normal $c\,v$, and proceeds in the direction $c\,d$. The same is true of the ray $a'\,b'$, which, directed to k_2, at b' passes through unrefracted, but at c' is bent from the normal $c'\,v'$, and proceeds as $c'\,d'$. Every ray, therefore, which is not refracted at the one surface, deviates at least at the other from its direction; and all rays which, while they are in the lens, are not directed to k_1 or k_2, are refracted at both surfaces.

In a lens, therefore, no nodal point exists, to be classed with the nodal point of a simple refracting surface, of such a nature that all rays directed thereto should pass through unrefracted.

VIII. *Every lens has two nodal points, k' and k'', to be found both by construction and by calculation.*

For every lens two points may be determined, k' and k'', which stand to each other in such a relation, that every ray directed before the first refraction to k', appears after the second refraction to proceed from k'', being at the same time parallel to its primitive direction.

These points are the nodal points of the lens, the first k' and the second k'' (Fig. 23). The ray $a\,b$, before the first refraction directed to k', appears after the second refraction to proceed as $c\,d$ from k'', while $c\,d$ is also parallel to $a\,b$.

The points k' and k'' are easily found for every lens, both by construction and by calculation.

Let k_1 (Fig. 24) be the centre of curvature of the surface h_1, k_2 of

---

* English writers would say concavo-convex, with a positive focal length.—S. H.

the surface h_2. Let an arbitrary normal $k_2 v_2$ now be drawn on the surface h_2, and parallel thereto the normal $k_1 v_1$ on the surface h_1. Let a ray of light, moreover, be imagined in the direction $b_1 b_2$, proceeding in the

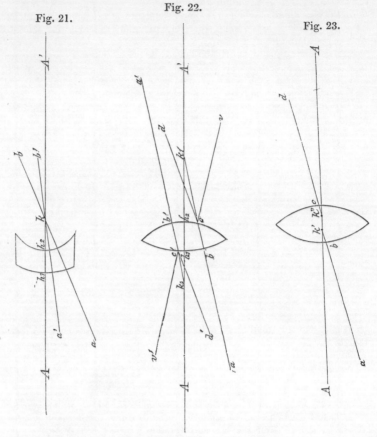

Fig. 21.

Fig. 22.

Fig. 23.

lens, then the angles formed by this ray with the two *parallel* normals k_1 v_1 and $k_2 v_2$ will be equal.

If the angles be equal, the deviations which the ray $b_1 b_2$ undergoes at b_1 and b_2 will also be equal, and as these deviations take place in opposite directions, $b_2 c$ is parallel to $a b_1$. The points k' and k'', to which $a b_1$ and $c b_2$ (respectively before and after the refractions) are directed, are therefore the nodal points of the lens.

In order to calculate the position of these points, first seek the point o, where the ray $b_1 b_2$ cuts the axis; if the radii $k_1 b_1 = \rho_1$, and $k_2 b_2 = \rho_2$ are parallel to one another, the triangles $k_1 b_1 h_1$ and $k_2 b_2 h_2$ are similar.

Consequently $\rho_1 : h_1\, b_1 = \rho_2 : h_2\, b_2.$

As, moreover, the triangles $h_1\, b_1\, o$ and $h_2\, b_2\, o$ are similar,

$$h_1\, b_1 : h_1\, o = h_2\, b_2 : h_2\, o\,;$$

and, consequently, $\rho_1 : h_1\, o = \rho_2 : h_2\, o\,;$

that is, the distances from h_1 and h_2 to o are proportionate to the radii of curvature ρ_1 and ρ_2 of the refracting surfaces h_1 and h_2. If the two radii of curvature are equal, o will therefore lie midway between h_1 and h_2.

If the point o be determined, we can easily, by calculation, find k' and k'': they are, in fact, the points whereon the rays which in the lens pass through o, or proceed from o, are directed without the lens—in other words, they are the images of o.

All the rays proceeding from o (Fig. 25), as $o\, b$ and $o\, c$, are, after refrac-

Fig. 24.

Fig. 25.

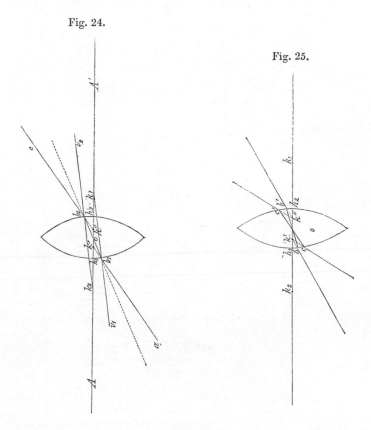

tion at the anterior surface h_1, directed to k', the rays $o\, b'$, and $o\, c'$ to k''. Consequently k' and o are the conjugate foci by refraction on the

surface h_1; k'' and o those for refraction on the surface h_2. Both are calculated according to the formula 3 c; it is therefore sufficient to apply
this formula to one of the two surfaces.

For the anterior surface of the lens (Fig. 26) $h_1 \phi'$ is $= F'$, $h_1 \phi'' = F''$
and $h_1 o = f''$. For $h_1 k' = f'$ we now find

Fig. 28.

Fig. 26.

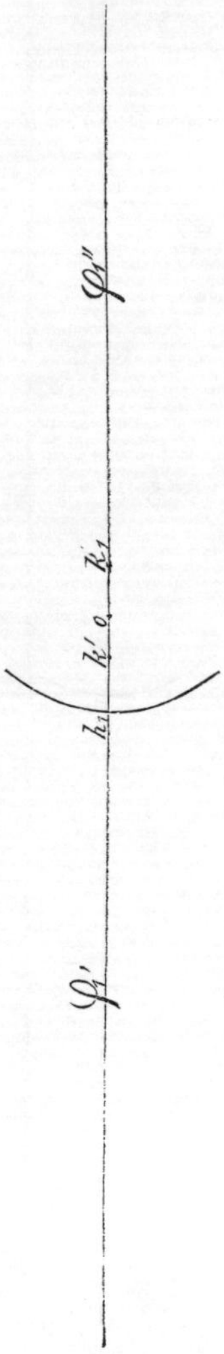

Fig. 27.

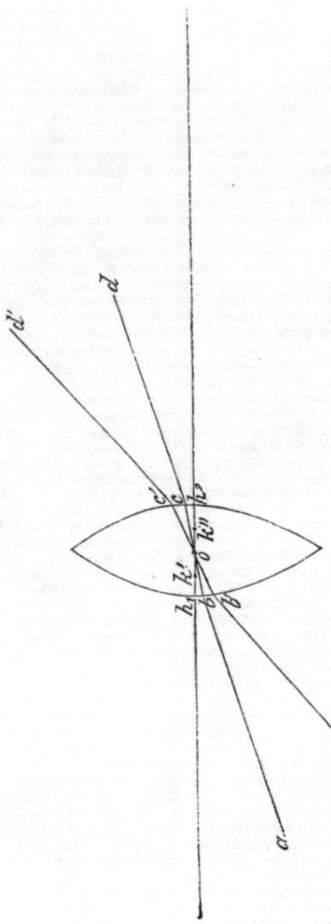

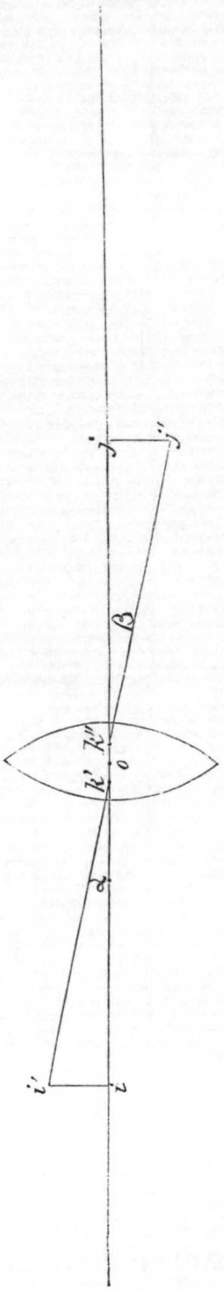

$$f' = \frac{F'f''}{F'' - f''}.$$

In this formula $f'' - F''$ has given place to $F'' - f''$, because the point of light o lies between h_1 and ϕ_1'' (compare Fig. 26), and k' is therefore a *virtual* image. In like manner, k'' is found for the surface h_2 of Fig. 25.

We have called k' and k'' the images of o. They are really so. Were there a little point in o in the lens (Fig. 25), it would, seen through the anterior surface of the lens h_1, appear to be in k', and, seen through the posterior surface h_2, in k''.

Now if the rays proceeding from o (Fig. 27), are, after refraction on the anterior surface h_1, at b and b' directed as $b\,a$ and $b'\,a'$ to k', after refraction on the posterior surface h_2, as $c\,d$ and $c'\,d'$ are directed to k'', the rays $a\,b$ and $a'\,b'$, which before the first refraction are directed to k', pass in the lens through o; and appear, after the second refraction as $c\,d$ and $c'\,d'$ to be derived from k'', $c\,d$ being, moreover, parallel to $a\,b$ and $c'\,d'$ to $a'\,b'$. The points found k' and k'' therefore correspond to the definition of nodal points above given.

IX.—*To make use of the nodal points.*

Of these nodal points we can make the same use as of the single nodal point (centre) of a single refracting surface (compare Fig. 10), with this difference, that between a point (Fig. 28) i' and its image j' we have to distinguish two rays of direction: the first, namely, $i'\,k'$, and the second $k''\,j'$. These are, however, parallel to one another, and the angles α and β are therefore equal. Consequently, the image $j\,j'$ is seen from k'' under the same angle, under which the object $i\,i'$ exhibits itself from k'. For the magnitudes of the object $i\,i' = B$ and the image $j\,j' = \beta$ we therefore find:

$$\beta : B = j\,k'' : i\,k'.$$

If the object lies at a great distance from the lens we may set down $i\,k' = i\,k''$, and the formula then becomes:

$\beta : B = j\,k'' : i\,k''$, whence the posterior nodal point results as sole nodal point, and we have to do with only one ray of direction.

X.—*Optical centre.*

The point o (Fig. 28, compare also Fig. 25) is known under the name of optical centre. Usually we assume that the rays directed to this optical centre, pass through unrefracted. The formula

$$\beta : B = j\,o : i\,o \text{ is then applied.}$$

We have already seen that this is not perfectly correct.

For thin lenses, with a long focal distance, this method, it is true, gives rise to no notable error. But for thick lenses, with a short focal distance, the deviation may be considerable, and the two nodal points must be taken into calculation. If either object or image be situated at an infinite, or at least at a very great distance from the lens, we may for these lenses, too, assume

4

one nodal point, namely, that on the side of the shorter conjugate focal distance (Compare IX.),—but in no case the optical centre.

XI.—*Every lens has two principal points, h' and h''.*

As a lens has two nodal points, it has also two principal points: If there exists only one refracting surface, the refracted ray is directed to the same point of that surface as the incident, and from this point, where the refraction takes place, we calculate the principal focal distance as well as the conjugate focal distances. The principal point lies then in the surface of curvature. If there be more than one refracting surface, a ray is after the last refraction evidently no longer directed to the point, where it underwent the first refraction. But we can, however, find two surfaces, perpendicular to the axis, which stand in such a relation to each other, that the rays before the first and after the last refraction are directed to exactly corresponding points of these two surfaces. This is, in fact, attained, if the two surfaces are images of one another, of equal size and like direction (situated on the same side of the axis). The two surfaces which fulfil these conditions, are the *principal surfaces*, and where they are cut by the axis, lie the *principal points*. From the first principal point h' the anterior, from the second h'' the posterior focal distance is calculated.

XII.—*Mode of finding the principal points.*

To find the principal surfaces, we must in the system, for example in a lens, determine in what position an object must be, in order to form similar images on both sides, these are then, also, images of one another, and therefore represent the principal surfaces. We immediately see that in a biconvex lens the place sought must be found, between the two refracting surfaces, *in* the lens. The magnitude of the virtual images, formed by each of the surfaces of an object situated here, we find by the formula (4 *b*),

$$\beta : B = F'' - f'' : F''.$$

In this each surface is considered, as if the other were not present.

Now in Fig. 29 let $h_2 \ \phi_2'' = F_2''$ be the posterior focal distance of the surface h_2 in glass for rays falling parallel in the direction $A' A$ on h_2, $h_1 \ \phi_1'' = F_1''$, the focal distance of the surface h_1, likewise in glass. Now if an object be at s, $sh_2 = f_2''$ and $sh_1 = f_1''$. If the images are of equal size, then since

$$\beta : B = F_2'' - f_2'' : F_2''$$

and

$$\beta : B = F_1'' - f_1'' : F_1''$$

the formula

$$f_2'' : F_2'' = f_1'' : F_1'' \ \ \ldots \ldots \text{ (b)}$$

must hold, which signifies, that in order to find the point s, $h_1 h_2$ must be divided into two parts, proportional to the focal distances $h_2 \ \phi_2'' = F_2''$ and $h_1 \ \phi_1'' = F_1''$.

The correctness of this result appears immediately from the construction (Compare Fig. 30).

Fig. 30.

Fig. 29.

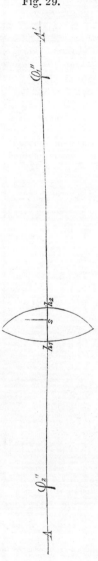

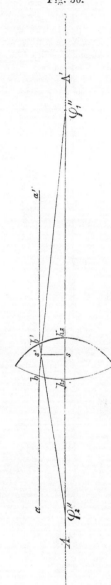

Each surface is here again considered, as if the other were not present.

The ray drawn from ϕ_1'' to s', becomes, as derived from the second focus of h_1', at b as $b\,a$, parallel to the axis, likewise that drawn from ϕ_2'' to s', in b' as $b'\,a'$. The distances from b and b' to the axis are therefore the magnitudes of the images of the line $s\,s'$, and these, $b\,h_1$ and $b'\,h_2$ assumed as vertical to the axis, are equally large, when $h_1\,h_2$ is divided proportionally to the focal distances. Then, since $\phi_2''\,s'$ and $\phi_1''\,s'$ are prolonged to b' and b proportionally, they will therefore in b' and b again have come to similar heights above the axis, just as was the case in s'.

If we now know the position of the point s, we find the positions of its images by the same formula 3 c,

$$f = \frac{F'f''}{F'' - f''},$$

according to which the position of the nodal points from o is determined (Compare VIII.).

XIII.—*Signification of the principal surfaces.*

The signification of the principal surfaces is this, that each ray, for example, $a\,b\,c\,d$ (Fig. 31), after the second refraction as $c\,d$, is directed to a point of

Fig. 31.

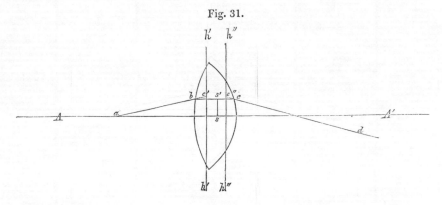

$h''\,h''$, removed as far from the axis as the point of $h'\,h'$, to which the ray $a\,b$ before the first refraction was directed. And that this must be the case, appears when we see that the ray in the lens passes through s', and remember that all rays passing through s' at the one side of the lens appear to come from e', and on the other side appear to come from e''.

XIV.—*Condition for the coincidence of the principal points and nodal points.*

In a lens bounded on both sides by the same medium, for example, air

($n' = n'''$), s and o coincide, and therefore also h' coincides with k', and h'' with k'' (Fig. 32).

Fig. 32.

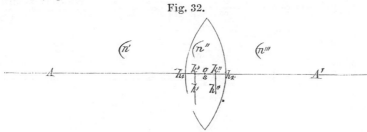

The point s is, namely, found by dividing the axis of the lens, into two parts, which are as the focal distances belonging to the principal points; the point o, by dividing the same axis into two parts, proportiona to the radii of curvature of the two surfaces. Now, since the focal distances are proportional to the radii of curvature, the division of the axis is in both cases the same, and therefore o and s coincide. The same must be true of their respective images, k' and k'', and h' and h''.

XV.—*Condition for the non-coincidence of the principal and nodal points.*

On the contrary, when the lens is not bounded on both sides by a medium whose refractive coefficient is equal ($n' \gtrless n'''$), s and o no longer coincide and therefore the images k' and k'' (of o) no longer coincide with h' and h (those of s).

For the principal points, also when $n' \gtrless n'''$, the formula still finds application: s lies always at the point where the distance $h_1 h_2 = D$, is divided proportionally to the principal focal distances. Then, namely, the two images of s s' continue, as a glance at Fig. 30 immediately shows, of equal size.

Now, in proportion as $\dfrac{n''}{n'''}$ becomes smaller, the second focal distance $h_2 \phi_2''$ of the surface h_2 becomes longer, and s' approaches more and more to h', whose focal distance $h_1 \phi_1''$ has remained unaltered. Lastly, if $\dfrac{n''}{n'''} = 1$, $h_2 \phi_2''$ is infinitely large, and s therefore lies in h_1. Then two images of s are no longer formed, but s coincides with its image in the point h_1: the lens is changed into a single refracting surface, of which I have in IV. shown how to recognise the cardinal points.

While in the case that n''' becomes greater than n', the point s is removed forward, the point o deviates in the opposite direction, backwards. This appears already from the fact, that, when $\dfrac{n''}{n'''}$ has become $= 1$, and consequently only one refracting surface has remained, s comes to lie on the surface of curvature h_1, and o, on the contrary, in the centre of curvature k_1 (Fig. 33) (compare Fig. 17). It must, however, be more accurately

Fig. 33.

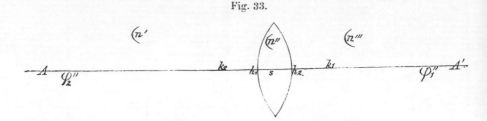

proved, and at the same time shown, how the position of o may in this case also be found.

In Fig. 34 $\frac{n''}{n'''}$ is much smaller than $\frac{n''}{n'}$, as it thence appears, that the focal distance of rays, parallel in the lens and refracted on the posterior surface, as $h_2 \phi_2' = F_2'$, is three times greater than that of the same rays refracted on the anterior surface, as $h_1 \phi_1' = F_1'$; while the radius of curvature $h_2 k_2$ is only $1\frac{1}{2}$ times greater than $h_1 k_1$.

If we draw from the point a, situated in the focal surface of h_1, a ray $a\,b\,c$, directed to k_1, this passes through at b unrefracted to c. If, moreover, we draw in the lens a second ray $c'\,b'$, parallel to $a\,b\,c$ and directed to k_2, and prolong this to a' in the focal surface of h_2, we have in the lens two parallel rays $b\,c$ and $b'\,c'$. All the rays parallel in the lens now unite in each of the focal surfaces into one point, whence it follows that $a\,b\,c$ is refracted at c and proceeds as $c\,a'$; $a'\,b'\,c'$ refracted at c' continues in the direction $c'\,a$. Now it appears that at the surface h_1 the ray $c\,b$ passes through unrefracted, the ray $b'\,c'$, on the contrary, experiences a deviation, $c'\,a\,b = \gamma_1$; that, on the contrary, at the surface h_2 the ray $c'\,b'$ passes through unrefracted, but $b\,c$ undergoes a deviation $= c\,a'\,b' = \gamma_2$.

Now, the deviation of rays, parallel to $b\,c$, increases on the surface h_1, between b and c', regularly from zero to γ_1; on the surface h_2, between b' and c, from zero to γ_2. Between $b\,c$ and $b'\,c'$, therefore, lies a ray parallel to both, which, at the two sides, at h_1 and h_2, has an equal deviation. It is evident that we shall have found this ray, if $a\,e$ is parallel to $a'\,e'$, or, in other words, if the angle $e\,a\,b$ is equal to $e'\,a'\,b'$. For that purpose let us consider the triangles $a\,b\,e$ and $a'\,b'\,e'$: these have the side $a\,b$ parallel to $a'\,b'$, $a\,e$ parallel to $a'\,e'$, finally, $b\,e$ parallel to $b'\,e'$, because both are perpendicular to the axis. They are consequently similar, and therefore

$$b\,e : b'\,e' = a\,b : a'\,b',$$

but because $a\,b$ has the same inclination, with respect to $h_1 \phi_1'$, that $a'\,b'$ has with respect to $h_2 \phi_2'$, we may write,

$$b\,e : b'\,e' = h_1\,\phi_1' : h_2\,\phi_2' = F_1' : F_2'.$$

Fig. 34.

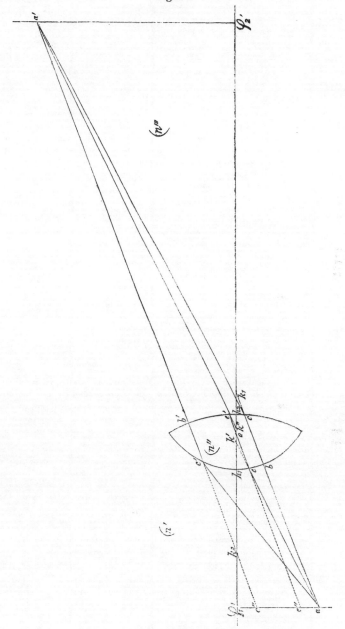

Finally, because the three lines $a'\, b'\, c'\, c''$, $e'\, o\, e\, e''$ and $k_1\, c\, b\, a$ are parallel,

$$k_1\, o : k_2\, o = e''\, a : c''\, e'',$$

and as

$$e''\, a = e\, b \text{ and } c''\, e'' = b'\, e'$$

$$k_1\, o : k_2\, o = b\, e : b'\, e' = F_1' : F_2'.$$

The point o is therefore found, by dividing the distance $k_1\, k_2$ between the centres of curvature of the two surfaces into two parts, proportional to F_1' and F_2', or (compare 2b and 2d) to the focal distances G_1'' and G_2'' belonging to k_1 and k_2.

This expression is the more general: it is applicable to all cases, and therefore also in the case where $n''' = n'$, for which above (VIII.) another expression was found.

Now, if the point o be known, the positions of the two nodal points k' and k'', the images of o (as well as that of the two principal points h' and h'', the images of s), are calculated according to the formula $3\, c$, as is pointed out in VIII. By construction k' and k'' have already been ascertained in Fig. 34. The anterior nodal point k' lies, namely, where the ray $a\, e$, prolonged as a right line (dotted), should cut the axis; the second k'', where the ray $e'\, a'$ should cut it. Every ray, which before the *first* refraction is directed to k', is after the *first* refraction directed to o, and after the *second* refraction to k'', and is again parallel to its original direction.

XVI.—*Foci.*

It now remains to define the *foci* of a lens (Fig. 35).

For this it is necessary to know the thickness of the lens $h_1\, h_2 = D$, and the focal distances of the two surfaces separately.

The foci of the surface h_1 lie in ϕ_1', and ϕ_1''; those of h_2 in ϕ_2' and ϕ_2''. Let us call the focal distances $h_1\, \phi_1'$ and $h_1\, \phi_1''$ F_1' and F_1''; the focal distances $h_2\, \phi_2'$ and $h_2\, \phi_2''$ are F_2' and F_2''.

They are found according to formulæ $1a$ and $1b$. If rays now come in the direction $A\, A'$, parallel to the axis, they are at the surface h_1 refracted towards the point ϕ_1''; if they arrive at h_2, their focal distance $h_2\, \phi_1''$ is $= F_1'' - D$. Here they are again refracted at a surface with focal distances F_2' and F_2''. They will therefore unite in ϕ'', and $h_2\, \phi''$ will be found according to the formula $3\, d$.

The second principal focal distance, which is calculated from the second principal point h'', is now $F'' = h_2\, \phi'' + h_2\, h''$.

In like manner we find $h_1\, \phi'$, by letting the rays fall, parallel to the axis, in the direction $A'\, A$ on h_2, and undergo a second refraction at the surface h_1. Moreover, F' is $= h_1\, \phi' + h_1\, h'$.

If the first and last media be similar, $n''' = n'$, then $F' = F''$, and therefore needs not to be separately sought. Of this the proof is simple.

For, let $h''\, \phi''$ be found $= F''$ (Fig. 36), then from the point a, situated in the posterior focal surface, let two rays proceed: the first $a\, h''$, directed to the nodal point, is at the other side of the lens in (n', as $h'\, a'$, parallel to $a\, h''$; the second $a\, b\, b'$, proceeding from the same point a, must in (n' be parallel to $a\, h'$, and since it in (n''' is parallel to the axis, it must in (n' cut the axis in the anterior focal point ϕ'.

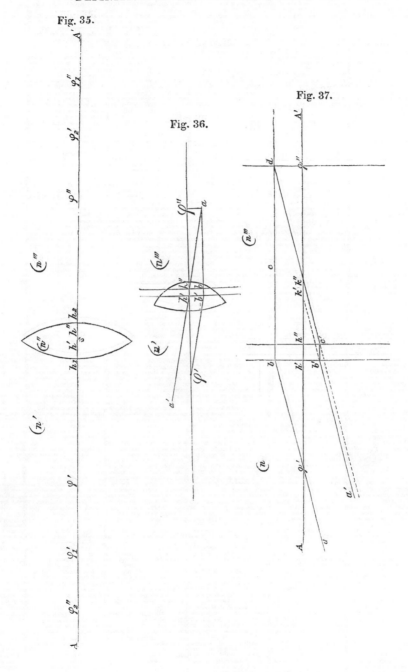

Fig. 35.

Fig. 36.

Fig. 37.

As in the triangles $a\ h''\ b$ and $\phi'\ b'\ h'$, $h'\ \phi'$ is evidently parallel to $a\ b$, and $b'\ \phi'$ to $a\ h''$, and, moreover, $h''\ b = h'\ b'$, the two triangles are equal and similar, and $h'\ \phi' = h''\ \phi''$, that is $F' = F''$.

XVII.—*Reciprocal dependence of the position of the principal points and nodal points in reference to the foci.*

In §§ XIV. and XV. it was shown, in what manner, when n''' is $\diagdown\diagup$ n', and, consequently, the principal points and nodal points do not coincide, these points may be separately found. This was done in order to exhibit clearly the signification of these points, and to afford a proof, that in a compound dioptric system points are to be found, having the already explained signification of principal points and nodal points. Now we may proceed from this signification, to show their reciprocal dependence in position, whence it will appear that the foci being known, from the position of the nodal points that of the principal points, or *vice versâ*, may be deduced.

We may remember that for a single refracting surface, where only one principal point and one nodal point exists (Fig. 17),

$$k\ \phi'' = h\ \phi'$$
$$F' = F^v \frac{n'}{n''} \ \ldots\ldots 1\,c$$
$$F^v = F' + \rho \ \ldots\ldots 1\,d$$

In agreement with this we shall show, that in a compound dioptric system,

$$h'\ \phi' = k''\ \phi'', \text{ that is, } F' = G'' \ \ldots\ldots 5\,a$$
$$h'\ h'' = k'\ k'' \ \ldots\ldots\ldots\ldots\ldots\ldots\ldots\ldots\ldots 5\,c$$
$$h''\ \phi'' = k'\ \phi', \text{ that is, } F'' = G' \ \ldots\ldots 5\,b$$
$$F^v = F' \frac{n_m}{n'} \ \ldots\ldots\ldots\ldots\ldots\ldots 5\,d.$$

It is first to be proved that $h'\ \phi' = k''\ \phi''$.

The ray $a\ b$ (Fig. 37), cutting the axis in the anterior focus ϕ, falls upon the first principal surface in b, and now runs in (n''' as $c\ d$ parallel to the axis. All rays, in (n' parallel to $a\ b$, unite with $a\ b$ in the same point d of the posterior focal surface. *Vice versâ*, therefore, every ray proceeding from d runs in (n' parallel to $a\ b$.

One of these rays, namely $d\ c'$, is in (n''' already parallel to $a\ b$, and must therefore in n', as $b'\ a'$, continue parallel to $a\ b$, that is, to itself. Now the distinctive mark of the nodal points is, that rays, in (n''' directed to k'', in n' are directed to k' and parallel to themselves. Consequently, where $d\ c'$ cuts the axis, lies k'', and the point of the axis, whereon $a'\ b'$ is directed, is k'. Now it immediately appears that the triangles $\phi'\ b\ h'$ and $k''\ d\ \phi''$ are equal and similar, and consequently,

$$k''\ \phi'' = h'\ \phi', \text{ that is, } G'' = F' \ \ldots\ldots 5\,a. \text{ Q. E. D.}$$

It is at the same time included in this construction, that

$$k'\ k'' = h'\ h''.$$

For $k' k''$ $b' c'$ is a parallelogram, and $b' c'$ h' h'' a rectangle,

Therefore $h' h'' = b' c' = k' k''$............5 c,

Now, if $k' k'' = h' h''$, it follows further that

$$h' k' = h'' k'',$$

and since

$$k' \phi' = h' k' + h' \phi'$$
$$h'' \phi'' = h'' k'' + k'' \phi''$$
$$k' \phi' \text{ is } = h'' \phi'', \text{ that is, } G' = F'' \ldots\ldots 5 \, b.$$

Moreover, we see that ϕ', h' and k' have a relation to the direction of the rays in $(n'$; ϕ'', h'' and k'' to the direction of the rays in $(n'''$.

XVIII.—*The principal focal distances are proportional to the coefficients of refraction of the first and last media.*

In order to prove this important proposition, we must make use of a well-known law, which connects the magnitude of the images with the divergence of the rays, independently of the position and the focal distance of the refracting surface.

In Fig. 38, let i be a point, j its image, h the refracting spherical surface; consequently, $i\,h = f'$ and $h\,j = f''$. For small angles $h\,b$ may be regarded as perpendicular; and if this perpendicular be short, the opposite angles $h\,i\,b = a$ and $b\,j\,h = a'$ are inversely proportional to their distances from $h\,b$.

Consequently, $f' a = f'' a' \ldots \ldots A.$

Moreover, we know, that

$$\frac{F''}{F'} = \frac{n''}{n'} \text{ and } \frac{\beta}{B} = \frac{f'' - F''}{F''} \ldots\ldots 2\,c \text{ and } 4\,b.$$

By multiplication we obtain:

$$\frac{\beta}{B} \cdot \frac{n''}{n'} = \frac{F''}{F'} \cdot \frac{f'' - F''}{F''} = \frac{f'' - F''}{F'}$$

Now likewise (as follows from 3 c),

$$\frac{f''}{f'} = \frac{f'' - F''}{F'},$$

consequently,

$$\frac{f''}{f'} = \frac{\beta}{B} \cdot \frac{n''}{n'}.$$

This value, placed in the above equation A, gives

$$B \, n' \, a = \beta \, n'' \, a' \ldots\ldots\ldots 6\,a,$$

which formula expresses the law above mentioned.

Let us now consider a compound dioptric system (Fig. 39), in which the object, $i\,i' = B$, is equal in size to its image $j\,j' = \beta$. In order to construct this, let us first place the nodal points k' k'', and draw the line $i'\,k'$, and $k''\,j'$ parallel to it $= k'\,i$. At some distance from k' k'' let us now place k' $h'' = k'\,k''$. All rays, proceeding from i', unite in its image j'; one of these rays, namely $i'\,b$, proceeding from i' parallel to the axis, shows the position of the posterior focal point ϕ''; and as $b\,h'' = i'\,i = j\,j'$, the triangles $h''\,\phi''\,b$ and $j\,\phi''\,j'$ are equal and similar, consequently $h''\,\phi'' = \phi''j$, or $h''\,\phi'' = \frac{1}{2}\,h''j$, that is, $F'' = \frac{1}{2}\,f''$.

Fig. 39.

Fig. 38.

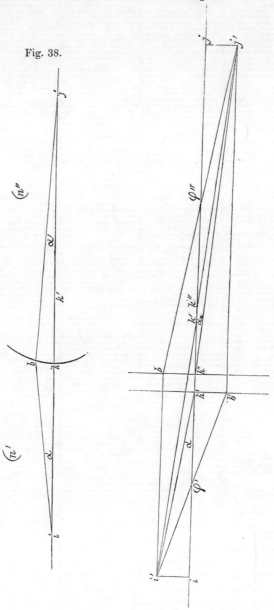

Likewise the ray $j'\,b'$, proceeding from j' parallel to the axis, shows, where it cuts the axis, the position of the anterior focal point in ϕ', and in like manner it appears, that $h'\,\phi' = \frac{1}{2}\,h'\,i$, that is $F' = \frac{1}{2}f'$.

Let us now consider the ray, which, proceeding in the direction $i'\,h'$ from i, arrives in the direction $h''\,j'$ in j', but on its way, refracted at various surfaces, has so many times acquired another unknown direction. We know only the angle $i'\,h'\,i = a$, which it forms before the first refraction in the medium with index $(n'$, and the angle $j\,h''\,j' = a_m$, which it makes after the last refraction in the medium with index n_m, with the axis.

In the first place it appears that $\dfrac{a}{a_m} = \dfrac{F''}{F'}\cdot$

For, since $i\,i' = j\,j'$, the little angles opposite each are inversely proportional to their distances from $i\,i'$, or $j\,j'$. Consequently:

$$\frac{a}{a_m} = \frac{j\,h''}{i\,h'} = \frac{f''}{f'};$$

and since, in the supposed case,

$$F' = \tfrac{1}{2}\,f' \text{ and } F'' = \tfrac{1}{2}f'',$$
$$\frac{F''}{F'} = \frac{f''}{f'} \text{ and } \frac{a}{a_m} = \frac{F''}{F'}\cdot$$

Secondly, we shall show that

$$\frac{a}{a_m} = \frac{n'}{n_m}.$$

Let us call the angles, which the ray proceeding from i under the angle a, and arriving at j' under the angle a_m, in its course successively makes with the axis, a', a'', a''', etc. With the magnitudes of the angles the magnitudes of the images also every time alter: let the magnitude of the image in the first principal surface be β, and that of the series of images after each refraction β'', β''', etc.; lastly, in the second principal surface, after the last refraction $\beta_m = \beta'$. Now, as two successive images may each time be considered related as object B to image β, we may apply the formula $(6\,a)$.

$$B\,n'\,a = \beta\,n''\,a',$$

to the series of images, formed in the compound system, and thus we obtain

$$\beta'\,n'\,a = \beta''\,n''\,a'$$
$$\beta''\,n''\,a' = \beta'''\,n'''\,a''$$

etc.

Whence follows:

$$\beta'\,n'\,a = \beta_m\,n_m\,a_m;$$

and as $\quad\quad\quad\quad \beta' = \beta_m$

so $\quad\quad\quad\quad n'\,a = n_m\,a_m,$ or

$$\frac{a}{a_m} = \frac{n'}{n_m}\cdot$$

Now if, as we have above shown for the particular case,

$$\frac{a}{a_m} = \frac{F''}{F'}, \text{ so also,}$$

$$\frac{F''}{F'} = \frac{n'}{n_m}\text{ Q. E. D.}$$

and which, of course, holds good for all cases.

XIX.—*Application to the crystalline lens.*

All the foregoing may be applied to the crystalline lens. In the non-accommodated eye the radius of the anterior surface (Fig. 40 h_1) is about $= 10$ mm.; that of the posterior surface $h_2 = 6$ mm.; its thickness $h_1 \, h_2 = 3.6$ mm.; and the coefficient of refraction is stated to be, for the lens 1·455, for the vitreous and aqueous humours 1·3366.

Hence the cardinal points are to be calculated. The optical centre o lies $(3.6 \times 6 : 6 + 10 =) \ 1.35$ mm. from the posterior, and therefore $(3.6 - 1.35 =) \ 2.25$ mm. from the anterior surface of the crystalline lens. From this optical centre let rays pass forwards into the aqueous humour, and backwards into the vitreous humour, and calculate (according to formula 3 c), from what points in the lens they shall appear to proceed. These points appear to be k' situated at 1·4927, and k'' at 1·2644 mm. from the posterior surface of the lens, and therefore less than $\frac{1}{4}$ mm. from each other. By the method pointed out in XVI., we calculate $h_2 \, \varphi''$, and add $h'' \, h_2$, then we have the posterior principal focal distance $h'' \, \varphi'' = F'' = 43.707$ mm., and to this the anterior is equal, because the vitreous and aqueous humours may be considered similar. Therefore, also, k' and k'' coincide with h' and h''.

Our knowledge of the crystalline lens, however, leaves much to be desired. Probably the index of refraction is somewhat too great, and thus the focal distance as assumed is too small.

The use which may be made of our knowledge of the six cardinal points, in the determination of the magnitude and position of the images, is included in the foregoing, but will be still more evident when we shall have studied:—

C.—Refraction through a compound system, consisting of a spherical surface and a biconvex lens.

XX.—*General indication of the cardinal points of the eye.*

The dioptric system of the eye consists of a spherical surface and a biconvex lens. We shall at once make the cornea and crystalline lens, with which we are now acquainted, the foundation for finding the cardinal points of this compound system. Let system A (Fig. 41) represent the position of the cardinal points of the cornea; system B that of the lens; system C that of the eye. The distances are taken as they occur in a well-constructed eye. System C must be found from the systems A and B. From the diagrammatic representation which the figure gives us, we are directly led to the conclusions: 1. That the principal points and nodal points in system C cannot coincide, for, just as in system A, the first and last media, $(n'$ and $(n'''$, are dissimilar. 2. That as the nodal point of system

A nearly coincides with k' and k'' (or h' and h'') of system B, k' and k'' of system C come to lie nearly at the same height, at least undoubtedly in the posterior part of the crystalline lens. 3. That while the principal point h of system A lies on the anterior surface of the cornea, and the principal points h' and h'' of system B lie in the lens, at 5·7073 and 5·9356 mm. behind that of system A, those of system C must fall in the aqueous humour. 4. That ·by the combined action of A and B the focal distances $h' \phi'$ and $h'' \phi''$ in system C are much shorter than in system A and system B.

XXI.—*Calculation of the position of the principal points in the eye.*

If we now wish to determine the situation of h' and h'' in system C, we have nothing else to do (compare XII.) than to seek for the point s, and to calculate the positions of the two images from this point ; the two images are then the principal points $h' h''$ of system C. Now the point s lies between h (system A) and h' system B : and indeed at distances proportional to the principal focal distances of each of these systems. For this being the position of s, the image of the perpendicular $s s'$ (Fig. 42) formed by the cornea C, is of equal size with the image formed by the crystalline lens L. The magnitudes are easily found by construction (compare Fig. 30). In Fig. 42 $h \phi''$ is the posterior focal distance F_c of the cornea, $h' \phi'$ the anterior F_l' of the crystalline lens. Supposing the crystalline lens away, the cornea forms an image of $s s' = h a$; supposing the cornea away, the lens forms an image of $s s' = h' a'$. These two images $h a$ and $h' a'$ are of equal size (compare XII.), when

$$\phi'' s' : s' a = \phi' s' : s a',$$

in which case

$$h \phi'' : h s = h' \phi' : h' s.$$

At the same time it appears that the point s lies where $h h'$, and not where $h h''$ is divided proportionally to the focal distances $h \phi'' = F_c''$ and $h' \phi' = F_l'$; for already from the point a, situated in the surface h', the ray $\phi'' a'$ is continued as $a' b$ parallel to the axis. Furthermore, it appears that if the first system A, as well as system B, had two principal points, the distance between h'' of system A and h' of system B must be divided proportionally to the focal distances, in order to find the point s.

Now, in the eye, h lies in the curve of the cornea, h', on the contrary, 5·7073 mm. behind the cornea ; F_c'' is $= 31·692$, $F_l' = 43·707$ mm. Consequently s lies $5·7073 \times 31·692 : 31·692 + 43·707 = 2·399$ mm. behind the cornea, that is, $5·7073 - 2·399 = 3·3083$ before the anterior principal point of the crystalline lens. The position of the images of s we now further find as h' and h'' (system C), according to the formula $(3 c)$:

The position of $h' = \dfrac{2·399 \times 23·692}{31·692 - 2·399} = 1·9403$ behind h (the anterior

surface of the cornea), and the position of $h'' = \dfrac{3·3083 \times 43·707}{43·707 - 3·3088} = 3·5793$

before the posterior principal point of the lens. This lies 5·9356 mm. behind the cornea, and consequently, h'' at $5·9356 - 3·5793 = 2·4563$ behind the anterior surface of the cornea.

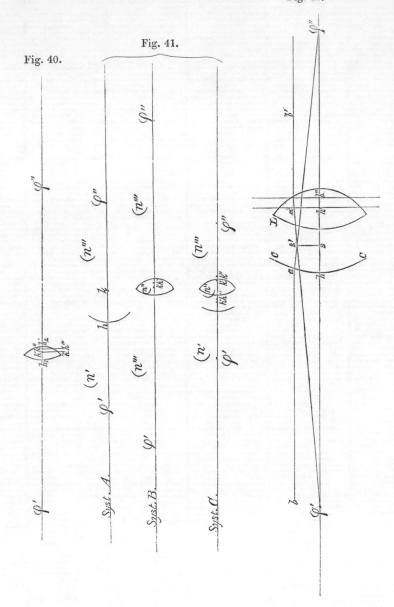

Fig. 40.

Fig. 41.

Fig. 42.

XXII.— *Calculation of the position of the nodal points in the eye.*

In order to find the positions k' and k'' of system C, we should remember (VIII.), that they are the images of the point o, which divides the distance between the nodal points of system A and system B (compare XV. and Fig. 41) into two parts, proportional to the focal distances G_1'' and G_2'' belonging to the nodal points.

The focal distance belonging to h, system A, is $\phi'' k = \phi' h' = 23\cdot692$. The focal distance belonging to k', system B, $= 43\cdot707$. Moreover, k lies at 8, k' at $5\cdot7073$ behind the cornea. Their mutual distance amounts to $2\cdot2927$. This is to be divided in the proportion of $23\cdot692$ and $43\cdot707$. We now find $\dfrac{2\cdot2927 \times 43\cdot707}{43\cdot707 + 23\cdot692} = 1\cdot4867.$

So much does o lie behind h' of system B, and consequently,

$$5\cdot7073 + 1\cdot4867 = 7\cdot194 \text{ mm., behind the cornea.}$$

The image k', formed of o by the cornea, is found at

$$\frac{23\cdot692 \times 7\cdot194}{31\cdot692 - 7\cdot194} = 6\cdot957 \text{ behind the cornea.}$$

The image k'', formed of o by the crystalline lens,

lies at $\dfrac{43\cdot707 \times 1\cdot4867}{43\cdot707 + 1\cdot4867} = 1\cdot4376$ behind the second principal point of the crystalline lens, and consequently $1\cdot4376 + 5\cdot9356 = 7\cdot3732$ behind the cornea.

The distance $k' k''$ of system $C = 7\cdot373 - 6\cdot957 = 0\cdot416$ mm. = the distance $h' h''$ of system C.

If we first determine the position of the foci, that of the nodal points will follow without separate calculation.

$$k'' \phi'' = h' \phi'$$
and
$$k' k'' = h' h''$$

which has already been proved (XVIII. and XVII.).

XXIII.— *Calculation of the position of the foci in the eye.*

Lastly, the focal distances of system C are easily calculated.

Parallel rays, refracted by h of system A, converge to the point ϕ, situated at $31\cdot692$ behind the cornea. On their way lies system B, and of it they meet h' at $5\cdot7073$ behind the cornea, that is, while they converge to a point situated $31\cdot692 - 5\cdot7073 = 25\cdot9847$ behind h'. Calculated from h'', F'' of system B is $= 43\cdot707$.—We therefore find (according to form. 3 d) the posterior focus ϕ'' of system C at $\dfrac{25\cdot9847 \times 43\cdot707}{25\cdot9847 + 43\cdot707} = 16\cdot296$

behind h'' of B, and consequently $16\cdot296 + 5\cdot936 = 22\cdot23$ behind the cornea, that is, $22\cdot231 - 2\cdot3563 = 19\cdot875$ mm. behind h_2 of system C. The posterior principal focal distance F'' of the eye therefore amounts to $19\cdot875$ mm.

5

To calculate the anterior focal distance, we start from rays parallel in the vitreous humour. Refracted by the lens, these converge at 43·707 before h' of system B; consequently they arrive at the anterior surface of the cornea at $43·707 — 5·7073 = 37·9997$, and are there refracted at

$$\frac{23·692 \times 37·9997}{31·692 + 37·9997} = 12·918$$

before the cornea, that is, $12·918 + 1·9403 = 14·8583$ before h' of Syst. C.

Fig. 43.

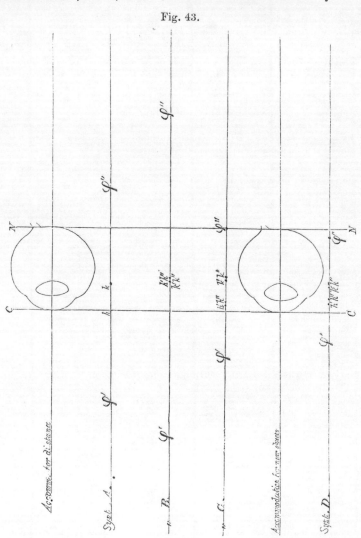

The anterior principal focal distance F' of the eye therefore amounts to 14·8583 mm.

A similar separate calculation is not, strictly speaking, necessary for F', because we may apply the formula ·5 d.

XXIV.—*Review of the position of the cardinal points in the eye.*

We are now enabled to combine in a table the positions of the cardinal points, first separately of the two component systems of the eye, system A, the cornea, system B, the lens; and subsequently of the compound system C, the eye itself. We have prefixed the computed position and curvature of the refracting surfaces, and represented the values found, in their true magnitude for each system in a diagram (Fig. 43). Above system D is placed a scheme of the form of the lens and of the position of the cardinal points in the eye accommodated for near objects. The line $C\,C$ represents the position of the cornea ; $N\,N$ that of the retina. The lengths are given in millimètres, and the position is calculated from the anterior surface of the cornea. The refractive coëfficients are assumed as $\dfrac{103}{77}$ for the aqueous and vitreous humours, and $\dfrac{16}{11}$ for the crystalline lens.

We have placed the values which obtain in accommodation for near objects, next those for the eye in a state of rest :

	Accommodation for Distance.	Accommodation for Near Objects.
Radius of curvature of the cornea	8	8
Radius of curvature of the anterior surface of the lens	10	6
Radius of curvature of the posterior surface of the lens	6	5·5
Position of the anterior surface of the lens	3·6	3·2
Position of the posterior surface of the lens	7·2	7·2
The refracting numbers, represented by the diagram, are the following :—		
Anterior focal distance of the cornea	23·692	23·692
Posterior focal distance of the cornea	31·692	31·692
Focal distance of the lens	43·707	33·785
Distance of the anterior principal point of the lens from its anterior surface	2·1037	1·9745
Distance of the posterior principal point of the lens from its posterior surface	1·2644	1·8100
Distance of the two principal points of the lens from each other	0·2283	0·2155
Posterior focal distance of the eye	19·875	17·756
Anterior focal distance of the eye	19·875	13·274
Place of the anterior focus	12·918	11·241
Place of the first principal point	1·9403	2·0330
Place of the second principal point	2·3563	2·4919
Place of the first nodal point	6·957	6·515
Place of the second nodal point	7·373	6·974
Place of the posterior focus	22·231	20·248

Hence it appears, that $h'\ \phi' = k''\ \phi''$, $k'\ k'' = h'\ h''$, $k'\ \phi' = h''\ \phi''$, and $F'\ n'''$ $= F''\ n'$; that is, 103 $F' = 77\ F''$ (compare XVII. and XVIII.).

XXV.— *Use to be made of the knowledge of the cardinal points.*

After we have learned the cardinal points in the eye, it remains to show what use is to be made thereof, in order to find by construction the course of each ray, and the situation and size of the dioptric images.

For the sake of clearness, we take, in the following figures, all measurements at double the size of those in the eye, and the mutual distance of the two nodal and of the two principal points as somewhat greater than it really is. The line $C\ C$ represents the anterior surface of the cornea, $V\ V$ the anterior surface of the vitreous humour.

Let us briefly recapitulate (compare Fig. 44): 1. That every ray, for

Fig. 44.

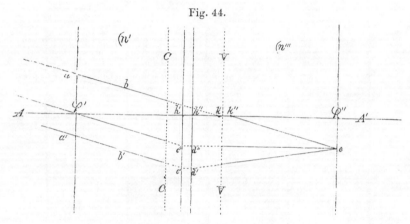

example $a\ b$, which in the first medium (n' is directed to k', in the last medium (n''' is parallel to its primitive direction, but is directed to k''. 2. That every ray, for example $e\ d'$, in (n''' is directed to a point (d') of the surface $h^{\varepsilon}\ d''$, removed as far from the axis $A\ A'$ as the point (c') of the surface h' c'', to which it, as $b'\ c'$, was directed in the first medium: that is, $c'\ d'$ is parallel to the axis. 3. That all rays which are parallel in (n', for example $a\ b$ and $a'\ b'$, unite in one point in the second focal surface $\phi''e$ (and indeed in the axis in the point ϕ'', when they are parallel to the axis). 4. That all rays, parallel in (n''', unite in one point in the anterior focal surface $\phi'\ a$, and if they are parallel to the axis, as $e\ d''\ c''$, in the point ϕ'.

By the application of these rules we can out of each given ray in (n', ascertain its course in (n'''. What deviations it undergoes at the several refracting surfaces, we do not in this mode trace. The lines, therefore, represent only the course of rays, so long as they are in the air (n', or in the vitreous humour (n'''. To denote this they are dotted between the cornea and the vitreous humour, where the ray leaves the course of the line.

Now let a ray, $a\,b$ (Fig. 45) in $(n'$, be given; it is desired to ascertain

Fig. 46.

Fig. 45.

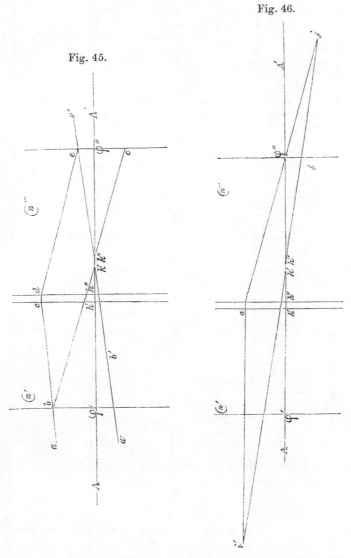

its course in $(n'''$. This object can be obtained in two modes. First, let the ray be produced to the first principal surface, which it cuts in c; the ray will thus in $(n'''$ be directed to the point of the second principal surface, corresponding to c, that is to d (rule 3). Let the ray now cut the anterior focal sur-face in b. All rays, proceeding from b, are parallel in (n''' (compare 4); the direction of one of these rays, $b\,k'$, is known, for it continues as $k''\,c$ parallel to its primitive direction ; but we thus need only, proceeding from d, to draw a line parallel to $b\,k'$ or $k''\,c$: to find the direction of the line $d\,e$, which the ray follows in (n'''.—We may equally make use of rules 1 and 3 to find the course. All rays parallel to $a\,b$ unite in the posterior focal surface ϕ'' into one point. Of one of these rays $a'\,b'\,k'$ we know the direction, which, namely, continues as $k''\,e'$ parallel to $b'\,k'$. Where this ray cuts the focal surface ϕ'', the ray $a\,b$ must also cut the focal surface, and the line $d\,e$ drawn from d therefore gives the direction of the ray $a\,b$ in (n'''.

Let a point i' (Fig. 46) be given : it is desired to ascertain its image j'. For this purpose it is necessary only to determine the course in (n''' of two rays proceeding from i', and to see where they cut one another. The ray $i\,k'$ passes as $k''\,b$ through the vitreous humour (compare 1), the ray $i'\,a$, parallel to the axis, cuts the axis in the posterior focal surface at ϕ'' and intersects $k''\,b$ in j'. In j', therefore, the image of i' should lie, if the vitreous humour extends so far : its virtual image lies there.

XXVI.—*Calculation of the position and magnitude of the dioptric images of the eye.*

From the foregoing constructions it appears, that the cardinal points of a compound system being known, the position and magnitude of the dioptric images of the eye are to be calculated according to the same for-mulæ, as in the case of a simple refracting surface.

$h'\,\phi' = k''\,\phi''$ (Fig. 47) is the anterior focal distance $F' = G''$,

$h''\,\phi'' = k'\,\phi'$ is the posterior principal focal distance $F'' = G'$.

Fig. 47.

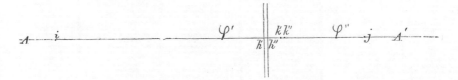

Let i now be a point of light, j its image, then

$$h'\,i = f'$$
$$h''\,j = f''$$
$$k'\,i = g'$$
$$k''\,j = g''.$$

According to the formula (3 d or b) we can now calculate the position of j, if f' or g' be given, and *vice versâ* (according to the formula 3 a and 3 c) the position of i, if f'' or g'' be known.

Of this formula we shall here make use, in order to calculate at what distance g' (reckoned from k), the diagrammatic eye, accommodated for near objects, sees accurately.

In this eye (compare XXIV.) ϕ'' lies $20\cdot248 - 6\cdot974 = 13\cdot274$ mm. behind k''. Consequently $G'' = 13\cdot274$. The retina lies $22\cdot231 - 6\cdot974 = 15\cdot257$ mm. behind k''. Hence $g'' = 15\cdot257$, $G' = 6\cdot515 + 11\cdot241 = 17\cdot756$

Now we find $g' = \dfrac{G' \, g''}{g'' - G''} = 1136\cdot6$ mm. $= 5\cdot047$ Parisian inches. This is the nearest point of distinct vision; the farthest (diagrammatic eye, accommodated for distance) lies at an infinite distance. This range of accommodation of $1 : 5\cdot047$ corresponds to that of the age of about 20 years.

In the eye the two nodal points lie so close to one another, and in ordinary vision g' is so much larger than g'', that, just as in a single refracting surface, we may draw the lines of direction of the object immediately through the posterior nodal point, without taking the anterior into consideration. The magnitudes of object and image are therefore proportional to their distances from the posterior nodal point k''. In the diagrammatic eye the last distance amounts to $14\cdot858$ mm. Now if the object lies $14\cdot851$ mètres from the eye, the image is a thousand times smaller than the object.

XXVII.—*Comparison of R and P, deduced from measurements on the eye and optometrically determined.*

In XXVI. we calculated the farthest and nearest points of distinct vision of the diagrammatic eye. Now Dr. Knapp has in four eyes, from the radii of curvature and the position of the refracting surfaces, together with the two limits of accommodation, calculated the position of the cardinal points, and thence deduced the nearest and farthest points of distinct vision with the range of accommodation. Now it was extremely important to see how far these results of measurement and calculation agreed with those of the simple optometrical investigation in the same persons. The result is, that in three of the four persons the agreement is as great as could be expected in the difficult and complicated mode of determining the surfaces of curvature. There was found (compare *Archiv f. Ophthalmologie*, Bd. VIII. 2. 138) :

	Accommodation determined by	
	Measurements of the s of Curvature.	Optometrical Investigation.
I.	1:6·207	1:3·953
II.	1:4·227	1:4·064
III.	1:3·883	1:4·248
IV.	1:3·581	1:3·214

If it were necessary, we might in this agreement find a fresh argument in favour of the view, that the accommodation depends exclusively upon

an alteration of the system of the crystalline lens.   If no further arguments are necessary to this end, this agreement establishes the correctness
of Dr. Knapp's measurements.

SECOND PART.

Range of Accommodation.

XXVIII.—*Foundation and definition of the range of accommodation.*

The measure of the range of accommodation must be connected with the
change which takes place in accommodation in the eye.   If the power of
accommodation depended, as was formerly supposed, on a prolongation of
the axis of vision, the numerical expression of the range of accommodation
should be sought in the amount of this prolongation.   The alteration which
takes place in the eye in accommodation is, however, of a wholly different
nature, and is confined, as we have seen, to the system of the crystalline
lens: the anterior surface increases considerably in convexity, and at the
same time advances more forward, the posterior surface becomes a little
more convex, without going backward, and with these complicated modifications the position of the cardinal points of the lens, and, at the same time,
that of the cardinal points of the whole eye, is altered. The chief point, therefore, which presents itself is: the shortening of the focal distance of the lens;
that is, as if the crystalline received the addition of a positive lens.   Now
from the focal distance A, of such an auxiliary lens, is the range of accommodation to be determined, and as the power of a lens is inversely proportional to its focal distance, the numerical expression of the range of accommodation becomes $1 : A$.   We can by investigation determine the distance
R of the farthest point r, and the distance P of the nearest point p, both
reckoned to the eye.   From these distances $\frac{1}{A}$ must be deduced, and if the
position and radius of curvature of all refracting surfaces of the eye, in
accommodation for r and for p are not known, we have no other data.   Now
we have assumed $\frac{1}{P} - \frac{1}{R} = \frac{1}{A}$.   Rays, namely, proceeding from the
nearest point of distinct vision, shall appear to proceed from the far-
thest point, when (P and R being reckoned to the cornea) they are refracted by a lens l with focal distance A (compare formula, p. 28). Thus, if
such a lens be placed immediately before the cornea, it represents the range
of accommodation so far, that without the lens the rays proceeding from r,
with the lens, those proceeding from p, come to a point upon the retina. But
by this the expression $\frac{1}{P} - \frac{1}{R} = \frac{1}{A}$ is not yet justified. The lens, namely,

which is added to the eye in accommodation for p, lies *in* and not *before* the eye, and it thus produces other modifications in the position of the cardinal points than accommodation for near objects.   Moreover, with the difference of position a difference of focal distance of the auxiliary lens will be combined, and consequently $\frac{1}{A} = \frac{1}{P} - \frac{1}{R}$ is by no means the lens, which the crystalline of the eye adds to itself in accommodation for p. The question therefore is, whether we may consider this formula as the numerical expression of the range of accommodation.

Evidently we here deal only with proportional magnitudes.   The formula must serve us, to compare reciprocally the different values of the range of accommodation under various circumstances.   Now if the alteration of the crystalline lens, although not altogether equal, be at least sufficiently proportional to $\frac{1}{A} = \frac{1}{P} - \frac{1}{R}$, this formula fulfils all requirements and represents also the changes in the eye.   It shall be shown that this is actually the case.

XXIX.—*Determination of the range of accommodation by the focal distance of a lens, with its nodal point situated in one of the nodal points of the eye.*

In XXVI. the distance g' from the first nodal point to the object, for which the eyes were accommodated, was calculated from the position of the retina and of the cardinal points in given eyes.   *Vice versâ*, we may from g' and g'' deduce the position of the cardinal points of the system. We start from the formula (3 b).

$$\frac{G''}{g''} + \frac{G'}{g'} = 1, \text{ and since,}$$

if

$$\frac{n''}{n'} = n,$$

$$G' = n\,G'',$$

we have

$$\frac{G''}{g''} + \frac{G''\,n}{g'} = 1$$

$$\frac{1}{g''\,n} + \frac{1}{g'} = \frac{1}{G''\,n}$$

$$G''\,n = \frac{g''\,n\,g'}{g''\,n + g'}$$

$$G'' = \frac{g''\,g'}{g''\,n + g'}.$$

Knowing G'' and g'', it now immediately follows, what lens the eye has added to itself, to be accommodated to the distance g'.   In this we suppose that the nodal points of the eye have continued unaltered, which, as is evident from what has been above advanced, is the case, when the infinitely thin auxiliary lens stands in the vitreous humour and its nodal point coincides with the posterior nodal point of the eye, or stands in the air, its nodal point coinciding with the anterior nodal point of the eye. We start from a system represented in Fig. 48, system A, whose posterior focus $= \phi''$ lies in the retina $N\,N$. In this system the foci change, and indeed so (compare system B) that the image j of the point i now comes to lie in $N\,N$, where, in system A the focus ϕ'' lay. The question therefore is, what is the focal distance L'' of the auxiliary lens in the vitreous humour which should remove the posterior focus from j to ϕ''. Evidently this lens must make the rays, which, arrived at k'' converge to j, converge to ϕ'' Now $k''\,\phi'' = G''$, $k''\,j = g''$. Consequently $\dfrac{1}{G''} - \dfrac{1}{g''} = \dfrac{1}{L''}$. Therefore the auxiliary lens which changes system A into system B is $\dfrac{1}{L''}$.

The question is, further, in what relation does $\dfrac{1}{G''} - \dfrac{1}{g''}$ stand to g $(= k'\,i)$. As we have seen

$$\frac{1}{g''\,n} + \frac{1}{g'} = \frac{1}{G''\,n}.$$

Consequently,

$$\frac{1}{g''} + \frac{n}{g'} = \frac{1}{G''}$$

$$\frac{1}{G''} - \frac{1}{g''} = \frac{n}{g'}.$$

Hence it appears that $\dfrac{1}{L''} = \dfrac{n}{g'}.$ Consequently, to bring an eye which is accommodated for infinite distance, to the distance g', an auxiliary lens of $L'' = \dfrac{g'}{n}$ focal distance is required. If R be not infinite, we may suppose that an auxiliary lens $\dfrac{n}{R}$ was already present, and that in accommodation for the nearest point an auxiliary lens of $\dfrac{n}{P}$ is required, in which case the difference between these two auxiliary lenses $\dfrac{n}{P} - \dfrac{n}{R}$ expresses the range of accommodation. We thus obtain, as a general formula,

$$\frac{1}{L''} = \frac{n}{P} - \frac{n}{R} \ldots \ldots B,$$

and if

$$R = \infty$$

$$\frac{1}{L''} = \frac{n}{P}.$$

The formula B, in agreement with our formula, makes the range of accommodation dependent on the factor $\dfrac{1}{P} - \dfrac{1}{R}$ But we have assumed $\dfrac{1}{A} = \dfrac{1}{P} - \dfrac{1}{R}$, and find

$$\frac{1}{L''} = \left(\frac{1}{P} - \frac{1}{R} \right) \times n,$$

consequently

$$L'' = \frac{A}{n}.$$

The focal distance of the lens required, placed in the vitreous humour, is therefore n times shorter than was assumed in the formula for the range of accommodation.

We may, however, also suppose the auxiliary lens to be situated in air, and its nodal point to coincide with k' of the eye. It is indeed true that there is no air in k'; but a system might be constructed, whose cardinal points should have the same position as those of the eye, and wherein air should really be present in k'. Moreover, there are lenses (although *not* infinitely thin) whose nodal points lie without the mass of the glass, and of such we therefore may suppose, although they are placed before the eye, that the nodal point coincides with the anterior nodal point of the eye. But apart from this, we may imagine the eye away, and the auxiliary lens placed in air, its nodal point coinciding with k'. Refracted by this lens, the rays are altered as to their direction. We may now suppose the direction to be prolonged backwards, and that the rays already had this direction when they fell upon the cornea. If, therefore, R be the distance from the farthest point to k', P that of the nearest point to k', L' the required focal distance, then

$$\frac{1}{L'} = \frac{1}{P} - \frac{1}{R} = \frac{1}{A};$$

and

$$L' = A.$$

The focal distance of the lens may therefore be n times greater, when in air, than when it is present in the vitreous humour. The correctness of this is easily seen. In order to make the focal distances of the eye accommodated to the farthest and nearest points equal, the auxiliary lens, standing in air, must displace the focus of parallel rays coming from behind from g' to G': it must be $\dfrac{1}{L'} = \dfrac{1}{G'} - \dfrac{1}{g'} = \dfrac{1}{A}.$

If it be in the vitreous humour, it must displace the focus of rays coming from before from g'' to G''. It must therefore be

$$\frac{1}{L''} = \frac{1}{G''} - \frac{1}{g''} = \frac{n}{G'} - \frac{n}{g'} = \frac{n}{A}.$$

XXX.—*Comparison of the obtained formula* $\dfrac{1}{A} = \dfrac{1}{P} - \dfrac{1}{R}$ *with the results of observation.*

In the foregoing consideration (XXIX.) it was assumed that, in accommodation of the eye for p, while the focal distances become shorter, the nodal points maintain their place unaltered. System A (Fig. 49) should be changed into system B. In both systems $k' \phi'$ must be $= n \, k'' \phi''$, that is, $G' = n \, G''$. In this is included that the principal points $h' \, h''$ likewise change their position. In fact $h' \phi'$ must be $= k'' \phi''$ and $h'' \phi'' = k' \phi'$. If we call ij the approximation of ϕ'' to k'', that of ϕ' to h' will be $= n \, ij$. Now in order that $\phi' \, h' = \phi'' \, h''$, h' must recede, and the amount of this recession $= n \, ij - ij$ or $ij \, (n - 1)$ is pretty considerable.

Hence it appears, that the change produced by placing an auxiliary lens with its nodal point in the nodal point of the eye, differs not in-

considerably from the change in accommodation for near objects.   Yet
in this the principal points are scarcely displaced backward, the nodal

Fig. 48.

Fig. 49.

Fig. 50.

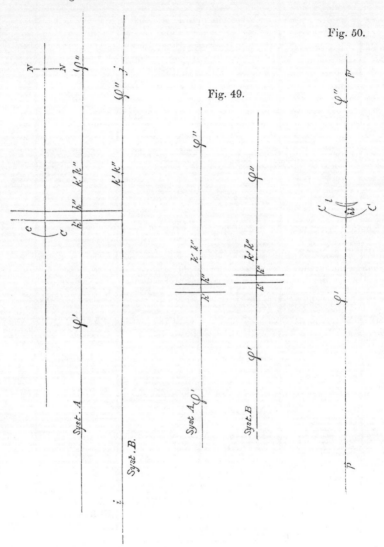

points, on the contrary, advance pretty considerably, and the anterior focus at the same time acquires a different position (compare systems C and D of Fig. 43).

It therefore appears doubtful whether the change in focal distance which the crystalline lens undergoes in accommodation is nearly proportional to the focal distance of the supposed auxiliary lens, that is to the value of A in the formula $\dfrac{1}{A} = \dfrac{1}{P} - \dfrac{1}{R}$. This we must therefore investigate. We employ for this purpose the diagrammatic eye assumed by Helmholtz, and the results of the measurements obtained by Knapp in four eyes.

| | Focal Distance of the Crystalline Lens in Accommodation for | | $1 : Fa$ $= \dfrac{1}{Fp} - \dfrac{1}{Fr}$ | P | R | $\dfrac{1}{A} = \dfrac{1}{P} - \dfrac{1}{R}$ | $Fa : \dfrac{1}{A}$ |
	Distance. $Fr.$	Proximity. $Fp.$					
I.	38·176	31:971	1:196·7	172·4	∞	1:172·4	0·8763
II.	37·706	29·222	1:129·9	118·6	∞	1:118·6	0·9132
III.	41·449	30·944	1:122·1	109·16	∞	1:109·16	0·894
IV.	43·133	30·939	1:112	100·97	∞	1:100·97	0·9016
Diagrammatic Eye.	43·707	33·785	1:148·8	136·6	∞	1:136·6	0·918

It appears that the value $\dfrac{1}{Fa} : \dfrac{1}{A}$, it is true, is no fixed coëfficient, that consequently no perfect proportion exists between the calculated auxiliary lens, corresponding to our formula of the range of accommodation, and the actual alteration of the crystalline lens, but that nevertheless we come sufficiently near the truth in assuming that the crystalline lens in accommodation has received the addition of a lens, having $\dfrac{9}{10}$ of the power of $\dfrac{1}{A}$, the focal distance of which consequently amounts to $\dfrac{10}{9} A$. This result is not without importance. The formula $\dfrac{1}{P} - \dfrac{1}{R} = \dfrac{1}{A}$ thus becomes more than a mathematical fiction, it acquires a physiological signification.

§ 37. If we observe that the change in the lenticular system consists almost exclusively in the application of a positive meniscus to the anterior surface of the crystalline lens, we readily arrive at the conclusion that an auxiliary lens, placed before the crystalline, should alter the cardinal points of the eye in such a manner as actually takes place in accommodation, and should therefore most accurately express the range of accommodation. This last we can easily test. Let, namely (Fig. 50), ϕ'' be the posterior focus of the cornea $C\,C$ for rays proceeding from the farthest point; p' for rays, proceeding from the nearest point, then the auxiliary lens l must make the rays converging to p' converge to ϕ'', before they reach the crystalline lens. If d be the distance from the principal point h of the auxiliary lens of the cornea, $h\ \phi'' = F''$, $h\ p' = f''$ then $\dfrac{1}{l} = \dfrac{1}{F'' - d} - \dfrac{1}{f' - d}$.

For d let us put two millimètres. It is true, the anterior surface of the crystalline lens lies farther removed from the cornea; but the auxiliary lens l, which in a certain sense places itself before the crystalline, has the form of a positive meniscus, whose principal points are situated in front of the convex surface, and the infinitely thin lens, which is supposed to contain the meniscus, must, in order to have such an action, stand in its second principal point. Now, in the diagrammatic eye, the radius of the cornea = 8 mm., the focal distances of the cornea $F' = 23 \cdot 692$ and $F'' = 31 \cdot 692$ mm.; p lies, in accommodation for near objects, as we have seen, 136·6 mm. from the nodal point, therefore $136 \cdot 6 - 6 \cdot 5 = 130 \cdot 1$ mm. ($= f'$) from the cornea.

The focus p', of rays proceeding from p consequently lies at

$$\left(f'' = \frac{F'' f'}{f' - F'} \right)$$

$$f'' = \frac{31 \cdot 692 \times 130 \cdot 1}{130 \cdot 1 - 23 \cdot 692} = 38 \cdot 75.$$

The rays proceeding from the farthest point r converge in ϕ'' at $31 \cdot 692$; those proceeding from the nearest point p in p' at $38 \cdot 75$ behind the cornea. At 2 mm. behind the cornea, therefore the distance of the points of convergence amounts to $29 \cdot 692$ and $36 \cdot 75$ mm. To direct rays converging at $36 \cdot 75$ to $29 \cdot 692$, an auxiliary lens of $\dfrac{29 \cdot 692 \times 36 \cdot 75}{7 \cdot 058} = 155$ mm. is necessary.

We may make the same calculation for all the four eyes measured by Knapp. In doing so, we should come nearest the truth, by taking into account, in each particular case, the found radius of the cornea and the depth of position of the crystalline lens. But if we start also from fixed focal distances of the cornea, the anterior surface of the lens being situated at 2 mm. from the cornea, the auxiliary lens found by calculation comes really very near the alteration of the crystalline. This appears from the following numbers:

	$= \dfrac{1}{Fp} - \dfrac{1}{Fr} = 1 :$	F'' Posterior focal distance of the cornea.	$P.$	f'' Focus of the cornea for rays proceeding from p.	$1 : (F'' - 2) - 1 : (f'' - 2)$
I.	196·7	31·692	165·9	36·97	196·6
II.	129·9	31·692	112·5	40·15	133·9
III.	122·1	31·692	103·3	41·22	121 9
IV.	112	31·692	95·06	42·21	113·5
Diagrammatic Eye	148·8	31·692	130·1	38·75	155

It thus appears, that an infinitely thin auxiliary lens, placed 2 mm. behind the cornea, in the four eyes measured by Knapp, almost exactly corresponds to the alteration of refraction of the lens. If it were now desired to express by such a lens the range of accommodation, a table may easily be prepared of the value of f'' for the different optometrically-found values of p. But in fact it must be called an accident, that in the assumption of a position of the auxiliary lens, unaltered at 2 mm. behind the cornea, so much agreement is found. The position has, in fact, a very great influence. If, for example, the auxiliary lens lies at 4, instead of at 2 mm. behind the cornea, the numbers change—

$$\left.\begin{array}{c} 196\cdot6 \\ 133\cdot9 \\ 121\cdot9 \\ 113\cdot5 \\ 155 \end{array}\right\} \quad \text{into} \quad \left\{\begin{array}{c} 172\cdot9 \\ 118\cdot3 \\ 107\cdot8 \\ 100\cdot6 \\ 136\cdot3 \end{array}\right.$$

Therefore it is not strange that the diagrammatic eye does not answer when d is assumed $= 2$ mm. In this case d should amount to about $2\frac{3}{4}$. In the second eye, also measured by Knapp, some deviation appears. In both instances this is to be ascribed principally to the fact, that the anterior surface of the crystalline lens lies more deeply, and thus the distance of 2 mm. for the auxiliary lens is not quite sufficient.

Hence it appears, that if it were desired from r and p to calculate the auxiliary lens at the crystalline, we must likewise determine the place of the anterior surface of the crystalline, and this involves a difficulty of time and means, without leading to more accurate knowledge than is attainable by the application of the simple formula $\dfrac{1}{A} = \dfrac{1}{P} - \dfrac{1}{R}$. We keep therefore to this formula, which for the determination of the range of accommodation supposes only the optometrical determination of p and r (calculated to the nodal point at about 7 mm. behind the cornea), and thus recommends itself for practical utility. If we wish to know what auxiliary lens has been applied to the crystalline, we multiply the result obtained $\dfrac{1}{A}$ by the coëfficient 0·9. We thus come certainly very near the truth. The influence of ametropia, and of the use of spectacles and eye-glasses on the range of accommodation, shall hereafter be examined.

CHAPTER II.

DEFECTS OF REFRACTION AND ACCOMMODATION IN GENERAL.

§ 6.—Distinction between defects of refraction and of accommodation.

Hitherto the defects of refraction and of accommodation have been more or less mixed up one with another. This confusion was an impediment to the clearness of description, which in this department particularly, is absolutely necessary to the correct appreciation of the subject. The ideas of refraction and of accommodation must therefore in the first instance be accurately distinguished from one another. It will then not be difficult subsequently to recal the connexion, so far as may be necessary, between the two.

By *refraction of the eye*, we understand its refraction in the state of rest; that is, the refraction which the eye possesses in virtue of its form and of that of its component parts, independently of muscular action, independently of accommodation. The term, therefore, applies to the refraction of the eye whose muscles of accommodation are inactive or paralysed (for example under the influence of atropia), to the refraction also of the dead, but as yet otherwise unaltered eye.

To begin with refraction, in the condition of relaxation proper, the eye possesses a power of accommodation. The farthest point of distinct vision, therefore, corresponds to the state of rest of accommodation. Now, so soon as the action of accommodation occurs, the eye becomes adjusted to an adjoining point, and it is by diminution of this active operation that it is subsequently capable of seeing a more remote point. Hence, accommodation for an adjoining object alone is an active operation (compare § 3). The stronger this action is, the nearer is the accurately seen point. *Accommodation is, therefore, the voluntary action whereby the eye becomes adjusted to a nearer point than is the case in the state of rest of accommodation.*

Hence it appears, that refraction is dependent on the anatomical condition of the component parts of the eye; accommodation, on the contrary, depends upon the physiological action of muscles.

With regard to refraction, we call the structure of the eye normal, when, in the state of rest, it brings the rays derived from infinitely distant objects to a focus exactly on the anterior surface of the layer of rods and bulbs; in other words, when parallel incident rays unite on that layer (in φ' Fig. 51). The farthest point of such an eye lies at

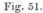

Fig. 51.

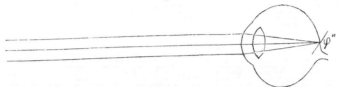

an infinite distance. If convergent rays are also capable of being brought to a focus, the eye possesses something which it does not need: for from all objects proceed divergent or at most parallel rays. If on the contrary, the farthest point lies not at an infinite, but at a finite distance, vision is indistinct throughout a great part of the space. Consequently the *refraction* of the media of the eye at rest can be called normal in reference to the situation of the retina, only when parallel incident rays unite on the layer of rods and bulbs. Then, in fact, the limit lies precisely at the measure; then there exists emmetropia (from ἔμμετρος, modum tenens, and ὤψ, oculus). Such an eye we term *emmetropic*.

This name expresses perfectly what we mean. The eye cannot be called a *normal* eye, for it may very easily be abnormal or morbid, and nevertheless it may be emmetropic. Neither is the expression *normally constructed eye* quite correct, for the structure of an emmetropic eye may in many respects be abnormal, and *emmetropia* may exist with difference of structure. Hence the word *emmetropia* appears alone to express with precision and accuracy the condition alluded to.

Emmetropia then is met with, when the principal focus of the media of the eye at rest falls on the anterior surface of the most external layer of the retina (compare Fig. 51). This is the simplest definition.

The eye may deviate from the emmetropic condition in two respects: the principal focus φ'' of the eye at rest may fall *in front of*

6

(Fig. 52) or *behind* (Fig. 53) the most external layer of the retina.

Fig. 52.

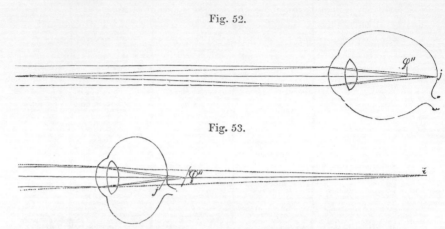

Fig. 53.

In the former case divergent (dotted in Fig. 52), in the latter convergent rays (dotted in Fig. 53) come to a focus on the retina. In the first case, therefore, in the condition of rest, objects are accurately seen which are situated at a definite finite distance (Fig. 52 *i*); in the second they are at no distance accurately seen, for the rays in falling upon the cornea must, in order to unite in the retina, already converge towards a point situated behind the eye (Fig. 53 *i*). In the first case the farthest limit lies *within* the normal measure: the measure is too short, and the condition might, therefore, be called *brachymetropia*. In the second case, the boundary lies *beyond* the measure, and I have, therefore, called this state *hypermetropia*.

Hence it is perfectly clear, that brachymetropia and hypermetropia are two opposite conditions.

The definitions are now extremely simple : the posterior principal focus ϕ'' of the media of the eye at rest falls :—

in EMMETROPIA *on* the most external layer of the retina ;

in BRACHYMETROPIA *in front of* ,,   ,,   ,,

in HYPERMETROPIA *behind*   ,,   ,,   ,,

In order to express that the eye is not emmetropic, we may use the word *ametropia* (from ἄμετρος, extra modum, and ὤψ, oculus). Brachymetropia and hypermetropia are both, therefore, referrible to ametropia.

Brachymetropia is evidently nothing else than *myopia*, and it appears preferable to use the word myopia, as being an established term. The word brachymetropia was formed only in contrast to hypermetropia, to which expression I thought it right to adhere.

Hence it is evident that myopia and hypermetropia are opposite conditions. That myopia is of very frequent occurrence, and is to be considered as an important condition, has long been admitted. Still more common, however, and more important in its results is hypermetropia, which has hitherto been for the most part either overlooked, or confounded with other states.

I repeat, what, in consequence of its importance, I have already put prominently forward, that *myopia and hypermetropia are the opposite conditions of ametropia*.

From the definitions given of anomalies of refraction, it has been shown, that the distance R of the farthest point of distinct vision is the foundation on which they rest. The shortening of the focal distance, whereby adjoining points become accurately visible, is the work of the muscles of accommodation. Under the maximum action of these muscles the eye is adapted to the distance P of its nearest point. Now we found as a numerical expression for the range of accommodation $\dfrac{1}{A} = \dfrac{1}{P} - \dfrac{1}{R}$. The range of accommodation diminishes, as shall hereafter be more particularly pointed out, with advancing years. At the same time R may remain almost unaltered, and P thus becomes greater. The result of this is, that in the emmetropic eye the nearest point is at a certain period of life removed so far from the eye, that more minute operations can no longer be well performed with near objects. This condition of the eye is called *presbyopia*. *Presbyopia therefore exists, when, in consequence of the increase of years, with diminution of the range of accommodation, the nearest point has been removed too far from the eye.*

Formerly writers were in the habit of contrasting presbyopia with myopia. Apparently this was quite correct. But in myopia only near, and in presbyopia only distant, objects can be distinctly seen. In myopia they found "the mean distance of distinct vision" to be situated too near the eye, in presbyopia too far from it. Thus they would feel obliged, while they either overlooked hypermetropia, or confounded it with presbyopia, to place myopia and presbyopia directly against one another, to regard them as deviations, similar in nature, but opposite in direction.

On closer examination it appears, however, that such opposition is illogical. The fact is, that both in an anatomical and in a physio-

2

logical point of view, myopia and presbyopia belong to very different categories.   Myopia is based upon an abnormal construction of the eye; presbyopia is the normal condition of the normally constructed eye at a more advanced period of life.   In myopia the power of accommodation possesses the normal range; presbyopia on the contrary is based upon diminished range of accommodation, as the natural result of advancing life.   Myopia, finally, rests upon an abnormal situation of the *farthest* point of distinct vision; presbyopia, on the other hand, on an altered situation of the *nearest* point.   So little are myopia and presbyopia opposite conditions, that they may both occur simultaneously in the same eye.   An eye, for example, which can see accurately only from 20″ to 14″, is at the same time myopic and presbyopic : the farthest point of distinct vision is situated at too short, the nearest point at too great a distance.

Hence we may consider it to be fully proved and demonstrated :—

1. That myopia and hypermetropia are to be regarded as opposite conditions.

2.   That it is illogical and unpractical to contrast myopia and presbyopia with one another.

With respect to presbyopia, this state is no anomaly, but rather the normal condition of the normally constructed, emmetropic eye, at a more advanced period of life.   Were presbyopia an anomaly, it should not be looked upon as an anomaly of refraction, but of accommodation.   It should not be classed with myopia and hypermetropia, but, on the contrary, with the disturbances of accommodation.   As, however, it is no disturbance, but a diminution of the range of accommodation, it must be treated of in considering the influence of the time of life upon the eye.

Accommodation is, as we have seen, based upon a change of form of the lens, produced by contraction of the internal muscles of the eye.

Hence it follows, that anomalies of accommodation may be dependent :—

    a. On disturbance in the lenticular system.

    b. On disturbance of the internal muscles.

Of the disturbances in the lenticular system the condition of total absence of the lens, which I have termed *aphakia,* comes almost exclusively under observation.

The disturbances of the muscles of accommodation are of a very varying nature.   Principally we shall have to distinguish :—

1. The weakness which not unfrequently manifests itself by definite phenomena after different exhausting illnesses.

2. The more or less complete paralysis, which, probably without exception, is connected with a similar condition of the M. sphincter iridis, and often occurs only as a part of the paralysis of the oculo-motor nerve.

3. The spasm, which occurs much more rarely than the paralysis, and, like the latter, is based upon a direct or indirect abnormal action of the nervous system.

Besides these rare forms of spasm, we shall observe, as a very ordinary phenomenon in hypermetropia, a persistent increase of contraction of the muscles of accommodation dependent upon habit. This subject shall, therefore, be treated of in speaking of hypermetropia.

Moreover, it is here to be noticed in general, that the condition of refraction exercises an important influence on the ordinary use of the range of accommodation, and consequently upon accommodation itself. The modifications so produced cannot be separated from the states of refraction on which they depend, and they therefore come with them under consideration. For this and other reasons it was necessary to give an idea of the subject of accommodation, before passing to the description of the anomalies of refraction.

From the foregoing, it appears that our principal distinction is based upon the situation of the farthest point of distinct vision. Thus we obtain a classification of the anomalies of refraction, which of itself excludes a confusion of the latter with the anomalies of accommodation.

The question naturally arises, whether a classification resting on the nearest point of distinct vision, that is upon P, may not also be observed. On a little reflection it will, however, be seen, that this would lead to constant confusion of the anomalies of refraction and of accommodation. Indeed P depends upon both factors, both on the refraction of the eye at rest, and on the range of accommodation. Consequently two eyes, in which P is similar, may, with respect to refraction and accommodation, present great differences : it is only necessary that the differences compensate one another in the two factors. A myopic eye with a small, and a hypermetropic eye with a great, range of accommodation, may have their nearest point at the same distance as an emmetropic eye, with an average range of accommodation. Now, if they were classified according to their nearest point, all these different eyes should be referred to the same category. Moreover, how should we, on this basis, determine the categories? It should evidently be done quite arbitrarily. We should, for example, distinguish—

A category with P less than 2″,

      ,,   ,,   ,,   4″,

      ,,   ,,   ,,   8″,

etc., or choose other arbitrary numbers. Lastly, the same eye should, in proportion as the power of accommodation diminished, belong each time to a different category. This is enough to prove that a classification of eyes, based upon the shortest distance of distinct vision, is entirely unpractical, and almost leads to the absurd. A classification according to the mean distance of distinct vision, which it has been attempted to make by contrasting myopia and presbyopia, is an illusion; for a mean distance of distinct vision does not exist, and what does not exist is certainly not to be defined. (Compare *relative* range of accommodation.)

On the contrary, a classification founded on the greatest distance of distinct vision is simple and logical. With the knowledge of R we perceive, in the first place, whether an anomaly of refraction exists. Taking the time of life into consideration, we can, moreover, thence nearly determine what P ought to be; and if P does not actually correspond thereto, we may infer the existence of an anomaly of accommodation.

§ 7. Causes of the Defects of Refraction in General.

In defining the anomalies of accommodation, their cause is at the same time assigned. For although very different morbid conditions or morbid processes, may give rise either to paralysis, or to spasm of the muscles of accommodation,—we know that, in the first case the phenomena are always dependent on diminished or wholly arrested, in the second on involuntarily exalted action of the muscles of accommodation.

On the cause of the anomalies of refraction, on the contrary, the dioptric definition laid down does not throw any light. They are defined simply as disturbances of connexion in the relative position of principal focus and retina. On what anatomical or physiological deviation these disturbances of connexion may depend, is thus left undecided.

This would seem to be the place to treat of this subject in general. However, we here state only what is the rule. Deviations, of a peculiar nature, which occur only sometimes as exceptions, will come under consideration first in speaking of each of the anomalies in detail.

The rule is expressed in the annexed three figures. Fig. 54 is an emmetropic, Fig. 55 a myopic, and Fig. 56 a hypermetropic eye. It immediately strikes us, that in the myopic eye the axis of vision is longer, while in the hypermetropic eye it is, on the contrary, shorter, than in the emmetropic. To this almost exclusively it is to be attributed, that parallel incident rays in the myopic eye, come to a focus in front of, in the hypermetropic, behind the retina. Of this difference in length of the axis of vision we can even in life satisfac -

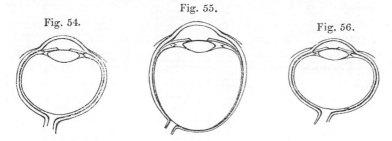

Fig. 54.   Fig. 55.   Fig. 56.

torily convince ourselves.   Thus if we cause the axis of vision to be as strongly as possible directed outwards, we shall observe the slow alteration of the arching of the oval myopic, and the rapid change of the direction of the arching in the anteriorly situated equator of the hypermetropic eye.   Moreover, the other axes of the myopic eye appear to be longer, while those of the hypermetropic are shorter than those of the emmetropic eye.

Myopia and hypermetropia might also be supposed to be dependent on many other causes.   Anomalies of refraction might depend upon the curvature of the different refracting surfaces (compare p. 38), as well as on the relative coëfficients of the refraction of light. Theories have not been wanting in reference to this subject.

The opinion has in the first place been rather generally entertained, that in myopia the cornea is more convex.   So far as hypermetropia was known, it was supposed to be connected with too great flatness of the cornea, which was positively assumed to exist in presbyopia.   And on external inspection it would really appear, as if in myopic individuals the cornea was more convex, while in those who are hypermetropic and presbyopic it is flatter than in emmetropic persons.   This appearance proceeds from the fact, that in myopia the iris and the crystalline lens lie far behind the cornea, while in hypermetropia and presbyopia they are situated nearer to it.   An observer is still further misled to assume a difference in the curvature of the cornea, as in a myopic subject the entire globe of the eye is more prominent, while in the hypermetropic it is more sunk in the orbit, as is often seen.   But in truth, the curvature of the cornea in ametropia does not essentially differ from that of emmetropia, and the time of life also exercises scarcely any influence.   Numerous measurements of the curval radius of the cornea have satisfied me on this point. They have shown me that, quite contrary to what it was thought should be expected, the cornea at an advanced period of life rather becomes a little more convex, and that in the extreme degrees of myopia, on the contrary, a somewhat flatter cornea is met with. Moreover, the radius of the cornea of both eyes of the same individual seemed in general to present no difference, or at least a much less difference than usually occurs between corneæ of different persons; while, lastly, the radius (as well as the whole eye) is in women somewhat shorter than in men.

Though in ordinary myopia the cornea is not more convex, it is evident that, *ceteris paribus*, a greater convexity of the cornea must give rise to myopia, and we shall hereafter see that in diseases of the cornea myopia is occasionally produced in this way.

Moreover, it naturally occurs to us to consider the principal focal distance of the lens as a cause of anomalies of refraction. In connexion with it both the curvature of the refracting surfaces and the coëfficient of refraction may come under notice. In advancing years the lens becomes externally especially firmer, and thus the coëfficient of refraction of the outer layers appears to increase. If this actually takes place, and if the coëfficient of the cortical layers thus approaches more to that of the nucleus, the focal distance becomes greater (compare p. 39). On this the diminution in advanced life of the refractive condition of the eye appears really to depend. But beyond this no facts exist, which give us a right to assume, that definite changes in the focal distance of the crystalline lens usually occur in definite anomalies of refraction. In some measurements of the surfaces of curvature of the lens from eyes of myopic persons, after death, I found no deviation; it would rather appear as if, in strongly hypermetropic individuals, a flatter lens were to be expected. Determinations of this kind during life take up a great deal of time, still they ought to be made. Of the eyes measured by Helmholtz, as well as among those measured by Knapp, there was by accident one myopic eye. The values found by these observers do not indicate that the lens in myopic subjects should present a shorter focal distance; nor do the results of the removal of the lens in myopic patients lead to this conclusion, as shall be more fully shown in treating of aphakia.

Now if the lens in myopic individuals evidently lies (compare Fig. 55 with Fig. 54) in general farther from the cornea than in emmetropic persons, the focus of the dioptric system must in the former lie even somewhat deeper than in the latter; and it is in spite thereof, that in consequence of the elongated axis of vision, myopia exists. In hypermetropia, the lens being situated more anteriorly (compare Fig. 56 with 54), must, *ceteris paribus*, bring the principal focal distance nearer to the cornea; but, the axis of vision being much shorter, the principal focus still lies behind the system. In both cases, therefore, the anomaly of refraction is rather compensated than promoted by the lenticular system.

As to modifications in the coëfficients of refraction nothing is known. From a theoretic point of view we must say, that the index of the cornea and aqueous humour being greater, and that of the vitreous humour being on the contrary less, the principal focus should be removed forwards (compare p. 39).

The final result, therefore, remains what we laid down in starting : that *myopia usually depends upon an elongation, and hypermetropia upon a shortening, of the axis of vision.*

The measurements of the radius of the cornea were made with the assistance of the ophthalmometer (compare p. 17). They were recorded in the *Verslagen en mededeelingen der Koninklijke academie van Wetenschappen* (Reports and Communications of the Royal Academy of Sciences), Afd. *Natuurkunde*, D. xi. p. 159, and subsequently in the *Archiv f. Ophthalm.*, B. viii. The principal results are here appended :—

1. The radii of the two eyes of the same individual are in general nearly equal. In the statistics, therefore, when two eyes of the same person were examined, only one mean eye was taken into account.

2. The *radius in the line of vision* ρ° amounted in mm. to—

	Maximum.	Minimum.	Average.
In men	8·396	7·28	7·858
In women	8·487	7·115	7·799

3. As to the influence of time of life—

In 79 men, average $\rho^\circ =$			$= 7\cdot858$
„ 20 „	under 20 years, average		$= 7\cdot932$
„ 51 „	„ 40 „	„	$= 7\cdot882$
„ 28 „	above 40 „	„	$= 7\cdot819$
„ 11 „	„ 60 „	„	$= 7\cdot809$
In 38 women, average ρ°			$= 7\cdot799$
„ 6 „	under 20 years		$= 7\cdot720$
„ 22 „	„ 40 „ average		$= 7\cdot799$
„ 16 „	above 40 „	„	$= 7\cdot799$
„ 2 „	„ 60 „	„	$= 7\cdot607$

4. As to refraction—

Men. { In 27 emmetropic persons, ρ° .... $= 7\cdot785$
„ 25 myopic   „   „   .... $= 7\cdot874$
„ 26 hypermetropic „   „   .... $= 7\cdot96$

Average.

Women. {
In 11 emmetropic persons, ρ° .... $= 7\cdot719$
,, 12 myopic   ,,   ,, ... $= 7\ 867$
,, 15 hypermetropic ,,   ,, ... $= 7\cdot767$
}

5. Influence of the degree of myopia (M)—

Men. {
M. greater than $\frac{1}{4}$, ρ° .... $= 7\cdot930$
M.   ,,   ,, $\frac{1}{10}$,   ,, ... $= 7\cdot829$
M. less   ,, $\frac{1}{10}$,   ,, ... $= 7\cdot867$
(Emmetropic .... $= 7\cdot785$)
}

Women. {
M. greater than $\frac{1}{4}$, ρ° .... $= 7\cdot935$
M. less   ,, $\frac{1}{10}$,   ,, ... $= 7\cdot780$
(Emmetropic .... $= 7\cdot719$)
}

6. Influence of the degree of hypermetropia (H.).

Men. {
$H = \frac{1}{5}$ to $\frac{1}{10}$, ρ° .... $= 7\cdot935$
,, $= \frac{1}{10}$ to $\frac{1}{20}$,   ,, ... $= 8\cdot010$
,, $= \frac{1}{20}$ to $\frac{1}{60}$,   ,, ... $= 7\cdot939$
(Emmetropic .... $= 7\cdot785$)
}

Women. {
$H = \frac{1}{6}$ to $\frac{1}{20}$, ρ° .... $= 7\cdot876$
,, $= \frac{1}{20}$ or under,   ,, ... $= 7\cdot692$
(Emmetropic .... $= 7\cdot719$)
}

§ 8. Diagrammatic representation of the range of accommodation, and of the anomalies of refraction and accommodation.

In § 5 we have seen what is to be understood by range of accommodation. We described the faculty of accommodation as the power of the eye to add to itself a positive lens, and the strength of this lens was for us the measure of the range of accommodation. We further showed, that the focal distance of this auxiliary lens was immediately found by ascertaining the distances from the nearest and farthest points of distinct vision to the nodal point of the eye. These distances we called P and R, and the range of accommodation was then :—

$$\frac{1}{A} = \frac{1}{P} - \frac{1}{R}.$$

If $\frac{1}{A}$ be the range of accommodation, A is the focal distance of the auxiliary lens, which the eye is capable of adding to itself.

All this is very clear. But it was still a desideratum, by means of a drawing, to make it easier. An attempt in this direction succeeded beyond expectation. Not only can we in a diagram express

Eye.	Age.	A=
Emmetropia	12 years	1: 2⅔
id.	25 „	1: 4
id.	45 „	1: 8
id.	60 „	1: 24
Myopia 1/12	16 „	1: 3
id. 1/4	40 „	1: 8
id. 1/24	65 „	1: 24
Hypermet. 1/24	20 „	1: 4
id. 1/2	30 „	1: 6
id. 1/2	20 „	1: 6
id. 1/4	60 „	1: 6
id. 1/8	60 „	1: 24
Aphakia (without the lens)		1: 24

1: 2 2 2/7 2 3/7 2 2/3 3 3 3/7 4 4 3/5 6 8 12 24 ∞ 24 12 8 6 4 3/5 4 3 3/7 3

W. West lith.

the range of accommodation, proportional to the length of lines, but the beginning and end of the lines at the same time show p and r, and thus at once make us acquainted with the degree of myopia and hypermetropia of the eye so represented. A glance at the appended table will demonstrate this. The lengths of the thick horizontal lines represent the ranges of accommodation. Above the slighter vertical lines the distances from the eye, at which acute vision takes place, are noted: the numbers exhibit (in Parisian inches) the distances whence rays must *diverge,* in order to come to a focus on the retina. The explanation of a couple of these lines may serve to elucidate this.

The first transverse line represents the boundaries and range of accommodation in a child of twelve years. The latter begins at ∞, that is, at an infinite distance, and terminates at $2\frac{2}{3}''$. This indicates that the distance of the farthest point $R = \infty$, while that of the nearest $P = 2\frac{2}{3}''$. The eye is therefore emmetropic, and has a range of accommodation of $\dfrac{1}{2\frac{2}{3}} - \dfrac{1}{\infty} = \dfrac{1}{2\frac{2}{3}}$. All this is seen at once from the first line.

The fifth transverse line represents the boundaries of accommodation, and the range of accommodation of a young man, aged sixteen. The farthest point lies at 18, the nearest at $2\frac{2}{3}$, inches from the eye ($R = 18$, $P = 2\frac{2}{3}$). He is therefore, in the first place, near-sighted, and his near-sightedness is of that degree, that it may be corrected by glasses of $-\dfrac{1}{18}$ (that is of $18''$ negative focal distance). Such glasses give, to the rays derived from infinitely remote objects, a direction as if they came from a point $18''$ from the eye. Therefore, the degree of myopia is also expressed by $\dfrac{1}{18}$, $M = \dfrac{1}{18}$. Now if, moreover, the nearest point lies at $2\frac{2}{3}$, we find as the range of accommodation $\dfrac{1}{2\frac{2}{3}} - \dfrac{1}{18} = \dfrac{1}{3}$. All this is included in the fifth line.

The principle involved in this diagrammatic representation is this, that by the mutual distance of two vertical lines a definite range of accommodation is each time expressed; for this $\dfrac{1}{24}$ is here assumed. If we now begin at ∞, and reckon to the left, we find:—

above the first line 1 : 24, corresponding to $\dfrac{1}{24}$ range of accommodation.

above the second line 1 : 12 .... $2 \times \dfrac{1}{24}$

  „   third   „   1 : 8 .... $3 \times \dfrac{1}{24}$

  „   sixth   „   1 : 4 .... $6 \times \dfrac{1}{24}$

  „   seventh „   1 : $3\frac{3}{7}$............ $7 \times \dfrac{1}{24}$

etc.

The difference between the range of accommodation of two adjoining lines is, moreover, always $= \dfrac{1}{24}$; for example :—

$$\frac{1}{6} - \frac{1}{8} = \frac{1}{24}, \quad \frac{1}{2\frac{2}{3}} - \frac{1}{2\frac{2}{3}} = \frac{1}{24}, \text{ etc.}$$

If we now have the nearest and farthest points united by a transverse line, we need only to reckon how many intervening spaces of vertical lines the latter runs through, in order to ascertain how much $\times \dfrac{1}{24}$ the range of accommodation amounts to.   The first transverse line passes through nine intervening spaces, and therefore represents $\dfrac{9}{24} = \dfrac{1}{2\frac{2}{3}}$ range of accommodation; the sixth, runs through eight intervals, corresponding to $\dfrac{8}{24} = \dfrac{1}{3}$ range of accommodation, etc.

From this representation it is now very plain, that as much power of accommodation is necessary to come from an infinite distance to 8″, as from 8″ to 4″; as much, to come from 6″ to 4″ as from 4″ to 3″, etc. In a word, the distance of each pair of vertical lines corresponds to the same $\left(= \dfrac{1}{24} \right)$ range of accommodation, and therefore in order to come from one to the other, the same action of the power of accommodation is each time required, that is, the eye must each time add to itself a positive lens of $\dfrac{1}{24}$.

Moreover, we observe, that also to the right of ∞ vertical lines occur, above which numbers are placed. These all belong to the domain of hypermetropia. The numbers show, namely, in Parisian inches, at what distance behind the eye the incident rays must converge to a point, in order to unite upon the retina. The eighth transverse line therefore represents the eye of an hypermetropic person. In total relaxation of its accommodation, the rays must, in order to unite upon the retina, converge at 24 inches behind the eye. In order to see accurately at an infinite distance, the individual will therefore require glasses of $\frac{1}{24}$, with which parallel rays acquire the convergence just mentioned. This hypermetropia is consequently neutralised by glasses of $\frac{1}{24}$; in his eye a lens of $\frac{1}{24}$ falls too short, and therefore we define the degree as $H = \frac{1}{24}$. With the strongest possible tension of the power of accommodation, the same eye sees accurately at the distance of $4\frac{4}{5}''$, from which point the rays must therefore in this case diverge, in order to come to a focus upon the retina. The range of accommodation of this eye therefore reaches, in the first place, to $\frac{1}{24}$, in order to come to ∞, and, moreover, to $\frac{1}{4\frac{4}{5}}$, in order to come to the nearest point of distinct vision. It is therefore

$$\frac{1}{24} + \frac{1}{4\frac{4}{5}} = \frac{1}{4}.$$

In accordance with this result, we see that the transverse line extends over six intervening spaces, corresponding to $\frac{6}{24} = \frac{1}{4}$ range of accommodation.

In an hypermetropic condition of the eye the distances are negative, that is, they lie behind the eye. Therefore we also find in the table to the right of ∞, 1 : 24, etc., marked; and therefore, too, in the formula for the range of accommodation $\frac{1}{P} - \frac{1}{R} = \frac{1}{A}$, the terms are negative, so far as the distances expressed by P and R lie on the negative side. In the example above adduced of the eighth transverse line, this was the case with R.

The formula therefore became

$$\frac{1}{P} - \left(-\frac{1}{R} \right) = \frac{1}{A},$$

and consequently the range of accommodation must be calculated as $\frac{1}{4\frac{4}{5}} + \frac{1}{24}$ and not as $\frac{1}{4\frac{4}{5}} - \frac{1}{24}$.

The other eyes, represented in the table, need no further explanation. The above has, however, fully shown how to deduce from the transverse lines the nature and the degree of the ametropia, as well as the range of accommodation.

It need not be remarked, that by the method here described, we can rapidly and easily register a series of eyes, whose accommodation we determine, and that on a definite principle we can easily compare with one another cases classified in this manner. We shall hereafter repeatedly make use of this method.

The range of accommodation is expressed by the dioptric power of an infinitely thin auxiliary lens, which is supposed to be placed in air, and to have its nodal point in the anterior nodal point of the eye.

I have chosen the same mode of expression for the different degrees of myopia and hypermetropia. To this I was led by the following reasoning:—If we could place in the hypermetropic eye a positive, in the myopic eye a negative corrective lens, these might thereby be converted into emmetropic eyes. The optical power of the required lens therefore represents the degree of ametropia. With the knowledge of R the lens is given. In the emmetropic eye, R is $= \infty$; in the myopic, R is a finite magnitude; in the hypermetropic eye this magnitude is negative. In both cases $\dfrac{1}{R}$ is the dioptric power of the infinitely thin lens, which, placed in air, and having its nodal point in the anterior nodal point of the eye, should make the ametropic eye emmetropic, without altering the situation of the nodal points (compare p. 73 *et seq.*). Consequently, $\dfrac{1}{R}$ is the numerical expression of the ametropia itself. The myopic eye has a lens of $\dfrac{1}{R}$ too much, the hypermetropic has a lens of $\dfrac{1}{R}$ too little. We may therefore consider myopia M., in reference to emmetropia, as a positive, hypermetropia H., as a negative condition. Therefore, too, as the negative is included in the word hypermetropia, we need not write $H = -\dfrac{1}{R}$, but for the sake of simplicity we may use the expression $H = \dfrac{1}{R}$, as well as $M = \dfrac{1}{R}$.

Against this method of expressing the degree of ametropia by the dioptric power of a lens, the objection may be raised, that in ametropia the dioptric system is, by a corrective lens, by no means made similar to that of the emmetropic eye. Ametropia does not, in fact, depend upon a deviation in the power of the crystalline lens, but rather on a deviation from the normal length of the axis of vision. With a positive lens we therefore obtain, in hypermetropia, a stronger dioptric system with a shorter axis of vision; with a negative lens in myopia we obtain a weaker system with a longer axis of vision.

This objection is not without some foundation. Still, what applies to range of accommodation does not hold good for ametropia,—that it is in the eye actually represented by a lens. Nevertheless, I have not hesitated to use this measure also for ametropia. In the first place, it recommends itself by its practical utility: not only is the degree of ametropia thus easily found by the definition of R, but with its expression is at the same time given the focal distance of the glasses by which it may be neutralised. In the second place, no other measure is possible. Were we, in order to fix the actual deviation, to take the length of the axis of vision as a measure, we should be met with the difficulty, that during life it cannot be directly determined, and, could we determine it, it would not afford an immediately practical indication. Besides, nothing is easier than to calculate the length of the axis of vision, which about corresponds to different degrees of ametropia, and thence to make tables such as shall be found in the Chapters which treat of Myopia and Hypermetropia.

Thus I consider the method I have pursued to be fully justified. It is, indeed, new only in form, not in reality. What I term $M = \dfrac{1}{R}$ would formerly, if it were desired to express the degree of myopia, have been described as *a degree of myopia, for which glasses of R — x Parisian inches' negative focal distance are required, in order to adjust the eye for parallel rays.* The value $R - x$ still needs some explanation. R is the distance from r to the nodal point k'. Consequently the corrective lens is supposed, in ametropia, to lie in k', as well as the auxiliary lens, which expresses the range of accommodation. This is done on purpose, in order to admit of the distances of distinct vision of ametropic and emmetropic eyes being compared with one another, and registered in the same diagrams. If it be desired to neutralise the ametropia by an actual corrective lens, that is, by an eye-glass, we must always take into account the distance x between the nodal point of the corrective lens and the nodal point of the eye, as shall hereafter be more fully explained.

A not unimportant question still remains to be solved. The range of accommodation we have set down as $= \dfrac{1}{P} - \dfrac{1}{R}$. We found, however, that the actual change of the crystalline lens is not quite equal thereto (compare p. 75 *et seq.*). Now the query arises, whether the length of the axis of vision has influence on the value of $\dfrac{1}{P} - \dfrac{1}{R}$, in other words, whether, on a given change of the crystalline lens, a difference in range of accommodation shall be found, according as the eye is emmetropic, myopic, or hypermetropic. The question is easily investigated. We take the diagrammatic (*schematisch*) eye of Helmholtz, in accommodation for distant and near objects, as our basis, and calculate R and P, and thence deduce the range of accommodation for different supposed lengths of the axis of vision.

	Length of the axis of vision.	R P in millimètres.	$\dfrac{1}{P} - \dfrac{1}{R}$.
Emmetropic - - - -	22·231	∞ 136·62	1 : 136·62
Myopic - - - - - -	25·231	118·31 65·056	1 : 144·54
Hypermetropic - - -	20·231	— 177 505·73	1 : 131·11

Hence it appears that an equal change of the crystalline lens produces, where the axis of vision is longer (myopia), a less, and where the axis of vision is shorter (hypermetropia), a greater value of $\dfrac{1}{P} - \dfrac{1}{R}$. By calculating the eyes determined by Knapp, I obtained the same result. The difference is, however, but slight. With the supposed lengths of the axis of vision, R was, for the myopic eye $= 4''$; for the hypermetropic eye $= - 6''$; so that the myopia amounted to $\frac{1}{4}$, the hypermetropia to $\frac{1}{6}$; and with these high degrees of ametropia the deviation in the values of $\dfrac{1}{P} - \dfrac{1}{R}$ amounted only, in the case of myopia, to about 6 per cent., and in that of hypermetropia to 4 per cent. For practical purposes these differences present no difficulty.

In this comparison of ametropic eyes with emmetropic, we started from the supposition that the dioptric system of the former agrees with that of the latter. This is, however, not quite correct. In general the crystalline lens lies, in the hypermetropic eye, closer to the cornea, in the myopic, farther from it. Now a change of form of the crystalline lens will have less influence on the distance of distinct vision, in proportion as the lens is situated farther behind the cornea (compare p. 62 *et seq.*). Consequently this influence will be less in the myopic, and greater in the hypermetropic eye, than in the emmetropic. In this we have therefore a second reason why a definite change of the crystalline lens shall represent in. the myopic individual a less, and in the hypermetropic, a greater range of accommodation than in the emmetropic. Now if, notwithstanding, a greater range of accommodation be found in myopic than in hypermetropic individuals, the inference is evident, that the former can produce a much more decided change in their crystalline lens than the latter.

§ 9. Clinical determination of Ametropia in General.

As we have already seen, and as shall hereafter more fully appear, both myopia and hypermetropia exercise a great influence upon the function of vision, and both are closely connected with numerous affections of the eyes of a different nature. Hence it is, that the ophthalmic surgeon must make it a rule, in every patient who applies to him, to determine the refractive condition of the eyes. But in acute inflammatory affections, it is quite allowable in the first instance to defer the determination; though, when the inflammation gives way, it ought not, even in such cases, to be neglected. I have long been accustomed to note this of all my patients: in the lists in the Ophthalmic Hospital a special column is provided for the purpose. I have in numerous instances found the great advantage of this rule.

The determination itself is effected, after some practice, with rapidity and certainty. Two methods have been employed. The first consists in testing the power of vision with glasses of known focal distance. The second in the determination of the refractive condition by means of the ophthalmoscope.

I. For the employment of the first method we require, in the first place, the necessary glasses from $\frac{1}{80}$ to $\frac{1}{2}$ and from $-\frac{1}{80}$ to $-\frac{1}{2}$; in the second place, the necessary objects for testing.

The pairs of glasses are kept loose in a box, with a spectacle-frame in which they can be placed.* It is also convenient to have a black plate of metal of the same size as the glasses, which, placed in the frame, closes one of the eyes; by closing the eye with the finger, the accuracy of vision is easily lost for some moments, so that we cannot make the examination of this eye follow immediately upon that of the other.

The most suitable objects are letters and numbers. Dr. Snellen has drawn up these in a regular system, and has thus supplied a want which had long been felt. The principles kept in view by Dr. Snellen are the following:—

1. Detached, separate letters, black on a white ground, in irregular sequence.

2. The letter, large Roman, square, the vertical strokes being $\frac{1}{4}$, the horizontal $\frac{1}{8}$ of the breadth of the letter.

---

* Paetz and Flohr, opticians, unter den Linden, Berlin, supply such boxes with the necessary positive and negative glasses. The boxes contain, moreover, prismatic and coloured glasses, with a spectacle-frame. Jaeger's spectacle-frame, prepared by Kraft und Sohn, mechanicians, Vienna, Stadt, Karrnerstrasse, 1043, im Bürgerspital, is convenient, in which the rings containing the glasses are movable, admitting of their distance being so regulated that the patient can look nearly through the centre of both glasses.

3. Exclusion of some letters which are much more difficult to distinguish than others.

4. Ascending magnitudes from I to CC, the magnitude being proportional to the number, so that CC is two hundred times larger than I; XX ten times larger than II, etc.

5. The several magnitudes distinguishable by a sharp eye, in good light, at the distance of so many feet as the number amounts to. Thus II at 2 feet, VI at 6 feet, XX at 20 feet, etc., all seen at similar angles (of 5 minutes), are equally easily distinguishable by the eye exactly accommodated to the distance.

By the application of these principles great advantages are obtained. In the first place, the existence of ametropia is at once apparent, when, with respect to the power of distinguishing, the proportion between distance and magnitude is destroyed: for example, if a person sees I at 1 foot, II at 2 feet, and cannot see XX at 20 feet distance, myopia exists, etc. If he sees XX at 20 feet, and does not see I at the distance of 1 foot, the nearest point lies at more than 1 foot from the eye, etc. In the second place, we can immediately with perfect accuracy determine the sharpness of sight. He who, having his eyes properly accommodated, distinguishes XX only at 10 feet, instead of at 20, has a sharpness of vision $S = \dfrac{10}{20} = \dfrac{1}{2}$, when he distinguishes III at 1 foot, his vision is $S = \dfrac{1}{3}$; when he sees C at 20 feet, it is $S = \dfrac{20}{100} = \dfrac{1}{5}$, etc. He who distinguishes C, LX, XII, III, only at the distance of 1 foot, has his vision equal respectively to $\dfrac{1}{100}, \dfrac{1}{60}, \dfrac{1}{12}, \dfrac{1}{3}$, etc.

In the examination for the determination of ametropia, we have to do only with R, and for this purpose we cause the patient to look at the distance of about 20 feet; while on the card intended for distance (as card 2 appended to this work), even CC still occurs, thus it appears applicable as far as $S = \dfrac{1}{10}$. If S be still less, we bring the card nearer to the eye; finally, reckoning the fingers may be conveniently substituted for distinguishing letters.

For persons who cannot read, we may substitute reckoning vertical strokes. By this method, however, it is difficult to obtain results, and they are, moreover, not capable of comparison with those ob-

tained with letters. It is therefore better to teach such patients to recognise a couple of letters and a couple of figures, which is easily done.

The mode of quickly recognising the ametropic condition, is best
learnt by means of practical instruction. We must here, however,
endeavour to give some general indications on the subject. For this
purpose let us assume a clinical point of view. Minuter details will
be given in treating of the several forms of ametropia and modified
accommodation.

A PERSON AGED TWENTY PRESENTS HIMSELF.

The question is :—does ametropia exist ? *We give him small print*
—I to IV of Snellen's test-types *to read.*

A. *He reads* I *without difficulty at a distance of from* 6 *to*
12 *inches;* II *at the distance of* 2 *feet.* We in the first place
infer, that his power of vision is sharp, secondly, that he is either
emmetropic or at least but slightly ametropic. We show him
XX at 20 feet. He reads it likewise. Is he then emmetropic? is
still the question.

1. *With* $-\frac{1}{40}$ *he does not see* XX *at the distance stated, better de-*

fined; he is not myopic. *With* $\frac{1}{40}$ *he sees the letters fainter, less*

black, although somewhat larger : he has no *manifest* hypermetropia.
May he, nevertheless, be hypermetropic? *Latent* hypermetropia
might exist, which, so long as accommodation is active, cannot
appear. This may manifest itself only after the instillation of sulphate of atropia (gr. i to dr. ii), paralysing the accommodation; if
it exists, the eye should now see much more sharply at a distance with
$\frac{1}{40}$, perhaps even with $\frac{1}{24}$ or $\frac{1}{16}$.

Must we then, in order to satisfy ourselves of the existence or
non-existence of latent hypermetropia, in each of our patients, paralyse the power of accommodation by means of atropia ? By no means ;
this ought to be done only when there is reason to suspect hypermetropia, and even then we should warn the patient, that, for some days,
impairment of vision, particularly for near objects, with dimness, and
probably with intolerance of light, will remain. When, therefore, are
we justified in assuming or suspecting in a youthful individual the
existence of latent hypermetropia ? We may assume it when manifest hypermetropia exists; a portion is then always latent through

2

the action of accommodation. We may with great probability suspect it: 1, when convergent strabismus is present; 2, when there are complaints of asthenopia; 3, when P is much too great for the time of life. If, for example, the person examined at the age of 20 years says he cannot read accurately at the distance of 6″, we shall in 19 cases out of 20 detect latent hypermetropia. As shall hereafter appear, it may then become desirable to give him glasses.

2. *If with* $-\dfrac{1}{40}$ *he sees more accurately at a distance,* he is very slightly myopic.

3. *If with* $\dfrac{1}{40}$ *he sees as accurately as without glasses,* there is manifest hypermetropia. Let us take glasses of higher power: $\dfrac{1}{36}, \dfrac{1}{30}$, etc. So long as he continues to see equally well, the manifest hypermetropia is not corrected. The highest glasses, with which he sees accurately, indicate the degree. If he still sees accurately with $\dfrac{1}{24}$, his manifest hypermetropia is $= \dfrac{1}{24}$. In this case we should also determine the total hypermetropia (manifest + latent), after paralysis with atropia.

B. *He reads* I *best at* 6″, *No.* II *at* 9″, *both, indeed, much nearer, but not farther off. From* 6″ *and* 9″ *reading becomes somewhat more difficult.* The dilemma is: either myopia or diminished sharpness of vision. At 20 feet distance he does not see No. XX, nor XL, nor LX, which last are three times larger than XX. Myopia almost certainly exists. We try with $-\dfrac{1}{9}$. Now he sees much more accurately and reads No. XXX or even XX at a distance of 20 feet: the myopia is proven. Its degree is, however, not exactly known. Why did we try glasses of $-\dfrac{1}{9}$? Because the farthest point, at which tolerably acute vision still existed, lay at about 9″. By attending to this, we come tolerably near the degree of M. If he sees with $-\dfrac{1}{9}$, the parallel rays acquire a direction, as if they came from a point situated 9″ in front of the glass. By comparison with glasses of $-\dfrac{1}{8}$ it appears, that with the latter he sees still more accurately; with $-\dfrac{1}{7}$ not better than with $-\frac{1}{8}$, with $\frac{1}{10}$ decidedly less accurately. M therefore exists

$= \frac{1}{8}.$

C. *He cannot, or at least can only with difficulty, read No.* I (*or even larger letters*), *at whatever distance the book be held.* His time of life excludes presbyopia. But three cases are still possible : there exists either diminished accuracy of vision, or H, or paresis of accommodation. Where the pupil is freely movable, with normal diameter, the last is almost with certainty excluded. The shortest way is, however, immediately to make him read with $\frac{1}{10}$. Spectacles with these glasses should always lie on the oculist's table. It is in very many cases the first number which he tries in order to arrive quickly at a conclusion. If with $\frac{1}{10}$ No. I be read at 12 inches, even at 16″ I$^\mathrm{I}$ ($= 1\frac{1}{2}$) be read : we can no longer suspect diminished accuracy of vision, and H has become very probable. At the distance of 20 feet XL is distinguished, also XXX, but XX, on the contrary, is not. But with $\frac{1}{30}$ the patient sees them more accurately ; with $\frac{1}{20}$ he distinguishes XX, with $\frac{1}{16}$ he still sees them as well; with $\frac{1}{13}$ the letters begin to be diffused : the existence of H and indeed of H $= \frac{1}{16}$ is thus established : S is at the same time perfect. If positive glasses produce a considerable improvement, but if none can be found, with which XX is distinguishable at 20 feet, H is complicated with diminished sharpness of vision, as often is the case. In either instance, the total H should now, by the artificial production of paralysis, be determined. Had paresis of accommodation existed, without H, the naked eye should have seen accurately at a distance, and even weak positive glasses should have diminished the accuracy of vision with respect to remote objects. The condition would have been immediately distinguishable from H from the fact, that with $\frac{1}{10}$ at more than 10″ the letters would have become somewhat diffuse, and consequently I$^\mathrm{I}$ could not have been read at 16″. Where complication with diminished accuracy of vision exists, examination of the media and of the fundus oculi with the ophthalmoscope is necessary. In H this investigation is frequently negative, although the accuracy of vision is diminished. Not unfrequently astigmatism is at the same time present, the consideration of which I must defer to a subsequent chapter.

D. *The patient reads* II, *or at least* IV *and* VI *at* 3″, 4″, *or* 5″ *from the eye, but not at a greater distance.* Here either myopia with diminished accuracy of vision, or a high degree of hypermetropia exists. If he reads No. VIII at 2 feet, it can scarcely be anything else than hypermetropia. If at a distance he sees only LX, with glasses of $\frac{1}{6}$, No. XXX with those of $\frac{1}{5}$ less well, it is hypermetropia, and indeed H$m = \frac{1}{6}$; a portion is still latent. Had myopia existed, with greatly diminished accuracy of vision, the patient would have seen worse at two feet distance, and, what is decisive, the vision of remote objects would have diminished with positive glasses; with negative, on the contrary, it would have increased. Why in high degrees of H letters of a definite size are seen better very close to the eye than at a distance of 1 foot, shall be explained in the Chapter upon Hypermetropia.

E. *He says he can see quite well and accurately, particularly at a distance, but that his vision is also good for near objects. But the eye soon becomes tired; close work he cannot keep up.* This is asthenopia, to be treated of, in detail, in a separate chapter. Here I may just observe, that in the great majority of cases H is the ultimate cause of it. We should try whether the patient can read at 6″, 5″, and 4″; whether it is difficult or not. We cause him to look to a distance : weak positive glasses of $\frac{1}{40}, \frac{1}{36}$, etc., improve or at least do not diminish the accuracy of vision. Thus the presence of H is demonstrated, and it now remains only to determine its increase by artificial paralysis (the latent H). But sometimes, notwithstanding the existence of asthenopia, the letters at a distance are rendered somewhat diffused by weak positive glasses, for example of $\frac{1}{40}$. Can we thence infer the absence of H ? By no means, it is almost certain that latent H exists. We must, therefore, in such cases determine P, and afterwards have recourse to artificial paralysis of accommodation. Should it thus appear that no H exists, $\frac{1}{A} = \frac{1}{P} - \frac{1}{R}$ will be found particularly small, and we thus come to the question of paresis of accommodation, which is infinitely rarer than H.

All these cases hang upon the determination of R. With it the existence or non-existence, and at the same time the degree of ametropia are given. Moreover, we could in the simple manner already described determine the nearest point; with it the range of accommodation $\frac{1}{A} = \frac{1}{P} - \frac{1}{R}$ is known. With the increase of years it diminishes (compare the Third Chapter, p. 126), and vision is consequently considerably modified. Therefore it was necessary in the foregoing examples to suppose a definite time of life, and we chose a young man of 20 years. It will be advantageous to bring forward some persons of more advanced age.

A MAN AGED FIFTY PRESENTS HIMSELF.

A. In good light he easily recognises No. II at 20, and even at 24 inches, No. I¹ doubtfully at either distance, No. I not at all. At the distance of 16 feet he recognises the letters of XX. The accuracy of vision is therefore practically perfect. With $\frac{1}{40}$ he sees less accurately at a distance, but near objects with much greater ease. Our conclusion is: there exists only Pr, and for close work he had already been obliged to use spectacles.

B. *He cannot read without spectacles. Even ten years ago he began to experience difficulty at his work. At a distance, however, he then saw accurately, but now he sees less sharply: No. XX he does not recognise, at the distance of 20 feet, No. XXX doubtfully, and the letters are not black.* We may be nearly certain, that in this case Pr has been superadded to H. With $\frac{1}{10}$ he reads No. I at about 12″, closer with greater difficulty: the accuracy of vision is perfect; the existence of H has, properly speaking, been already proved by seeing at 12″ with glasses of $\frac{1}{10}$. Let us determine it by looking at a distance; with $\frac{1}{30}$ vision is acute as well as with $\frac{1}{40}$, with $\frac{1}{24}$ it is less good. H exists $= \frac{1}{30}$. At fifty years of age the latent H is very trifling; we need not determine it. Glasses of $\frac{1}{30}$ may be constantly worn by this patient; for reading and writing something stronger is required.

C. "He has always had excellent sight, saw distant and remote objects exceedingly well, boasts conceitedly of his eyes, but has for some weeks observed that he no longer sees at a distance so accurately with the right eye." *He reads* I *from* 6" *to* 12", No. II. *at* 2, *but not* No. III *at* 3 *feet distance*. We infer near-sightedness. The patient denies it; is surprised that he cannot recognise Nos. XX and XXX at a distance, and still more that he accurately distinguishes them with glasses of $-\dfrac{1}{30}$. The eye with which he could still read, but could see less accurately at a distance, appeared to be affected with a trace of cataract.

These examples may suffice to point out in general the mode of looking for ametropia. As important for the first indication, I shall add only, that many hypermetropic persons complain of asthenopia; myopics for the most part know, that they see comparatively less accurately at a distance; that, moreover, the first have usually a shallower, the latter a deeper eye-chamber, while, lastly, the age for presbyopia affords an indication.

In the determination of R with the aid of glasses, the distance x from the glass to the nodal point k of the eye is neglected. In using glasses with a long focal distance x has less influence; but when those with a short focal distance are employed, x must be taken into account. If we have to do with positive glasses, x must be deducted from the focal distance; if with negative, it must be reckoned with it. This has already been explained (pp. 32 and 35). Thus, if myopia be neutralized by glasses of $-\dfrac{1}{6}$, and if $x = 1''$, M $= \dfrac{1}{7}$; if hypermetropia be corrected by glasses of $\dfrac{1}{8}$, and if $x = 1''$, then H $= \dfrac{1}{7}$.

The influence of x may also help us in the determination of the degree of ametropia. If, namely, an equally accurate or even a more accurate image was obtained with the glass employed, by moving it further from the eye, the negative was too weak or the positive too strong. We thus know what glass we should subsequently try. It might, perhaps, be supposed that we should have only to determine with the glass first tried, x, and to take its value into account. This might, however, lead to an incorrect result. Myopic individuals, in fact, will often prefer to hold a glass, though it is too strong, close before the eye: the image is then larger, and by some tension of accommodation they prevent its being diffused. Therefore we must, as a final determination, with the myopic always try what is the weakest glass, which, held close before the eye, gives a defined image.   In the hypermetropic we run less risk in taking a great value of x into account; but it is better in this case also, to make the final determination with a glass, which, held close to the eye, gives defined images.   In high degrees of myopia, and where uncertain answers are given, the investigation is often shortened by ascertaining the influence of weak glasses, for example, of $\frac{1}{40}$ and $-\frac{1}{40}$, alternately held before the stronger negative glass placed in the spectacle frame.

II. In the second place, we may in a certain sense determine more objectively the refractive condition by means of examination with the ophthalmoscope.   The great inventor of the instrument has not only pointed this out, but has also communicated the application of this method.   It may be explained in a few words.   According to well known laws, the rays proceeding from a point of the retina, refracted by the media of the eye, shall have, on entering the air, a direction similar to that of the rays which, falling on the cornea, unite in the same point of the retina.   If M exists $=\frac{1}{8}$, the point r, whose emitted rays unite in the retina, lies 8″ in front of the nodal point, and in the same point r will the rays emitted by the retina, converging in front of the eye, unite.   If H exists $=\frac{1}{10}$, there unite upon the retina rays, which, converging to a point r, situated 10″ behind the nodal point, fall upon the cornea; and, *vice versâ*, the rays emitted by the retina, having reached the air, are diverging, and appear to have proceeded from the said point.   Lastly, the emmetropic eye at rest, which has its focus for parallel rays in the retina, gives to the rays proceeding from the retina, when they reach the air, a parallel direction.   Consequently the eye of the observer, in order to see accurately a non-inverted image of the retina of the emmetropic eye, must be adapted for parallel rays; on the contrary, it must be adapted for converging rays, in order accurately to distinguish that of myopic persons; and for diverging, in the case of hypermetropic individuals.   Therefore, if the observer knows the condition of his eye, with which he sees accurately the retina of another, he can form an opinion as to the refractive condition of the observed eye.   It is best to practise one's self in voluntarily seeing with accommodation for one's farthest point (ascertained by investigation), and to try what glass we must place before one's eye, so as accurately to see the vessels in the retina of another.   In order to be able to bring the most different glasses before the eye, I have had a ring made on the ophthalmoscope, adapted to hold the glasses of the spectacle box.   My eye is emmetropic and is accustomed, in the use of all optical instruments, to adapt itself for parallel rays.   Now, if I need a glass of $-\frac{1}{8}$, to see a retina accurately, myopia of $\frac{1}{8}$ exists; if for this purpose I require a glass of $\frac{1}{10}$, H of $\frac{1}{10}$ is present.   Some correction, negative for M, positive for H, is necessary, both for the distance between the observing and the observed eye, and for that between the glass and the observing eye (pp. 32 and 35); but if we approach as much as possible, this may be reduced to about 1″: by introducing this correction, therefore, in the above quoted examples, M may have been $=\frac{1}{9}$ and H $=\frac{1}{9}$. Moreover, in the alteration of the distance between the observing and the observed eye we have a means of estimating whether we should try a stronger or a weaker glass.—If the eye of the observer be ametropic, the degree thereof is easily taken into account. If, for example, the same glasses as above had been necessary for an eye with M $=\frac{1}{18}$, the eyes examined should have given M $=\frac{1}{9}-\frac{1}{18}=\frac{1}{18}$, H $=\frac{1}{9}+\frac{1}{18}=\frac{1}{6}$. *Vice versá*, where the same glasses were required for an observing eye with H $=\frac{1}{18}$, the M found should have amounted to $\frac{1}{9}+\frac{1}{18}=\frac{1}{6}$, the H $=\frac{1}{9}-\frac{1}{18}=\frac{1}{18}$.

In observing with the ophthalmoscope in the inverted image the estimation is more difficult, because the influence of the objective glass to be held before the eye and the position of the image cannot be well defined.   High degrees of myopia, however, manifest themselves immediately, as, without holding a convex glass before the observed eye, we see the inverted retinal image stand before this eye. So far as we can determine the distance from this image to the eye, we know also the degree of myopia.

I have thus given the principles of the determination of ametropia with the aid of the ophthalmoscope.   Generally speaking, this method is inferior in accuracy to the determination of vision with glasses of known focal distance.   1. It is for many observers difficult, in the use of the ophthalmoscope, entirely to relax their power of accommodation : if they are not certain of this, the method is inapplicable to them.   He who, on the contrary, has by practice attained so far that he can not only wholly relax his power of accommodation, but also justly estimate the degree of voluntary action, can very often usefully employ it.   I know this by my own experience.

2. Without producing paralysis of accommodation, we are never perfectly sure that we determine the refraction in the condition of rest.

3. It is sometimes difficult, at least when strongly negative glasses are required, with a narrow pupil accurately to see the vessels of the retina.

4. The vessels which lie at different depths in the fibrous layer afford no perfectly correctly situated object for estimation.

5. Moreover, such a vessel is not a suitable object to determine with precision whether we see accurately.   Consequently, the method in each case requires a great degree of attention.

6. The determination in the line of vision, which it chiefly concerns, is for the most part difficult of execution, because the place of the yellow spot is not well seen, or our estimation of the accuracy of seeing it is particularly difficult.

If this second method, therefore, is not equal to the first in accuracy of results, it nevertheless deserves our attention, because it is applicable in cases where the first wholly or partly fails us.   This is, in the first place, true in all young children, likewise in the blind, and even in high degrees of amblyopia, where the knowledge of the refractive condition is sometimes of great importance.   Further, by this method we can better and more easily ascertain the degree of ametropia for indirect vision than by the first : in many instances I have by it alone succeeded in satisfying myself that the myopia for indirect vision was less than when the patient looked in the line of vision.   Besides, the want of fixation of a hypermetropic eye examined with the ophthalmoscope, sometimes gives rise to more complete relaxation of the power of accommodation, whereby hypermetropia, latent in trials of vision, may manifest itself.   Finally, this method may be of great use in simulated ametropia.

NOTE TO CHAPTER II.

In the commencement of this Chapter much stress was laid upon the necessity of drawing an accurate distinction between the anomalies of refraction and those of accommodation. Each eye has a definite refraction; according to this the first distinction is to be made. Now, whether the eye be emmetropic or ametropic, in either case it has a power of accommodation, and this may be normal or abnormal. Abnormal accommodation is, therefore, as independent of refraction as any other disease of the eye.

In my work upon Ametropia and its results (*Ametropie en hare gevolgen*), Utrecht, 1860, as well as in my papers in the *Archiv f. Ophthalmologie*, B. iv., vi., und vii., I had prominently put forward, as the basis of a correct description and of a scientific explanation, the distinction just alluded to. Stellwag von Carion now thinks (*Zeitschrift der k. k. Gesellschaft der Aerzte zu Wien*, 1862) that I should have mentioned his merits respecting this point. I am quite prepared to do so.

In his Essay, entitled *die Accommodationsfehler des Auges*, to be found in the *Sitzungsberichte der kaiserlichen Akademie der Wissenschaften, Mathem.-naturwissenschaftliche Klasse*, B. xvi., pp. 187-281, he calls natural visual line (*natürliche Sehlinie*) the line of accommodation, to which the eye in absolute inactivity of the muscle of accommodation is adapted. His natural visual line is, therefore, the farthest point of distinct vision, considered as a Czermackian line of accommodation. "Inasmuch as the degree of the greatest possible accommodation-pressure, which the eye can exercise," he says, "in every case is limited, so must the natural visual line determine the position of the nearest point of distinct vision, that is, of the nearest final point of the shortest line of accommodation" (p. 200).

"This degree," he continues, "of the available pressure-exciting power of the muscle of accommodation, on the one side, and the natural visual line on the other, are, therefore, the factors which determine the absolute visual distance of the eye, the length of the line connecting the farthest and the nearest points, as well as the position of the latter in the elongated optic axis. But the length and position of this line constitute the measure according to which alone the form and degree can be determined, wherein the dioptric part of the visual function deviates from the normal proportions. It is, therefore, evident that the defects of accommodation of the eye, *from a scientific point of view*, can be divided only into those depending upon anatomical disproportions of the whole eyeball or of the several light-refracting media; further into those, caused by limitation of the function of the muscle of accommodation; and, thirdly, into those depending upon both causes." In this is, in fact, contained the first indication of a distinction between the anomalies of refraction and the disturbances of accommodation. Nevertheless, the hint was lost upon Stellwag von Carion just as it was upon others. He immediately adds: "Such a division, however, renders treatment difficult, and prevents a proper view of the subject under consideration." Had he tried it, perhaps he would have seen, that his second and third class (in order not again to mix up accommodation and refraction) must be reduced to one, comprising the anomalies of accommodation *in general*, independently of refraction, and perhaps he would then also have strictly adhered to the ideas of myopia and hypermetropia, or would, at least, not have included them among the defects of *accommodation*. But he adopts a quite different (more practical ?) method. He opposes presbyopia to myopia, and subsequently passing over to hypermetropia (N.B., by him termed hyper-presbyopia), he begins by calling the latter a higher degree of presbyopia.

I regret not to find in Stellwag's work the merit to which he thinks he has a claim. Those of my readers who take an interest in the matter will please to consult his treatise. They may pass over the less successful mathematical introduction (compare with reference to it : Zehender, *Anleitung z. Studium der Dioptrik des menschlichen Auges*, Erlangen, 1856. p. 166), which deterred so many, myself among the number, from the earlier perusal of this essay.

The diagrammatic sketch of the anomalies of refraction and accommodation, in which the commencement and termination of the lines represent r and p, and the lengths of the lines the range of accommodation, I first applied in the *Nederlandsch tijdschrift voor geneeskunde*, D. II., 1858. The idea of expressing the range of accommodation by a lens of definite focal distance, is to be met with so early as in the masterly work of Young (*Philosophical Transactions*, 1801).

CHAPTER III.

Fuller Development of the Different Meanings of Range of Accommodation.

§ 10. *Relation between accommodation and convergence of the visual lines; Meaning of* $1 : A$, *of* $1 : A_1$ *and of* $1 : A_2$. So far as the range of accommodation for both eyes extends, the state of accommodation of the eye corresponds to a definite convergence of the visual lines. Thus the emmetropic eye, with parallel visual lines, is accommodated for infinite distance; with a convergence at 8″, for a distance of 8″, &c. Unmistakably, therefore, a connexion exists between convergence of the visual lines and accommodation, to which Porterfield* and John Mueller† already directed attention. Both these observers, however, appeared to assume, that this connexion is absolute and causal ; that a definite convergence is necessarily attended with a definite accommodation, and admits of no other; it was thought that only *beyond* the limits of accommodation a greater or less convergence was possible, to which the accommodation, respectively for the nearest and farthest point of distinct vision, should then still correspond. Now this is incorrect. Even Volkmann showed,‡ that also *within* the limits of the range of accommodation such absolute dependence does not exist, and I § gave further proofs of this by simple experiments, which were capable at the same time of determining the degree of independence. The experiments were made partly with convex and concave, partly with weak prismatic glasses. It is easy to convince one's self that both eyes together, as well without as with slightly concave or convex glasses, can accurately see an object at a definite distance, and that, consequently, without change of convergence, the accommodation can be modified. With equal ease, we observe that, in holding a weak prism before the eye, whether with the refracting angle turned in-

---

* *A Treatise on the Eye*, Vol. I., pp. 410 *et seq.* Edinburgh, 1759.

† *Vergleichende Physiologie des Gesichtssinnes*, 1826, p. 216.

‡ *Neue Beiträge zur Physiologie des Gesichtssinnes*, 1836, p. 148.

§ *Holländische Beiträge zu den anat. u. physiol. Wissenschaften* herausgegeben von van Deen, Donders u. Moleschott, 1846, B. 1, p. 379.

wards or outwards, an object can be accurately seen with both eyes at the same distance, and that, consequently, the convergence may be altered, without modifying the accommodation. When, therefore, it is required for the sake of distinct vision with both eyes, the connexion between convergence and accommodation can be, at least partially, overcome. I early stated the method of determining how far the independence existed. Some time afterwards it was applied with the requisite accuracy.*

The question is very simple: it is only necessary to know R_1 and P_1 with parallel visual lines and with a series of converging degrees (to the maximum), and these we find, by a calculation from the nearest and farthest points, discovered by means of different convex and concave glasses. For accurate determination, however, a special optometer is required, which shall be described at the end of this section.

The results of the examination of the emmetropic eyes of a person aged 15, are represented in the annexed Figure (57).

Fig. 57.

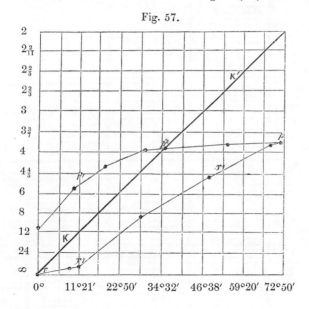

At different points of the diagonal $k\ k'$, intersection takes place between the transverse lines, before which, in Parisian inches,

* Conf. Mac Gillavry, *Onderzoekingen over de hoegrootheid der Accommodatie.* Diss. inaug., Utrecht, 1858.

the distances are placed; and the longitudinal lines, under which the degrees of convergence of the visual lines corresponding to the distances are noted. The mutual distance of the visual lines of the two eyes in the parallel state amounted to $28\frac{1}{2}''$, in which case (compare the figure), at a distance of $12''$, a convergence of $11° 21'$, at a distance of $6''$, a convergence of $22° 50'$, etc., exists. The line $p_1 p_2 p$ represents, in the consecutive convergence, the course of the nearest point, the line $r r_1$ that of the farthest point. The dots in these lines are the points determined by investigation.

Now the figure shows that the eyes here supposed with parallel visual lines can accommodate from infinite distance up to $11''$, with $22° 50'$ convergence from about $12''$ to $4''.16$, etc. At p_2, where the line of nearest points cuts the diagonal $k\,k'$, we attain the shortest binocular distance P_2 of distinct vision. With still stronger convergence, for example, $46° 38'$, the line $p_2 p$ remains under the diagonal $k\,k'$, so that accommodation can no longer take place for the point of convergence which here lies only $3''$ from the eye: the nearest point with that convergence lies, namely, as appears from the figure, at about $3''.8$. The absolute nearest point p lies somewhat closer still, and in fact at $3''.69$, but for this a convergence of about $70°$ is required, that is at a distance of about $2''$. With this maximum of convergence all space for accommodation is lost, and therefore the lines $p_2 p_1$ and $r r_1$ cut one another.

From the foregoing it appears, that in every one who has two sufficiently equal and movable eyes, we may distinguish :—

1. The greatest distance of distinct vision R, (in figure 58 as ∞ at r).

2. The shortest binocular distance of distinct vision P_2 (in the figure = 3.9 at p_2).

3. The absolute shortest distance of distinct vision P, with the maximum of convergence (in the figure = $3''.69$ at p).

4. Relatively shortest distances of distinct vision P_1, at each given convergence (for example, in the figure at $22° 50'$, $P_1 = 4''.16$).

5. Relatively greatest distances of distinct vision R_1, at each given convergence (for example, in the figure, with $22° 50'$ convergence, $R_1 = 12''$).

By the determination of these several distances, three different meanings with as many values of accommodation are to be obtained.

I. The absolute,

$$\frac{1}{A} = \frac{1}{P} - \frac{1}{R}.$$

II. The binocular,

$$\frac{1}{A_2} = \frac{1}{P_2} - \frac{1}{R_2}.$$

III. The relative,

$$\frac{1}{A_1} = \frac{1}{P_1} - \frac{1}{R_1}.$$

They are all to be deduced from Fig. 57.

Now in the foregoing sections we spoke only of the *absolute* range of accommodation, comprising the accommodation from the absolute farthest point r to the absolute nearest point p, for each eye in particular: in the figure this is $\dfrac{1}{A} = \dfrac{1}{3 \cdot 69} - \dfrac{1}{\infty} = \dfrac{1}{3 \cdot 69}$.

The binocular comprises the accommodation from the farthest point r_2, for both eyes at once, to the nearest point p_2 for both eyes at once. In the emmetropic eye, r_2 coincides with r, and the binocular range of accommodation, to be deduced from Fig. 57, is consequently,

$$\frac{1}{A_2} = \frac{1}{3 \cdot 9} - \frac{1}{\infty} = \frac{1}{3 \cdot 9}.$$

Finally, the *relative* is the range of accommodation over which we have control at a given convergence of the visual lines. It represents the degree in which accommodation is independent of convergence, and is, for every convergence, measured by the distance between the lines $p_1 \, p_2 \, p$ and $r \, r_1$. On referring to the figure it now appears that, with increasing convergence, the relative range of accommodation becomes at first greater, then less, until at the maximum of convergence, where the lines mentioned meet one another (in p) it is $= 0$. On consulting the figure in detail we see that, with parallel visual lines,

$$\frac{1}{A_1} = \frac{1}{1 \cdot 1} - \frac{1}{\infty} = \frac{1}{11},$$

and that, with a convergence of $11^\circ \, 21''$,

$$\frac{1}{A_1} = \frac{1}{5 \cdot 33} - \frac{1}{72} = \frac{1}{5 \cdot 76}.$$

already attains the maximum. Throughout some degrees $\dfrac{1}{A_1}$ now continues nearly unchanged, at the convergence of $22^\circ \, 50'$ it is

8

diminished to $\dfrac{1}{6\cdot4}$, and at the binocular nearest point, with a convergence of about 38°, still amounts to $\dfrac{1}{9}$.

It is of importance further to observe, that the relative range of accommodation consists of two parts: a *positive* part and a *negative*. The diagonal $k\,k'$ represents the convergences of the visual lines: the part situated above this diagonal is the positive, that situated beneath it is the negative. The first represents what, reckoning from the point of convergence, we can accommodate still nearer, the latter what we can accommodate still farther off. For example (compare Fig. 57): the emmetropic eye is, under a convergence of 11° 21′, that is at 12″, in ordinary vision accommodated for this distance of 12″; but the accommodation may, with the same convergence, be made more tense, for a distance, namely, of 5·33″, and it may likewise be relaxed to distinct vision at a distance of 72″. The first is evident, since with negative, the second, since with positive glasses of definite strength, at the distance of 12″, with both eyes at once, accurate vision can be attained. At 11° 21′, therefore, $p_2\,k_1$ is the positive, $k_1\,r_1$ the negative part of the relative range of accommodation. They are calculated as

$$\text{the positive} = \frac{1}{5\cdot33} - \frac{1}{12} = \frac{1}{9\cdot6},$$

$$\text{the negative} = \frac{1}{12} - \frac{1}{72} = \frac{1}{14\cdot4},$$

so that at 11° 21′, in the case investigated, we find

$$\frac{1}{A_1} = \frac{1}{9\cdot6} + \frac{1}{14\cdot4} = \frac{1}{5\cdot76},$$

that is, as above.

A glance at the figure now shows further, that in the emmetropic eye at ∞ (parallel visual lines) $\dfrac{1}{A_1}$ is wholly positive, that, with increasing convergence, the negative part rapidly increases, soon also at the expense of the positive, and that at 36° convergence $\dfrac{1}{A_1}$ has become entirely negative.

The distinction here made already acquires practical importance from the fact, *that the accommodation can be maintained only for a distance, at which, in reference to the negative, the positive part of the relative range of accommodation is tolerably great.*

It is not in every one that we can satisfactorily determine the ranges of accommodation corresponding to different degrees of convergence. For this purpose two freely moveable, accurately seeing eyes of nearly equal refraction, and equal accommodating power, are in the first place required, and, in addition, some talent for observation. Each of these requisites was perfectly met with in the person aged fifteen, who supplied the data for Fig. 57. The determination requires special care. As object we may take wires, which are to be finer in proportion as the point to be defined is nearer to the eye. Accurate results may also be obtained by the use of little holes (from $\frac{1'''}{20}$ to $\frac{1'''}{6}$ in diameter) in a black metal plate, with a background of dull glass turned towards the clear daylight. Soon the accommodation for the holes is no longer perfect, they lose their round form and rapidly emit rays. With different glasses of known positive and negative focal distance, at different degrees of convergence, the greatest and least distances of distinct vision are now to be determined. At the same time, in order to obtain correct results, care must also be taken that the distance of the glasses from the eye shall remain unalterably the same; lastly, that at each degree of convergence the axis of the glass shall nearly coincide with the axis of vision. In order to fulfil these conditions, an optometer has been constructed (Fig. 58), partly in imitation of that of Hasner, Edlem

Fig. 58.

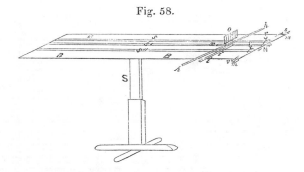

von Artha (*Prager Vierteljahrschrift f. praktische Heilkunde*, 1851. B. xxxii., p. 166). Our optometer consists of a horizontal, oblong, quadrangular board *B B*, placed on a stand *S*. The board is nearly five feet long, nine Parisian inches in breadth (compare particularly Fig. 59, representing a part of the board); it possesses three parallel grooves *s s′ s″*, in which, by means of a couple of copper handles (*h h*), a well-fitting rod, *x*, with perpendicular bar can be inserted, bearing the wire-optometer *o*, or the plate with fine openings. The mutual distance of the two external grooves amounts to 28½‴, and therefore corresponds to that of the parallel visual lines; if the object moves, as in Figs. 58 and 59, in the middle groove, then both eyes contribute equally to the convergence. The one extremity of the board has a notch *N* for the nose of the person under examination; in

2

front of his eyes are two half-rings *r r*, supporting the glasses. Each of these rings is moveable in an arched groove (*a a*) (whose centre of curvature

Fig. 59.

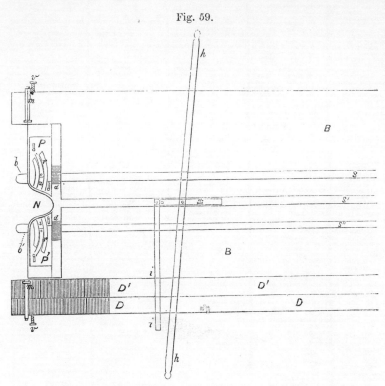

lies in the centre of motion of the eye, while the anterior surface of the cornea coincides with the crossed lines), present in the small microscopes *m m*, which are applied at both sides. The position of the eyes is fixed by two wooden rods (*b b*), which, drawn out at pleasure, are fastened by screws under the board, and against which the cheeks rest. The ring-bearing grooves are in two copper-plates *P P'*, which by means of the screws *v v* can be brought to one another and are kept separate by springs. The mutual distance of these plates is read off on the scale *d*. During observation the distance of these plates must correspond to the mutual distance of the two parallel visual lines. (This distance can be determined with an instrument, described under the name of visuometer by Alfred Smee (*The Eye in Health and in Disease*. London, 1854), and constructed upon the principle laid down by Hawkins. We make use of a similar instrument: two short cylinders of small diameter are moveable along a divided bar ; the head being fixed, one eye sees a distant object in the centre of one of the cylinders ; the second cylinder is now moved until the other eye sees the same object in its centre. Each eye is then alternately closed a few times, in order to make sure that the object stands in the centre of the cylinders, afterwards the person looks once more with both eyes, and the mutual distance of the cylinders is read off on the divided bar. This distance is then transferred to the plates P P' of the optometer). If the half-rings in the grooves a a be now placed at $0°$, the eyes see remote objects through the axes of the glasses placed in the rings. In this position the absolute farthest point r and the nearest point p, with parallel visual lines, are determined. With these determinations we begin; the optometer-object is taken away, and an object some metres distant is employed, whether vertical black lines on a white surface, or an opening of about $1'''$ diameter, in a black plate turned towards dull glass, according as a wire-optometer, or a plate with fine holes is thought preferable for the determination at different degrees of convergence. We find r with the weakest negative or the strongest positive glass, with which the remote object is accurately seen; on the contrary p_1 with the strongest negative or weakest positive. It is only necessary, in addition, to take into account the distance at which the glasses are from the eye; in this case, where the object remains fixed in its place, the distance in question may be modified as necessary, by pressing in, or drawing out, the rods b b from the optometer.

If, now, r and p, the visual lines being parallel (compare Fig. 57), be known, we place the object on the optometer, and determine, without glasses, the nearest point of binocular vision p_2; only in old people, and in high degrees of hypermetropia are glasses required for the determination of p_2. For the further determination of p_1 and r_1, at different degrees of convergence, I formerly— (conf. Mac Gillavry, *over de hoegrootheid van het accommodatie-vermogen* (on the extent of the power of accommodation), Utrecht, 1858)—placed the optometer-object at such a distance, that it was seen at a convergence of precisely $10°$, $20°$, $30°$, etc.; and removing *each* of the two rings respectively $5°$, $10°$, $15°$, etc., we found by experiment the strongest positive and the strongest negative glasses with which the object could be accurately seen at each of these distances. Apparently this method was simple and good; but it nevertheless gave no accurate results: by the long-continued trial, the muscular system for accommodation becomes fatigued, and along with the sacrifice of much time, we obtain too great a distance. We acquire a sufficient number of points with much greater rapidity and certainty by successively determining with some suitably chosen positive and negative glasses, the nearest and farthest points, by moving the optometer object, according to whose distance the lens-bearing rings must be moved in the arched grooves. The distances thus give directly the convergence at which vision took place, and by taking the glasses, wherewith this was possible, into account, p_1 and r_1 are found for the convergence. By this method I mark for each glass first the nearest, and then (if the distance is positive and occurs on the optometer) the farthest point, and afterwards wait a few minutes before passing to the determination with another glass. Lastly, the absolute nearest point p is sought. This is not unfrequently attended with difficulties. In those who voluntarily converge very strongly, it often succeeds best by looking with each eye separately, while the other eye is covered with a disc, at the maximum of convergence ; in doing so we may also use positive glasses.   Where there is less mobility of the eyes inwards, and in general in those who are strongly myopic, p coincides with p_2, or the necessary convergence for p_2 is even not obtainable.

After this general description, the mode of calculation may be still more accurately indicated in a couple of plain selected examples.   Having determined r and p_1 with parallel visual lines, and p_2, for which no calculation is necessary, let us find : with $-\dfrac{1}{12}$ the binocular nearest point at 6″ from the eye, that is with a convergence of 22° 50′ ; the question now is, what p_1 at that convergence actually amounts to ?   We find : the rays from the accurately seen object diverge from a point situated 6″ in front of the eye, 6″ — 0″.5 = 5″.5 in front of the glass.   Refracted by the glass of $-\dfrac{1}{12}$, they appear to diverge from a nearer point, namely :

$$\left(\frac{1}{5\frac{1}{2}} + \frac{1}{12} = \frac{1}{3.77}\right)$$

from a point 3″·77 from the glass, and therefore 3·77 + 0·5 = 4″·27 from the eye.   With a convergence of 22°50′ therefore p_1 = 4″·27.   Let this distance be noted on the fourth line, under which 22°50′ stands.

A farthest point r_1 is not to be determined with $-\dfrac{1}{12}$, because the eye at the same time becomes hypermetropic and r thus comes to lie behind the eye. With $\dfrac{1}{12}$, on the contrary, both r_1 and p_1 are to be found at a certain convergence.   Let us begin with p_1.   Let us find with $\dfrac{1}{12}$ the binocular nearest point precisely at 3″, that is at 2″·5 from the glass.   In front of the glass therefore the rays diverged from a point 2″.5 distant ; refracted by the glass, on the contrary, they appear to proceed from a point situated

$$\left(\frac{1}{2·5} - \frac{1}{12} = \frac{1}{3·16}\right)$$

3″.16 before the glass, 3″.66 before the nodal point of the eye.   With a convergence of 3″, that is of 46° 38′, p_1 lies therefore at 3″.66.

Now, further let the binocular farthest point be found with the same glasses $= \dfrac{1}{12}$ at 8″.   Thence r, with a convergence to 8″, can be calculated : the rays diverge from a point situated 7″.5 from the glass ; after having passed through the glass, they diverge

$$\left(\frac{1}{7\frac{1}{2}} - \frac{1}{12} = \frac{1}{20}\right)$$

from a point situated 20″ in front of the glass, 20″·5 before the nodal point of the eye.   We therefore make, under the point where the distance of 8″ cuts the diagonal, a dot corresponding to the distance of 20″·5.   It represents r_1 at a convergence to 8″.   By making similar calculations with some other glasses, we soon have dots enough to deduce p_1 p_2 p and r_1, and thus all questions respecting the range of accommodation in an individual are answered.

§ 11. *Difference of the relative range of accommodation* 1 : A₁, *according to the refractive condition of the eye.*

We closed the preceding section with a practical result, namely : that accommodation can be maintained only for a distance, when, in reference to the negative, the positive part of the relative range of accommodation is tolerably great.

In connexion with this point it is of special importance to show, that the relative range of accommodation in ametropic eyes is something quite different from that in emmetropic. The difference is of a twofold nature. In the first place, with a given convergence, the relation of the positive to the negative part of $1 : A_1$ is not the same; in the second, the lines $p_1\ p_2\ p$ and $r\ r_1$ have another form.

We shall first treat of the relation of the positive to the negative part of $1 : A_1$. We may also thus express what we have said on this point : the relative range of accommodation has, in reference to the refraction of the eye, a totally different position with reference to the line of the convergences $k\ k'$. Fig. 60 illustrates this in detail. This

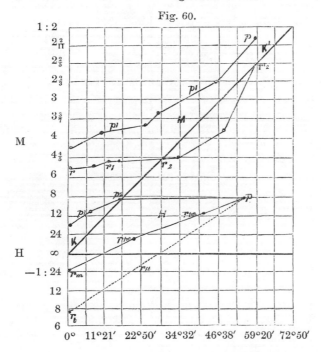

Fig. 60.

diagram contains the curves of the nearest and of the farthest points
in a myopic eye M, and in a hypermetropic H. Both require
further explanation. First as to M. The beginning of the line $r \, r_1$
shows, that we have to do with a myopia of $\dfrac{1}{5.33}$; the farthest binocular point r_2 is found at 5″. Up to this distance, that is up to a
convergence of about 28°, $1 : A_1$ is altogether positive. Now, however, a negative part is rapidly developed, which even at 34°
amounts to half the positive. So far $1 : A_1$ was always increasing,
and here attains as a maximum, $\dfrac{3}{24}$, while the total range of accommodation amounts to $1 : A = \dfrac{7}{24}$. Henceforth, however, $1 : A_1$ diminishes a little; but the negative part becomes, meanwhile,
greater and greater, and indeed up to about 50°, where, the
difficulties of convergence increasing, the farthest point begins so to
approach, that at about 58° it coincides with the point of convergence. At this *maximum* convergence still stronger tension of
accommodation is, however, possible, as the perpendicularly ascending line $r_2 \, p$, here still representing about $1 : A_1 = 1 : 18$,
shows. Hence we see, that in high degrees of myopia, at the maximum of convergence also, a certain range of accommodation still
remains, and the more so in proportion as the convergence itself is
more limited. Moreover, this diagram shows, that in myopia in the
domain of binocular vision, the negative part of $1 : A_1$ is very slight.
On the contrary, the convergence is often very limited. Hence,
therefore, it follows, that *in the higher degrees of myopia, the difficulty
of maintaining binocular vision does not proceed from tension of
accommodation, but rather from difficulty of convergence.*

In those degrees of myopia where, as in the above diagram, Fig.
60, p lies closer to the eye than the nearest point of convergence of
the visual lines, p_2 is wanting and gives place to r'_2. As binocular
range of accommodation nothing else can be assumed than

$$\frac{1}{A_2} = \frac{1}{R'_2} - \frac{1}{R_2},$$

where R'_2 represents the distance from the point r'_2 to the nodal
point of the eye.

We now pass over to the consideration of the hypermetropic eye
H of Fig. 60. Here we find, just as in the emmetropic eye (Fig.
57), $p_1 \, p_2 \, p$, as the curve of the course of the nearest points,

and r_m r_{1m} as that of the course of the farthest points, both in relation to the convergence. But besides these, we find a dotted line r_t r_{1t} ; the latter requires further explanation. Thus, as has already been observed, the hypermetropic individual does not completely relax his power of accommodation. In looking at a distance in the case of a hypermetropic subject, aged 16, registered in the scheme, the preference was given to glasses of $\frac{1}{28}$ above stronger ones ; consequently there existed $\frac{1}{28}$ manifest hypermetropia H_m, represented by the point r_m. But after artificial paralysis of the power of accommodation (by sulphate of atropia), glasses of $\frac{1}{8}$, at $\frac{1''}{2}$ from the nodal point, were required in order to see accurately at a distance, so that the total hypermetropia H_t amounted to $\frac{1}{7\cdot5}$. Now this is expressed by the point r_t. In this state of paralysis the refraction remains, on convergence, unaltered ; we cannot, therefore, investigate where the farthest point, at different degrees of convergence should lie, if the involuntary spasmodic contraction did not exist, and r_t r_{1t} p is consequently only an imaginary line, connecting the absolute farthest point r_t with the absolute nearest point. It appears that the total range of accommodation amounts to

$$\frac{1}{A} = \frac{1}{8} - \left(- \frac{1}{7\frac{1}{2}} \right) = \frac{1}{3\cdot87}.$$

As to the relative, we see it is particularly great, diminishes tolerably uniformly as the convergence is increased, and that its positive part, which, when the visual lines are parallel, is not inconsiderable, on convergence to 9″ (with p_2) under an angle of from 16° to 17°, becomes completely negative, and, moreover, remains negative. If we reckon from the absolute farthest point r_t, the positive part amounts, the visual lines being parallel, to only half of the negative ; if we reckon from the manifest farthest point r_m, the positive part is at first, it is true, greater, but we observe that even at a convergence of 5° the relation is inverted. In connexion with the practical result expressed above, we thus come to the conclusion, that with this degree of hypermetropia, eyes cannot long consecutively accommodate themselves to the point of intersection of their visual lines. With still higher degrees of hypermetropia, as shall hereafter appear, binocular, and with the highest degree (absolute hypermetropia) even monocular vision is never acute.

The foregoing applied to thé position of the range of accommodation, with reference to the convergence of the visual lines.—We must now take the form of the curves into closer consideration. Even in Fig. 60, we see that the curves of M are concave upwards, while those of H are convex upwards. If with this we compare Fig. 57, it appears, that the curves for the emmetropic eye keep the mean between M and H. The reason of this lies in the fact that, with slight convergence, a myopic eye can accommodate proportionally less; a hypermetropic, on the contrary, more (but also must so accommodate) than the emmetropic. The diagram Fig. 61,

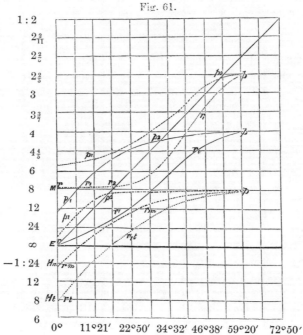

Fig. 61.

will make this plain. It contains the curves of the nearest and farthest points, as function of the convergence, both for the emmetropic eye E (the middle ordinary lines), and for the myopic M (the dotted lines), and for the hypermetropic, H (the striped and dotted lines) ; $\frac{1}{A}$ is, in order to facilitate comparison, assumed $= \frac{1}{4}$; and the maximum of convergence is taken at 59° 20'. The letters E, M, and H are placed before the farthest points, as defining the refraction; H_m (manifest hypermetropia) stands before r the *manifest* farthest point, H_t (total hypermetropia), before r_t the *absolute* farthest point. In other respects, the letters have the same signification as in Fig. 60. Now the study of this diagram shows:—

1. That with parallel visual lines, the emmetropic eye can bring into action about $\frac{1}{3}$, the myopic only $\frac{1}{4\cdot5}$, the hypermetropic, on the contrary, $\frac{3}{5}$ of its total power of accommodation.

2. That, with slight convergence, the myopic eye can accommodate much less, the hypermetropic on the contrary, much more. (but also must do so) than the emmetropic. Compare particularly the curve $r\ r_1$, which for the myopic eye at first runs nearly transversely, for the hypermetropic strongly ascends.

3°. That with stronger convergence, the accommodation of the myopic eye can still increase much, that of the hypermetropic only a little. We see, with a convergence of 18°, the curve $p_1\ p_2\ p$ of the hypermetropic eye keeping nearly a transverse direction, while the curves of the myopic now begin decidedly to ascend.

The diagram will readily answer any further question which may suggest itself; it appears therefore to be superfluous to expatiate at greater length upon the subject.

The difference ascertained is practically of great importance. Thence it follows, namely, directly, that when the ametropia is neutralised by glasses (r brought to ∞), the eye by no means becomes equal to an emmetropic eye of similar range of accommodation. This is easily deduced from the above figures. It appears still more distinctly on reference to Fig. 62, where the curves of Fig. 61 are repeated (as Ep and Er, as Mp and Mr, and as Hp and Hr_m and Hr_t) but so that in all, r is brought to ∞.* The diagram shows that the neutralised myopic eye has its binocular nearest point at 16″, so that $1 : A_2$ amounts only to the fourth of $1 : A$; and that *vice versá* for the hypermetropic eye the binocular nearest point p_2 is nearly equal to the absolute. Moreover, in the myopic, $1 : A_1$, even at from 8° to

---

* As shall appear in § 13, the reduction of the ametropia is not entirely without influence on the form of the curves. This influence is, however, so slight, that here it may be altogether disregarded.

9° of convergence, becomes wholly negative; in the hypermetropic, $1 : A_1$ is at more than 30° of convergence entirely positive. Hence

Fig. 62.

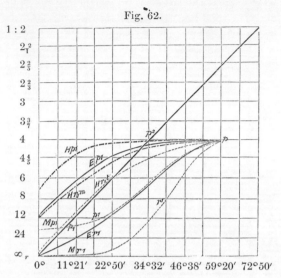

proceeds for both eyes difficulty in binocular vision, under moderate convergence; for the reduced myopic, because, under these circumstances it accommodates too weakly, for the reduced hypermetropic, because it accommodates too strongly.

The cause of this difference is at once apparent; it is the result of practice. The myopic eye has learnt to converge in a certain degree, without bringing its power of accommodation into action in the same proportion as the emmetropic eye. Thereby the binocular farthest point (Fig. 61, Mr_2), although seen at a tolerably considerable convergence, remains almost as far from the eye as the absolute farthest point Mr. But on the other hand, the eye has not practised itself with slight convergence, to bring a relatively great part of its accommodation into action, because it has had no necessity to do so. The hypermetropic eye, on the contrary, found itself obliged, in order to see accurately, even with parallel visual lines, to put its power of accommodation on the stretch, and it has brought itself so far in that respect, that it is no longer in a position to become completely relaxed, that at least on every effort to see, the act of accommodation takes place involuntarily. As further, with increasing convergence, a disproportionately great part of the range of accommodation must always come into action, it is not strange, that the relative range of accommodation has been considerably displaced.

That practice really may produce the difference just described, we have the following proofs.

1. The use of positive or negative glasses has, even after the lapse of a few hours, an influence on the range of accommodation of the emmetropic eye. Fig. 63 exhibits the effect of practice in look-

Fig. 63.

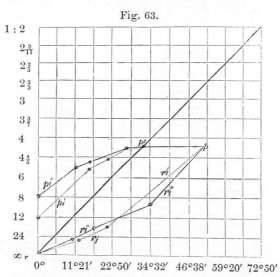

ing with negative glasses. It relates to a young emmetropic subject, aged 21 years, who with slight convergence can accommodate somewhat less than usual. The dotted curves represent the course of his nearest and of his farthest points. After having occasionally practised for some days with negative glasses, he obtained, by repeating the investigation, the linear curves, which, at least $p''_1\ p_2\ p$, approach much more closely to those of hypermetropic persons than the dotted ones. Had he continued the practice longer, permanent contraction would, just as in the hypermetropic, have occurred, and r would not have stood at ∞. For some minutes after the removal of the negative glasses, this was the case. On the other hand, the use of positive glasses rapidly makes the power of accommodation, with a certain amount of convergence, less: it is well known that, particularly when positive glasses are used too soon, reading much without their aid quickly becomes more difficult than before.

2. The relative range of accommodation is displaced in ametropic individuals when they have for a long time worn correcting glasses. That of myopics, as well as of hypermetropics, gradually tends to that of emmetropics.

3. In the diminution of the range of accommodation in advancing age, even before proper presbyopia has begun, the curves of the emmetropic eye approach to those of the hypermetropic. Fig. 64 is

Fig. 64.

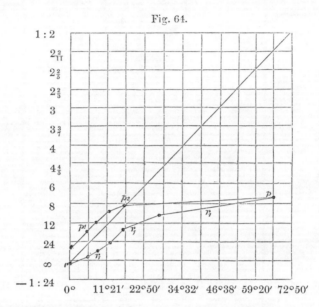

the faithful expression of the range of accommodation of an emmetropic individual aged 44. For vertical lines he has a trace of hypermetropia, so that r is found beneath. Further, to convince one's self that, with the required practice, the curve p_1 p_2 p especially has approached to that of a hypermetropic eye, we need only observe that with a convergence to 9″, nearly the maximum of accommodation is attained.

In the following Chapter, treating of Spectacles; and also in speaking of each of the forms of ametropia, I shall revert to the important distinction made in the foregoing section.

CHAPTER IV.

SPECTACLES AND THEIR ACTION IN GENERAL.

§ 12. *Different kinds of spectacles.*—In ophthalmic surgery different kinds of spectacles are in use, which are employed for very different purposes.

I. *Protecting spectacles.*—Of these we distinguish two varieties: *a,* those which serve only to keep off the mechanical influence of foreign bodies, dust, fragments of metal, stone, coal, etc. They have nothing to do with the refraction of light in the eye, and call for no further comment here.

b. Spectacles for warding off light.—These consist mostly of coloured glass, green and especially blue, which is less hurtful to the eye. In general, however, at least in daylight, the grey, so-called neutral glasses, deserve the preference. The white sunlight, reflected by different objects in their particular colours, is the natural adequate stimulus to the retina, and by good neutral glasses these rays are tolerably uniformly diminished. The same end opticians formerly attempted to attain (Fischer) by combining two glasses of complementary colours. It is desirable in every case that, so far as possible, the whole field of vision should be uniformly obscured, which is accomplished, with tolerable accuracy by the use of large, round glasses, resembling watch-glasses, but more perfectly by lateral flaps of silk or some other semitransparent substance, or else by glass of the same colour as the spectacles, the objection to the latter being, however, the increase of weight. The light falling in from the side has a doubly unpleasant action, when *coloured* glasses are applied in front of the eye, for the lateral parts are then seen by contrast in the complementary colour of the glasses, and in the remaining part of the field of vision the complementary colour appears still stronger as a secondary image, so soon as the spectacles are taken off. In persons affected with irritation of the retina, or with photophobia in general, we may recommend the use of light-absorbing glasses, when these patients are obliged to expose themselves for a certain time to a bright light. In the house, with moderate light, they ought to lay them aside.   We should not forget that these glasses when worn in the sun, become heated in proportion to the amount of rays they absorb, and that very dark glasses may, therefore, be considered to be specially injurious to the eye.   In women, moderating the light, when necessary, by means of veils, is to be recommended.

II. *Stenopæic spectacles, stenopæic lorgnette, stenopæic apparatus.* —Slight obscurations of the light-refracting media, especially those of the cornea, often produce great disturbance of the accuracy of vision.   The cause of this is to be sought not so much in the reflection or absorption of a portion of the rays, as in the diffusion of the light passing through them.   This is easily explained.   From the entire field of vision rays fall on each local obscuration, and from the latter they spread further in all directions through the whole eye. Consequently in the region of the yellow spot also, an image is not merely formed of the object lying about in the direction of the line of vision ; but over this image is spread, with the existence of semi-transparent spots, a uniform light, derived from the whole field of vision.   This diffused light is very disturbing.   Indeed the differences of illumination of the image formed by regular refraction are in consequence much more faintly distinguishable.   Just as in looking through a real mist, the diffused light is added to the relatively weaker image, and therefore also spots give the impression, as if one were looking through an actual mist : the only difference is, that a mist is more perceptible for more remote objects, and that misty vision, produced by a spot, affects all objects alike, independently of distance.   It is well known that obscurations produce much less disturbance, when the eye, turned from the light, contemplates a certain object.   If a picture or another object be hung against the pier between two windows, and if it be illuminated through a window behind the observer, the latter will see the object much more accurately, and with more contrast of light and shade when the two windows are closed than when they are open.   The explanation of this fact is to be found in the foregoing.   In both cases (supposing that the open windows throw no light upon the object) the object sends, in an equal degree, rays into the eye, which, regularly refracted, form a good image in the region of the yellow spot ; but if light falls upon the eyes through the windows placed at the sides of the object, numerous rays proceed, in that case, likewise from the illuminated spots over the image of the yellow spot, which thus becomes covered as with a white crape.   Even if there be no spots, some light is always diffused in the eye, and thus even the normal eye will, especially if the time of life be somewhat advanced, perceive, as it were, light crape, when, in the experiment just described, the windows are opened. We know further, that where obscurations exist, exclusion of the peripheric light with the hand, looking through a tube, etc., increases the accuracy of the images. Again, it is the warding off of the laterally incident light diffusing itself from the spot throughout the whole eye, which here acts beneficially. The practical rule hence deducible is this : *in order, where obscurations exist, to distinguish with relative accuracy, let the small portion of the field of vision, over which the observation is to extend, be properly illuminated, and let the remaining portion be kept as dark as possible.* These reflexions on the injurious effect of obscurations led me to the application of stenopæic remedies. Their object is to cut off the light which should reach the obscurations, and through an opening to give, so far as possible, entrance only to the light which is subjected to a regular refraction on the normal part of the refracting surface. The narrow opening is in them the essential part : hence the denomination stenopæic (from στενός, narrow, and ὀπή, a peephole). In order not to limit the field of vision more than is necessary, the opening must be as close as possible to the eye, and with a view still better to keep off all lateral light, it may be surrounded with a wall widening like a funnel. The opening may in general have the form and nearly the size of the clearest part of the portion of the refracting surface corresponding to the pupil : it may, according to circumstances, be round, oval, or slit-like. Rarely will the diameter be less than a millimètre ; often it will amount to two or more millimètres.

The stenopæic apparatus, which is an indispensable item in the ophthalmic surgeon's means of investigation, is a very short cylinder, furnished with a handle, open at one end and indented towards the eye, and provided at the other with an opening, in front of which is a diaphragm, containing different smaller openings of various diameters, and capable of turning round, so that each of these openings can be seen in turn. There are also stenopæic apparatus provided with a slit capable of being widened and narrowed.* With the aid of this apparatus we can examine whether the stenopæic principle increases the accuracy of vision, which is often of importance in a diagnostic

* They are, as well as the stenopæic spectacles and eyeglasses, prepared, among others, by Paetz and Flohr, opticians, unter den Linden, Berlin.

point of view; moreover, we may acquire an indication whether it may be advantageously applied, and what size of opening is the most useful. Of the result obtained we may then make use in prescribing a stenopæic spectacle, or eyeglass. To spectacles for use in the streets, the stenopæic principle is in general not applicable, as the field of vision is too limited. On the other hand, such spectacles to which the requisite glasses have been fitted, are sometimes very serviceable for reading. The chief application of the principle, however, is to the stenopæic eyeglass. Many persons suffering from opacity have recourse to it of their own accord, by warding off the peripherically incident light with the hand, by voluntarily narrowing the slit between the eyelids, etc., in order to increase the accuracy of vision, but this object is always much more perfectly attained by means of a stenopæic eyeglass.

If the part which has remained clear has an oblong form, a slit-like opening will be most suitable. In general, it is a great advantage in reading, when a horizontal slit effects the object; this should, therefore, always be tried. If the opacity is only on one side, we may obtain a great advantage by making an ordinary spectacle-glass opaque over the obscured part (for example, by applying a black lacker). In general the simplest stenopæic spectacles are those in which the preferable form of opening is left as the only part of the glass not obscured, in which also by opaque matter on the outside che light incident from that point can be warded off. The glass may in ordinary cases be flat, but otherwise according to the necessities of vision it should have a certain focus. In some cases, among others, after the extraction of cataract, I have found great advantage from partially covering the glass with black. It is not uncommon, when the flap-section was made downwards, for the inferior part of the cornea to become somewhat turbid, particularly if the iris has attached itself to the wound, or is even slightly prolapsed. The disturbance is the greater, because the pupil too is thereby drawn downwards, and probably the curvature of the cornea is somewhat irregular, so that reading with an ordinary convex glass is attended with great difficulty, or is even quite impossible. But it is in the most surprising manner relieved, when the glass is covered to a definite height with an opaque black matter over which the eye sees, while the rays which should reach the inferior non-transparent and irregular part of the cornea, are cut off. This mode of using the glass limits the field of vision only inferiorly, and is therefore attended with no impediment whatever to reading, nor even to vision in general.

Lastly, it may be mentioned (what has reference more especially to anomalies of refraction), that the stenopæic eyeglass has also rendered me very essential service in the highest degrees of myopia, particularly when the accuracy of vision had at the same time suffered comparatively much. If it were only for this reason, therefore, the stenopæic apparatus ought not here to be passed over in silence. In such cases vision of near objects, at least with one eye, is attended with no other inconvenience than that the object must be brought very near the eye, to 3″ or less. But distant vision is extremely imperfect, and is comparatively little improved by concave glasses, which correct the myopia. If, with their aid, the images are more accurately seen, they at the same time become so much smaller, that an amblyopic eye still distinguishes little, and is, therefore, by no means satisfied. In such cases then, a stenopæic eyeglass with a small opening yields very good service. It here acts in a well-known manner, quite different from that treated of above, by diminishing the circles of diffusion. It is manifest that, in imperfect accommodation, the magnitude of the circles of diffusion increases with the magnitude of the base of the cone of light (the surface of the pupil). Now in high degrees of myopia the pupil is usually very wide, and the disturbance in looking at distant objects is, therefore, relatively very great. Precisely for this reason it is that a stenopæic eyeglass produces so great improvement. If a myopic individual looks through an opening of from $\frac{1}{2}'''$ to 1″ in diameter, he distinguishes at a distance as accurately as through glasses, which imperfectly neutralise his myopia, and he has the advantage that the objects appear larger. If an emmetropic person wishes to convince himself of this, let him hold a positive glass before his eye, so that it becomes myopic, and he will, on looking through an opening, obtain the effect described, and can estimate the partial neutralisation of the artificial myopia. In like manner we may also within the nearest distance of distinct vision, by diminution of the circles of diffusion, with the aid of a small opening, distinguish with tolerable accuracy, and thus view small objects much nearer to the eye, that is under a much greater angle. However, in either case we lose both in light and in extent of the field of vision. As to light, we lose the more, the smaller the opening is, and in myopia it is therefore often advisable not to have the opening very small, but with the stenopæic

2

eyeglass to combine a glass, which partially corrects the myopia. With respect to the extent of the field of vision we lose the more, the farther the opening is from the eye. In combining a negative glass with the stenopæic eye-piece, the patient will therefore turn the small opening towards the eye, when his principal object is to increase the field of vision; on the contrary the negative lens, when he chiefly desires to obtain greater distinctness of vision.

III. *Prismatic glasses, prismatic spectacles.*—Prisms are used, in order by refraction of the light upon two surfaces, to obtain the well-known spectrum. The angle, which the two refracting surfaces make with one another, is the angle of refraction of the prism. For the object mentioned a large angle is taken: most prisms are triangular, and each of the three angles then amounts to 60°. They are usually made of flint glass, in order, with considerable declination, at the same time to obtain a decided dispersion. For ophthalmological purposes, on the contrary, only slight declination is required, and we therefore use prisms with a smaller angle of refraction, from 3° to 24°; moreover, it is necessary to select a kind of glass, which, with reference to its refracting power, presents but slight dispersion, for example, crown glass. Such prisms are given in the boxes for ophthalmological use, usually in sixteen numbers. The numbers from III. to XXIV. indicate the refracting angles, 3° to 24°. In the position of least declination, the angles of declination, for the low numbers, are nearly the half of these refracting angles: for the higher numbers, they are somewhat more. If we wish to know these accurately, it is necessary to determine the deviations for each glass separately.

The declination of the light by prismatic glasses is the cause why objects, seen through such glasses, exhibit themselves in another direction. Let *i* (Fig. 65) be a point of light, *i a* a ray falling at *a*

Fig. 65.

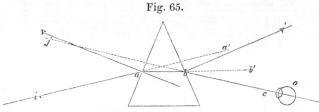

on one of the refracting surfaces of the prism, this approaches the perpendicular *v a*, instead of continuing in the same direction *a a'*, and runs as *a b* in the prism; arrived at *b* it again alters its direction, now in passing from glass into air, declining from the normal v' b, and as $b\,c$ reaches the eye O. Evidently, therefore, the point i is seen in the direction $b\,c$, about in j. In this, however, the more refrangible rays, those on the violet side, undergo a greater, the less refrangible, those on the red side, undergo a less declination. Hence proceeds a disturbance by coloured margins to the objects, which is greater in proportion to the strength of the prism, and which, precisely in powerful prisms, it is hard to remove. In order to obtain a declination without dispersion, the prism must be made achromatic by being compounded of two prisms, C (Fig. 66) of crown glass, F of flint glass, which, acting in opposition, com-

Fig. 66.

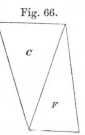

pletely remove each other's dispersion, but only partially destroy each other's refraction. Such achromatic prisms, however, soon become, when a declination of some degrees is required, too thick and too heavy to be worn. This objection might perhaps be partly met, by having the prisms very small (to have large prisms as eye-glasses is of no use), because in order to see rather distinctly, we must not look obliquely through the glass, but about at the angle of least declination. So far, however, the achromatic prisms have not yet come into use.

What led to trying prismatic glasses, was a declination of the visual lines. The idea of making it possible to look with both eyes, in spite of this declination, occurred first to my friend Krecke, Doctor of Natural Philosophy, of Utrecht, whose idea I endeavoured to realize and to explain physiologically.* On experimenting with the glasses, three remarkable phenomena immediately presented themselves. In the first place it appeared, that one feels involuntarily impelled, by changing the direction of the visual lines, to remove the double vision which has taken place. If we hold the glass with the refracting angle inwards, then, in order to bring the double images into one, stronger convergence is required, and this is immediately almost involuntarily effected. On removing the glass, double images again exhibit themselves, which, by diminishing the convergence, are once more forthwith thrown together; only, if the prism has been long held before the eye, a tendency to increased convergence continues for some time. In the second place it seemed, that the

* *Nederlandsch Lancet*, uitgegeven door F. C. Donders, G. L. H. Ellerman en J. H. Jansen, 2ᵉ Ser. D. III., pp. 227 and 233, 1847.

visual lines are usually capable of only very slight divergence, and that they can scarcely decline upwards and downwards, even under the pressure of the necessity of rendering the vision single. In general the prism, when the refracting angle is turned to the outside of the eye, ought to be very weak, in order to allow the observer still to see remote objects single; and the same weak prism, when the refracting angle is turned upwards or downwards, produces double images, which cannot be overcome. If, finally, the observer has, after long-continued efforts, succeeded in throwing into one the double images standing (in the last case) above one another, the double images which now arise on removing the prism, do not immediately run together again. Thirdly and lastly, we can convince ourselves of what has been stated above (p. 110), that under the influence of a prism with the angle turned towards the inside or outside, the observer can converge more or less strongly, without being able to alter the tension of his accommodation.

These results, obtained with the aid of prismatic glasses, are of essential importance for the physiology, and for many points in the pathology of the eye. But beyond this, these glasses serve different useful purposes in ophthalmic surgery, which, partly previously foreseen, have been, especially by von Graefe, practically tested. Thus they may be applied in the diagnosis of different anomalies of the muscles, and of the degree of these anomalies. Thus they may be used to correct slight incurable declinations of the visual lines, outwards, upwards, or downwards, whereby confusing double images are produced, or to remove the muscular asthenopia, depending on insufficient power of the musculi recti interni. Thus we may further, in paresis of a muscle, so far meet the disease by means of a prism, that in order to make the double images which have been brought near one another, run together, the muscles will become powerfully tense, which, for the alleviation of the paresis, appears to be no matter of indifference. Finally, what deserves to be here particularly mentioned, these glasses are also of importance in anomalies of refraction. They show, that hypermetropic individuals distinguish accurately with greater ease, when they, looking through a prism with the angle turned inwards, for the sake of single vision, can converge more strongly, a fact by which the origin of strabismus, in consequence of hypermetropia, is explained; and it will hereafter appear that we sometimes advantageously apply the principle of the prismatic glasses, by modifying the mutual distance of either the convex or concave glasses of spectacles, so that the eyes look through these glasses *at the side* of the axes, which, just like the use of a prismatic glass, modifies the direction in which an object is seen.

Glasses with spherical surfaces, ordinary convex and concave spectacle-glasses.—Glasses, which modify the limits of distinct vision, are called lenses. Of these we have two kinds, both of which are used as spectacle-glasses: converging lenses (Fig. 67 *l*), which cause

Fig. 67 *l.*

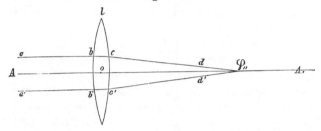

parallel rays *a b* and *a' b'* to converge as *c d* and *c' d'*; and diverging lenses (Fig. 68 *l*), which cause *a b* and *a' b'* to diverge as *c d* and

Fig. 68 *l.*

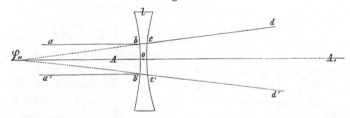

c' d'. A converging lens has its focal point ϕ'' on the other, a diverging lens on the same side as that whence the rays come. The first unites the rays into a real focus; the latter does not actually unite them, but causes them to assume a direction as if they had proceeded from the point ϕ'', in which the prolongations of *c d* and *c' d* (the dotted lines) cut one another: hence this point is called also a *virtual* focus.

Besides the above *biconvex* lenses, we have, as converging lenses, the *plano-convex* and the *concavo-convex* or *positive meniscus (with shorter radius of the convex surface)*, as well as, in addition to the *biconcave*, as diverging lenses, the *plano-concave* and the *convex-con-*

cave or *negative meniscus* (with shorter radius of the concave surface). The plano-convex and plano-concave have, for equal degrees of power, the greatest aberration, and they are consequently to be rejected as spectacle-glasses. The biconvex and biconcave answer better. To the menisci the advantage is attributed, beyond these, that, as Wollaston showed, the images suffer less, when the observer looks obliquely (under an angle with the axis) through them, so that the eyes can move more freely behind these glasses. They are therefore, also called *periscopic* (from περισκοπειν, to look around). However, we can also see satisfactorily in an oblique direction through biconcave and biconvex glasses, provided they are not too strong, and if high numbers are required, the periscopic glasses have again the disadvantage of greater weight. Were it only for this reason, therefore, the latter do not unconditionally deserve the preference. When we add that under some circumstances the periscopic glasses are more liable to produce disturbance by reflexion on the concave surface turned towards the eye, and that they are, moreover, somewhat more expensive, we shall not be surprised that they have not wholly supplanted the biconvex and biconcave glasses.

Biconvex and biconcave spectacle-glasses are ground with equal radii of the two surfaces. The optical centre *o* (Figs. 67 and 68) lies then in the middle of the lens in the axis A A$_1$. Now the distance from the focus ϕ'' to this optical centre *o* is usually called the focal distance F. This is, however, not quite correct; F is, in fact, the distance from focus to *principal point*. For ordinary, not very thick lenses, with equal radii of the two surfaces, that is, for the ordinary biconvex and biconcave spectacle-glasses, this inaccuracy is of no importance; but in the case of menisci, we must ascertain the principal points, in order to know the position of the foci, and to be able to take into account the distance from focus to principal point as F.

The subjoined figures (69, a biconvex, 70, a biconcave lens; 71, a

Fig. 69.

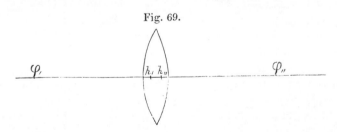

positive, 72, a negative meniscus), show, for these different forms of lenses, the position of the first and second principal points h_1 and h_2, and of the first and second focus ϕ_1 and ϕ_2. The rays which, parallel

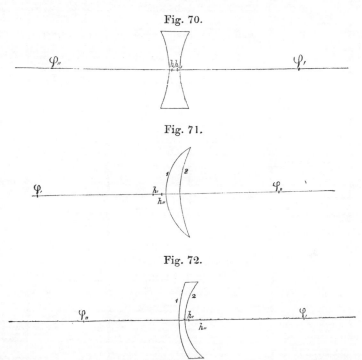

Fig. 70.

Fig. 71.

Fig. 72.

to the axis, fall on the surface 1, have their focus in ϕ_2; those which, coming from the other side, fall parallel to the axis on the surface 2, unite in ϕ_1. For a lens standing in air $h_1 \phi_1$ is always $= h_2 \phi_2$, both $= F$. If now, as in Figs. 69 and 70, the two surfaces of curvature be equal, the points $h_1 \phi_1$ and $h_2 \phi_2$ will evidently lie symmetrically in the axis. But if the surfaces of curvature be not equal, if even one of them be concave, the other convex, as in Figs. 71 and 72, the points $h_1 h_2$ may have another position, and may even be external to the mass of the glass, and the foci ϕ_1 and ϕ_2 will then also lie at different distances from the lens. It will be understood that, even for these reasons, it is by no means indifferent which surface of these lenses is turned towards the eye. In speaking of the influence of the distance of the glass from the eye, I shall return to this point. The reader who may wish to examine more closely into the signification of the principal points, will find the explanation thereof at pp. 44 and 50.

The power (the converging or diverging power) of a lens is inversely proportional to its focal distance F. It may, therefore, be expressed by $\frac{1}{F}$ for converging, and by $-\frac{1}{F}$ for diverging lenses. The value of F we state, just as in the numerical expression of the range of accommodation, in Parisian inches: glasses of $\frac{1}{6}$, of $-\frac{1}{8}$, etc., are therefore glasses of 6″ positive, of 8″ negative focal distance, etc.

Besides the spectacle-glasses above described, there are others with a difference of focal distance in the superior and inferior parts. Franklin was slightly myopic and had little power of accommodation; for seeing at a distance he had need of negative, for seeing near objects he had need of positive glasses. Now, as in looking at near objects we look through the lower, in looking at a distance we look through the upper half of the spectacle glasses, he combined two halves, the one of a negative, the other of a positive glass, turned the negative halves upwards, the positive downwards, and in this manner provided very well for his want of accommodation. These spectacles have, after the philosopher who first used them, acquired the name of Franklin's glasses. Recently it has been attempted to attain the same object which Franklin proposed to himself, by grinding in the upper part of the spectacle-glass, the surface turned from the eye, with another radius. The glasses are prepared in Paris under the name of *verres à double foyer*. Fig. 73 *a* represents a

Fig. 73.

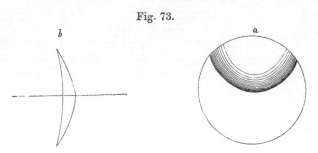

superficial view of such a glass (slightly positive above and strongly positive below); *b* exhibits a section of the same. I stated only, what focal distance I desired for the upper and lower part, and found that my directions were always accurately carried out, both when I requested only a different positive or negative focus in the two halves; and when I required a negative focus above, and a positive focus below. In general these spectacles answered well. It is indispensable that they be placed at the proper height before the eyes, so that in looking at a distance the rays may fall upon the organ only through the upper, and in looking at near objects, only through the lower part. It is also necessary that the difference in the direction of vision be determined more by moving the eyes, than by moving the head. If the pupil be opposite the boundary between the two parts, vision will, of course, be very confused.

It is by no means a matter of indifference of what material the spectacle-glasses are made. Flint glass and especially rock-crystal are harder, and glasses made of them are not so easily scratched. This is particularly a recommendation in the case of convex glasses which are so much more liable to be scratched. Against the advantage just mentioned as being possessed by flint glass and crystal, must be set down the disadvantage of greater power of dispersion. Hence it would appear that for *strong glasses* the preference ought to be given to *crown glass*. This is especially true of concave glasses, and as to convex glasses of crown glass, their low price makes it easy, if they are scratched, to replace them with others.

Achromatic glasses are not available for spectacles; if glasses of short focal distance be required, achromatism is attended with too great weight, and if glasses of long focal distance be sufficient, even with the use of crystals, glasses do not prevent the dispersion of colour.

As the ophthalmoscope is important for the objective diagnosis of defects of the eye, so is a collection of spectacle-glasses for their subjective investigation. Such glasses are at once indispensable, not only for the determination of anomalies of refraction and accommodation, but also in many cases for that of the accuracy of vision, so that without them the examination of the functions of the eye is impossible.

The usual boxes contain :—

1. Twenty-eight pairs of biconvex glasses, namely of 2, $2\frac{1}{4}$, $2\frac{1}{2}$, 3, $3\frac{1}{2}$, 4, $4\frac{1}{2}$, 5, $5\frac{1}{2}$, 6, 7, 8, 9, 10, 12, 14, 16, 18, 20, 22, 24, 28, 36, 40, 48, 60, 72, and 100 inches positive focal distance.

2. Twenty-eight pairs of biconcave glasses of the same focal distances, but negative.

3. Twelve (or sixteen) prismatic glasses with refracting angles of 3°, 4°. 5°, 6°, 7°, 8°, 9°, 10°, 12°, 14°, 16°, 18° (or to 24°).

4. A frame with elastic rings, in which these glasses can be used.

5. Some quadrangular pieces, 6 inches long, $1\frac{1}{2}$ inches broad, of different shades of blue glass, capable of being held before both eyes at once.

6. A glass of carmine-red, well adapted, in case of a false position of the visual lines, to colour one of the double images.

On the convex and concave glasses the focal distances are inscribed with a diamond.   The same is the case with many spectacles met with in trade.

Fig. 74.

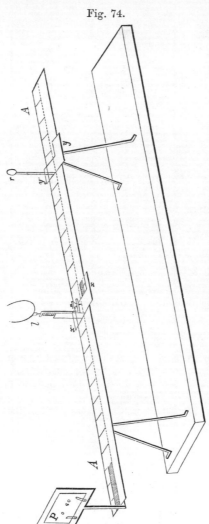

With respect to these last, however, we must not depend upon the mark, but must always determine the focal distance by comparison with the standard glasses. The method is extremely simple. We examine with our own eye, with what glass they agree in diminishing or magnifying power. As object we employ two slight parallel lines. We hold the glass tolerably far from the eye (about a foot), and so far from the paper, that we see the two lines accurately through the glass. We now hold the standard glasses for comparison in the same plane with the glass to be examined, and we shall then be able to determine, with sufficient precision, to which of these it corresponds.

The direct determination of the focal distance of a glass is more difficult. The simple measurement of the distance, at which, behind a convex glass, the solar image is exhibited upon a screen, gives the value only approximatively. The same is of course true of the determination of the conjugate focal distances of a flame and its image, whence the principal focal distance can then be calculated. Different other methods are stated which lead to a more correct result. I obtained very accurate determinations by measuring the magnitudes of an object and of its dioptric image, both with the aid of the ophthalmometer (compare p. 17).

As object I employed three small openings in a very thin blackened metallic plate (Fig. 74 P), behind which was placed, in front of an opening in a large screen, the globe of a brightly burning lamp. This plate is fixed to the extremity of a flat copper ruler (A A') resting on a pedestal, and furnished with an accurate scale, and on which a small plate (x x'), provided with a lens-bearer (l), is movable. This little plate has at x' a nonius, with which the twentieth part of a line can be read off. On the same ruler (A A') a second plate (y y') is movable, carrying a small ring (r). The centres of the two rings, and the centre of the image (the three openings in the plate P) lie in one horizontal line, which must be so placed as to coincide with the axis of the ophthalmometer. By adjusting the ophthalmometer consecutively for the three different distances, we can ascertain whether this condition is fulfilled. The axis of the ophthalmometer being fixed they must appear, on moving the eyepiece, successively and accurately in the centre of the field of the ophthalmometer.

We now first measure the magnitude of the object. As the reader is aware (compare p. 18), measuring with the ophthalmometer is accomplished by doubling the image and reading off the degrees on the ophthalmometer, when the double images are removed from one another by the breadth of the object to be measured. Now no object is capable of more accurate measurement than three small points of light (Fig. 74 $P \ldots$). Thus we can very perfectly determine (method of Bessel, in use in astronomy), when, on doubling (Fig. 75), $1'$ of the one image ($1'$, $2'$, $3'$) comes to stand exactly in the centre between 2 and 3 of the other image (1, 2, 3), and the distance x y is then measured as object. For the same reasons we use three points of light, namely, the three reflex images of three distant flames, when

Fig. 75.

we wish to determine from the magnitude of the reflected image, the radius of curvature of the cornea, or of any other reflecting surface.

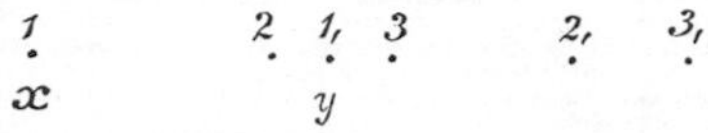

Now knowing the magnitude of the object, which we have been able to measure accurately by the method just described, we next seek the magnitude of the dioptric image formed of it by the lens, whose focal distance we wish to ascertain. For this purpose we place the latter in the lens-bearer l (Fig. 74), bring this to a distance from the object (the plate P) equal to the double of the nearly known focal distance of the lens, and make the distance r l equal to l P. The ophthalmometer we have permanently fixed, after having measured the object (the three small openings) in the centre of the field. We now move the eyepiece so as to see the ring r accurately, and we shall then at the same time perceive the dioptric image of the three openings. But the axis of the lens will then coincide, as it ought, with that of the ophthalmometer, only when the dioptric image falls *exactly in the centre of the ring* r. Hence we must take care to effect this, and precisely on the accuracy with which this can be accomplished, depends the validity of the method here pursued. While we see the dioptric image, we at the same time observe, whether it coincides in magnitude with the object. In this case the points of light will occupy the same place in reference to one another (Fig. 75), as that at which the object was measured, that is, $1'$ will stand in the middle between 2 and 3. If it appears that the dioptric image is larger, we remove the plate x x' from P; if on the contrary it is smaller, we approximate x x' to P, until the position of the images is precisely the same as it was in measuring the object. When this has been attained, we have only with the nonius x' to read off the exact distance of the lens from the thin plate P, in order to know the double focal distance of the lens. Indeed, when object and dioptric image have the same magnitude, both are at an equal, and in fact at the double focal distance from the respective principal points of the lens, and if the latter be a biconvex lens, with equal radius of its two surfaces, likewise at an equal distance from its optical centre.

In the manner proposed we can conveniently make only one measurement of the dioptric image. More accurate results are obtained when, irrespectively of equality of magnitude of object and dioptric image, the first being known, and the lens being arbitrarily placed, we simply measure the latter, and of different determinations take the mean. The magnitudes of the object B and the dioptric image β are to one another as the conjugate focal distances f' and f'', whereof f', being the distance between the lens and the object, is known by reading off.

Hence we find

$$f'' = \frac{B}{\beta} f'$$

and, further,

$$F = \frac{f' \quad f''}{f' + f''}.$$

If we repeat the calculations with some different values of f', the average will be extremely accurate.

The focal distance of concave glasses can be ascertained with tolerable accuracy, by selecting the convex glass, which when combined with the concave, removes all effect of the latter. But in doing this, it is not a matter of indifference which of the two glasses is turned towards the eye. By the above-described method I have, in connexion with Dr. Doijer, determined the focal distances of the spectacle-glasses (those with shorter focal distances directly, those with longer by combination) in my box, furnished by Paetz and Flohr at Berlin, and I found that the focal distances are all shorter than is stated. This is in great part to be attributed to the fact, that the distances are expressed in Prussian inches, which are somewhat less than the French. If we calculate a reduction in the ratio of 15 : 16, the deviation will be slight enough to prevent any practical inconvenience. My proposal to make Parisian inches the basis of the formulæ of the numerical values of the range of accommodation, of anomalies of refraction and of the glasses, is generally enough followed, to make it highly desirable that boxes should be obtainable, the focal distances of whose glasses should be accurately expressed in Parisian inches. I feel confident that Nachet et fils, opticians in Paris, will bring them into the market.

The nature of the material of which the glasses are prepared can be best ascertained by determining the cöefficient of the refraction of light. In order to calculate this, according to the simple formulas (compare p. 40), we must know the focal distance and the radius of the two surfaces of curvature. The mode of determining the focal distance, with the aid of the ophthalmometer, has been accurately explained. The same instrument may serve for deducing the radius of curvature from the magnitudes of the catoptric images. The method is the same as that used for the determination of the radius of the cornea (compare p. 18). If in this mode we determine the cöefficient of refraction, we shall find, that many lenses are considered to be pebbles, which consist of flint glass, or even of simple crown glass.

§ 12. *Direct influence on vision, of glasses with spherical surfaces.*

When such glasses are held before the eye, they are to be considered as an integral constituent of the dioptric system of the organ. We shall now, *in the first place*, consider the glass to be centred with this system, that is, that the centres of curvature of its surfaces lie in one axis with the centres of the surfaces of curvature of the eye. If this be not the case, certain deviations will result, which we shall consider at the end of this section.

Now the immediate consequences of placing a glass, with positive or negative focus, before the eye, are these :—

1°. The greatest and least distances of distinct vision, P and R, undergo a modification.

2°. The range of accommodation is altered.

3°. The region of accommodation changes in position and extent.

4°. The magnitude of the retinal images does not continue the same.

5°. The determination of the distance, magnitude and form of the objects, undergoes a change.

6°. Stereoscopic vision with two eyes suffers some modification.

I shall investigate and explain these results consecutively.

The direct influence of glasses with negative or positive focus is :—

1°. *The greatest and least distances of distinct vision, P and R, undergo a modification.* To prove this we need only follow the action of the glass on the course of the rays of light.

For the eye O (Fig. 76) without a glass, let p be the nearest

Fig. 76.

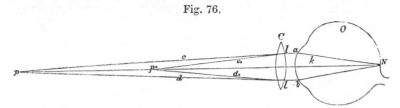

point of distinct vision, then the rays $p^c\ l\ a$ and $p^d\ l\ b$ unite in the retina N. Now if the lens L be placed before the eye, the rays $p_o \, c_o$ and $p_o \, d_o$ refracted by the lens, will acquire the same direction as $P \, c$ and $p \, d$; that is, they will proceed as $l \, a$ and $l \, b$ and fall into the eye, and will, therefore, in the same manner unite in the retina : $p \, k =$ P, has therefore given way to $p° \, k =$ P°. The calculation is very simple. Let F be the focal distance of the lens; x the distance of the lens from k, then $P - x$ is the distance of the lens L from P, and

$$\frac{1}{P - x} + \frac{1}{F} = \frac{1}{P° - x}$$

Thus we find P° — k, in which we have only to number k, in order to find P_o.

In like manner R° should be found from the formula

$$\frac{1}{R - x} + \frac{1}{F} = \frac{1}{R° - x}.$$

If L were a negative lens (compare Fig. 77), the rays $p_o \, c_o \, l$ and

Fig. 77.

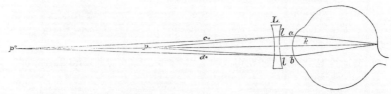

$p_o \, d_o \, l$, refracted by the lens, should have acquired the directions $l \, a$ and $l \, b$, as if they had proceeded from P, and an accommodation for the distance $p \, k =$ P should, through the lens have given way to an accommodation for $p° \, k =$ P°. In this case P° is found by the formula $\dfrac{1}{P - x} - \dfrac{1}{F} = \dfrac{1}{P_o - x}$. In like manner we find the modi-fication for the distance R, and for that of every other point, for which the eye is accommodated.

If we neglect the distance x, the formulæ become simplified respectively to

$$\frac{1}{P} + \frac{1}{F} = \frac{1}{P°}, \text{ and } \frac{1}{P} - \frac{1}{F} = \frac{1}{P°}.$$

But it is only in the use of weak glasses that this is in practice un-attended with inconvenience. If in a presbyopic individual P = 24″, then with a glass of $\dfrac{1}{12}$, $\dfrac{1}{P°}$ becomes about $= \dfrac{1}{24} + \dfrac{1}{12} = \dfrac{1}{8}$, and P° therefore = 8″.

If in a myopic, $R = 10''$, then we find with a glass of $-\frac{1}{12}$, neg-lecting x, $\frac{1}{R^\circ} = \frac{1}{10} - \frac{1}{12} = \frac{1}{60}$, $R^\circ = 60''$; while the exact calcu-lation, assuming $x = \frac{1}{2}$, gives, in the first case

$$\frac{1}{P^\circ - x} = \frac{1}{23\frac{1}{2}} + \frac{1}{12} = \frac{1}{7\cdot944}$$
$$P^\circ = 8\cdot444\,;$$

in the second case

$$\frac{1}{R^\circ - x} = \frac{1}{9\frac{1}{2}} - \frac{1}{12} = \frac{1}{45\cdot6}\,,$$
$$R^\circ = 46\cdot1.$$

In these cases the values of R° according to the two calculations differ too much to allow of our neglecting x.

2°. *The range of accommodation is altered.*—By the use of negative glasses it becomes greater, by the use of positive, on the contrary, it becomes less. Much more still does it diminish, with reference to the actual distance of the objects observed, in using microscopes and telescopes.

With respect to the absolute range of accommodation $\frac{1}{A} = \frac{1}{P} - \frac{1}{R}$, it changes into $\frac{1}{A^\circ} = \frac{1}{P^\circ} - \frac{1}{R^\circ}$. If $\frac{1}{P} - \frac{1}{P_0}$ were $= \frac{1}{R} - \frac{1}{R^\circ}$, then $\frac{1}{A^\circ}$ should be $= \frac{1}{A}$. This is, however, the case only when we can leave x out of the cal-culation. In this case the scheme of the accommodation (Fig. 78 a) with

Fig. 78.

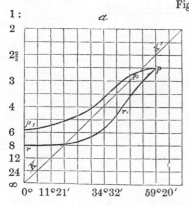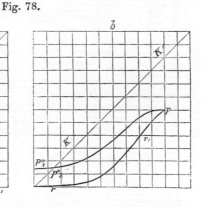

$M = \frac{1}{8}$ should by glasses of $-\frac{1}{8}$ (or rather of $-\frac{1}{7\cdot5}$ at $\frac{1''}{2}$ distance from k),

10

simply be so altered, that the lines $p^1\, p^2\, p$ and $r\, r'$ should fall only $\frac{1}{8}$, maintaining the same form, and should then be changed into Fig. 78 b.

We should thus obtain :—

$$\frac{1}{A} = \frac{1}{P} - \frac{1}{R} = \frac{1}{A^0} = \frac{1}{P^0} - \frac{1}{R^0}.$$

This is, however, applicable only in slight degrees of ametropia, and with the use of weak glasses. This may be seen from the following consideration.

We wish completely to correct the myopia of $\frac{1}{8}$, represented in Fig. 78 a, therefore, to make the dioptric system emmetropic, by the addition of a lens. Now, if x be $= \frac{1}{2}$, this lens must be $-7\frac{1}{2}$. Then, in fact, parallel rays, refracted by the lens, acquire a direction, as if they had proceeded from a point situated at $7\frac{1}{2}$ inches in front of the L, and therefore $8''$ before k (compare Fig. 76), and R_0 becomes $= \infty$.

Now what is P^0, assuming that $\frac{1}{A} = \frac{1}{4}$, and that P therefore amounts to $2\frac{2}{3}''$, as in Fig. 78 a ?

The calculation shows :—

$$\frac{1}{P\, -x} = \frac{1}{P^0\, -x} - \frac{1}{7\frac{1}{2}} = \frac{1}{2\frac{1}{6}} - \frac{1}{7\frac{1}{2}} = \frac{1}{3\cdot 05};$$
$$P^0\, - x = 3\cdot 05 \text{ and } P^0 = 3\cdot 55.$$

Consequently $\dfrac{1}{A^0} = \dfrac{1}{3\cdot 55} - \dfrac{1}{\infty} = \dfrac{1}{3\cdot 55}$,

While $\dfrac{1}{A}$ was $= \dfrac{1}{4}$,

and the absolute range of accommodation has therefore become greater. In place of by simple reduction obtaining Fig. 79 a (the same as Fig. 78 b) we obtain Fig. 79 b.

Fig. 79.

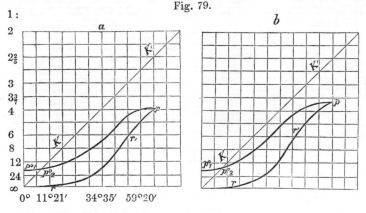

1 :
2
2⅔
3
3³⁄₇
4
6
8
12
24
∞

0°   11°21′   34°35′   59°20′

What is the effect of the glass on the binocular range of accommodation ? The binocular farthest point is by the glass brought to infinity, therefore, $R_2^0 = \infty$. In order to ascertain P_2^0, we must know where the line $p_1^0\, p_2^0\, p^0$ shall cut the line of convergence $k\, k'$. This should be discoverable only by an experimental calculation. But in determining the relative range of accommodation the farthest and the nearest binocular points were also ascertained with $-\frac{1}{7\frac{1}{2}}$, and thence it appeared that this point (p_2^0 of Fig. 79 b) lies at 14″. The binocular range of accommodation of the reduced myopic eye therefore amounts only to :—

$$\frac{1}{A_2^0} = \frac{1}{14} - \frac{1}{\infty} = \frac{1}{14},$$

and is therefore much less than $\frac{1}{A_2^0} = \frac{1}{2 \cdot 75} - \frac{1}{7 \cdot 5} = \frac{1}{4 \cdot 361}$, being the binocular range of accommodation of the myopic eye, without a negative glass (Fig. 78 a). However, $\frac{1}{A_2^0}$ is still *greater* than in the simple reduction, expressed by Fig. 79 a $\left(\text{whereby } \frac{1}{A_2^0} = \frac{1}{16}\right)$; and this favourable circumstance makes it at least somewhat easier to many myopic individuals, to see near objects with a reducing glass (whereby $R = \infty$), than would have been inferred from the impossibility of, with slight convergence, bringing into action a proportionate accommodation. Besides, the range of binocular accommodation in reduced myopia usually proves considerably more favourable than in the case represented by Figures 78 and 79.

The above is applicable in the use of glasses with a negative focus ; those with a positive focus have precisely the opposite influence. The subject is, in its further application, important enough to justify its illustration by an example.

Let us suppose, that in a case of hypermetropia $H = \frac{1}{8}$, p at 12″, therefore, $\frac{1}{A} = \frac{1}{8} + \frac{1}{12} = \frac{1}{4\frac{4}{5}}$.

Through a glass of $\frac{1}{8\frac{1}{2}}$, placed at half-an-inch from the eye, R^0 becomes $= \infty$ and P^0 is found as

$$\frac{1}{P^0} - x = \frac{1}{11\frac{1}{2}} + \frac{1}{8\frac{1}{2}} = \frac{1}{4 \cdot 88}.$$

Consequently $P_0 = 5 \cdot 38$, so that, with $\frac{1}{A} = \frac{1}{4 \cdot 8}$,

$$\frac{1}{A_0} \text{ has become } = \frac{1}{5 \cdot 38},$$

and the total range of accommodation is therefore decreased. In hypermetropia, however, the great advantage is always obtained by reducing glasses, that the useless part of $\frac{1}{A}$, namely, that of the accommodation for converging rays, is removed. Moreover, the increase of the range of accommodation, by the reduction acts favourably on $\frac{1}{A_2^0}$, in so far that thereby the too strong accommodation, peculiar to slight convergence, is partially corrected.

The same influence which has here been spoken of is likewise exercised

2

by positive glasses, when they are used by emmetropic individuals against presbyopia, or as magnifying glasses (even by myopic persons). If the emmetropic eye, with $\frac{1}{A} = \frac{1}{4}$, uses a magnifier of $\frac{1}{3}$, at $0 \cdot 5''$ from the nodal point,

$$R_0 \text{ becomes } = 3\tfrac{1}{2}$$
$$P^0 \text{ becomes } = 2\tfrac{3}{26}$$
$$\text{and} \frac{1}{A^0} = \frac{1}{5 \cdot 84}.$$

If the magnifying glass has only $1''$ focal distance, $\frac{1}{A^0}$ becomes $= \frac{1}{12}$, that is three times less than $\frac{1}{A}$. Hence we see how much the range of accommodation is reduced by the use of a magnifier. The reduction is greater, the farther the glass is held from the eye. With a magnifier $= \frac{1}{3}$ and $x = 1''$, $\frac{1}{A^0}$ becomes $= \frac{1}{6 \cdot 66}$; with the same magnifier, x being $= 3''$, we find $\frac{1}{A^0} = \frac{1}{10}$. With the strong lenses of simple microscopes $\frac{1}{A^0}$ becomes still less, on account of the stronger system, but continues greater, because the eye is usually held closer to the lens.

In the use of the compound microscope we see an aërial image (formed by the object-glass) through a lens (the eye-glass). This aërial image possesses, as a simple calculation shows, an extraordinary depth in relation to the slight depth of the object. Since it, moreover, lies very close to the eye, and is seen through a lens, the accommodation of the eye in relation to the difference in depth, that we can see of the observed object, is reduced nearly to *zero*. The great depth of the aërial image possesses, however, this advantage for microscopic observation, that of the object a definite surface is accurately seen, and what lies only a little above or beneath appears very diffused, and therefore has no disturbing influence.

In the use of telescopes also, the accommodation of the eye is almost entirely removed. For with a telescope which enables us to see an infinitely remote object, with relaxation of accommodation, we can, with the greatest tension, see only at a very great distance; and this difference requires of the eye without any glass scarcely any change of accommodation. But even the accommodation, of which the telescope itself is capable, by altering the distance between the eye-glass and the object-glass, represents, in the difference in distance of the objects which are distinguished, only an extremely slight range of accommodation. A simple calculation will easily show, that an eye behind a telescope finds its accommodation almost entirely annihilated. A positive lens, like the object-lens, forms images behind it, at a distance varying from F to ∞. At the distance F lie those of infinitely remote objects, at an infinite distance lie those of objects situated at the distance F before the object-lens. If a more or less myopic eye be now placed so far behind the object-lens, that accommodating for R, it sees accurately the dioptric image of infinitely remote objects, the objects, whose dioptric images are seen with accommodation for P, will also lie at a tolerably great distance. Consequently the range of accommodation is very much limited, even by the object-lens alone. Now, this limitation increases considerably, when the eye looks in addition through an eye-piece, and is thus much nearer to the focus of the object-lens. If the eye-piece consists of positive lenses, as in the proper telescope, this is so close behind the focus, that the images formed by the object-glass of even rather remote objects fall without the instrument, and thus vision will extend only from infinite to very remote distances. If the eye-piece be a negative lens, as in the Dutch telescopes, this is immediately in front of the focus of the object-lens, so that the strongly convergent incident rays through this eye-piece acquire a (slightly diverging) direction, whereby they come to a focus on the retina. But of less remote objects the image lies so much farther from the object-glass, that the rays reach the eye-piece comparatively less converging, and by this negative lens are, therefore, rendered so highly divergent, that the strongest accommodation is no longer capable of bringing them to a focus upon the retina.

The reduced range of accommodation $\dfrac{1}{a}$, in looking through microscopes and telescopes may be calculated, when are given :

$\dfrac{1}{A}$ the range of accommodation.

F_1 the focal distance of the object-glass.
F_r the focal distance of the eye-piece.
x the distance from the object-glass to the eye-piece.
y the distance from the eye-piece to k in the eye.

It may suffice to explain this further for the Dutch telescopes.

If the eye (Fig. 80, O) be adjusted for infinite distance, the rays $a\,b$ and $a'\,b'$ falling parallel on the object-glass $l\,l$, are, after refraction, directed as $c\,d$ and $c'\,d'$ upon ϕ; rendered parallel by the eye-piece $l'\,l'$, they now further impinge as $e\,f$ and $e'\,f'$ upon the cornea, and unite after refraction on the retina N. The relaxed emmetropic eye in this manner sees, with the telescope, infinitely remote objects. If the eye now ac-

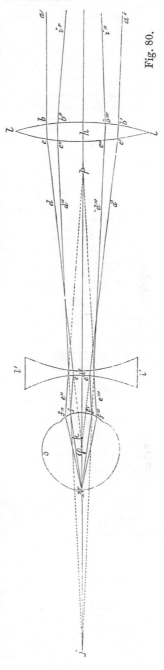

Fig. 80.

commodate itself for the point p, the rays $e'' f''$ and $e''' f'''$, directed to p, come to a focus on the retina. In order to acquire this direction, they must, as i, $b_{,}$ and $i_{,} b_{,,}$, have proceeded from such a point (i, not visible in the figure) in front of the object-glass $l\,l$, that after refraction through the object-glass they are directed as $c_{,} d_{,}$ and $c_{,,} d_{,,}$, upon j. In the supposed point i the prolongations of $b_{,,} i_{,}$ and $b_{,,,} i_{,,}$ intersect, and the point i is therefore the reduced nearest point of distinct vision. Consequently the distance from the point i to the nodal point k of the eye (O) is the reduced shortest distance of distinct vision, which, since the farthest is infinite, is in this case $= a$, and thus shows the reduced range of accommodation $\frac{1}{a}$.

In the telescope adjusted for infinite distance and emmetropic eyes:
$$h \ \phi = F_{,}$$
$$h_{,} \phi = F_{,,}$$
$$F - F_{,,} = ij.$$

Moreover,
$$p \ k = A$$
$$h_{,} k = x, \quad p \ h_{,} = A - x.$$

We now seek, in the first place, $h_{,} j = J$, according to the formula of the conjugate focal distances,
$$\frac{1}{J} = \frac{1}{F} - \frac{1}{A - x}.$$

We now know $h\,j = J + ij$, and calculate $h\,i$ again according to the same formula
$$\frac{1}{h\,i} = \frac{1}{F} - \frac{1}{h\,j}.$$

Therewith are known
$$h\,i + ij + x = i\,k = a,$$

and therefore also the reduced range of accommodation $\frac{1}{a}$.

$3°$. *The region of accommodation alters in position and extent.*

By *range* of accommodation (accommodatie-*breedte*) we understand a dioptric value, as being proportional to the focal distance of the lens, which expresses the difference of accommodation for P and for R. The *region* of accommodation (het accommodatie-*gebied*), on the contrary, is only the expression of the distance between r and p, and is therefore $= R - P$. The accommodation rules this distance in every direction, and we might therefore call it also the radius of the region of accommodation. Evidently a completely different region of accommodation may correspond to the same range of accommodation, and *vice versâ*. If R $= \infty$, P $= 6$, the range of accommodation is $\frac{1}{6}$; the region of accommodation on the contrary extends from infinity to six inches before the eye. If R $= 6$, P $= 3$, the range of accommodation is likewise $\frac{1}{3} - \frac{1}{6} = \frac{1}{6}$, and the radius of the region of accommodation is reduced to $6'' - 3'' = 3''$. There is consequently no proportion whatever between range and region of accommodation.

The above is sufficient to remind us what region of accommodation, in relation to range of accommodation, signifies. We now see at once, that, while the absolute range of accommodation undergoes only a slight modification by spectacles, the region of accommodation is quite altered by them. A myopic individual, for example, with $R = 6''$ and $P = 3''$, whose region of accommodation has a radius of only $6'' - 3'' = 3''$, sees through glasses of $-\frac{1}{5\frac{1}{2}}$, placed at $\frac{1}{2}''$ from the eye, r brought to ∞, and p to about $6''$: his range of accommodation has continued about the same, and his region of accommodation has become infinitely greater. A hypermetropic person of $\frac{1}{8}$, with range of accommodation $= \frac{1}{6}$, sees from ∞ to $\left(\frac{1}{6} - \frac{1}{8} = \frac{1}{24} \right)$ $24''$; through glasses of $7\frac{1}{2}$, at $\frac{1}{2}''$ from the eye, he sees from ∞ to not much less than $6''$, — again without change of the range of accommodation, save only in so far as the useless $\frac{1}{8}$ is rendered useful range of accommodation. The presbyopic subject, on the contrary, who, with a range of accommodation of $\frac{1}{24}$, has a region of accommodation from ∞ to $24''$ from the eye, loses, by the use of glasses of $\frac{1}{24}$, a considerable part thereof: the accessory modifications being omitted, his region of accommodation is limited to $24'' - 12'' = 12''$, although his range of accommodation was scarcely modified by these glasses.

The examples here given have certainly been sufficient, to deduce the general rule:

that glasses increase the region of accommodation, when they make r approach to ∞, and on the contrary diminish it when they remove r from ∞.

Hence it follows, that if for a certain object a definite distance of distinct and easy vision was not usually required, it would in general be indicated to give myopic and hypermetropic individuals command over the greatest possible region of accommodation, by the complete neutralisation of the ametropia, and thus to put them on a par with emmetropic persons. Frequently, however, this cannot be done, because for a definite object we must also attend to the distance of the nearest point, as in presbyopic persons.

4°. *The magnitude of the retinal images does not continue the same.*

A comparison of the angles, under which objects, accordingly as they are viewed with or without auxiliary glasses, exhibit themselves to the eye, can without further determination, take place only so far as the object at the distance at which it is, can be accurately seen both with and without these glasses. To a certain extent this is indeed very possible. An emmetropic person, for example, with sufficient power of accommodation, can accurately see an object situated at 8″ from his eye, not only without, but also with glasses, whether of $\frac{1}{12}$ or $-\frac{1}{12}$. A myopic person can do the same with respect to a near, a hypermetropic with respect to a more remote object. In all these cases we can easily satisfy ourselves, that glasses with negative focus diminish the images, while those with positive focus magnify them. The demonstration of this is very simple. The relation between the magnitude of the retinal image

Fig. 81.

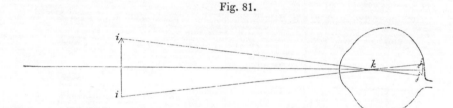

$j\,j'$ or β (Fig. 81), and the object $i\,i$ or B, is dependent on the position of the nodal point k. The more the latter moves forwards, the larger does β become, in relation to B; the more backwards, the smaller it becomes. What the eye can now do by accommodation, that is, by alteration of its crystalline lens, scarcely displaces the nodal point, because the latter lies in the crystalline lens itself. On the contrary, so soon as an auxiliary lens is placed before the eye, k moves forwards, if it be a positive, backwards if it be a negative lens,—and the more so for the same lens, according as the latter is further removed from the eye. The amount of this displacement is easily calculated (compare p. 56 and p. 65). Therefore, the retinal image is larger when the object is accurately seen without tension of accommodation through a positive lens, than when it is accurately seen without this lens by tension of accommodation of the eye; and on the contrary, it is smaller when, by very strong tension, it still exhibits itself distinctly through negative glasses.

With glasses of shorter focal distance (common magnifying glasses), the amount of enlargement cannot be in this manner determined. The object must then be held closer to the eye than it can be accurately seen without the lens, and the magnitudes of the images are consequently no longer comparable. In this case we are, therefore, compelled to start from an accommodation for a definite point, and to calculate how large the retinal image under the circumstance is; this magnitude we can then compare with that of the accurate retinal image obtained with the aid of the lens, while the object is brought to the distance of distinctness of the eye armed with the lens. In this comparison the enlargement now proves less, in proportion as the distance of distinct vision of the naked eye is shorter; to this distance, in fact, the retinal image is nearly inversely proportional, while, on the contrary, the magnitude of the image seen with a strong lens increases but little in proportion to the increase of the distance of distinct vision of the unaided eye.

5°. *The determination of the distance, magnitude, and form of the objects undergoes a change.*

In order to demonstrate the influence which positive and negative glasses exercise on our estimation of distance, magnitude and form, it is necessary to trace, in what manner, without the use of glasses, this estimation is established.

With differences in the distances, magnitude, and form of objects, are connected peculiar modifications in the requisite movements of the eyes, in the accommodation and chiefly in the retinal images; and in the changes, which these undergo by accommodation, and by movements of the eyes or of the head, and of the whole body. It is exclusively from these modifications, that the mind is in a position to form an opinion as to distance, magnitude, and form. This, however, for the most part takes place spontaneously, quite involuntarily, or at least without consideration. The rapidity of the judgment, without analysis of the elements on which it is based, is the result of practice, partly of the individual, partly of his parents, and is, in the latter sense, innate.

In the first place, we observe that the estimation of distance and that of magnitude are correlative. Three cases are to be distinguished. 1. We know the true magnitude of the object, and thence form, by the magnitude of the retinal image, our opinion as to the distance; 2. We know the distance and base thereupon our opinion of the magnitude; 3. Distance and magnitude are both imperfectly known, and through reciprocal influence an idea ·is developed, which brings both into connexion with one another, and thus at the same time more accurately defines them. The connexion just mentioned between our estimation of distance and of magnitude is particularly striking when we project the ocular spectrum of a flame upon a wall, in which case we suppose the flame larger, in proportion as we withdraw from the wall, and smaller in proportion as we approach it, notwithstanding that the retinal image of course remains unchanged.

In order thoroughly to investigate how our judgment is established, we must examine, what and how we are able to distinguish, first under the simplest, and subsequently under more and more complicated conditions of vision, whereby new means are each time added to those already obtained, confirming our opinion with greater certainty, and sometimes modifying it.

The following are to be distinguished as conditions of vision:—

a. An eye, without motion, seeing figures in a plane, to which the visual line stands perpendicular; *b,* the same eye, looking freely into space; *c,* an eye with movable visual line looking on a surface or into space; *d,* an eye, by movement of the head or even of the body, changing its place; *e,* two eyes at rest; *f,* two eyes in motion; *g,* two eyes with movement of the head or of the body.

We should, however, be led too much into detail, were we fully to follow out this scheme. We must confine ourselves to a succinct and elementary development of the intricate question, and shall also even pass over almost completely in silence the literature of the subject, which has attained to a wholly disproportionate extent.

Here, under 5°, we speak of our judgment in seeing with one eye; under 6°, stereoscopic vision with two eyes comes under consideration. We begin by supposing, that the figures are all situated in one plane, which is viewed only from one point with one eye, whose visual line is perpendicular to this surface. In this manner we have no means of directly judging of the true magnitude, *if this is not otherwise known to us.* It is only with respect to the distance that the consciousness of our accommodation gives some idea. Let a person, through a tube perforating a wall, so that he cannot estimate its length, read print placed behind the tube ; in this way many will form a not very incorrect idea of the distance, and consequently also of the magnitude. If we now place in the tube a weak positive glass, so that less tension of accommodation shall be required, the print will appear to the observer to be at a greater distance, and he will therefore suppose it to be really larger, even though a print so much smaller has been substituted, that the retinal image has retained the same size. If, on the contrary, we place in the tube a negative glass, whose action can still very well be overcome by tension of accommodation, the observer will suppose that the print is closer to the eye, and the actual magnitude is thus set down as less, even if a type have been taken so much larger, that the retinal images, notwithstanding the diminishing influence of the negative glass, have maintained the same size.

But if, on the contrary, *the magnitude of the object be known,* the judgment in general yields from the consciousness of accommodation of the eye having taken place, and the object, seen through a negative glass, is supposed to be more remote, because the retinal image is smaller,—seen through a positive glass, on the contrary, it is supposed to be nearer, because the retinal image is larger.—Exceptionally, however, the consciousness of the required accommodation comes into play, even when we look round in nature, where there is no want of objects of known magnitude, and where numerous other means of deciding are at the service of the mind. I observed this, many years since, in myself.* As a phenomenon, namely, of diminished power of accommodation, in consequence of the instillation of a weak solution of belladonna, I saw all objects too small, because I supposed them nearer to me, and Warlomont has also communicated an example of the same.† In paresis of accommodation too, produced by other causes, the same has once occurred to me. The determination of the distance from the accommodation required, appears to me besides *in looking with one eye* to be accomplished chiefly through the fact, that the other (covered) eye, in connexion with the tension of accommodation, alters its convergence,

* *Nederlandsch Lancet,* 2ᵉ Serie, D. VI , p. 607, 1851.
† *Annales d'Oculistique,* 1853, T. xxix., p. 277.

in which alteration we, in looking with both eyes, possess so accurate an aid in the comparison of distances.

In looking at objects in space, with one eye from one point, the estimation of magnitude and distance for an infinite number of successive planes can be effected in the same manner as above for one plane, and positive and negative glasses can also in the way described modify our estimation. Thus, then, an idea of the form of a body could be developed as well without as with the use of glasses. Under these circumstances, however, the reasoning is often inverted; we know the form, and thence deduce the relative distances of different points.

This must be further explained.

Many objects have for us known forms, and on their distance it depends, what the form of the perspective image on the retina shall be. An example may illustrate this:—

Let the observer place himself before the middle of a square table A B C D (Fig. 82 I). In order to know how large A B and C D are represented on the retina, we have only to draw lines from the points A B C and D, through the nodal point k of the eye, which we suppose here to be placed *above* the horizontal plane of the table. We then find the respective magnitudes $a\,b$ and $c\,d$ on the retina R. While the distance from A B to the eye amounts to the double of C D, the image $c\,d$ is nearly double as large as $a\,b$. The retinal image has therefore the form of Fig. 82 II. This form leads us to infer, that the nearest edge of the table A B is about as far from us as the table itself is long. If we now move the eye from A B to C D, the accommodation required helps us in our decision, and if we know the height of the table, the angle under which the lines A B and C D are seen beneath the horizontal plane, in which the eye lies, assists in determining our opinion as to the distance. The same table, placed at double the distance from the eye, gives another perspective image, in which $a\,b : c\,d = 2 : 3$ (compare Fig. 83 I), and in which the angles at a, b, c and d deviate less from the right angles (II). We, however, consider the dimensions to be equally great, and the angles to be right angles, only because such is usually the case with tables, and we infer that the length of the table amounts to about half the distance from C D to the eye. If there be now only some object, whose true magnitude or distance is known, this serves as a standard whence to judge of all other objects, whose relative magnitude and distance are inferred upon the same principle (the perspective projection).

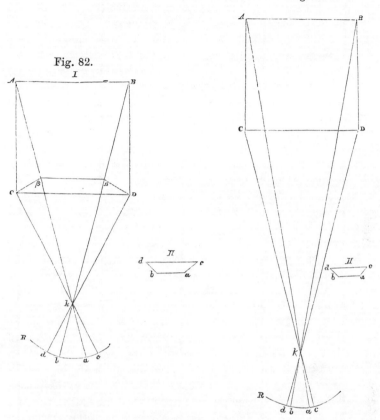

Fig. 82.

Fig. 83.

In the foregoing we assumed a knowledge of the true form of some objects, and the direction of some lines or surfaces. This knowledge, indeed, is scarcely ever wanting. In a room we see surfaces, which we may consider to be nearly horizontal or perpendicular, and numerous objects which present to us vertical and horizontal lines. From the angles which these surfaces and lines form on the perspective retinal images, we deduce our judgment. In nature the ground we walk upon, the horizontal water surface, ascending trees, houses with their frames and windows, lastly, man himself, are sufficient starting-points. Therefore also we judge tolerably correctly even what is seen only with one eye from one point.

Properly speaking our judgment can fail only through an intentional arrangement. For example, the table (Fig. 82 a) would have produced the same retinal image, if the edge A B had had only the breadth α β, but at the same time had been proportionally raised, so as to make the edges α C and β D coincide perspectively with A C and B D. Thus we can on one surface (a drawing) represent a number of objects in perspective projection, of which the retina then receives an image, such as the objects themselves would produce, and if the effect of light and shade be added, this image may be very deceptive, when seen with one eye from one point. However, if the surface be not too remote, the consciousness of tension of accommodation will even still teach us, that all lies in one and the same plane. But, moreover, these are artificial circumstances, which do not invalidate the rule, *that the form of the perspective projection on the retina is sufficient to enable us to judge of the relative, and even of the absolute magnitude and distance, provided only the magnitude or the distance of some object be known.*

Now on this judgment, deduced from the perspective projection, the use of positive and negative glasses exercises an influence. The cause of this is easily seen. In fact, in using positive glasses, the objects appear to us not only larger but nearer, and the distance in depth between two objects, and likewise between two lines of the same object, is thus shortened, there is, therefore, an enlargement of the object with diminution of its depth; the reverse takes place in the use of negative glasses. We can explain this still more fully. With actual difference in distance of objects the angles, as we have seen, change, and the proportions of the perspective images alter (compare Figs. 82 and 83). But proportions and angles remain the same, when by means of glasses the retinal images are magnified and diminished, and we consequently suppose the objects to be at other distances. The form which our judgment connects with the perspective image, must therefore be different.

Most remarkable is the influence of the magnitude of the retinal image on the estimation of the depth, provided that we know the angles of a surface. If, for example, the latter be the horizontal quadrangular leaf of a table, the relation between depth and breadth will be connected with a definite magnitude of the retinal image; in other words, the estimation of that relation will be different, when the retinal image, retaining the same form, becomes larger or smaller. A simple construction will demonstrate this. In Figs. 84 I, and 85 I, *a b* and *c d* are projected in the same proportion upon the retinas R: they stand to one another as 2 : 3. As the adjoining retinal images II show, *a b* lies lower than *c d*, but still in the same proportion. The retinal images, therefore, do not differ in the least in form, and nevertheless we are compelled to suppose the relation between length and breadth in the objects to be different (compare A B D C of Figs. 84 I and 85 I), and on this relation, different for each magnitude of the image, the distance at which we project it, has no influence (compare Fig. 85 I. A B C D with A′ B′ C′ D′). That we do

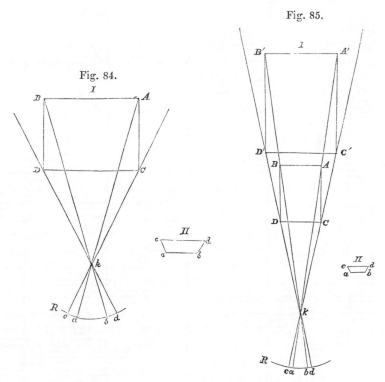

Fig. 85.

Fig. 84.

not connect similar forms of the objects (unless they lie in the same plane perpendicular to the visual line), with similar forms of the retinal images, but of different magnitudes, cannot surprise us, when we see on the other hand, that objects of similar form, but of different magnitude, do not give uniform retinal images (unless those, with difference in distance of the objects, are also equally large). If we place in the middle, or in whatever part we think well, of a quadrangular leaf of a table, a square sheet of paper, uniform with this leaf of the table, the projected retinal images will be dissimilar : the difference in dimension of the superior and the inferior boundary will, for the table, be relatively greater (for this relation depends on the relative distance from the eye), and with it the four angles differ.

Hence, it most clearly appears, how positive and negative glasses, which cause us to estimate the distance differently, and alter only the magnitude, not the form of the retinal images, modify our estimation of the depth. Hypermetropics observe this most distinctly, who, armed with positive spectacles, see the objects larger, which they before, through tension of accommodation, also saw distinctly, but smaller, and most of all persons, who replace the lost crystalline lens with positive spectacles. They suppose all distances to be less, and therefore see objects less deep.

Myopic individuals experience the opposite influence, but somewhat less distinctly, because without the negative glass they did not see remote objects accurately, and the comparison is therefore less perfect. It becomes more evident when they take a too strong negative glass, which they, however, overcome by accommodation; and in like manner emmetropic persons may in these experiments make use of a negative glass proportionate to their accommodation. But the phenomena appear much more striking in using the Dutch telescope, for instance, when we look through an ordinary double opera-glass with one eye, and close the other. Let us thus look at a small table as above. The retinal image of course preserves its form : if the glass magnifies n times, the image is only n times larger in all its dimensions. But we see the table broader and shorter at whatever distance we endeavour to suppose it to be. Often we have difficulty in supposing it to be short enough. Then it is, of course, too broad behind : A B (Fig. 83) appears to us larger than C D. This we sometimes correct by, in our thoughts, making C D rise a little; and those persons also do this, who in aphakia wear a convex glass, so that on flat ground they suppose they are running up a hill.

The phenomenon is particularly striking when we look with the opera-glass at an ordinary book, lying at a short distance on the table. The book immediately becomes square, although the retinal image retains the same form, it often remains somewhat broader at the upper edge, loses this when in our imagination it acquires an inclination, and the letters of the title are now broad and low, while before they were decidedly oblong.

If we now turn the opera-glass round : the retinal images, while retaining the same form, have become diminished, and the dimensions in depth, contrary to our former observation, are very considerably increased; even the leaf of the table and the book appear to become narrow above.

All this takes place in using one eye.

The estimation of relative distances, in monocular vision, becomes still more correct and certain when the head, or even the body moves, so that the objects are seen successively from different points.	In this manner, in fact, a parallax is created between objects placed at different distances, which apparently change their relative places, whereby the relative distances even of simple free points can be estimated.

6°. *Stereoscopic vision with two eyes is modified.*—From what has been said under 5°, it is evident, that the estimation of distance and of solidity of objects, even using only one eye, is tolerably perfect. This must here be remembered, for the beautiful discovery of Wheatstone has been found so important,* that it finally appeared to make us forget what a single eye can do. Two eyes, however, can certainly do more. At least when near objects are concerned, the solidity of the object can be estimated with more certainty; we cannot, in binocular vision, so easily be deceived by an artificial arrangement, and a peculiar

* Not to speak of the older literature, which is to be found everywhere, that on binocular vision has of late years been increased by the following great essays and works:—

Panum, *Physiologische Untersuchungen über das Sehen mit zwei Augen.* Kiel, 1858.

Recklinghausen, Netzhautfunctionen, *Archiv f. Ophthalmologie,* B. v. S. 2, 1859.

Volkmann, Die Stereoscopische Erscheinungen in ihrer Beziehung zur Lehre der identischen Netzhautpunkten, in *Archiv f. Ophthalmologie,* B. v. Abth. 2.

Nagel, *Das Sehen mit zwei Augen und die Lehre von den identischen Netzhautpunkten.* Leipzig und Heidelberg, 1861.

Wundt, a series of articles reprinted from the *Zeitschrift f. rationelle Medicin,* collected under the title of *Beiträge zur Theorie der Sinneswahrnehmung,* 1862.

Fechner, *Ueber einige Verhältnisse des binocularen Sehens,* from the *Abhandlungen d. k. s. Gesellschaft der Wissenschaften* vii., Leipzig, 1861; and numerous short articles, by Dove and others, in Poggendorf's *Annalen.*

sensation of the solid is developed in us, which the monocular person seems not to be acquainted with.

This depends upon two causes.

The first is, that in connexion with the distance between the two eyes, in fixing a definite point of an object, in which the two visual lines intersect, the retinal images of the two eyes are not equal and uniform, in consequence of which most points are seen as double images, whose deviation corresponds, for every direction, to the difference in distance of those points. With this the idea of the solid arises in us; but often, if all movement be avoided, and if no adjoining bodies guide us in the estimation, confounding of the stereoscopic with the pseudo-stereoscopic is possible: that is, the point seen under double images may as well be nearer, as more remote than the fixed point.

The second cause is: the successive fixing of the different points of the object (Bruecke). In fact we are perfectly conscious (at least, if the movement does not run through large angles), whether, in passing from one point to another, single vision requires more or less convergence, according as the fixed point is less or more remote than that previously fixed. At the same time, in examining the object, that is, in running through different points in different directions, the two retinal images constantly change, and their dissimilarity every time alters, which necessarily forces upon us a definite bodily form, and almost makes us touch and feel—which is precisely the characteristic of binocular vision. If, in fixing some point, we already have a tolerably accurate idea of the position of the point indirectly seen, which we now wish to fix, we even modify, with the simultaneous movement of the visual lines, the convergence of the axes. If we miss this idea, we see the double images disappear only when the visual lines have about reached the desired point. We shall best satisfy ourselves of this, if by holding a carmine glass before one eye, it colours one of the double images, and if we now look in succession at points of light situated at different distances. We then observe also, that with a rapid movement of the visual lines, the required change of convergence is for a moment exceeded, and is then quickly corrected.

Now the use of convex and concave glasses modifies the two factors of stereoscopic binocular vision.

As concerns the first factor, we observe, that the glasses modify the magnitude, and consequently the apparent distance, without producing a corresponding modification of the difference between the retinal images of the two eyes.   This difference decreases, accordingly as the distance of the objects increases.   While, namely, the angle, under which an object exhibits itself, is inversely proportional to its distance, the parallax of stereoscopic vision, and therefore also the difference between the two retinal images, are, at great distances, inversely proportional to the *square* of the distance.   If on the line $k'l$ (Fig. 86), standing perpendicular to the line $k\,k'$, connecting the nodal points of the two eyes, two points a and a' be moved without altering their mutual distance, then, as a simple calculation shows, at great values of $k'\,a$, with respect to $k\,k'$ and to $a\,a'$, the angle $a\,k\,a'$ is inversely proportional to the square of $k\,a$.   Now, this angle is evidently the parallax of the stereoscopic vision.

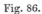

Fig. 86.

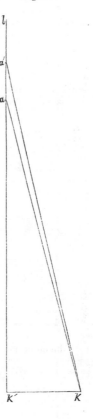

Thus it is proved, that the retinal images of the two eyes differ less, accordingly as the distance from the object is greater.   With convex glasses, and especially with an opera-glass, the object is now seen larger and apparently nearer ; but the difference between the two retinal images appears only equal to what it was in looking with the naked eyes.   Consequently the object exhibits, in reference to its magnitude, too slight a depth.   The reverse takes place in the use of concave glasses, which exhibit the objects smaller, and therefore apparently at a greater distance.   Thus the first factor is altered.

As to the second factor, it is dependent on the first : the difference in the retinal images is precisely that which requires a difference of convergence, accordingly as we view one or other point of the object, and therefore there is no necessity to treat separately of it.

From these considerations it appears, that, in the use of glasses, stereoscopic vision with two eyes modifies our judgment in the same sense, as takes place for each eye separately.   An apparent magnifying, namely, of the dimensions, perpendicular to the axis of vision, in both cases, causes us to estimate the depth as relatively less, and *nice versá ;* on a diminution of these dimensions, we are led to

2

infer a relatively greater depth.   However, in this the modification of the perspective projection for each eye separately is of much greater importance than the modification in the binocular vision.

Attention must still be directed to a few subordinate points, relating to the influence of glasses.   I allude, in the first place, to the apparent movement of objects, when the observer, *by moving his head*, passes from one object to another.   If we see, namely, through the glass, the objects under a smaller angle than with the naked eye, we must turn the head to a comparatively great degree, in order, by so doing, to direct the visual line alternately to the one or to the other edge of the object, and thus the latter appears to fly before the movement of the head.   On the contrary it comes in this movement to meet the glance of the beholder, when the visual angle is magnified, and therefore, in reference to the latter, little movement of the head is required.   If the same does not take place *in moving the eye* behind the glass, this is to be ascribed to the fact, that a person, in looking obliquely through the glass, no longer sees the object in the direction in which it actually is, whereby the want of harmony between the magnitude of the retinal images and the movement required to make them pass over a point of the retina, is compensated: without this compensation, we could not have said, on the preceding page, that the second factor of stereoscopic vision lies included in the first.   Finally, it deserves here to be mentioned, in a single word, that glasses limit, if not the magnitude, at least the symmetry of the field of vision; that behind glasses the movements of the eyes are not free in all directions; and that by reflection on the two surfaces of refraction some light is lost.

In the above (under the 6th head), our views were based upon the doctrine of the identical or corresponding retinal points.   Of late this has been much disputed.   It therefore appears necessary here to explain myself upon this subject.   In eyes whose visual lines exhibit no morbid deviation, the existence of points which project the impressions received upon each other into space, is not to be denied.   In this sense the points in the same meridians equally remote, upwards or downwards, to the right or to the left, from the fovea centralis of the yellow spot, may be considered as sufficiently corresponding.   The identity, however, is not absolute.   The images of two circles, of somewhat different magnitude, the one received on the right, the other on the left retina (whether through the stereoscope or by convergence), so that the lines may coincide in the fovea centralis, project a circle, whose magnitude is the mean between the two actually present.   On the contrary, no matter how the observer may draw the smaller in the larger, and what point he may now fix, he will, with one eye, still always recognise the two circles, and certainly see none of medium magnitude.   So far Wheatstone was undoubtedly right, when his discovery made him reject the theory of the identical retinal points.   So far, also, the statement made above, that every variation in the form of the retinal images gives rise to double vision of the points not falling upon corresponding parts, is to be corrected.

But the controversy of the identical points has been carried still further.

Some began by wholly denying the mental projection of the retinal images into space. This denial would not have been made, if observers had always distinguished between two different things: the projection of the *field of vision* and the projection of *a point in* the field of vision (Conf. *Ueber die Bewegungen des Auges*, von F. C. Donders, in *Holländische Beiträge zu den anat. und physiol. Wissenschaften*, herausgegeben von J. v. Deen, F. C. Donders und Jac. Moleschott; B. 1. pp. 105 *et seq.*, 1848). The projection of the field of vision depends on the position of our eye and the direction of the visual line, which we assume to be present; and the assumption is tolerably accurate, when the eye, in normal movement, is voluntarily brought into this position, and the visual line has been voluntarily given this direction. In what part of the field of vision thus projected we project a certain point, is, on the contrary, determined by the place which its image occupies on the retina.

In this manner every projection in the normal condition is explained. Thus it is also understood how, with accurately directed eyes, of which direction the observer is conscious, corresponding points of the retinas project the impressions received on each other. This may still continue under abnormal circumstances. In recent paralysis, for instance, of a muscle, we estimate the direction of the visual line incorrectly, and we consequently project the field of vision, and with it each point of the field of vision, in a false direction. We suppose that the deviating visual line intersects that normally directed in the point that we wish to see. Consequently we project the image falling on the fovea centralis of the deviating eye on the projected image of the fovea centralis of the properly-directed eye. These two different images thus appear to cover one another. If the deviation is not great, we speedily find the directly-seen object of the properly-directed eye as indirectly seen on the deviating one, and thus *double vision* is the result. But in every case confusion arises also in direct vision, which becomes particularly great, if accidentally a strongly illuminated part of the field of vision forms its image on the yellow spot of the deviating eye. However, we occupy ourselves almost always with the more illuminated parts of the field of vision, and the result thereof is, that in general the image on the yellow spot of the properly-adjusted eye excels in clearness that of the deviating eye. This makes it easier to neglect the image of this last eye; and it is very remarkable that this psychical abstraction, always increasing, is attended with physiological torpor, that is, with want of sensibility.

So far the law of the identical points holds good. But now it happens, particularly in cases of strabismus divergens, that we become conscious also of the direction of the deviated eye. This is the case when one continues to use this eye in its turn. In these cases, an object is still fixed in general with the eye, whose muscles act normally. If we now hold a second object in the visual line of the deviated eye, and request the person to fix it, the eyes sometimes remain completely at rest. The patient can thus occupy himself alternately with the one or with the other object, which respectively forms its image on the one yellow spot or on the other, and he knows perfectly in what direction each is. In this case, it is in the first place remarkable with what certainty he distinguishes with which eye he observes anything: he who has two good, regularly-moving eyes, is not at all aware of this; we can ascertain in which eye we have muscæ volitantes, only by closing one. But, in the second place, it hence appears most distinctly, that in such a person the corresponding points have lost their mutual relations. Indeed, what impinges on the two yellow spots is projected in very different directions, and likewise what touches on similarly directed meridians in points equally removed from the yellow spot. Now the reason why originally corresponding points are projected in different directions is clearly none other than *that the whole field of vision is projected in another direction:* the projection of the different points of the same retina has, with respect to one another, continued the same. This relation alters only when the retina is plaited or irregularly extended ; and I should not venture to assert, that if the accuracy of vision were maintained, the projection should not again by observation and trial gradually come to correspond to the actual position of the objects. In treating of progressive myopia I shall revert to this point. But from the foregoing thus much has appeared, that the deviation of the visual line, produced by muscular anomaly, which originally gives rise to false projection, may become known to us by experience, with which each eye begins its independent projection ; and no further proof is needed that, consequently, double images which, according to the theory of the identical points, we should see intersected, may be changed into homolateral ones. An organically necessary similarity of impression of corresponding points of both retinas, which should lead to an equally necessary similarity of direction of projection, is therefore out of the question. But, nevertheless, what we at first put forward remains true, whether it be congenital or the result of practice, that in eyes whose visual lines exhibit no morbid deviation, certain corresponding points of the retinas project the impressions received on each other into space.

The assertion, that by merely fixing a point with both eyes, confusion of the stereoscopic with the pseudo-stereoscopic is possible, I have above noted, after having also taken cognizance of the most recent articles of Dove and of Recklinghausen (Poggendorff's *Annalen,* B. 110, p. 491, and B. 114, p. 170, 1861). This is not the place to enter into the subject at greater length.

In the beginning of this section I stated, in investigating the action of glasses, that I provisionally assumed, that the axis of the glasses coincided with the visual axis. This is certainly almost never exactly the case. Firstly, the glasses in a pair of spectacles are not placed precisely so, that the distance of their two axes should be exactly equal to that between parallel visual axes, and, moreover, in being placed before the eyes they easily come to stand somewhat higher or lower than the visual axes; or the glasses, and therefore also the axes, have, when the head is perpendicular, a certain inclination. Secondly, every movement of the eye immediately alters the relation between the visual lines and the axes of the glasses.

The question now is, what is the result of this deviation?

In the first place, when the axis of the glass is parallel to the visual axis, but is displaced in one or other direction, we obtain also a displacement of the object seen through the glass. We satisfy ourselves of this, by pushing a convex or concave glass before the eye, so as to look always parallel to the axis, but alternately through the centre, and through the edges of the glass. If the glass be convex, the displacement occurs in the opposite direction to that of the glass, if it be concave, in the same direction.

The explanation is simple. Let k be the centre of the surface at h, representing the dioptric system of the eye, i a point situated in the elongated axis k h, this point will then find its image in the axis, for example in j. If a lens, whose centres of curvature fall in the line k j, be placed before h, the image of i will also remain in the same line. If, on the contrary, a refracting surface as h', with its centre of curvature in o, be placed before h, this is no longer the case. If we imagine, for instance, h h' to be a reflected ray, this will, refracted at h', deviate from the vertical v o, and proceed in the direction h' i'; consequently a ray must, *vice versâ*, come from a point situated in the line, for example, from $\ddot{i}$, in order, after refraction at h', to enter the eye as h' h, and to proceed as h j. Evidently, therefore, a point, situated in i', is seen in i, that is, displacement occurs in the direction opposite to that in which the axis of a convex glass is pushed before the visual axis.

Fig. 87.

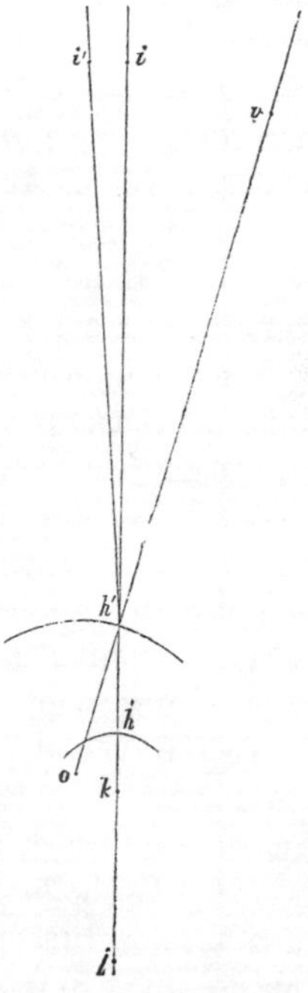

Hence it follows, that, if the two convex glasses of a pair of spectacles stand too close to one another, the objects are for both eyes displaced more outwards, and thus less convergence is required; the reverse is the case, when the glasses stand too far from one another. The opposite, of course, takes place, when concave glasses are in question. In either case the change of convergence required is less, the weaker the glasses are, and the less they are pushed to the side. For many years I have advantageously made use of such eccentric placing of the glasses, where otherwise, in insufficiency of one or other muscle, combination with a weak prism was indicated. Nor will it easily happen, that, in doing so, we exceed the limits, whereby the acuteness of the images suffers too much. If, however, we desire to encroach as little as possible upon the convergence of the visual lines, corresponding to the distance, we must, as has been correctly shown by Giraud-Teulon and Knapp, regulate the distance of the glasses according to the reciprocal distance of the visual lines. We have then, as Knapp has remarked, to attend particularly to the axes of the glasses, for these do not always correspond to the centre. In order now to find the axis, we have only to ascertain what part of the glass we have to hold before the eye, in order to see a vertical line, even when the glass is made to revolve, unrefracted as well through, as under or above the glass. However, we need not be too careful in regulating the axis. Whether, in order to see an object, a little more or less convergence must be employed, is often rather a matter of indifference; and if this is not the case, we accordingly involuntarily regulate the distance between eye and object. Against this no difficulty is to be expected from the accommodation: indeed, its limits, under the influence of the spectacles selected, are not defined so precisely, that we could approve or disapprove of a slight modification of the convergence under which the accommodation for a certain distance is required. We have only to take particular care, that in spectacles worn out of doors, we have not so short a distance of the axes of the concave, nor so great a distance of those of the convex glasses, that in looking to a great distance a divergence of the visual lines should be required, which might easily cause difficulty. A difference in height of the axes, which should cause a mutual deviation of the visual lines in a vertical direction, we must above all avoid.

In the second place, as to looking through the glass under an angle with the axis, we have already observed that this is unavoidable in the use of spectacles. The deviation thence proceeding is of two kinds. In the first place, the object directly seen exhibits itself in another direction than that in which it actually is. A construction as above (Fig. 87), modified so far, that the axis of the lens makes an angle with the visual axis, shows this directly. This altered direction is, as we have already remarked, of that nature, that the disturbance in harmony between the angle under which we see a dimension through convex or concave glasses, and the turning of the eye required in order to traverse them, is sufficiently compensated: moreover, this deviation causes no difficulty. But, in the second place, the objects are seen less accurately. Besides the ordinary aberration, in fact, a new and very important one occurs. Of this we may convince ourselves, by looking at a point of light through a convex or concave glass held obliquely before the eye, and, better still, by receiving on a screen the dioptric image of a point of light formed by an obliquely-placed convex lens. This image has a clear eccentrically-situated point, whence the light spreads chiefly to one side in the form of a fan, so that it reminds one of the appearance of a comet. In treating of astigmatism I shall return to this subject. Here it may only be remarked, that the diminished accuracy of the images, especially when strong glasses are in question, renders it imperatively necessary to attend to the direction of the axes. If spectacles be used only for distance, the axes must be placed nearly parallel and horizontally; on the contrary, in spectacles used only for near objects they require to converge proportionally, and to be directed downwards. This, when strong glasses are required, produces a difficulty of making use of the same frame for every distance, even in these cases, where the range of accommodation still admits of the use of the same glasses. The inclination of the axes can be sufficiently modified by placing the spectacles. But the convergence of the axes cannot be altered, without bending the frame. Therefore convergence must correspond to the mean distance, at which the spectacles are used, whereby, during their use, a certain margin in the convergence of the visual axes is least excluded.

NOTE TO § 12.

In this section we have spoken only of the immediate effects of convex and concave glasses. What results are mediately produced by them, with respect to refraction, accommodation, movements of the eye, &c., will be better discussed in connexion with the anomalies in which particular spectacles are indicated.

I have also thought it right here to pass over in silence the action of simple and compound cylindrical glasses. It is only in astigmatism that they are applicable, and they will more properly come under consideration in the chapter on this anomaly.

Respecting the different forms of spectacle frames, the desirable distance of the glasses from the eye, the use of spyglasses for one and for two eyes, the employment of reading-glasses, of magnifiers and of opera-glasses, &c., some remarks will be found in speaking of the different anomalies of refraction and accommodation, in connexion with which these instruments come under observation. In general, on this subject, among other writings, the following deserve to be compared :—

Szokalski, in *Prager Vierteljahrschrift*, B. v., 1, 1848, and Smee, *The Eye in Health and in Disease*, London, 1854, pp. 44, *et seq.*

NOTE TO CHAPTER IV.

The chief literature on the subject of spectacles is to be found in Ruete (*Lehrbuch der Ophthalmologie für Aerzte und Studirende.* B. I., p. 238, Braunschweig, 1853). Spectacles are among the most indispensable instruments for man. For many they extend the power of vision to an infinite distance, and others should, for want of spectacles, at a certain time of life see themselves completely shut out from the occupations to which, in a busy society, they are called. If we add that spectacles laid the foundation for the invention of the microscope and telescope, whose mighty influence is powerfully exemplified in the development of most natural sciences, we shall not view these simple instruments without respect. The history of the ordinary concave and convex glasses, which we here have exclusively in view, is somewhat obscure. Any who take a special interest in the matter will find the most essential points briefly collated in the work on the Microscope by my colleague Prof. P. Harting. (See the German translation by Theile, under the title of *Das Mikroskop*, p. 585. Braunschweig, 1859.)

W. Krecké, Ph. D., Vice-Director of the Royal Meteorological Observatory, suggested the use of prismatic spectacles in strabismus. To his communication I added my investigations of the physiological action of these glasses (*Nederlandsch Lancet*, D. III., pp. 227 *et seq.*, 1847). Von Graefe (*Archiv f. Ophthalmologie, locis diversis*) especially showed how still more advantage was to be derived therefrom, both in diagnosis and in treatment.

The use of stenopæic apparatus was introduced by me (compare van Wijngaarden, *over stenopæische brillen*. Diss. inaug., Utrecht, 1856, and *Archiv f. Ophthalmologie*, B. I., Abth. 2). It is true, that in mydriasis use was sometimes made of small openings; but it did not occur to any one to remove, by their means, the injurious effect of obscurations. How these by throwing diffused light into the eye, disturbed the power of vision (compare pp. 128, 129), was also first explained by me in Wijngaarden's paper. The explanation given is quite in harmony with the law developed by Fechner for the senses in general (*Ueber ein wichtiges psycho-physisches Grund-Gesetz*, Leipzig, 1859, and *Elemente der Psycho-physik*, Leipzig, 1860).

Green and blue glasses, for moderating the light, are highly valued. In a work recently published by Professor Dr. Ludwig Boehm, of Berlin, under the title of *Die Therapie des Auges mittels des farbigen Lichtes*, Berlin, 1862, blue glasses, of different shades, are particularly recommended in numerous, especially functional, disturbances of the retina.

SPECIAL PART.

I.—ANOMALIES OF REFRACTION.

CHAPTER V.

THE EMMETROPIC EYE.

THE emmetropic eye presents, both in its structure and in its functions, the standard by which the anomalies of refraction must be estimated. As such the knowledge of the emmetropic eye must here occupy a prominent place. But, in other respects, this eye, which as little as any part of the body escapes the influence of age, must also not be passed over in silence. The range of accommodation early diminishes; soon the accuracy of vision lessens, and lastly the emmetropia is converted into ametropia, giving way to hypermetropia acquisita. The emmetropic eye, in its retrogression, in its yielding to the advance of years, is our task. To the latter we are called, the rather because art can protect the eye against the senile metamorphosis, and by suitable means can help to maintain it in a position to discharge its functions.

§ 13. DEFINITION OF THE EMMETROPIC EYE; THE DIAGRAMMATIC EYE; THE SIMPLIFIED EYE.

The emmetropic eye is that, the principal focus of whose dioptric system is, in rest of accommodation, found in the retina (Fig. 88).

Fig. 88.

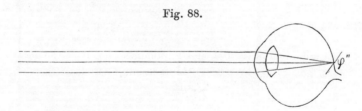

Of infinitely remote objects, which send out parallel rays, this retina therefore receives *accurate images*, to be improved neither by convex nor by concave glasses, and by means of its accommodation it sees equally accurately at relatively short distances. No other refraction of the eye is capable of giving to the region of accommodation so great an extent.

That this condition is to be regarded as the normal, we have already (page 81) shown. Singularly enough, for a long time the opinion was rather generally entertained, that almost every eye is more or less myopic; that at an infinite distance, apart from the imperfect transparency of the air, it is only exceptionally that objects can be distinguished under the same least angle of vision as at a moderate or short distance. This opinion is an error. By far too often does the eye deviate in the opposite direction from the standard, and can, with hypermetropic structure, bring converging rays to a focus on the retina.

If the emmetropic eye is to be considered as the typically normal eye, another question is, whether it is at the same time the ordinary eye, and whether, therefore, ametropia is the exception.

In an absolutely mathematical sense no single eye is perhaps to be called emmetropic. In the first place, I have never met with an eye whose focal distance in the different meridians was absolutely the same; in general, as shall be more fully shown in the Chapter on Astigmatism, the focal distance is shorter in the vertical meridian of the eye than in the horizontal. But, apart from this, here, if anywhere, we must allow a certain latitude to the rule. Slight degrees of M, for example $M = \dfrac{1}{120}$, in which, at the distance of 10 feet ($= 120''$) vision is still perfectly accurate, are almost always unobserved. Slight degrees of H are in youth not even to be proved, much less to be reduced to their numerical value: indeed, whenever a deficiency of refractive power exists in the eye, when in a state of absolute rest, it is supplied by the accommodation. And even if the eye in paralysis of accommodation should be emmetropic, the tone of the accommodation alone effects a slight degree of M. Consequently, the actually emmetropic vision requires, in a certain sense, a minimum of H, and that minimum is capable of no accurate taxation, because to the tone itself a certain latitude, perhaps from $\dfrac{1}{100}$ to $\dfrac{1}{40}$, must be allowed.

In this sense, and it is practically the only correct one, the majority of eyes of young persons are undoubtedly emmetropic.

Finally, should the question be proposed, whether E is the most desirable condition: as concerns myself, I should give the preference to a slight degree of M, and I shall subsequently state my reasons for doing so.

The emmetropic eye is dioptrically to be realized in various modes. Apart from the possible differences of the coefficients of the refraction, a compensating action may take place between

a. The radius of the cornea : the less this is, the shorter is the focal distance.

b. The form of the crystalline lens : the more convex its surfaces, the shorter is its focal distance.

c. The position of the crystalline lens : the more anteriorly it lies, the more, *ceteris paribus,* has it a shortening influence upon the focal distance of the whole system.

d. The length of the visual axis : it needs only to correspond to the condition, resulting from *a, b,* and *c,* to make the eye in each case emmetropic.

However, each of the factors mentioned, by itself presents in the emmetropic eye, comparatively little difference. With respect to the cornea, this is directly seen from a large number of measurements.* For the other factors it may be assumed for reasons, the development of which would here lead me too far. Hence we are completely justified in assuming a diagrammatic eye, and for the sake of different calculations, starting therefrom. The values assumed by Listing were somewhat modified by Helmholtz, who considers the crystalline lens to be a little flatter, and its position to be rather more anterior. With these modifications I have adopted them at page 67, where they are collated with those of the accommodated eye.

Following Listing's example,† we may go still a step further in the simplification : it is, in fact, allowable to reduce the compound dioptric system of the eye to a single refracting surface, bounded anteriorly by air, posteriorly by aqueous or vitreous humour, and this reduced eye, where the greatest accuracy is not required, may be made the basis of a number of considerations and calculations. With this simplification we can, with the greatest ease, form a satisfactory idea of the magnitude of the retinal images, of the position of the conjugate foci, of the extent of the circles of diffusion in imperfect accommodation, in astigmatism, &c., and of numerous other points.

The right to this simplification we derive from the minuteness of

* Conf. *Verslagen en Mededeelingen van de Koninkl. Akademie van Wetenschappen.* 1860. D. xi., page 159.

† *Dioptrik des Auges,* in Wagner's *Handwörterbuch der Physiologie,* B. iv. page 493. Braunschweig, 1833.

the distance between the two nodal points and between the two
principal points of the dioptric system of the eye; this distance
amounts to less than one-fourth of a millimètre.   It is evident that
neglecting this will cause only a very slight difference. We thus obtain, besides the two focal points, as cardinal points, only one principal
point, h, and one nodal point, the latter being the optical centre, k :
that is, we retain simply the cardinal points of one simple refracting
surface (compare pp. 40-44), whose centre of curvature is k. Fortui-
tously the radius of curvature for the human eye is 5 mm. ; the coefficient of refraction may further be assumed as $\frac{4}{3}$.   Hence results
such a simple position of the cardinal points, that we can without
difficulty imprint them on our memory, and make many calculations
even without the use of figures.   To this I attach great importance,
because our ideas thus gain so very much in clearness.

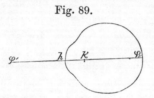

Fig. 89.

Fig. 89 represents the reduced eye in
its true dimensions.

k is the optical centre.

h is the principal point.

$k\,h=5$ mm. is the radius of curvature
of the refracting surface.

$\phi_{,\prime}$ is the *posterior* focus, that is, the
focus of rays, parallel in the air (compare Fig. 90).

ϕ' is the *anterior* focus, that is, the focus of rays, parallel in the
vitreous humour (compare Fig. 91).

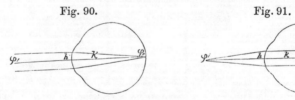

Fig. 90.   Fig. 91.

$h\ \phi_{,\prime}=$F$_{,\prime}$ is the posterior focal distance $= 20$ mm.

$h\ \phi_{,}=$F$_{,}$ the anterior focal distance $= 15$ mm.

Therefore the coefficient of refraction $\dfrac{n'}{n} = \dfrac{4}{3}$, as being $=$ F$_{,\prime}$: F$_{,}$ $=$
$20 : 15.$

The meaning of the reduction thus made is this : that for the
ordinary eye we substitute one with a cornea, whose radius of curvature is only 5 mm., while behind this is merely vitreous or aqueous

humour, without crystalline lens, and with a length of visual axis of 20 mm. In such an eye retinal images would have the same magnitude, the same distinctness, and the same position which they exhibit in the emmetropic eye with its cornea of nearly 8 mm. radius of curvature, its crystalline lens of a little more than 43 mm. focal distance, and its visual axis of a little more than 22 mm., and it can, therefore, really be substituted for this last.

That in the assumed reduction the system alters but little, we can render evident by reasoning. In the first place, the cornea is the principal refracting surface, where the rays deviate most: its focal distance is 31·7, while that of the crystalline lens amounts to 43·7. In the second place, in the crystalline lens the two principal points lie so close to one another, that they may be united into a single optical centre. If we now consider, that this optical centre of the lens lies about 16 mm., that of the cornea a little more than 14 mm. in front of the retina, we shall understand that the effect of both is combined in one point, situated 15 mm. from the retina. In order now further to combine in one surface of curvature the dioptric action of lens and cornea, the coefficient of refraction being $\frac{4}{3}$, a radius of curvature of precisely 5 mm. is required.

NOTE TO § 14.

The reduction assumed in round numbers scarcely differs from that found by calculation (see the method in Listing, *l. c.*, p. 493) from the diagrammatic eye of Helmholtz ; in place of the

calculated values,	we assumed,
$F_{\prime} = 15\cdot036$	15
$F_{\prime} = 20\cdot113$	20
$h\,k = 5\cdot077$	5.

In connexion herewith we assumed, as coefficient of refraction, in place of $\frac{103}{77}, \frac{100}{75} = \frac{4}{3}$, which values stand to another $= 308 : 309$. Listing's diagrammatic eye differs, it is true, somewhat more from the round numbers ; but still Listing has elsewhere (*Beitrag zur physiologischen Dioptrik.* Göttingen, 1845) found himself justified in substituting the same round numbers.

I now wish to show, by some examples, what use we can make of the numbers ascertained, in order to be able to form a quite satisfactory idea respecting several problems.

a. In the first place, a ray, directed to *k* (compare pp. 42 *et seq.*, Fig.

19), coincides with the radius of curvature, and thus passes through unrefracted : let $i\,i$ be an object B, $j\,j$ its image β ; let $k\,i$, the distance from the object to k, be g' ; $k\,j$, the distance from the image to k, be g''. Evidently now

$$B : \beta = g' : g''$$

We saw that $g' = 15$ mm. We have thus only to divide the distance g' of the object, expressed in mm., by 15, in order to find how many times the retinal image is smaller than the object : a mètre, placed at 15 mètres (15,000 mm.) distance, gives a retinal image 1,000 times smaller, and therefore one millimètre in size.

b. If the eye remains accommodated to infinite distance, the image j of a point i, placed at an infinite distance, falls behind the retina. How far does it lie behind it ? In other words, how large is $f_{\prime\prime} - F_{\prime\prime} = y$? Above (p. 44) we found the distance, $k\,j$, as

$$f_{\prime\prime} = \frac{f_{\prime}\,F_{\prime\prime}}{f_{\prime} - F_{\prime}},$$

If we put $\qquad f_{\prime} - F_{\prime} = \zeta,$

Then $\qquad f_{\prime} = \zeta + F_{\prime},$

and we may write $\qquad f_{\prime\prime} = \dfrac{F_{\prime\prime}\,(\zeta + F_{\prime})}{\zeta},$

$$f_{\prime\prime} = F_{\prime\prime} + \frac{F_{\prime\prime}\,F_{\prime}}{\zeta},$$

consequently $\qquad f_{\prime\prime} - F_{\prime\prime} = \dfrac{F_{\prime\prime}\,F_{\prime}}{\zeta}.$

In order, therefore, to find $f_{\prime\prime} - F_{\prime\prime} = y$, that is the displacement of j behind the retina, we have only to divide the fixed product $F_{\prime\prime}\,F_{\prime} = 20 \times 15 = 300$ by $\phi_{\prime}$, that is by the distance of the anterior focus ζ, to the object. If the point i lies 320 mm. from k, that is 300 from $\phi_{\prime}$, its image j will fall precisely 1 mm. $(300 : 300 = 1)$ behind the retina. The point i, situated at 1 metre in front of $\phi_{\prime}$, (1020 mm. in front of k), makes j fall only 0·3 mm. $(300 : 1000 = 0·3)$, the point i, situated at 100 mm. from $\phi_{\prime}$, makes j fall not less than 3 mm. $(300 : 100 = 3)$ behind the retina. Thus we can easily, without the use of figures, calculate y for each distance of i.

c. If we thus know y, we can further easily find the diameter of the circles of diffusion, and so obtain an idea of the degree of distinctness of vision. In the reduced eye the matter is simple. A cone of rays, derived from one point i, unites in j. On the retina, in $\phi_{\prime\prime}$, this cone has yet a certain section : that is, the circle of diffusion. The length $\phi_{\prime\prime}\,j = y$, we have only to divide by the length of the whole cone, calculated from the pupil, in order to find in what proportion the pupil, as circle of diffusion, is reduced. The distance from the pupil to $\phi_{\prime\prime}$ we may fix at 19 mm. Now if $y = 1$ mm., the circle of diffusion is $(1 : 19 + 1)$ $\dfrac{1}{20}$ of the diameter of the pupil; with $y = 2$ mm., we find $\dfrac{2}{21}$, with $y = 3$ mm. $\dfrac{3}{22}$, etc. The diameter of the pupil being taken at 4 mm., the diameter x of the circle of diffusion is in the first case $= \dfrac{1}{5}$, in the second $\dfrac{8}{21}$, in the third $\frac{4}{11}$ mm., etc. Evidently, with equal deviation of accommodation, the circles of diffusion become greater, and the accuracy of vision consequently diminishes the more, the larger the pupil is.

To be quite correct, we should make the position and the magnitude of the pupil, as they manifest themselves as the image of the crystalline lens, the basis of the calculation. The influence of the crystalline lens is, however, not great: with a true magnitude of 4 mm. its image of the crystalline lens is 4·23, and a position of 3·6 mm. changes into a position of 3·713 behind the cornea: with this the assumed distance = 19 mm. in front of the retina, agrees.

If we wish to make the calculations for Parisian inches and lines, we may, in place of 5, 15 and 20 mm., put down 2‴·2, 6‴·6, and 8‴·8, which values we can easily remember and use in the calculations.

We, can, moreover, in reference to the reduced eye, form a very good idea of the accommodation. In the first place, if we suppose this to occur through an imaginary auxiliary lens situated in air, the latter has only to make the diverging rays parallel : the focal distance of the auxiliary lens must then be equal to its distance from the point for which we accommodate. Thus understood, the imaginary auxiliary lens is equal to a spectacle-glass correcting according to the distance. In this, however, the position of the cardinal points changes in another mode than actually takes place in accommodation. If we wish to obtain the actually altered position, we must also reduce the accommodated eye in itself. We may assume :

$$r \ = 4\cdot5 \text{ mm.}$$
$$F_{\prime} = 13\cdot5$$
$$F_{\prime\prime} = 18.$$

Here, now, $\phi_{\prime\prime}$ lies at 2 mm. before the retina: the visual axis has, in fact, maintained its length of 20 mm., and this must happen, because the principal point has scarcely changed its position (compare p. 67). On the other hand, k has approached to h, as actually takes place in the accommodation. We find the distance to the object for which this eye is accommodated to be (13·5 × 18 = 243, and 243 : 2 = 121·5) 121·5 mm. from $\phi_{\prime\prime}$, and consequently 139·5 from k, that is about 5″, so that the reduced eye here assumed represents an emmetropic eye, using $\frac{1}{A} = \frac{1}{5}$.

The calculation of the altered position of k by the use of glasses is rather complicated. The method results from xv. p. 53, and xxii. p. 65. In the section on *aphakia* we shall be obliged to make use of it, and therefore to illustrate it with examples.

---

§ 15. Centre of Motion and Movements. Angle between the Axis of the Cornea and the Visual Line.

It would be going beyond the plan of the present work, here to enter into the whole doctrine of the movements of the eye. The great complexity of the subject, especially when taken in connexion with binocular, stereoscopic vision, would alone be sufficient to deter us from so doing.* But, besides, there is little application to be made thereof in reference to ametropia; and only so far as they are modified in ametropia, have we here to deal with the functions of the emmetropic eye. As to the mechanism of the movements, a modification with respect to two points is to be noted, which is of importance for our object: *a.* with reference to the position of the centre of motion; *b.* with reference to the extent of turning round the vertical axis.

Respecting the position of the centre of motion numerous investigations have been made, among others by Volkmann, Mile, Burow, and Valentin. These investigations yielded rather discordant results, but as the eye does not differ much from a globe, and is in great part contained in a globular cavity, these observers agreed that the centre of motion should be situated about in the middle of the visual axis. The discrepancy of the results obtained is attributable in part to the methods of investigation employed, but in part, no doubt, also to the difference of the eyes. Since, in fact, it was shown, that ametropia depends principally on a difference in length of the visual axis, it must even *à priori* have been supposed, that the distance at which the centre of motion lies behind the cornea, should, in ametropia undergo a modification, and I therefore thought it necessary to investigate that subject. The investigation took place in concert with my friend Dr. Doyer, according to a method described at the end of this section.

The results obtained in emmetropic individuals, are collected in the subjoined table. The subjects were all men. D. signifies the right, and S. the left eye.

* Compare Ruete, *Lehrb. der Ophthalmologie*, Bd. i. 1848, S. 8.
  F. C. Donders, *Zur Lehre der Bewegungen des menschlichen Auges* in *Holländischen Beitr. z. d. anat. und physiol. Wiss.* 1848, Bd. i., von van Deen, Donders und Moleschott.
  Von Graefe in *Archiv f. Ophthalm.* Bd. i.
  Meissner, *Die Bewegungen des Auges, Archiv fur Ophthalm.* Bd. iii.
  Fick, *Zeitschrift f. ration. Medicin* von Henle und Pfeufer, B. iv. und v. Neue Folge.
  Wundt, *Archiv f. Ophthalmologie*, B. viii., 1862.

Nos. of the Persons.	Age.	Eye.	Position of the centre of motion behind the apex of the cornea.	Angle between the axis of the cornea and the visual line.
1	23	D.	13·9	6°
"	"	S.	13·84	6°
2	23	S.	13·72	5°
3	30	D.	13·03	4°
"	"	S.	13·58	6°
4	31	S.	13·49	3°5
5	34	D.	13·27	6°
"	"	S.	14·04	6°
6	35	S.	13·55	4°5
7	35	S.	13·58	6°
8	40	S.	13·17	7°
9	43	D.	13·99	4°66
10	43	D.	13·32	3°5
"	"	S.	13·19	3°5
11	50	·D.	13·38	4°4

The length of the visual axis in emmetropic individuals is supposed to be equal to that in the diagrammatic eye, namely, 22·231 mm. Now by the method adopted we found the distance from the centre of motion to the base of the segment of the cornea; this base being 2·6 mm. from the apex of the cornea, 2·6 mm. must be added to the number obtained, in order to find the position of the centre of motion behind the apex of the cornea.

The same determinations were made in ametropia. They will be communicated in detail in the chapters upon H and upon M, where the importance of these results in the production of strabismus divergens and strabismus convergens will be shown. In this place I give in the subjoined table only the averages of the results obtained for emmetropic, myopic, and hypermetropic subjects.

		Position of the Centre of Motion.					
		a	*b*	*c*	*d*	*e*	*f*
		Length of the visual axis.	Behind the cornea.	Before the posterior surface of the sclerotic.	In per centage proportion.	Behind the middle of the visual axis.	Angle between the axis of the cornea and the visual line.
		mm.	mm.	mm.		mm.	
1. E.		23·53	13·54 :	9·99 =	57·32 : 42·46	1·77	5°·082
2. M.		25·55	14·52 :	11·03 =	56·83 : 43·17	1·75	2°
3. H.		22·10	13·22 :	8·88 =	59·8 : 40·2	2·17	7°·55

From this table it appears :—

1st. That in the emmetropic eye the centre of motion is situated at a considerable distance (1·77 mm.) behind the middle of the visual axis.

2nd. That in myopic individuals the centre of motion is situated more deeply in the eye, but also farther from the posterior surface, and indeed so that in the eyes of such persons the relation between the parts of the visual axis, situated before and behind the centre of motion, is nearly the same as in the emmetropic eye.

3rd. That in hypermetropic eyes the centre of motion is situated not so deeply, but relatively very much closer to the posterior surface of the eye.

In the above tables a column, *f*, is assigned to the angle between the axis of the cornea and the visual line. The subjoined figures,—Fig. 92, representing an emmetropic; Fig. 93, a myopic; and Fig. 94, a hypermetropic eye,—are intended to illustrate the meaning of that angle, and at the same time the position of the centre of motion *d*.

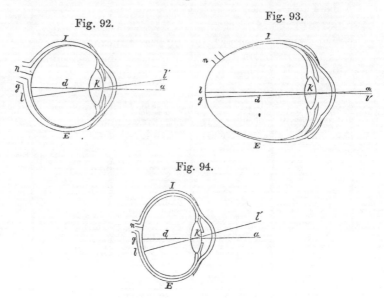

Fig. 92.

Fig. 93.

Fig. 94.

All are seen in horizontal sections, carried through the optic nerve, *n*. I is therefore the innermost, E the outermost part of the eye. The axis of the cornea, *g a*, cuts the cornea in the middle: to this, in fact, the apex of the ellipsoid of the cornea corresponds. Now this axis is by no means directed to the object fixed, which, as such, has its image in the fovea centralis of the yellow spot l. A line drawn from the retinal image of the fovea centralis towards its object is the visual line $l\ l'$, and this may be considered to cut the axis of the cornea in the united nodal point k. The angle, $l'\ k\ a$, is therefore the angle between the axis of the cornea and the visual line in the horizontal plane. In the vertical plane this is usually much less, and has no special bearing on our present subject. Now it appears that in the emmetropic eye the visual line cuts the cornea to the inside of its axis. This had already been ascertained by Senff, and was confirmed in a small number of eyes by Helmholtz and Knapp.* We found it as a rule in more than fifty eyes. I had, however, previously observed † that in myopic individuals the angle $l'\ k\ a$, is less than in emmetropic persons, and that in the highest degrees of M the cornea may be cut by the visual line, even on the outside of its axis. The investigation carried on with Dr. Doyer showed further, that, contrary to what was observed in M, the angle $l'\ k\ a$ is in H particularly large.

Hence, now, it follows, that in looking at distant objects, while the visual lines are parallel, the axes of the cornea in emmetropic individuals diverge about 10°, still more in those who are hypermetropic, but less in myopic persons, in whom they may even converge. This gives, considering the position of the eye in emmetropic subjects to be normal, in hypermetropics apparent strabismus divergens, in myopics apparent strabismus convergens, which, when once one is aware of it, is very evident, and contributes much to the peculiar physiognomy of myopic and hypermetropic persons.

Finally, as to mobility around a vertical axis, proceeding from the position in which the axis of the cornea stands perpendicular to a vertical surface carried through the centre of motion of both eyes, the normal emmetropic eye can in youth turn from 42° to 51° inwards and from 44° to 49° outwards. In myopic persons, as will appear, the movements are often limited.

* Knapp, *Die Krümmung der Hornhaut*, Heidelberg, 1859.
† *Verslagen en meded. der Koninkl. Akademie*, 1860, D. xi. p. 159.

NOTE TO § 15.

In the investigation of the mechanism of the movements of the eye, the knowledge of the position of the centre of motion is a primary requisite. It may therefore cause reasonable surprise, that in the numerous and elaborate researches carried on of late years respecting this mechanism, the determination of the centre of motion should have attracted so little attention. If observers started on the assumption, that the position of this centre had been determined by previous investigations with sufficient accuracy, they were mistaken. In the first place, as Ludwig, among others, observed, the methods employed left much to be desired; and in the second place, the influence of the length of the visual axis upon the position of the centre of motion was wholly left out of consideration. Now if the latter was found, as a result of observation, at a distance of from 11·9 to 14·1 mm. from the cornea, it was certainly extremely arbitrary hence to assume it as proved, that the centre of motion must be situated in the middle of the visual axis.

Some years ago I thought I had found, in the measurement of the displacement of a reflected image on the cornea, a simple and accurate mode of determining the centre of motion.

In the first place I ascertained, with the aid of Helmholtz' ophthalmometer (compare p. 17), the radius of curvature in the middle of the cornea. Subsequently I endeavoured, from the displacement just alluded to of a reflected image, to deduce how far behind the centre of curvature the centre of motion was situated.

The reasoning was as follows : —if the centre of motion of the eye should coincide with the centre of curvature of a spherical cornea, an image reflected in the axis of this cornea would, on movement of the eye, undergo no change of place whatever. If, on the contrary, the centre of motion, as was to be expected, should lie behind the centre of curvature, then, on turning the eye, the reflected image would be displaced in the same direction in space as that in which the eye was moved, and this displacement, as a simple construction shows, is the sine of the angle of motion, described from the centre of motion of the eye with a radius, equal to the distance between the centre of motion and the centre of curvature.

From this reasoning it followed that we should have to measure only this *displacement* at a *known angle*, in order, from the sine thus determined, to find the radius, and with it the distance between the centre of curvature and the centre of motion.

Now the angle was ascertained, by looking successively towards two sights (*visieren*) in a horizontal surface.

It was, moreover, easy to measure the displacement of the reflected image. Immediately before the opening, to which the eye, the head being fixed, corresponded, a hair was vertically extended. If, on fixing the first sight, the reflected image coincided with the hair, it appeared, on directing the eye to the second sight, to deviate therefrom, and this deviation was measured by making the double images, seen with the ophthalmometer, to separate so far, that the second image of the hair coincided with the first of the reflected image. Further, by repeatedly looking alternately to each of the two sights, the required distance of the double images could be still more nearly, and, indeed, very accurately, determined, while at the same time, the influence of slight movements of the head was excluded. The measurement was accurate when, on quickly and alternately fixing the two sights, the one image of the flame completely coincided alternately with the two hairs, or deviated therefrom by an equal comparative quantity.

If the accuracy of this determination left nothing to be desired, there was another difficulty. The cornea is not a spherical surface. Its curvature approaches much more nearly to the ellipsoid, and the eccentricity of the ellipse, obtained as a horizontal section, seemed great enough, to exercise an influence upon the position of the reflected image. Professor van Rees had the goodness to calculate this influence, and it appeared, that in consequence of actually established eccentricity of the elliptical meridians of the cornea, a deviation arises, which, in the calculation, may produce, for the position of the centre of motion, a difference of 2, or even of 3·6 mm. Hence the application of the method was very limited. Indeed, the ellipse of the horizontal section must always be determined, and this determination requires so much time, that it is difficult to apply it to a great number of eyes. The method is here communicated, because in those cases in which the ellipse is determined, it is not unserviceable in the control of other methods.

A similar method had, as I subsequently learned, been previously proposed by Professor Junge, of Petersburg. His results, obtained in Helmholtz' laboratory, were published by him in the Russian language. I became acquainted with them from the manuscript of the German translation of his valuable treatise. Junge's method depends, like that above described, on the displacement of the reflected image of the cornea, in movement of the eye. This displacement, however, he determined, by throwing the reflection of the same flame, both with parallel visual lines, and at a certain convergence of these lines, on the two corneæ, and by measuring the mutual distance of the reflected images, in the two positions of the eye just mentioned. In order to be able to use the ophthalmometer for this measurement, the images must, by reflection, be brought close to one another, for which purpose Junge made use of a sextant. He effected the determination on five eyes with great accuracy. But the numbers obtained have not a corresponding value, because he neglected to ascertain the eccentricity of the elliptical section, and therefore could not apply the requisite correction.

Subsequently I succeeded in discovering a method, in using which the form of the elliptical section of the cornea has not to be taken into consideration. In concert with Dr. Doyer, I have applied this method to a great number of eyes. We were, in fact, not satisfied with knowing the position of the centre of motion in the normal emmetropic eye ; we wished to inquire what differences in that respect myopic and hypermetropic eyes exhibit.

The method consists in this :—*That we determine how great the angles of motion (with equal excursions on both sides) must be, in order to make the two extremities of the measured horizontal diameter of the cornea coincide alternately with the same point in space.*

The horizontal diameter of the cornea was measured with the aid of the ophthalmometer. For this purpose the flame of a lamp was placed perpendicularly immediately above the ophthalmometer. The reflected image of this flame in the cornea was seen through the ophthalmometer. A second lamp, placed near the cornea, was covered towards the side of the ophthalmometer with a screen and served only to produce a bright illumination of the cornea to be examined. By giving to the eye to be investigated a definite direction, by making the patient look to a sight (we call this, moreover, the primary sight), which was movable along a scale,* it was not difficult to make the reflected image of the flame placed above the ophthalmometer fall precisely in the middle of the cornea. If this reflected image was really in the middle, the reflected images on both sides in fact, by doubling, reached at the same time the margins of the corneæ now half covering one another (compare Fig. 95; C the cornea, p the pupil, b the reflected image).

Fig. 95.

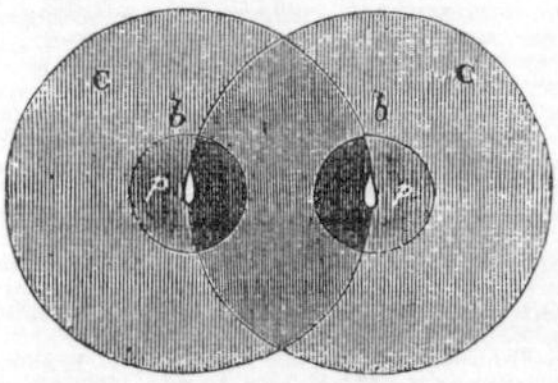

The result of this first investigation is evident. The number of degrees read off on the ophthalmometer, which was required to make the reflected images fall on the margins of the corneæ half covering one another, corresponded to half the breadth of the cornea, or rather to half the chord which subtends the cornea.

A second measurement, in which the glass plates were turned in the opposite direction, served to verify the first, and at the same time to avoid the error of collimation. In this manner we obtained, by reading off the ophthalmometer, above and below, four measurements. Of these four the average was taken.

A table expressly prepared now directly gave, from the ascertained number of degrees, the corresponding magnitude, whereby, consequently, the half-breadth of the cornea was known.

At the same time, the position of the primary sight on the scale showed what angle the visual line made with the axis of the cornea, assuming that this passes through the centre of the cornea.

In order further to determine the arc which the cornea must describe, in order to traverse the length of its own transverse diameter in space, a ring was suspended before the eye to be examined, in which a fine hair was perpendicularly stretched. It was now merely necessary to try how many degrees (starting from the position in which the axis of the cornea was directed on the cross of the ophthalmometer) must be sighted at each side, in order, while the head was immovably fixed, to make each of the margins of the cornea alternately coincide with the hair. The number of degrees ascertained corresponded to the angle which the eye had described

---

* In front of the eye to be examined a horizontal graduated arc was applied, with an arbitrary radius described from the centre of motion of the eye. In the middle of this arc, in the direction in which the eye saw the cross of the ophthalmometer, was the zero of the scale. Right and left of this zero the degrees were numbered.

from the centre of motion. It very soon appeared, that in normal eyes, this angle amounted to about 56°. We therefore began each time with one sight 28° to the left, to place another at as many degrees to the right of the primary sight. The head was placed so, that on fixing the one sight, the one margin of the cornea coincided with the hair; and it was tried whether, on fixing the second sight, the opposite margin of the cornea corresponded to the hair. Only rarely was this exactly the case; but it then, nevertheless, appeared, whether a greater or lesser arc must be described. Accordingly, the two sights were removed from, or approximated to each other, by an *equal* distance, which was repeated until at length the exact coincidence of the margins of the cornea with the hair was obtained. By making the eye look a few times in rapid succession alternately towards the one and the other sight, the influence of movement of the head was with certainty excluded.

The knowledge of the half-breadth of the cornea, and of the angle of motion, whereby that dimension in space was traversed, was sufficient to determine the position of the centre of motion. The subjoined figure illustrates this. It represents a horizontal section of the eye: o is the centre of the visual axis, or rather of the axis of the cornea $g\,a$; l is the yellow spot; $l\,l'$ the visual line, which in the posterior part of the crystalline lens (that is, in the nodal point) cuts the visual axis. If we now draw from the centre of motion x the lines $x\,y$ and $x\,y'$ to the margins of the cornea, and, moreover, the line $y\,y'$ as chord of the cornea, we obtain an isosceles triangle, of which the angle $y\,x\,y'$ is known to us. The perpendicular $x\,u$ divides this triangle into two equal and uniform rectangular triangles, (the acute angle of which, and, moreover, the side of the rectangle $y\,u$ the half-chord of the cornea) are known by measurement. The second side of the rectangle $x\,u$ is evidently the distance from the centre of motion to the base of the segment of the cornea. It is found by multiplying the side of the rectangle $y\,u$ by the co-tangent of the opposite angle $y\,x\,u$. By adding to this the height $u\,a = 2\cdot6$ mm. of the segment of the cornea, we obtain the distance $a\,x$, that is, the position of the centre of motion behind the anterior surface of the cornea.

Fig. 96.

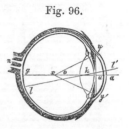

In many cases, especially in myopic persons, the mobility of the eye was too limited to make the cornea traverse the required space. In this case we used a ring, provided with *two* extended parallel threads, whose mutual distance was accurately determined. This usually amounted to 3·02 mm. The sights were now so placed that the one thread coincided alternately with the inner margin, the other with the outer margin of the cornea. In order to know the space traversed, it was now necessary only to substract the distance of the threads from the previously ascertained breadth of the cornea, and this value was further made the basis of the calculation.

The results we have comprised in three tables. The first contains the eyes of *emmetropic* individuals, the second those of *myopic*, the third those of *hypermetropic* persons. This distinction was made in order to exhibit the influence of the length of the visual axis. Above (p. 181), a table was given for emmetropic eyes ; and, moreover, one containing the average of the results obtained in E, M, and H.

We do not conceal from ourselves, that after this investigation, much remains to be done with respect to the determination of the centre of motion of the eye. In the first place, we have not yet examined how far the centre of motion may be regarded as a fixed, unalterable point. Our investigations extend only to horizontal motion, and almost always to an equal amount. We can therefore answer only for the accuracy of the direct determination—*that of the distance between the base of the segment of the cornea and the centre of motion, in rather extensive movements in the horizontal plane.*

---

§ 16. ACUTENESS OF VISION MODIFIED BY AGE.

With the increase of years, the eye undergoes a number of changes of different kinds. Some of these are recognisable on mere external inspection, as the diminished lustre of the cornea and of the con-junctiva, the smaller pupil, the changes of colour and less transparency of the sclerotic and of the iris, the diminished depth of the anterior chamber of the eye, the arcus senilis, etc. Some appear only on proper anatomical examination : to these belong, among others, the warty granulations of the structureless membranes, with secondary changes of the retina, calcareous deposits in the posterior part of the sclerotic, the peculiar metamorphoses of its anterior part, changes of the choroid, atrophy of the musculus ciliaris, greater firmness and a yellower tint of the lens, followed by turbidity of some layers, and lessened transparency of the vitreous humour. Even before anato-mical investigation can exhibit any trace of turbidity, the comparative ophthalmoscopic examination of sound eyes at different periods of life shows, that with the increase of years the perfect clearness and trans-parency are lost, in virtue of which the fundus oculi of the child is seen with such incomparable clearness.

With these anatomical changes, different disturbances of function are combined. The principal of these are diminution of the accuracy of vision and lessening of the range of accommodation. Both are to come under our consideration : the accuracy of vision, because it is not only the measure for the estimation of many morbid deviations, but is also effectively diminished in most anomalies of refraction ; lessening of the range of accommodation, because, although no

anomaly, it requires the interference of the oculist. We shall speak
first of the accuracy of vision. Lessening of the range of accommodation shall be the subject of the next section.

We have already (p. 97) seen, that the determination of
the state of refraction must go hand-in-hand with that of the
accuracy of vision. We there became acquainted also with the
test-types of Dr. Snellen, the utility of which has become more and
more evident to me. In the place alluded to, I have also illustrated
by examples, how, by means of these, the accuracy of vision may be
determined. The general formula is very simple. The letters bear
as number the distance D, at which they exhibit themselves under
an angle of 5 minutes, and are recognised in normal accuracy of
vision. If we now determine the distance d, at which they are seen,
we find the accuracy or *sharpness* of vision

$$S = \frac{d}{D}.$$

To this work is appended a table of Snellen's, extending from XX to
CC. If the room does not admit of making the examination at the
distance of twenty feet, lower numbers must be added.* In order to
be able to estimate also extraordinarily good accuracy of vision, it is desirable even, that the number in the table should go somewhat lower
than the number of feet, at which the observation can take place.

S = 1 was assumed by Snellen as sufficient accuracy of vision. This
held good for young subjects. It was to be anticipated, and indeed
was already known by experience, that even without extraordinary
defects, the accuracy of vision at a certain age begins to diminish. In
order to be able to use it as a standard in morbid conditions, it was
therefore necessary that the accuracy of vision proper to each period of
life should be known. This subject has been recently investigated by one
of my pupils, Dr. Vroesom de Haan.† S was determined in 281 persons
from seven to eighty-two years of age, by means of XX of Snellen.

* The tables are now published also with English tests, under the title of
Test-types for the Determination of the Acuteness of Vision, by Dr. Snellen.
These are to be had from Williams and Norgate, in London. Those with
French text may be procured from Germer-Baillière, in Paris; those with
German, from H. Peters, at Berlin; those with Italian, at Turin, and all
these, with the Dutch, are to be had together from T. Greven, Bookseller,
at Utrecht.

The publication was designed for the benefit of the Netherlands Ophthalmic Hospital, and was therefore made a monopoly.

† *Onderzoekingen naar den invloed van der leeftijd op de gezigtsscherpte.*
Diss. inaug. Utrecht, 1862.

Placed at first at too great a distance, the persons under examination approached until they correctly indicated V, A, C, and L.   These letters are the most easily recognisable, and de Haan could confine himself to them, because he usually had to make on each person only one good trial, and therefore needed no great variety.   Subsequently I determined the relation between the distinguishing of all the letters adopted by Snellen and of the four used by de Haan, found that it was as 5 : 6, and reduced accordingly the S found by de Haan. It is to be found thus reduced in Fig. 97.   The lengths of the ordi-

Fig. 97.

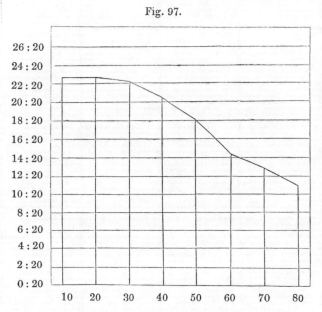

nates represent the acuteness of vision proper to the subjacent times of life: 20 is the mean of from 15 to 25 years ; 30 that of from 25 to 30, etc.   The value of S is given at the side as d : 20, d signifying the distance in feet at which XX is recognised.

Astigmatism $> \dfrac{1}{40}$ and ametropia were carefully excluded—the latter so far that M $> \dfrac{1}{50}$ and manifest H $> \dfrac{1}{60}$ are not taken in. At an advanced period of life, H $= \dfrac{1}{20}$ was still admitted, because it may in great part be considered as hypermetropia acquisita.   In each case the ametropia was corrected by a glass held close before the eye. All eyes were carefully examined externally, many also with the ophthalmoscope; all without exception being so examined in reference to which any suspicion of anomaly existed. If the slightest defect were found, they were excluded.

In the first place it was ascertained, that the individual difference is very great. Cases occur in which, after reduction, $S = 1\cdot6$ to $1\cdot7$; in youth very few where S is $< 0\cdot8$. With this great individual difference, it is not to be wondered at, that notwithstanding a rather considerable number of observations, the line drawn for the averages of each year of life makes many jumps. It is not until calculations are made for each decennial period that the course, as Fig. 97 shows, becomes more regular. Further, we see that at the thirtieth year, S is still almost unchanged; thenceforward, however, it diminishes rather regularly, and at the eightieth year has descended to about one-half.

The degree of illumination is, in the determination, not without influence. In order roughly to estimate this, in his observations made on different days, de Haan each time determined the accuracy of vision in himself, and found the limits to be $19\cdot5 : 20$ and $22\cdot5 : 20$. As the observations for the different periods of life were divided tolerably uniformly over the differences in illumination, the form of the line of curvature was not perceptibly altered by a reduction to uniform illumination. In general, in the experiments of de Haan, the illumination was something better than it usually is in the oculist's study. It therefore appears that Snellen has, for practical use, correctly selected the rule as $S = 1$, which in de Haan's observations is a little exceeded for young eyes. Snellen's idea is this: that when in youth S is $= 1$, we have no reason to suppose the existence of an anomaly. Moreover, the method is quite satisfactory where we have to do only with the determination of the relative accuracy of vision.

The cause of the diminution of the accuracy of vision with increasing age rests on a double basis: it is, on the one hand, to be sought in the media, on the other, in the apparatus of the optic nerve. The first gives rise to less accurate images on the perceptive layer of the retina; the second renders perception and conduction more imperfect.

As to the media, even examination with the ophthalmoscope in general shows that with the increase of years they lose the great transparency and homogeneousness in virtue of which the fundus of the young eye exhibits itself with such striking clearness.   The cornea indeed changes the least, if we exclude the arcus senilis, which, on account of its eccentric position, throws but little diffused light into the eye, and indeed less in proportion as the pupil becomes narrower in advancing years.   The crystalline lens, on the contrary, by degrees reflects much more light, which, thrown anew on the anterior surface of the cornea, returns partly into the eye : on focal illumination, the separation of its sectors becomes more distinct, its irregular astigmatism increases, the polyopia monocularis, in imperfect accommodation, becomes (notwithstanding the diminished diameter of the pupil) stronger and more irregular, the colour of the crystalline lens is yellower, and entoptic investigation exhibits, over the whole, more disturbance of homogeneousness.   The vitreous humour also loses some of its perfect clearness, at least at an advanced period of life ; it becomes richer in membranes collecting into folds, in corpuscles and filaments, as both microscopic and entoptic investigations have proved to me : in consequence of these we have an increased number of muscæ volitantes.   Finally, the diminishing transparency of the retinal layers comes under notice. The very appearance of the optic nerve proves that changes of its fibres are not wanting.   However, with respect to direct vision, this has, while the bulbs of the fovea centralis lie almost naked (compare p. 4), but little importance.   The senile changes of the apparatus of the optic nerve itself have been but little investigated, and it is difficult to estimate their influence. The best known is the formation of vitreous elevations, globules and groups of globules (warty granulation), on the anterior surface of the choroid, in connexion with the limiting structureless membrane of the same.   The formation in question was observed by Wedl,* then I accurately described it,†and discovered and represented the intrusion of the globules with pigment into the locally atrophying retina.   H. Mueller‡ considers these formations as simple thickenings of the structureless limiting membrane of the choroid. The function of the retina must suffer from them; they occur, however, only to a small extent in the region of the yellow spot, and scarcely before the sixtieth year, after which they soon become constant.

* *Pathologische Histologie.*   Wien, 1853, p. 330.
† *Archiv f. Ophthalmologie,* B. i., Abth. 2, 1854, p. 107.
‡ *Archiv f. Ophthalmologie,* 1855, B. ii., Abth. 2, p. 1.

Undoubtedly other less well-known changes in the retina, in the optic nerve, and in the brain itself, come under observation as causes of diminished acuteness of vision at an advanced period of life.

All the foregoing has reference to direct vision, that is, to vision of fixed objects. Outside the fovea centralis the acuteness of vision rapidly diminishes. Even the surface, which at the same time is seen with *perfect* acuteness, appears to be so small, that its image does not occupy the whole fovea centralis. The diminution of the acuteness of vision in the parts of the retina remote from the yellow spot, has been investigated by Aubert and Förster.* At a certain angle (12°.5 to 20°), they found that acuteness nearly inversely proportional to the angle of deviation; at greater angles S diminished much more rapidly. Rather strange and unexpected is the result, that smaller letters and numbers are indirectly distinguished under lesser angles than larger ones : in other words, that in looking at near objects, S is, in the peripheric parts of the retina, greater than in looking at some distance.

In different morbid states the acuteness of vision diminishes by no means in equal proportion, in direct and indirect vision. Not unfrequently the disturbance is confined to the region of the yellow spot, with perfectly normal S in the peripheric parts of the retina ; in other cases indirect vision alone has suffered, and even in the periphery limitation of the visual field may occur, without direct vision having suffered. It is therefore of much importance to have formed an opinion also as to the accuracy of vision in the lateral parts. For practical purposes the observer possesses the power of comparison with his own normal eye. On closing one eye, the observed eye looks to the left and the observing eye to the right, or *vice versâ*, at each other, and taking care that the observed eye does not deviate, the observer now exhibits, about in the plane which is perpendicular to the visual lines, in the middle between the observing and the observed eye, different objects—his fingers, cut-out letters and numbers, &c.—and thus by comparison in corresponding parts, he soon estimates the degree of disturbance in the periphery of the retina. In order to obtain accurate knowledge, we should be able to follow the method of Aubert and Förster (*l. c.*).—Limitation of the field of vision is determined by projection on a sheet

---

* *Archiv f. Ophthalm.*, B. III., Abth. 2, p. 1.

of blue or black paper, as shall be more fully described in treating of M.

In the foregoing, the method was stated of determining the acuteness of vision for *practical purposes*. The formula $S = \dfrac{d}{D}$ gives, however, neither the absolute measure of the distinguishing power of the retina, nor mutually comparable relative values. The absolute measure we shall learn immediately, when we come to speak of the determination of the acuteness of vision as a *physiological value*. That the relative values are not comparable, Snellen (*l. c.*) has already observed. If an image has double the magnitude, it has not at the same time double distinctness. This we should be allowed to infer only in case the acuteness of vision was equal over the whole retina, in case the larger letter, used for testing diminished S, was at the same moment equally accurately seen by the normal eye in all its parts. This, however, is not so. Therefore, also, when the image must have double the magnitude to be recognised, we cannot say that the acuteness of vision is really reduced to half. Perhaps it would be correct to assume that the acuteness of vision is inversely proportional to the number of percipient retinal elements which are required, in a linear dimension, to the distinguishing of the image. But, on the one hand, this prejudges the question, whether the accuracy of vision diminishing towards the periphery depends actually on the greater distance from one another of the several percipient elements; and, in the second place, the principle could not be practically applied, in consequence of the difficulty of determining the number of percipient elements. Hence the method adopted appears to me to be the only one available. The objection we made, based upon the unequal value of the parts of the retina, on which a larger image is formed, is in great part got rid of when we consider that this larger image is not seen with immovable eyes fixed upon one point, but is inspected consecutively in its different parts by the fovea centralis: the different impressions thus received by the most acutely seeing part of the retina are then combined, in order thence to deduce an idea of the form of the whole. The physiological value of the acuteness of vision being an angular distance, it is evident that the values of S are to be calculated as inversely proportional to the linear dimensions of the images required for the distinction, and, consequently, to the squares of their superficies.

In all times letters and numbers have been preferentially employed by ophthalmologists in the investigation of the power of vision. A regular system was, however, for a long time wanting. Stellwag von Carion[*] proposed very useful letter-tests, on a good principle. Smee,[†] too, in his often-

---

[*] *Die Accommodationsfehler des Auges*, in *Sitzungsberichte der kaiserlichen Akademie der Wissenschaften*. Mathem. naturw. Klasse. B. xvi., p. 187.

[†] *The Eye in Health and in Disease*, p. 70. London, 1854.

quoted work, adopted a series of letter-tests. Ed. von Jaeger* conceived that the ophthalmologist needs tests on a greater scale, and his well-known *Leseproben,* although not based upon correct principles, were soon generally adopted. But the need of a better system, which should admit of the acuteness of vision being expressed by a number, was still generally felt, and Dr. Snellen has the merit of having supplied this want. Neither has Giraud-Teulon been behindhand. He, led by about the same reflections, has devised a similar system, which he lately laid before the Ophthalmological Congress at Paris.

In contrast to this determination of S, suitable for practical purposes, I above placed the determination of S as a physiological value. In the first place, the smallest angle under which the presence of any object is still recognised, has been adopted as such. Thus, as Buffon† already remarked, and as has appeared most evidently from the determinations of Harting,‡ this smallest angle is determined by the illumination. To illuminated points on a dark ground there are scarcely boundaries. Small as such a point may be, its image has, on account of the imperfection of the dioptric system of the eye, a certain extent; and the question is now only whether this produces, on one or more percipient retinal elements, a difference ($\frac{1}{100}$ to $\frac{1}{50}$) of illumination from the others sufficient to be distinguished. Small dark points disappear, on the contrary, very rapidly through irradiation on a bright ground, precisely because the difference of illumination of certain percipient elements thereby becomes less, and, if the illumination is very strong, relatively much less perceptible. The question as to the smallest angle under which any object is still to be seen, is thus governed completely by the degree of illumination, and in a physiological point of view it has therefore no meaning. It is a very different thing to determine the influence of the illumination on the indistinctness of objects, with which Jurin§ and Job. Mayer‖ already commenced. Nor is the investigation with a definite illumination devoid of importance in a practical point of view (microscopical investigation), from which view Harting (*l. c.*) especially has worked it.

The first exact appreciation of the physiological question we find in Hooke's work.¶ He investigates the angular distance required to observe two fixed stars separately, and he found that, among a hundred persons, scarcely one is in a position to distinguish the two stars, when the apparent distance is less than 60 seconds. Subsequently, similar investigations were carried on by Mayer,** and in our own time by Volkmann,†† Harting,‡‡

---

* *Ueber Staar und Staaroperationen,* etc. Wien, 1854. The tests appended were subsequently published separately.

† *Histoire naturelle.* T. III., p. 323. Paris, 1749.

‡ *Het mikroskoop, deszelfs gebruik, geschiedenis en tegenwoordige toestand.* D. I., p. 87. Utrecht, 1848.

§ *Essay on Distinct and Indistinct Vision,* 1738.

‖ *Comment. Goetting.* iv. 1754.

¶ Hooke, *Posthumous Works,* 1705.　**　*Comment. Goetting.* iv. 1754.

†† Art. *Sehen,* in Wagner's *Handwörterbuch der Physiologie,* Braunschweig, 1846, III., pp. 331, 335.　‡‡ *l. c.,* pp. 97 *et seq.*

2

Weber,[*] Bergmann[†] and Helmholtz,[‡] for the most part with parallel lines
or with gauze. It is evident that, for two minute points of light to be
seen separately, the centres of their images must lie farther (about one and
a-half times) from one another than the breadth of a percipient retinal
element : if the said centres fall at both sides precisely on the boundaries
of the same element, this middle element alone will then receive as much
light as the two adjoining elements together, while, in order to see two separate points, a less illuminated point must remain between two more illuminated points. In using stripes and wires, not only the interspaces, but also
the thickness of the stripes or wires come under consideration, and in the
calculation Helmholtz has therefore (*l. c.* p. 218) assumed the angle, corresponding to the sum of a line and an interspace—that is, to the distances of
the central points of the two adjoining objects : the retinal elements must
then, at least, be less than the retinal images corresponding to this angle.
Harting and Bergmann have some measurements in which the angle thus
calculated is less than 60 seconds. Almost invariably, however, it amounts
to from 60 to 90 seconds. By using the extremely thin cobweb filaments,
the angle in Harting's experiments proved much greater (2 to 3 minutes)
than when metallic gauze with thicker filaments was employed. To this
cause, no doubt, it is also to be attributed that Volkmann, who made use of
cobweb filaments, found particularly high values. The cones in the fovea
centralis have, according to Schultze[§], when shrivelled, a thickness of
0.002 — 0.0025, in the recent state probably of 0.0028 mm. at the basis ;
according to H. Mueller[||], of 0.0025 — 0.003. An angle of 60 seconds gives
a retinal image of 0.00438. This is equivalent to the thickness of one and
a-half rods, and therefore completely confirms, in connexion with what has
been above remarked, the hypothesis from which we started, that each
cone of the fovea centralis can separately project the received impression ;
the peculiar undulating curves, too, represented by straight lines, before
becoming accurately recognisable,[¶] are explicable from this hypothesis.
Hence it follows also that each cone has its distinct nerve-fibre.

For practical use in those labouring under affections of the eyes, the
method here laid down for physiological objects is not applicable. In
practice it is absolutely required that the person examined should give a
proof that he actually distinguishes, as is done by the naming of known
figures, letters, numbers, etc. I formerly endeavoured to attain my object
in this respect by causing the patient to determine what direction the
stripes had on a card, which was turned, behind the opening of a diaphragm,
around its centre. The distance at which the determination was every
time effected with precision should, as I supposed, present a very simple
measure of the accuracy of vision. It appeared, however, that the inclina-

---

* *Verhandl. der Sachs. Gesellsch.* 1852. p. 145.
† *Zeitschrift f. rat. Medizin.* 3e serie. II., p. 88.
‡ *l. c.*, p. 217.
§ *Sitzungsberichte der niederrh. Gesellsch. in Bonn.* 1861, p. 97.
|| *Naturwiss. Zeitschrift*, B. 11, p. 217. Würzburg, 1861.
¶ Compare Helmholtz, *l. c.*, p. 217, Fig. 102.

tion of the lines had a great and insuperable influence on the distinctness of their direction, a fact undoubtedly connected with irregular astigmatism. This circumstance rendered the method useless.

The cause of the diminution of S with the advance of years, we have sought partly in increasing imperfection of the dioptric system. We have spoken of the entoptic method of becoming acquainted with the changes occurring therein. Of this method and its results it is the more important that we should here speak, because in treating of the morbid changes of the vitreous humour, connected with extreme degrees of myopia, we must again specially revert to it. The inspection of objects existing in our eye we call *entoptic observation* (Listing). In ordinary vision, only obscurities which lie close in front of the retina can throw circumscribed shadows on that membrane. Under certain circumstances, however, irregularities remote from the retina become definitely perceptible. This occurs, when homocentric, and especially nearly parallel light, passes through the vitreous humour. Such light we obtain when, in ϕ', (Fig. 98), about 13 mm. from the cornea, a very small source of light exists, a dioptric or catoptric image, or simply a very small opening (of about 0·1 mm.) turned towards the light: through the round pupil rays penetrate, which form a cylindrical and sufficiently homocentric bundle of light in the vitreous humour,

Fig. 98.

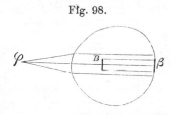

and cause an object B, to throw a shadow β, upon the retina. Thus, if we hold before the eye, at a distance of about 13 mm., a thin black metal plate, furnished with a small opening of 0·1 mm., and if we look through this opening towards the bright sky or the globe of a lamp, or if we cause the dioptric image of a flame to fall into the opening, the retina receives a circle of light of the form, and of about the magnitude of the pupil, without inversion, and therefore inversely projected, on which all irregularities are represented. Particularly shadows which are formed, but also diffraction-lines are to be seen thereon, and the effect of the refraction of light by some corpuscles is also not to be mistaken. We can distinguish:

1. The *muco-lachrymal spectrum*, dependent on tears, mucus, fat globules and bubbles of air, moving on the cornea; on the edges of the eyelids pushed before the pupil, whose lashes are also accurately represented, we see stripes, dependent on the layer of moisture.

2. The *spectrum of the vitreous humour.*—Particularly for the parts situated closer to the retina, the light needs less to be homocentric, and it is therefore advantageous, in order to be less disturbed by the spectrum of the crystalline lens (see 3), to take a somewhat larger opening. On an extremely finely granular ground (optical effect of the granular layers of the retina on the layer of rods?) every one sees with the greatest distinctness the movable *muscæ volitantes.* We distinguish, *a. Isolated little circles,*—some with dark, others with pale contours and bright in the centre, mostly sur-

rounded with a slender ring, from $\frac{1}{28}$ to $\frac{1}{120}$ mm. in diameter, from $\frac{1}{3}$ to 3 or 4 mm. from the retina. They appear particularly, and, it would seem, from the under side, on a rapid movement of the eye from beneath upwards interrupted by a sudden arrest, and they then again slowly descend : in the horizontal direction they have little, in the vertical they have $1\frac{1}{2}$ mm. or more mobility, and alter but little their distance from the retina.

b. Pearly strings, from 1 to 4 mm. in length, by from $\frac{1}{33}$ to $\frac{1}{190}$ mm. in breadth, the slightest close to, the broadest and darkest more remote from, the retina, all occurring at from ¼ to 3 mm. distance from this membrane. In the state of rest the same pearly string has for seventeen years always existed unchanged in form nearly in the visual line of my right eye. The most of them are, however, in rest, retracted upwards (apparently downwards), in order with the above-described movement to appear again, twisting in various modes. *c. Coherent groups of little circles of various sizes, some pale, some darker, more opaque than the other forms : these are, in ordinary vision, usually observed as muscæ volitantes.* Many are connected with short pearly strings, and move with these ; some have the appearance of convoluted pearly strings. *d. Plaits,* under the form of bright little bands, bounded by two rather dark, but not accurately marked, lines. They exhibit themselves either as twisted fibres, or as parallel little bands, connected to one another in some invisible mode, or as an irregularly rolled-up membrane of constant form. They hover and move chiefly in a vertical plane, at from 2 to 4 mm. from the retina. Besides this form, extended membranes occur, some situated close behind the lens, with plaits, which attain a breadth of $\frac{1}{23}$ mm., some removed only from 2 to 4 mm. from the retina, with slighter

plaits of $\frac{1}{60}$ mm , while at a distance of from 4 to 10 mm. from the retina, none whatever are met with. They appear when the visual axis is moved to the side, but especially on a powerful, suddenly-interrupted, movement from above downwards. Hereupon the membranes situated close behind the lens apparently rise upwards, while, on the contrary, those situated near the retina descend, so that in the visual axis they pass one another. But we now often see the plaited membranes become more and more indistinct, without its being evident that they recede from the field of vision, and yet, on repeating the movement, they each time appear afresh distinctly. Hence follows what on accurate study is more fully confirmed, that these membranes have only apparently an extensive motion, and that what, on superficial inspection, we should be inclined to look upon as a movement of the whole membrane, is merely the continuation of the folds, which on motion are formed at the periphery, and towards the extremity of the membranes lose their defined form. The cause of the difference in direction, in which the movement of the membranes and the propagation of the folds take place, is to be sought in the fact of location, in front of or behind, the centre of motion.—If we look with the pupil artificially dilated, or hold the illuminating point close before the eye, so that we can see tolerably well at the side of the visual line, we observe that, particularly on powerful lateral, suddenly interrupted movements, still more membranes appear tolerably close behind the lens, which rarely extend to the visual line, and here terminate with irregular points, sometimes torn off in rays. *These membranes increase and become less transparent in advanced life, especially where myopia exists.*

Having, in the manner to be stated hereafter, determined the position in depth of these different forms, I succeeded in finding, on microscopic examination, with Professor Jansen (*Ned. Lancet*, 2de Serie, D. 11, 1843), some, and subsequently with Dr. Doncan, all forms in the vitreous humour of the human eye. In the investigation the vitreous humour was transferred with the hyaloid membrane uninjured to a hollow glass; the vitreous humour soon becomes flat, and viewing it from different sides, we can, with tolerably strong lenses, search it all. Of the muscæ volitantes, which every one can see entoptically in himself, I have not here reproduced the representations. They are microscopically perceptible in the vitreous humour: *a*. pale cells, and débris of cells in a state of mucine-metamorphosis (Fig. 99 *a*, close to the visual axis in the posterior part of the vitreous humour; *b*, more laterally in the vitreous humour). These correspond to the isolated circles described under *a*. *β*. Fibres furnished with granules (Fig. 100), corresponding to the pearly strings; we found them less generally than the large number of those strings should have led us to suppose. *γ*. Groups of granules with adherent granular fibres (Fig. 101), corresponding to the groups described under *c*. *δ*. (Fig. 102) membranes, situated chiefly to the side, close behind

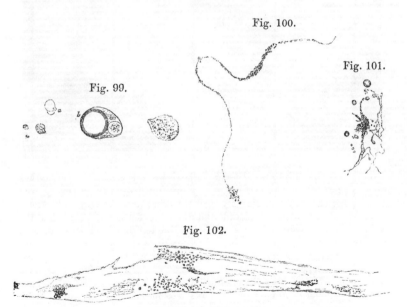

Fig. 100.

Fig. 101.

Fig. 99.

Fig. 102.

the lens, numerous in the vitreous humours of old persons, corresponding to those described under *d*.

3. *The spectrum of the crystalline lens.*—For observing this, more perfectly homocentric light, and therefore a very small opening, is necessary. The whole circle is then less illuminated, and covered, as it were, with a crape (Fig. 103, my right crystalline lens in mydriasis).   We find here : *a*.

Fig. 103

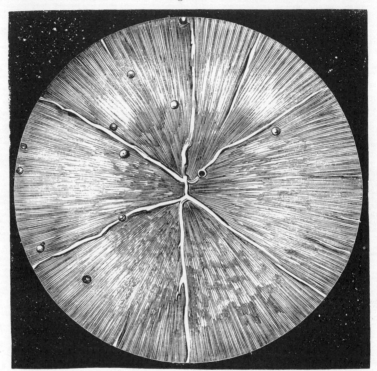

Pearl-spots, tolerably round disks with accurately circumscribed darker margins, but brighter internally, nearly universally occurring in every eye ; the majority are situated tolerably close to the surface of the crystalline lens, in great part eccentrically placed, and therefore appearing only when the pupil is artificially dilated.   Examining at different times, I on each occasion found others; they may be developed in a few days, and sometimes continue a year or longer ; in general their number increases with the advance of years. They are microscopically visible as large globules among the superficial fibres of the lens, which they, as it were, push out from one another.   *b. Black, or rather opaque spots*, usually round, but sometimes of irregularly angular, or oblong form, not so common as the pearl-spots.   I have also seen them, on microscopic examination, rather superficially, as white, granular, opaque corpuscles, almost always in the boundaries of the sectors of the crystalline lens. They appeared not to be dependent on fatty metamorphosis.   c.   A radiated figure, more or less regular, usually with ramifications proceeding about from the centre ; the rays exhibit themselves, sometimes as black, but ordinarily as white lines with dark boundaries.   If we remove the point of light from the eye, these lines pass into the well-known rays, exhibited by a star or point of light, for which the eye is not accommodated, and these correspond again to the manifold images, under which a point, for example, a fine white granule (such as of white-lead scraped off a visiting card), appears within the bounds of distinct vision upon a darker ground (for example, on black velvet).   These phenomena are connected with the composition of the lens of so-called sectors, which, as Helmholtz showed, can be very well seen with the magnifying-glass, with lateral focal illumination, in the living eye.   *All these irregularities of the lens increase with the time of life, and partly explain the diminished acuteness of vision.*

Of all the entoptic objects observed, we can easily determine the position in point of depth, according to a method, to which I was led by those of Sir David Brewster and of Listing.   Instead of looking through one, we look through two openings of 0·1 mm., placed at from 2·5 to 3 mm. from each other.   Two cylinders of light (Fig. 104, $a\,a'$, $b\,b'$, and $c\,c'$, $d\,d'$), each in itself homocentric, then penetrate the eye, under such an angle, that the circles of which $a'\,b'$ and $c'\,d'$, are the diameters, on the retina cover one another nearly by half.   We therefore see them as Fig. 105.   In each circle the entoptic

Fig. 104.

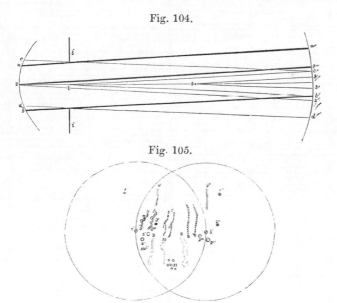

Fig. 105.

spectra are now to be seen. From a point 1, situated in the plane of the pupil $i i$, the two entoptic shadows lie precisely in the middle of the two circles, in the circle a' b', at c', in the circle c' d', at b', and therefore precisely as far from one another as the centres of the circles themselves: for each other point, situated in the plane of the pupil, the mutual distance of the two entoptic shadows, although now falling in other parts of the circles, is of course equal. On the contrary for a point 2, situated in the cornea, they fall farther from one another, as $2'$ and $2''$; for a point 3, situated behind the plane of the pupil, they fall closer to one another, as $3'$ and $3''$, as the lines drawn from these points, parallel to the rays of the two cylinders, signify. We now see also, without further demonstration, that the distance, d', of the double shadows, is in the same proportion to the distance D' of the entoptic objects from the retina, as the mutual distance d of the centres of the two circles, to the distance D from the plane of the pupil to the retina = from 18 to 19 mm. We have therefore only to project the mutual distance d of the two centres (= the breadth of the uncovered part of the circles), and that of the double shadows, d', of any object, in order to find for the same object, as distance from the retina, $D' = \dfrac{d' \times 19}{d}$.

The measurement of the projected images is most easily effected by the method à double vue, in use in micrometry: looking through the two small openings (which may for that purpose occupy the place of the object-glass in a microscope-frame) downwards on a mirror reflecting the light, we can with the other eye project and measure the forms on an adjoining sheet of white paper. In this manner the distances stated above were determined. In Fig. 105 we see, in the two circles of light, half covering each other, as c' and b', the centres; as $1'$, $1''$, the double images of the muco-lachrymal spectrum; as $2'$, $2''$, those of pearl-spots; as $3'$, $3''$, those of dark spots of the lens; as $4'$, $4''$, those of the anterior, as $5'$, $5''$, those of the posterior folds; as $6'$, $6''$, and as 7, 8, 9 and 10, those of smaller and smaller pearly strings; as 11 those of greater, as 12 those of smaller, isolated circles. Taking into account the distance at which we project, we also find easily the magnitude of the shadows, which, both on account of the diffraction-lines and of the imperfect homocentricity of the light, prove somewhat larger than the objects.

In conclusion, a word respecting the history of our knowledge of entoptic phenomena. Dechales (*Cursus s. Mundus Mathematicus*, Lugduni, 1690, T. III., pp. 393, 398, etc.), a Jesuit of the 17th century, saw, as being highly myopic, his entoptic spectrum in the circle of diffusion of remote points of light, and comprehended and described what he saw. He showed, on correct principles, that muscæ volitantes, observed during ordinary vision, must depend either on corpuscles situated near the retina, or on morbid parts of the retina itself. The observation of the true motion of muscæ volitantes by Andreæ (Graefe's und von Walther's *Journal der Chir. und Augenheilkunde*, vol. viii., S. 16, 1825), Prévôts (*Mem. de la Soc. de Phys. et d'Hist. Naturelle de Genève*, 1832, p. 244), Sotteau (*Ann. et Bull. de la Société de Méd. de Gand*, vol. xi. livr. 9, 1842), and others, should have been sufficient to solve the dilemma raised by Dechales; but, nevertheless, the truths and errors, taught by Morgagni (*Adversaria Anatomica*, vi., Ann. lxxv. p. 94, Lugd. Batav. 1722), were perpetually repeated. Since 1760, as we read in Mackenzie (*Edinburgh Med. and Surgical Journal*, July, 1845), observers had begun to study the muscæ volitantes both through a small opening, and with the aid of lenses. Mackenzie himself gave a very creditable description of the muco-lachrymal spectrum observed in this manner, and of that of the vitreous humour, but without making use of Brewster's method of determining the distance from the retina. Sir David Brewster had previously, however (*Transactions of the Royal Society of Edinburgh*, vol. xv. p. 374), by using two points of light (the dioptric images of two flames, towards which he looked through a powerful dioptric system), as an *experimentum crucis* doubled the shadows, and thus given a direct proof of the position of the objects in the vitreous humour producing muscæ volitantes, and even made a calculation of the position of one of his muscæ volitantes. This was followed by the treatise of Listing (*Beitrag zur physiologischen Optik*, Göttingen 1845), who fully developed the theory, discovered the spectrum of the crystalline lens, and deduced the position of the objects in the eye from their parallax in the motions of the eye: thus, as is easily conceived, the shadows of corpuscles, situated in the plane of the pupil, on movement of the visual line, maintain their place in the circle of light, while those in front of that plane thereupon exhibit a positive, those behind it, a negative parallax, which parallax is greater as the distance from the plane in question is greater. Listing's method is not very applicable to movable corpuscles. That of Brewster presented difficulties in the projection, and the calculation was uncertain and troublesome, until I pointed out (*Nederlandsch Lancet*, 2de Serie, 1847, D. 11, pp. 365, 432, and 537, and *Archiv f. physiologische Heilkunde*, viii. p. 30, 1849), that the centres of the two circles are nearly proportional (the crystalline lens causes a slight modification) to the distance between the pupil and the retina. In my method above described, I at first projected on a white paper on which the sun shone, subsequently, with Doncan (*De corporis vitrei structurâ*. Diss. inaug. Trajecti ad Rhenum, 1854), I used the *methode à double vue*. The corpuscles in the vitreous humour I had already partly found with my friend Prof. Jansen; subsequently I had discovered all forms with Doncan, who, under my direction, wrote his dissertation on this subject; I have also repeatedly seen those of the crystalline lens.—Elsewhere (*Ned. Lancet*, 2de Serie, D. iv. p. 638), I have also described how, by means of a lens with a pupil (an opening in a diaphragm) placed before it, and of two little lights in the focal plane of that lens, the phenomena, which apply to our method, can be made visible on a screen.

Sir David Brewster closes his paper with the following striking words: "And this is but one of numerous proofs, which the progress of knowledge is daily accumulating, that the most abstract and apparently transcendental truths in physical science, will, sooner or later, add their tribute to supply human wants, and alleviate human sufferings. Nor has science performed one of the least important of her functions, when she enables us, either in our own case, or in that of others, to dispel those anxieties and fears, which are the necessary offspring of ignorance and error." These words are drawn from life. Every oculist by experience knows their truth. "Few symptoms prove so alarming to persons of a nervous habit or constitution as muscæ volitantes, and they immediately suppose that they are about to lose their sight by cataract or amaurosis." Often, alas! this anxiety is even still kept up by ignorant practitioners. But nothing is easier than to convince such gloomy patients, who have usually already acquired some knowledge of the eye, that the seat of the phenomenon is to be met with in the vitreous humour, and not in the nerve: they readily comprehend the signification of the double shadows by comparison with an experiment with two lights, which can give double shadows of an object on a wall, only when the object does not lie against the wall. Under what circumstances complaints of muscæ volitantes may have a dangerous signification, shall be pointed out in treating of myopia.

I formerly wrote a detailed essay (*Ned. Lancet*, 2e Serie, D. 11) on the employment of entoptic investigation in the diagnosis of defects of the eye. Now that (thanks to the valuable invention of Helmholtz) the ophthalmoscope is in our hands, the importance of the entoptic mode of examination for diagnosis is thrown completely into the shade.

---

§ 16. Range of Accommodation, modified by Age.—Presbyopia. —Hypermetropia acquisita.

The refraction of the eye, and still more the range of accommodation, become modified with the increase of years. The diminution of the power of accommodation first takes place; it is perceptible long before the refractive condition of the eye in the state of rest has undergone any modification: for the distance R of the farthest point continues long unchanged, while P, that of the nearest point of distinct vision, becomes gradually greater and greater. Thus the range of accommodation diminishes.

The progressive removal of p is a fact of universal experience. People are, however, generally of opinion that this retrogression commences first about the fortieth year. But this is an error. Not until about that time of life, under some circumstances, does the retrogression of p make itself felt as a *disturbance* in the normal eye, and therefore attention is then first directed to this so-called weakness of the eye; but already in youth—nay, even before puberty—p moves considerably back. This change affects all eyes without distinction, as well the myopic (provided it be healthy) as the hypermetropic and the emmetropic eye.

In the first place, it may here be asked, in general, how and from what cause it is, that at so early a period of life, while all the functions, and especially that of the muscles, are in a state of progressive development, the power of accommodation, which depends upon muscular action, already loses in extent? As it must be admitted, that the ciliary muscle has continued normal, and is therefore still in full force, we come readily to the inference that, at least in the first instance, the diminution is to be sought exclusively in the condition of the parts, which in accommodation are passively altered, and by no means in the state of those whereby the change is actively produced. Now the organ which is passively altered is the lens. Is the early diminution of the range of accommodation $\frac{1}{A}$ to be explained from this? We know that at an advanced time of life the lens is firmer than in youth. I think I may even assert that the increase of firmness commences at an early period. Now, it is in consequence of this greater firmness that the same muscular action can no longer produce the same change in the form of the lens. It is therefore very probable that the early diminution of $\frac{1}{A}$ depends thereon.

After the power of accommodation has considerably decreased, a slight diminution of refraction gradually takes place. This appears from the fact that now also r begins to remove from the eye, and that, consequently, the posterior focus is transferred to a greater depth in the organ, or even to behind the retina. But, as I have already remarked, the diminution of refraction is not perceptible until a late period of life. At the fortieth year, it has not at all, or has scarcely commenced, and it is not until the sixtieth or seventieth year that it is distinctly present in an originally emmetropic eye. On account of the simultaneously diminished range of accommodation, the visual lines being parallel, the eye can then frequently not be accommodated, even for remote objects, and a positive glass is therefore required also for distance.

The doubt might be raised, whether the diminution in refraction is not only apparent,—whether in all those cases in which, at a later period of life, H is observable, an equal degree of latent H did not already exist in youth. If this were so, the change should be referrible exclusively to diminution of $\frac{1}{A}$. We are, however, justified in declaring this doubt to be unfounded. Sometimes a certain degree of

H is developed in relatively so short a time, especially when traces of obscuration arise, and, as it appears, also in glaucoma, that there is no ground whatever to assume the original existence of the same degree of H. Moreover, I have in myopia also occasionally satisfied myself of the presence of a diminution of refraction. Finally, and this in itself is convincing, at an advanced period of life H is much more common than in youth. The question therefore is, on what the diminution of refraction depends. Flattening of the cornea, and lessened circumference of the eyeball, the visual axis of which should thus have become shorter, have been suggested. It seems to me more probable that the cause is to be sought in the lens. It is generally known that, at a more advanced time of life the latter, together with the iris, moves forward, and this renders the cornea apparently flatter. But this displacement of the lens should in itself have precisely the opposite effect, and should move the focus somewhat forward. There must consequently be another cause, which, in spite of this influence, lessens the refraction. This, if I am not mistaken, is to be sought chiefly in a more uniform firmness of the several layers of the lens. Even Thomas Young remarked, and it has been more fully demonstrated by Senff, Listing, and others (compare p. 39), that with the laminated structure, with refractive power diminishing towards the periphery, the lens has a shorter focal distance than a lens of similar form, and composed wholly of a substance of the refractive power proper to the nucleus of the lens, would have. If, consequently, with the advance of years, the outer layers become more solid, a greater focal distance must be the result. Now, the existence of this increase of solidity is evident from the increasing reflection in advanced life on the anterior and posterior surfaces of the lens, a reflection which is proportional to the difference in refractive power between the outer layers of the lens and the aqueous or vitreous humour; and it is also capable of being established by anatomical investigation. But, in addition to this, in advanced life the lens appears to become flatter, on which account the radii of curvature of its surfaces, and its focal distance, are increased.—I have satisfied myself (see p. 89) that the cornea does not become flatter, and I have no reason to assume that the visual axis should become shorter, except in the most extreme old age. I therefore believe that the cause of the state of diminished refraction must be sought in the above-mentioned changes in the lens. In favour of this view is also the circumstance that the diminution of refraction at last goes hand in hand with the diminution of the power of accommodation: indeed this points to a common origin, and we have above seen that the latter depends upon a hardening of the lens.—The vitreous humour I have not compared, with reference to its refractive power, at different times of life. It is self-evident that, as its anterior surface is concave, an *increase* of its refractive power must move the posterior focus of the eye *backwards*.

As I have above remarked, the changes in accommodation and refraction occur in each form of the eye. We have here to subject to a more accurate examination only those which take place in the emmetropic organ.

Fig. 104 represents the course of the nearest *p p*, and of the

Fig. 104.

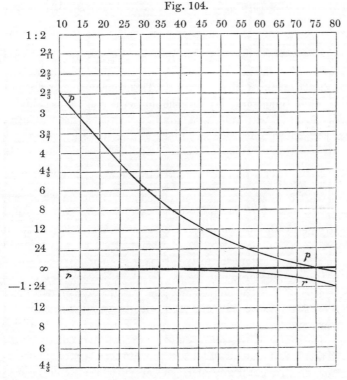

farthest points *r r*, and consequently that of the power of accommodation in the emmetropic eye, at different periods of life. The figure needs but little explanation. The numbers, to the left, indicate, as before, the distance in Parisian inches, for which accommodation can take place; those, which are lower than ∞, have, as in the previous figures, a negative signification: they represent the distance at which the converging rays, for which the eye is accommodated, come to a focus behind the nodal point. The numbers placed above the figure, indicate the age, expressed in years. On the lines $p\,p$ and $r\,r$ we can, therefore, for each year of life, read off the nearest and the farthest points of distinct vision, while, at the same time, the distance between these two lines exhibits the range of accommodation; the distance between two transverse lines is again $= \dfrac{1}{24}$ accommodation.

From the figure it directly appears, that, even from the tenth year, at which the observation becomes possible, p approaches the eye, and indeed with tolerably uniform rapidity, so that at the thirtieth year $\dfrac{1}{A}$ has fallen to about one-half what it was at the tenth year. From this time the descent appears to take place somewhat more slowly, but nevertheless to proceed incessantly to the most advanced time of life. The course of the farthest point is quite different. Up to the fortieth year it remains at the same height; but from that time an extremely slow descent occurs, the emmetropic eye becoming, at the fiftieth year, somewhat hypermetropic, which H at the eightieth year amounts to from $\dfrac{1}{24}$ to $\dfrac{1}{10}$. This acquired hypermetropia may, finally, become absolute, that is to say, that not only accommodation for divergent, but even for parallel, rays becomes impossible. I have not unfrequently met with this in persons at sixty years of age, who in their youth probably exhibited no H whatever. This was inferred when they did not before the forty-fifth year of their life, need spectacles in the evening for minute work.

The course of p in the emmetropic eye was deduced from a great number of observations. In Fig. 105 each observation is indicated by a point, and the position of these points shows at the same time that the deviations of the mean course are not particularly great. And still these must undoubtedly be in part ascribed to error in observation; in some a slight degree of H may also increase the deviations. In the preparation of this table, emmetropic eyes were, for the most part, used; but also eyes, affected with a slight degree of M ($= 1:40$

or less), were not excluded. These last even deserve to be preferred. Indeed, in these alone we have, without artificial paralysis

Fig. 107.

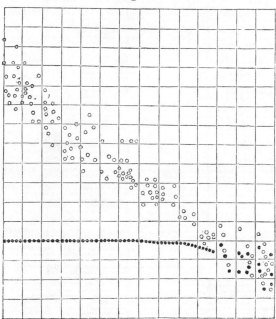

of accommodation, sufficient security that the nearest point is not influenced by a latent H, and we may safely assume that, with these degrees of M, $\frac{1}{A}$ is equal to that of the emmetropic eye. In proportion to the M ascertained, p was of course reduced. Lastly, I should observe, that when p appeared to lie at a greater distance than 8″, it was always calculated from a determination, made with the aid of positive glasses. It was thus brought to the distance of about 8″. If this were not done, then, on account of the absence of convergence, $\frac{1}{A}$ would, in advanced life, be computed too low.

On the diminution of refraction just described, and especially on that of the accommodation, depends a condition which has been termed presbyopia, Pr. Presbyopia has been set down as synonymous with *farsightedness*. By this we by no means wish to convey, that

14

the eye sees accurately at a great distance, for of this the young emmetropic and moderately hypermetropic eye is also capable. We wish only to express the fact, that it cannot see near objects accurately. In like manner we call a person near-sighted, not because he can distinguish small objects close to the eye,—for this too the young emmetropic eye enjoys in common with the near-sighted one, but because he does not see well at a great distance.

I will not, however, dwell upon the incorrectness of the English expression farsightedness. It is only the idea I would refer to, and this deserves to be more closely examined.

In this respect I would first observe, that only that farsightedness is to be considered as Pr, which is dependent on the diminution of $\frac{1}{A}$, as the result of advanced life. The very etymology of the word, compounded of πρέσβυς, old, and ὤψ, eye, indicates this. Were we to term every impediment to the accurate vision of near objects Pr, paralysis of the power of accommodation should be placed in the same category. Even H, so far as with it vision of distant, is easier than that of near objects, should be comprehended under the term, and we have made it clear enough to what great confusion of ideas we should, by so doing, give rise. (Compare § 6). *The term presbyopia is, therefore, to be restricted to the condition, in which, as the result of the increase of years, the range of accommodation is diminished and the vision of near objects is interfered with.*

From this definition it appears, that Pr is really included in the diminution of the range of accommodation dependent on advancing years. Still Pr is the normal quality of the normal, emmetropic eye in advanced age. It is, therefore, properly speaking, no more an anomaly than are grey hairs or wrinkling of the skin. Were it an anomaly, it should be much less one of refraction than of accommodation.

But where are we to place the commencement of presbyopia? If we consult the line pp' of Fig. 106, representing the emmetropic eye at different times of life, it appears that, from youth up to extreme old age, p removes with tolerable regularity more and more from the eye, and that, consequently, the vision of near objects becomes progressively more and more difficult. A stop in the line is nowhere observed.

Hence it follows, that in fixing a limit of Pr, we cannot avoid being arbitrary. In the eye itself, no reason is to be found, for making a definite distinction between presbyopic and non-presbyopic. Now, if the boundary be artificial, it must be conventional.

This, however, leads us to the question, whether it is necessary to speak of Pr, and whether we should not rather confine ourselves to fixing $\frac{1}{A}$, in connexion with the degree of M or of H, where these are found. Undoubtedly this mode would be scientifically satisfactory. Nevertheless we should, in my opinion, meet with but little response, were we to get rid of so generally known and extensively employed a word. I believe also that by so doing we should confer no favour upon practice. In practice, a word is required, which may indicate the condition in which the eye, at an advanced period of life, must, for ordinary close work, use positive spectacles, and this word is *presbyopia*.

However, with all this the commencement of Pr is not yet defined. That this must be done, is evident.

Our social condition requires that we should often be engaged in reading, writing, or other close work. It is plain that the average magnitude of the forms employed in such work, is closely connected with the accuracy of the power of vision, and with the distance of distinct vision for the normal eye. The same is true of the productions of art and of a number of trades. What the human eye, in the full power of life can do, has in general afforded the standard for this. Before the general application of spectacles the standard was undoubtedly different. If these instruments were no longer to be obtained by all, a larger type in general should replace that at present in use. The common employment of spectacles has, therefore, exercised an influence on the limits of distinct vision, with which we must allow presbyopia to commence. The changeableness of these limits thus appears most prominently. We have to investigate how long the eye fulfils the requirements of the assumed standard. Even in the thirtieth year the normal eye dislikes the small print, which the near-sighted person prefers and youth does not avoid. Still, in the fortieth year ordinary type presents no difficulty whatever to the emmetropic eye. In the forty-fifth year the notes, printed in smaller characters, are not unfrequently passed over, and the book is in the evening probably somewhat earlier laid aside. We now soon begin to observe, that an object, to be very accurately seen, is removed a little further from the eye; a clear light is also sought, rather for the purpose of

2

diminishing the circles of diffusion, in imperfect accommodation, by narrowing the pupil, than of obtaining more brilliantly illuminated images. Ordinary occupations are, however, even in the evening, still performed uninterruptedly without remarkable exertion. But where minute matters, which now and then occur, are to be accurately seen, comes the complaint, however unwillingly, from the lips, that our eyes are no longer what they were. The binocular nearest point p_2 now often lies at about 8″ from the eye. At this point I have already placed the commencement of presbyopia. I think too that I must now keep to it. In the following §, however, we shall see, that this does not always, and indeed not even in general, involve the use of spectacles.

If we have agreed upon a definite distance as the commencement of Pr, this may serve also to fix the degree of the presbyopia. This is done in a very simple manner. If, that is to say, p_2 be situated at n Parisian inches from the eye, then, assuming the above mentioned limit, $Pr = \dfrac{1}{8} - \dfrac{1}{n}$. Thus, if p_2 lie at 16 inches, $Pr = \dfrac{1}{8} - \dfrac{1}{16} = \dfrac{1}{16}$; if p_2 lie at 24″, $Pr = \dfrac{1}{8} - \dfrac{1}{24} = \dfrac{1}{12}$. For this glasses of about $\dfrac{1}{8} - \dfrac{1}{n}$ are required, and, in the examples given, glasses of $\dfrac{1}{16}$ and $\dfrac{1}{12}$, to bring p_2 to 8″, and so to neutralise the presbyopia. I say, about, for with the increased convergence, p_2 has somewhat approached the eye. But as, however, in presbyopia, the relative ranges of accommodation have approached much more to those of hypermetropia (Compare p. 126, Fig. 64), we may usually leave this out of the calculation. To be quite accurate, we should be able to determine the degree of Pr from the glass, with which, by means of direct experiment, p_2 is brought to 8″. But, it will be seen still more precisely in the following §, that the determination of the degree of Pr possesses only a subordinate value, on the one hand, because the commencement of Pr is conventional, on the other, because the accommodation complicates the condition, and this, as well as the accuracy of vision, influences the practical application: we should, therefore, take care to attach to the determination of the degree of Pr the great importance, which is connected with that of the degree of M and of H.

Thus far we have treated exclusively of the Pr of the emmetropic eye. But the hypermetropic and the myopic eye are also subject to the same. The first must be called presbyopic, so soon as in the use of glasses, which neutralise the H, p_2 lies farther from the eye than 8″. As to myopics, we hold to the definition given of Pr, and therefore let this first commence, when the distance of p_2 amounts to more than 8″. Hence it follows that it is only to the slight degrees of M, that Pr in the ordinary sense of the word, can belong, that with M $= \frac{1}{8}$ it is almost impossible, even with total loss of the power of accommodation. To this we must add, that in the slight degrees of M it occurs much later than in the emmetropic eye. Herein the myopic finds a compensation for what he loses, with reference to the vision of remote objects. The advantage is not small. Up to the sixtieth or even the seventieth year of our age, not to need spectacles, in order to see accurately whatever comes immediately under our eyes, is a great privilege. This privilege belongs to a M of from $\frac{1}{10}$ to $\frac{1}{14}$, in which degree the eye is not threatened with any special dangers. With slighter degrees of M a good deal of this privilege is still enjoyed. This is a condition which may well be envied by emmetropic eyes. I never found a normal eye which participated in the same advantage. Many persons, however, suppose that they are so highly privileged. Almost daily it occurs that at fifty-five years of age the distance of p_2 lies at only from 8″ to 10″, and spectacles are not yet thought of. Such people consider themselves a lucky exception. They are extremely proud of their sharp sight. The inquiry whether they are near-sighted is answered in the negative with a smile of self-complacency. At a distance of twenty feet hang Snellen's letter-tests : XX and XXX they do not recognise, XL not at all, or scarcely ; L and LX are the first which are easily recognisable to them. Not until they try glasses of $- \frac{1}{50}$ or $- \frac{1}{36}$ do they well distinguish XX, or at least XXX, with accurate contours. Reluctantly they acknowledge themselves beaten. They are consequently somewhat myopic ! It is true they had always attached a wholly different meaning to the idea of M. For the oculist it is, however, important to have proved the existence of this slight degree of M. He learns from it to recognise the unchangeable, the legitimate amount of the range of accommodation attached to each period of life, and he can sometimes also turn this knowledge to his advantage. Thus when we inquire into the hereditary nature of M, its existence in the parents is often denied, yet almost in the same breath it is added, as a proof of their excellent sight, that up to their fiftieth year, nay even longer, they still read and wrote in the evening without spectacles, and—we know what inference is to be drawn. If, on the other hand, a person comes to us, who in order to continue his close work, in his thirty-fifth or fortieth year evidently has need of positive spectacles, we shall almost always find, that a slight degree of H lurks in him. If its degree were somewhat greater, the difficulty would have earlier manifested itself more distinctly, under the character of asthenopia.

The more I investigate the subject, the more fully I am convinced, that at a given time of life the range of accommodation is an almost law-determined quantity. If there are no favourable exceptions, the unfavourable are connected with definite defects, the commencement of cataract or glaucoma simplex,* exhausting diseases, and paresis of accommodation. Of this we shall treat from a clinical point of view, in the following Section.

<hr>

NOTE TO § 17.

As was above remarked, an eye, affected in a higher degree by myopia, can never become presbyopic. It loses with the advance of years in range of accommodation ; the nearest point recedes, and this may be the case even with the farthest point; the physical changes which therewith go hand in hand in the myopic eye, are similar to those of other eyes. But presbyopia never arises : p_2 does not remove to more than 8″ from the eye. Hence appears anew the arbitrary, the conventional nature of the idea of presbyopia. At first I was inclined to attach a more extensive meaning to the word *presbyopia*. I wished to express by it the senile change affecting every eye. "The change," thus I reasoned, "indicated by definite anatomical properties, occurs in every eye without distinction. It gives rise to disturbance in vision, and, indeed, in each form of the eye, to one and the same disturbance, namely, that the eye, whether unaided, or furnished with definite glasses, cannot, at will, distinguish accurately at a great distance and close at hand. This disturbance, peculiar to old age, deserves the name of *presbyopia*."

From the scientific point of view this reasoning is perfectly correct.

* See, on the meaning of *Glaucoma Simplex*, Bowman, in the *British Medical Journal*, October 11, 1862.

Only so long as presbyopia was opposed to myopia, this extensive signification could not be applied to the former term; indeed, so long myopia must exclude presbyopia, and in old myopic individuals, whatever degree the senile change may have attained, the term presbyopia could not be applied. But now that this opposition has ceased, we readily see that the myopic eye also may become presbyopic; and the idea of expressing the senile change with diminished range of accommodation in every eye, without distinction, by the word *presbyopia*, occurs spontaneously to our mind. Moreover, its etymology is in favour of applying a more extensive meaning to the word presbyopia; indeed, since farsightedness occurs generally in old people, it has been called presbyopia; still more correctly should the latter term be connected with the state which is inseparable from advanced years.

On the other hand : *verba valent usu*. This has, finally, weighed more with me than the demands of logic and of etymology. I considered that *practice* has need of a word to signify, that without optical assistance ordinary close occupations can with difficulty be carried on, and I should be unwilling to propose another word to designate this condition. I have therefore retained the word presbyopia in its ancient signification. Only the idea was refined. Strictly was everything eliminated from it which belongs to hypermetropia or paralysis ; the senile change, with diminution of accommodation, was assumed as an essential requisite, and it was not difficult from this point of view to fix the limits of the application of the word presbyopia also to myopic and hypermetropic eyes.

§ 18. Treatment of Presbyopia.

Diminution of the power of accommodation leads, as we have seen, to presbyopia. To this, at a certain time of life, the emmetropic eye is inevitably liable. In youth it sees small objects, by preference and without perceptible tension, at a distance of about six inches. At a later period this distance becomes greater, in spite of powerful effort, in spite of more advantageous management of the still existing accommodation, even at relatively less convergence. Thus the time approaches that close reading and working are attended with difficulty. Presbyopia thus announces itself. Seldom do we hear at the same time that work fatigues. The complaint is rather that vision is not accurate : the letters *n* and *u* are not easily distinguished ; the numbers 3, 5, and 8 are confounded ; a stroke is seen double, a point sometimes multiple, etc. If we place small print in the hand of such a presbyopic person, he begins by holding the book too close to his eye, and does not distinguish; he subsequently very patho-gnomonically moves the book forwards and the head backwards, seeks a bright light, and — reads. The bright light is a principal point, not so much because the retinal images are by it more strongly illuminated, but because the pupil contracts, the circles of diffusion therefore become smaller, and the retinal images less diffused. Therefore, also the individual. first perceives some diffi-culty in twilight, unless it be particularly strong. Inconvenience would have arisen even earlier, if the diminution of accommodation had not been accompanied with diminution of the diameter of the pupil. Thus also the small pupil of the old man makes the loss of the power of accommodation lighter to him: to this he is indebted for the fact that, even at distances for which he is not accurately accommodated, he still distinguishes tolerably well. In full day-light, in the open air, a person can often, even in advanced pres-byopia, read ordinary type, and this always succeeds on looking through a small opening. But much earlier, even before the presbyopia manifests any disturbing influence, the small pupil is of importance, because in reading and writing the accommodation even then leaves something to be desired. To this I would expressly direct attention. The fact is significant, because hence it follows that in commencing presbyopia convex glasses are useful less by correcting the accommodation, than by increasing the sharpness of the retinal images. The eye already puts its accommodation rather strongly upon the stretch (still more powerful tension has no pro-portionate effect) without any hinderance or fatigue whatever. Aided by weak glasses, the eye continues the tension almost in the same manner. The result is therefore, that the eye now sees more accurately: the letters become black, confusion ceases, and the person rejoices in a distinctness of vision, of which he had almost lost the idea.

The correction, by means of positive glasses, in the commencement of the effort, of diminished accuracy of vision of near objects, is the characteristic mark of presbyopia.

From this, it may be stated in one word, the vision of hyper-metropics is evidently distinguished. These obtain perfect accuracy of sight, but only at the cost of so great a tension as they are not able to maintain, and therefore they obtain it only for a short time; weari-ness of accommodation (asthenopia) ensues. In the hypermetropic individual convex glasses aid the accommodation, in the presbyopic they at first rather increase the sharpness of the retinal images.

So soon as, by diminution of accommodation, in ordinary work the required accuracy of vision begins to fail, there is need of convex glasses. The test is, that with weak glasses of from $\frac{1}{80}$ to $\frac{1}{40}$, at the same distance as without glasses, the accuracy of vision is manifestly improved. The opinion is rather general that we should refrain as long as possible from the use of convex glasses. But is it not folly to weary the eyes and the mind together, without any necessity, condemning ourselves to guess with much trouble at the forms, which we could see pretty well with glasses? We have here to do with a prejudice which perhaps finds some support in vanity. It is asserted : practice of accommodation is desirable. Generally speaking, this is perfectly true. To look alternately at distant and at near objects, now to occupy one's self with smaller, now with larger objects, developes and maintains the functions of the eye. But we forget that we were obliged to practise more and more, as years have rolled on, and that by these efforts, increasingly necessitated by the diminishing range of accommodation, the power of using, with moderate convergence, a great part of the latter has already been acquired. The annexed Figures, 108 of a man of four-and-thirty (Dr. Doyer), 109 of a man of four-and-forty (myself), 110 of an emmetropic person aged sixty, compared with that of a person of fifteen (Fig. 111) demonstrate this most evidently. And is it not à

Fig. 108.

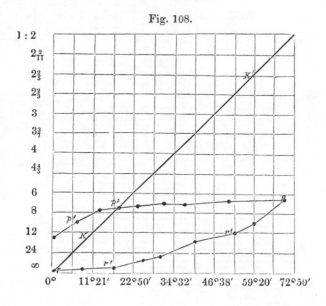

Fig. 109.

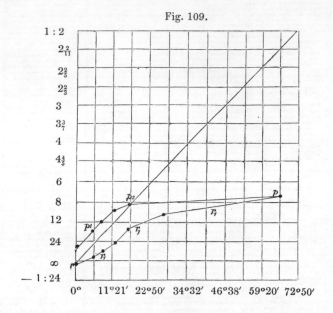

Fig. 110.

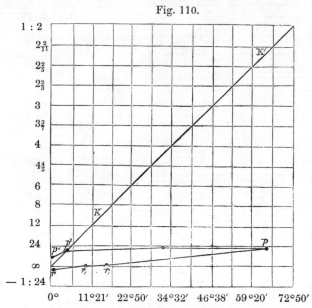

priori to be considered absurd, at nearly fifty years of age, to com-

Fig. 111.

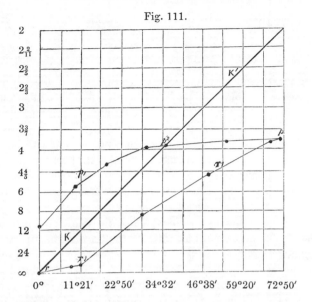

0°   11°21′   22°50′   34°32′   46°38′   59°20′   72°50′

mence a more powerful gymnastic system than youth was ever
called to?

Strangely enough! people have fallen also into the opposite
fault. Some have thought, by the early use of spectacles to be able
to preserve their power of vision: they have recommended and
employed "conservative spectacles." If I am not mistaken, self-
interest had something to do with this recommendation. So long as
the eye does not err, and remains free from fatigue in the work
required of it, its own power is sufficient, and it is inexpedient to
seek assistance in the use of convex glasses. Light blue spectacles
also, which have been sometimes recommended as "conservative
spectacles," are, under ordinary circumstances, objectionable for a
healthy visual organ. Most eyes find their soothing influence
agreeable, and people are therefore readily inclined to employ them.
But, while they withhold from the retina the ordinary stimulus of
white light, they increase its sensibility beyond the normal, and
create a permanent necessity for their employment. Now a more
than normal sensibility is an inconvenience, and at the same time
predetermines to disease.

Easy as it is to decide whether a necessity exists for the employment of convex glasses, so difficult is it to establish rules for ascer-

taining the degree of convexity required. This must, however, be tried here. It is well known, that at first, while as yet scarcely any disturbance has manifested itself, glasses of about $\frac{1}{60}$ are usually sufficient, and also that, in proportion as the time of life advances and the range of accommodation diminishes, stronger and stronger glasses are required. It was therefore natural to arrange convex glasses according to the time of life at which they become necessary. This old custom has been ridiculed, and in some degree with justice. It is true that eyes differ too much, to make age alone the criterion in the choice of spectacles. But, on the other hand, the regular diminution of the range of accommodation, already pointed out (§ 17) shows, that, in the case of emmetropic eyes, the time of life may in general be taken as a guide. Only, the many circumstances which modify the indication furnished by the time of life, are not to be neglected. Besides ametropia, which occupies the first place, diminished acuteness of vision and morbid disturbance of accommodation are to be noted, while, moreover, the nature of the work to be performed has some influence. Of these circumstances we intend to speak from a clinical point of view. But, in order to fulfil a practical object, we shall premise the empirical result: what glasses are required at different ages in emmetropia, with normal acuteness of vision and accommodation, for writing, and for reading ordinary type.

a Age.	Glasses required.		d Distance of Distinct Vision.	e	
	b In present E.	c In original E.		R_2	P_2
48	$\frac{1}{60}$	$\frac{1}{60}$	14″	60″	10″
50	$\frac{1}{40}$	$\frac{1}{40}$	14″	40″	12″
55	$\frac{1}{30}$	$\frac{1}{28}$	14″	30″	12″
58	$\frac{1}{22}$	$\frac{1}{20}$	13″	22ᶠ	12″
60	$\frac{1}{18}$	$\frac{1}{16}$	13″	18″	12″
62	$\frac{1}{14}$	$\frac{1}{12}$	13″	14″	12″
65	$\frac{1}{13}$	$\frac{1}{10}$	12″	13″	11″
70	$\frac{1}{10}$	$\frac{1}{7.5}$	10″	10″	10″
75	$\frac{1}{9}$	$\frac{1}{6.5}$	9″	9″	9″
78	$\frac{1}{8}$	$\frac{1}{5.5}$	8″	8″	8″
80	$\frac{1}{7}$	$\frac{1}{4.5}$	7″	7″	7″

This table needs, perhaps, some explanation. Column b gives the glasses required for E, proved at the moment; c for E in youth, and therefore for H acquisita at the time of observation; in both cases the diminished acuteness of vision belonging to the time of life is taken into account; d indicates the distance which is preferred for vision with these glasses; e, finally, the space through which they admit of acute vision, that is, from R_2 with the least, to P_2 with the greatest convergence $\left(\dfrac{1}{A_2} = \dfrac{1}{P_2} - \dfrac{1}{R_2} \right)$. In general it should be observed, that it is desirable to ascend but slowly with the numbers, to use the first spectacles in the beginning, only in the evening, and to keep these for day spectacles, so soon as stronger glasses are required for the evening, and thus, every time that stronger glasses are required, to continue using the former evening spectacles as day spectacles—finally, that, while stronger glasses are necessary for reading, the weaker are often sufficient for writing, and are to be preferred, since the person wearing them, being enabled to see at a greater distance, can avoid the bent position, which is so injurious to the eyes.

The above table holds good for emmetropic individuals. If ametropia be present, it must be taken into account. Therefore always, without exception, we should begin by determining the refraction, and at the same time S, according to the method described above (§ 9). With sufficient practice, this requires only a couple of minutes. The result obtained supplies the preliminary indication, which must then always be subjected to the control test. If the eye be emmetropic, the control is effected with the glasses mentioned above in column b; we ascertain, at what distance 2 and $2\frac{1}{2}$ are easily and by preference read, and we determine the space of $\dfrac{1}{A_2}$ by causing the patient to read 1 or $1\frac{1}{2}$ as close as possible, and larger type as far as possible. If we now obtain about the results to be found under d and e of the table, the glasses will usually answer. If the distance be too short, the margin for distinct vision too small and brought too near the eye, we must try weaker, and in the opposite case, somewhat stronger glasses.

If we find H, both this and the Pr must be corrected. Let, at 62 years of age, H be found $= \dfrac{1}{14}$, glasses of $\dfrac{1}{14} + \dfrac{1}{14} = \dfrac{1}{7}$ are indicated. $H = \dfrac{1}{20}$ at 55 years of age, indicates glasses of $\dfrac{1}{20} + \dfrac{1}{30} = \dfrac{1}{12}$, etc. Just as in E, we must then in this case

also further test, whether the glasses indicated are actually sufficient.
It will be easily understood that the rule here given for hypermetropic individuals, is applicable only to older hypermetropics,
that is to those who, when the H is neutralised, are presbyopic. It
is in great part H acquisita we have here to deal with; however,
also when H originally existed, the rule described is fully applicable,
provided the time of life have reached nearly fifty years, and, therefore, the range of accommodation, and especially the latent part of
the H, be reduced. If H originally existed, we usually find—at
least thus far I have found it so—that at a later period the eye has
continued to employ too weak glasses. In a couple of trials we then
reach the required strength. What glasses, under different circumstances, young hypermetropics need, shall be treated of in the Chapter
on H.

How far Pr is compatible with M, we have seen above (p. 213).
If $M > \frac{1}{8}$, Pr is, *per se*, excluded; but in slight degrees
of M it occurs at a later period. From the foregoing table
it appears that in emmetropic persons up to the 55th year
glasses of $\frac{1}{40}$, up to the 60th year glasses of $\frac{1}{22}$ are sufficient, etc. Now, if M. of $\frac{1}{40}$, of $\frac{1}{22}$, etc., exists, the necessity of
spectacles will be thought of first in the 55th and 60th years
respectively: indeed the glasses sufficient for these ages communicate to the eye in emmetropic individuals the degrees of M just
mentioned. Now where the myopia does not wholly compensate the
more advanced time of life, it must in each case be subtracted. If,
for example, at 65 $M = \frac{1}{40}$ exists, we shall, in place of glasses of
$\frac{1}{13}$, as in emmetropic persons, find glasses of $\frac{1}{13} - \frac{1}{40} = \frac{1}{19}$ or
$\frac{1}{20}$ sufficient. Generally speaking, I have found that myopics re-
quire convex glasses at a still later period than the degree of M
should have led me to expect, and that the glasses required for
emmetropics admit of a still greater reduction than that indicated
by the degree of myopia. In the above example, we shall often
have to give glasses, not of $\frac{1}{20}$, but only of $\frac{1}{30}$. The reason is,

that, on the one hand, in persons looked upon as emmetropic, a trace of latent H easily occurs, while, on the other, the limited distance (for example, 20 feet, representing $\dfrac{1}{240}$), at which the determination of M takes place, may make it appear somewhat too slight.

We have now to estimate the circumstances, which, both in ametropic and in emmetropic persons, may modify the degree of the glasses required. As such we mentioned

a. A range of accommodation not corresponding to the time of life. Those who are occupied almost the whole day in reading, writing, or other close work, usually accompany their demand for spectacles with the observation that their eyes have certainly suffered much, but that they have also exacted a great deal from them. I hasten to set such people right. Comparative observation has shown me that much close work does not essentially injure the eyes, at least those which are emmetropic, and that the range of accommodation diminishes scarcely, if at all, more rapidly under such circumstances, than it does in agriculturists, sailors, and others, who for the most part look to distant objects. It is true that eyes predisposed to M, are, by much reading and writing, easily rendered more myopic, but these occupations have no influence on the range of accommodation. The same is true of the frequent use of the microscope, or of a magnifying glass, as is required in the work of engravers and watchmakers: the regular course of $\dfrac{1}{A}$ is maintained despite of much or little tension. But there are morbid conditions which cause the range of accommodation, and sometimes also the amount of refraction, to diminish more rapidly than usual. In the first place, general debility, the result of exhausting diseases, is to be noted. Premature old age, in general also deserves to be mentioned. Of the influence of glaucoma I have already spoken. If a person has quickly and repeatedly to strengthen his glasses, we should suspect the existence of glaucoma simplex, and accurately examine the tension of the eyeball and other points connected with this affection. The commencement of cataract also appears to hasten presbyopia, probably through more rapid hardening of the crystalline lens interfering with its mutability of form. Emmetropic persons are then apt to complain that they can no longer accurately distinguish near objects, which is to be attributed partly to diminished S, partly to more rapidly lessening $\frac{1}{A}$, and they seek the aid of spectacles. The morbid condition, which especially interferes prematurely with the vision of near objects, is paresis and paralysis of accommodation. This is not the place to enlarge upon this subject, the last chapter of this work shall be devoted to it. Let it at present suffice to observe, that ordinary paralysis may occur at any time of life, but more particularly in youth, that it usually sets in suddenly, and that it is further characterised by a tolerably wide, immovable, or scarcely movable pupil : it is, therefore, hardly conceivable that it could be confounded with true presbyopia.

Now where, from whatever cause, $\frac{1}{A}$ is abnormally diminished, stronger glasses are required than where $\frac{1}{A}$ is normal. This is particularly true of a comparatively early time of life; but at a more advanced age $\frac{1}{A}$ is already, independently of special disturbance, so reduced, that its action in the convergence, whereby the spectacles produce accurate vision, has scarcely any influence, and that in no case has binocular vision, with the use of the required convex glasses, a margin of any extent. The knowledge of what glasses are necessary follows in this case, where we have not to take the accommodation into account, directly from the refraction and from the distance, at which we desire to see. In order, for example, to see at 12″ (which is sufficient with tolerably good S), the emmetropic person needs glasses of $\frac{1}{12}$; while with $M = \frac{1}{24}$ glasses of $\frac{1}{12} - \frac{1}{24} = \frac{1}{24}$; with $H = \frac{1}{24}$ glasses of $\frac{1}{12} + \frac{1}{24} = \frac{1}{8}$ are necessary. It is another question, whether these may be used. To this we can in general only answer, that the sole difficulty is when the morbid condition is such as to prevent tension of vision. In incipient senile cataract there is usually no difficulty ; in paresis of accommodation, tension of accommodation is, when the acute period is past, even desirable, and this is very much promoted by glasses, whereby the distance of distinct vision remains somewhat greater than the patient would wish ; but in threatening glaucoma,

prudence requires us to avoid tension of the eyes, and we are therefore recommended not to permit, unless exceptionally, the use of
spectacles with which the patient can read or work at near objects.

b. *Diminished acuteness of Vision.*—The distance of distinct vision
at different periods of life, estimated to be necessary, and therefore
to be obtained by means of convex glasses, is in close connexion
with S. Consequently with the increase of years, to which diminution
of S is related, we find this distance lessen (compare the table). Where
morbidly diminished S is concerned, we can take this also into
account in the determination of the glasses: we can cause the
retinal images to become greater about in the same proportion as
the acuteness of vision diminishes. This is to be attained simply by
means of stronger glasses. Not only do these bring the distance of
distinct vision nearer to the eye, but they also make the angle, under
which the object is seen, increase in a still greater ratio than the
distance diminishes (compare p. 152). They can thus render ordinary close work still possible with diminished S. The question
however, is: may this means be employed? We must admit that its
application is liable to great restrictions. In the first place, in acute
diseases of the eye, with diminished S, all tension is injurious, and
the eyes may, in the hope of improvement, be allowed to rest. And,
as to chronic diseases and defects, even in these diminished S cannot
unconditionally be compensated by stronger glasses. In general it
is to be considered that the limits, within which compensation is
possible, are rapidly attained through too great proximity, and that,
in proportion as we approach these limits, the survey of objects
becomes less, and the necessity increases, of keeping the same
distance unchanged, beyond, or short of which, with the range
of accommodation still diminished by glasses and the comparatively
wide pupil, objects cannot be properly distinguished. A peculiar
weariness, in consequence thereof, soon makes itself felt. Moreover
the bent position acts injuriously, which, if the distance of distinct
vision is very short, cannot well be avoided. Where the accommodation and refraction must be aided, convex glasses seldom give any
annoyance; but where the acuteness of vision fails, we must, so far
as practicable, rather meet the difficulty with larger objects than
with larger images, by abnormally diminished distance of the
objects. All this, finally, renders the cases rather rare, in which
the annoyance of diminished S can be met by the use of stronger
glasses. The latter is evidently unadvisable in chronic keratitis or

15

iritis, and even in apparent tendency to inflammation ; in deeper-
seated congestive affections tension is even to be considered dangerous.
It is connected with the least inconvenience in chronic opacity of
the cornea, in uncomplicated incipient cataract,* in congenital amblyopia from unknown causes, and finally in disproportionately
rapidly diminishing acuteness of vision in advanced years—senile
amblyopia.   We should, under these circumstances, recommend the
use of large type, and in general, occupation with coarser work ; but
if fine work cannot be avoided, the glasses required should be
strengthened so far, that the desirable degree of distinct vision should,
without too much effort, be obtained.   That we must sometimes

---

* Cataract or opacity of the lens is divided into primary and secondary :
the latter is developed secondarily, in consequence of diseases of the fundus
oculi (chorioiditis, retinitis, etc.), extending through the vitreous humour to
the lens.   The first is considered to arise independently and primarily in the
lens.   The secondary nature of cataract we may infer, when the preceding disease of the fundus oculi is recognised, or when the field of vision
is limited or the power of vision has evidently suffered more than is
to be explained by the obscuration.   To look upon all other cases as
primary is, however, an error.   Where the characters, just mentioned, are
wanting, the cataract is nevertheless often secondary.   I will go so far as to
assert, that in comparatively young persons spontaneous primary cataract
very rarely occurs.   Often we can, in the commencement, establish the presence of slight deviations in the fundus oculi ; not unfrequently also we find
turbidity of the vitreous humour, and rarely are the phenomena absent
which indicate a congestive condition.   The primary disturbance need not
therefore interfere much with the power of vision ; especially when it is
situated in the anterior part of the chorioidea, little or no inconvenience is
felt from it.   But that in many cases some disturbance of the function of the
retina is connected with it, is shown by the improvement of S, which is very
often obtained in the commencement of cataract, by therapeutic treatment,
—and even by the discharge of the aqueous humour, without the opacity
of the crystalline lens (it has been very ingenuously admitted) undergoing
the least change.   A practical observation may here be made :—Through
a certain charlatanophobia (*sit venia verbo*), which made charlatanism to be
seen where it did not exist, many have thought they ought to refrain from
all treatment in the commencement of cataract.   Now this is certainly not
for the interest of the patients.   To think of solution or diminution of senile
cataract, appears to me, from a physiological point of view, an absurdity.
Other morbid changes of the lens give way also only in exceptional cases.
But bearing in mind the frequent complications, treatment is here often
desirable, and hygienic prescriptions are absolutely necessary.   Therefore,
too, great caution is requisite with reference to allowing the use of convex
glasses.

at a very short distance, for the sake of binocular vision, have to contend with the difficulties of convergence, will immediately more fully appear.

c. The nature of the work to be performed.—Two points are here to be distinguished. In the first place, the minuteness of the objects, which renders it necessary that the work should be performed close to the eye, and therefore with relatively stronger glasses. For some work even the young normal eye is insufficient. Minute drawing, engraving, watch-making, and some anatomical operations, require the constant use of the magnifying glass. In other work the eye must at least, with normal S, be still accommodated for the distance of from 4″ to 6″. Hence convex glasses are even early necessary to render permanent accommodation for that distance possible. But, apart from its minuteness, the nature of the work sometimes requires a definite distance : in writing in large registers, in reading in the pulpit, in the use of certain musical instruments, it is often desirable that spectacles should bring the distance of distinct vision to one and a-half or two feet, and therefore weaker glasses are necessary than are given for writing, and particularly for reading. Guided by sound principles, we very soon find practically what glasses fulfil the object : an insuperable difficulty springs only from diminished S ; with this, as shall hereafter appear, we have to contend most in the case of M.

I have thus, I think, laid down the principal points which must guide us in the choice of spectacles for presbyopic persons. Some observations on the form of these auxiliary glasses may here not be out of place. In general, oval glasses in a frame, with wings resting on the ears, placed at a certain inclination, so that in work the axes of the glasses coincide nearly with the axes of vision, are to be preferred. The nasal portion should have such a form, that in looking at a distance, in the horizontal direction, the person wearing the spectacles should be able to look over the glasses ; and if this should be attended with any difficulty, the rings might be flattened above (the pantoscopic spectacles of Smee). Some men, from habit, wish for round glasses, which we may safely allow : they are usually old, quiet men, who, when they desire to look at distant objects, simply take off their spectacles. Others are not at all content with looking, thus unaided, at distant objects over their spectacles ; they prefer, as hypermetropics, wearing spectacles insufficient to read with, and they do not see accurately over their reading-glasses ; or

2

they have at the same time M and Pr, and desire with rapid alternation to read through their spectacles, and to see distant objects,
whether in their office, or as teachers in a school, or in the theatre,
or elsewhere. This wish may be gratified by means of glasses
à double foyer. With these some express themselves satisfied;
in the case of others, rays fall at the same time through both surfaces of curvature upon the eye, and these give them up again. I
found these glasses most satisfactory for presbyopic painters, who
require to look through the upper half, at a certain distance, at
persons or at nature, while the lower half is to bring the distance
of distinct vision on the canvass or on the paper. White Cooper*
states, that Sir Joshua Reynolds was much in the habit of using
such glasses when painting his inimitable portraits.

The stronger the glasses are, the more attention must be paid to their
mutual distance. Great accuracy is seldom required either in Pr—
where somewhat more or less convergence of the visual lines has so
little influence on the accommodation—or in youthful range of accommodation, which leaves a proportional space for the binocular. Therefore, it is usually sufficient to mention to the optician only when
either a particularly great or a particularly short distance of the
glass-bearing rings is necessary, and in the absence of such direction
to let the medium be used; in giving directions, let it be borne
in mind that the less the distance for which the glasses are to be
used, the closer they must be to one another. But, so soon as
insufficiency of the internal or external recti muscles in binocular
vision threatens to give rise to muscular asthenopia, it is of importance that the mutual distance of the glasses should not aggravate
this, but should rather counteract it. Now, less convergence of the
visual lines is required when convex glasses are placed nearer to one
another, and concave further from one another, and *vice versâ*.
If, therefore, the internal recti muscles are insufficient, we should
take care that the axes of the convex glasses are closer to one
another than the visual lines; in this manner we can, where strongly
convex glasses are necessary, very much assist the internal muscles,
and the images obtained are not perceptibly worse than those we
get with a similar effect through prismatic glasses. Whether
spherical glasses alone are sufficient, and how great their mutual
distance must be, we can ascertain best with the frame of v. Jaeger
(compare p. 97). If they are insufficient, we should give the com-

* *On Near Sight, etc.* London, 1853, p. 201.

binations with prismatic glasses, or perform tenotomy according to the indications laid down by von Graefe.* Nearly always, where strongly convex glasses are required to make binocular vision possible at a short distance, it is desirable, by placing the glasses comparatively near one another, to assist the internal recti muscles of the eye. Where very short distances are concerned, the *dissecting spectacles*, constructed and recommended by Bruecke,† with convex prismatic glasses, come into operation. Besides the spectacles, two kinds of *lorgnettes* are in use. Those ordinarily employed by ladies, where the glasses are at a fixed distance, are attended with no inconvenience when it is necessary to look for a short time, or to do anything for which both hands are not required, for one is occupied in holding the glass. But, for constant use, we should at the same time give a pair of spectacles. The glasses of the *lorgnette* may be somewhat stronger: during the short time they are used, no injury is experienced, and the advantage is gained of being able, when necessary, to distinguish smaller things. In the so-called nipping spectacles, used particularly by gentlemen, the distance of the glasses, determined by the thickness of the nose, is usually too short. Therefore, if the glasses are strong, the person wearing them sees with too slight convergence, unless the short distance of the rings be compensated by the axes being placed to the outside of the centre.

Reading-glasses, which magnify the visual angle, and are thus in some cases useful, give at the same time to the rays proceeding from a point a direction, as if they proceeded from a more remote point. Myopics can therefore make use of reading-glasses only when they come nearer to the object than the distance at which their farthest point lies. The recession of the objects increases with the increase of the distance between object and glass. So soon as the distance is equal to the focal distance of the glass, the rays proceed in a parallel direction, and the object appears to be at an infinite distance. Thus far therefore emmetropics can, provided the accommodation be totally relaxed, see through the reading-glass, and thus attain the highest degree of magnifying power; simple presbyopics, who put their accommodation little upon the stretch, always keep the glass nearly at this distance, because they soon see less accurately when the glass approaches the object. At what distance the eye is from

* *Archiv*, B. viii., Abth. 2.
† *Archiv*, B. v., Abth. 2, p. 180.

the glass, is of little consequence: only the field of vision becomes less, in proportion as the eye removes. If the distance between the object and the reading-glass becomes greater than the focal distance of this last, the rays fall convergingly into the eye, and it is in this manner that hypermetropics, and especially hypermetropic presbyopics, make use with much advantage of a reading-glass, and by its means obtain a high magnifying power.

In the use of reading-glasses binocular vision is usually sacrificed: the one eye looks through, the other close to the reading-glass, best with nearly parallel visual lines; on account of their indistinctness the images have no disturbing influence on the second eye, and the spectator even fancies that he sees binocularly.

If no great magnifying power be desired, we can also see binocularly through one glass, for which purpose the latter must then be held closer to the object. In doing so less convergence of the visual lines, and at the same time less tension of accommodation, is required, than in looking at the same object without the intervention of a reading-glass, and the object therefore appears, according to the laws of stereoscopy, to lie further off. However, even in the commencement of presbyopia, the tension of accommodation required is, in reference to the necessary convergence, quite too great, so that binocular vision through the same glass is possible only for young persons, and for older individuals, who are somewhat myopic. It is best attained, even in incipient presbyopia, when we begin by holding the glass at first near the object, and then gradually remove it. In general, however, it must be stated, that binocular vision through a reading-glass is possible to presbyopics only when they are, in addition, aided by weak convex spectacles.* Consequently these glasses in general serve only for monocular vision, and they are especially to be recommended for the purpose of magnifying minute objects of art. For reading their use is seldom advisable. They come, however, under notice where diminished S renders a magnifying power necessary, which is obtainable by means of spectacles only for a short dis-

---

* It may, in passing, be observed, that an emmetropic person (the myopic and the hypermetropic, of course, also, when their ametropia is reduced) can combine two figures stereoscopically through a reading-glass. The figures must, however, lie closer to one another than for ordinary stereoscopy, and as, with too strong convergence, we see the image situated to the right with the left eye, and *vice versâ*, the figures must also be changed, the left for the right, and *vice versa*, if we wish not to see them pseudo-stereoscopically.

tance from the eye. For the special purpose of reading, broad glasses, ground above and below, are the most suitable, and in particular bicylindrical convex glasses, with intersecting axes, deserve to be recommended : the dioptric action of these glasses (compare *Astigmatism*) is nearly equal to that of spherical glasses ; but they are distinguished by the fact that they have the greatest field of distinct vision in the direction perpendicular to the axis of the surface turned towards the eye, so that by turning the surface with vertical axis towards the eye, we possess in reading the advantage of having a good image over an extensive field in the horizontal direction.

No particular results are observed from the use of convex glasses. It is, however, true, that when a person with still sufficient $\frac{1}{A}$, in ordinary work regularly employs them—in other words, renders himself myopic, the relative $\frac{1}{A}$ will change, and be modified in the same direction as in myopic individuals, and that, consequently, although $\frac{1}{A}$ should not subsequently be changed, he will have difficulty in accommodating himself permanently for the distance of the point of convergence. For this reason also, I gave my opinion against the so-called conservative spectacles, that is, against the premature use of convex glasses : they then soon become a necessity, and hasten in emmetropic persons the difficulty of seeing accurately at the distance in the point of convergence. Even after a single trial this may be observed, but of course it then soon disappears again. In using optical instruments with one eye, we generally lay it down as a rule, that in order to avoid injuring the organ, it must be relaxed to its farthest point. I have for many years kept this in view in employing the microscope and in the use of magnifying glasses. However, the idea of the proximity of the object easily produces a slight convergence ; and if I have, avoiding all tension of accommodation, continued this for some time, I experience difficulty, on discontinuing it, in accommodating for the point of convergence : this difficulty continues longer, the longer I had, at a certain convergence, relaxed my power of accommodation as much as possible. I cannot, therefore, recommend to the emmetropic to totally relax his accommodation in using the microscope, the less so, because by doing this, he will soon find difficulty in applying, in measuring, the method à *double vue*, which in so many respects commends itself to our adoption.

Essential injuries to sight, which are often, with so much exaggeration, predicted, I have never seen arise, even from an undue use of convex glasses. On the contrary, as will appear in the Chapter on M, an inconsiderate use of concave glasses may be very dangerous.

NOTE TO § 18.

I have thought it well to exemplify the application of the precepts I have laid down respecting the use of convex glasses, by some cases taken from life. The reader will excuse me if this, for him, is quite superfluous.

1. *Commencement of simple presbyopia.*—D., a clerk, aged 48, asks for spectacles, because he begins gradually to find greater difficulty in distinguishing small writing in the evening, and sometimes makes mistakes in figures. His work does not otherwise fatigue him. He has $S = \dfrac{20}{20}$ (he sees No. XX at 20' distance), is emmetropic (sees XX at 20' not so well through either $\dfrac{1}{60}$ or $-\dfrac{1}{60}$), and by daylight reads 1½ with greater ease at 16″ than at 10″. He receives glasses of $\dfrac{1}{60}$, which give a space of from 7″ to 5′, to use in the evening, and also by day in dark weather, and subsequently when he experiences difficulty, regularly. When the necessity has become constant, the period will have approached at which the advisability of strengthening the evening glasses must be considered.—After some weeks, he states that he can no longer dispense with the spectacles in the evening. We readily believe him.

2. *Moderate Pr, with a desire to see at more than the usual distance.*—Mr. R., aged 58, is emmetropic, has $S = \dfrac{17}{20}$ and uses spectacles of $\dfrac{1}{16}$, which give him in reading a binocular space of from 16″ to 11″. With these spectacles he sees well, with the book in his hand; but his handwriting, which, while he is lecturing, lies at 20″, he does not easily distinguish, and his auditors are in a mist. He gets periscopic glasses of $\dfrac{1}{24}$, with rings flattened above, which he finds to meet all his requirements. He may use the same glasses in writing and for ordinary reading by day. For reading small print in the evening, his glasses of $\dfrac{1}{16}$ are to be recommended.

3. *Advanced Pr, with H. acq. and diminished S.*—L., aged 73, has

$H = \frac{1}{36}$, $S = \frac{11}{20}$, is fond of reading ("the only thing which remained to him"), and cannot do so correctly with his spectacles, particularly in the evening; he is soon tired. He has glasses of $\frac{1}{10}$, which make P_2 nearly $=$ $R_2 = 13''$. He gets glasses of $\frac{1}{7}$, sees with them at $9''$, and is quite satisfied. Large print is recommended to him. With the ophthalmoscope we see, when the axes of vision are directed downwards, traces of radiating opacity, which, however, are not the cause of the diminished S. I do not hesitate to permit him the free use of the spectacles, nor shall I hesitate to give him stronger glasses, when, with diminishing S and increasing H, the latter shall be more agreeable to him.

4. *Commencement of Presbyopia, with myopia.*—Prof. S., aged 56, cannot sufficiently praise the excellence of his sight. "I see admirably at a distance, read, write, and draw without difficulty, even in the evening." "Go on," is my answer. Prof. S., aged 62 : "I still usually see very well, but the work is sometimes difficult to me in the evening. Should I also need spectacles?" He reads $1\frac{1}{2}$ by preference at $14''$, deciphers it still at $18''$, and therefore has $S =$ about $\frac{1\cdot5}{1\cdot5}$; on the contrary, without spectacles, only $\frac{16}{30}$, and with $-\frac{1}{10}$, to his amazement, $\frac{18}{20}$. "Was I then really myopic?" He gets $\frac{1}{60}$, with a recommendation to use them in the evening. "These glasses magnify, and at a moderate distance, for example $2'$, I see by no means so well with as without glasses." I answer : "That is unavoidable, at 60 years of age we can with no glasses in the world see both distant and near objects, but set the spectacles somewhat lower, so that at pleasure you can see over them, or use rings flattened above."

5. *Slight H, requiring convex glasses before the usual age.*—Madame v. L. complains : "I have done much work, and spoiled my eyes ; I am only 36 years of age, and I can no longer see anything in the evening." "Not read?" "O yes, but I can do no fine work, and reading also tires me ; I get terrible neuralgic headach, for which my doctor, and also Dr. K., the homœopath, have given me all sorts of things in vain." She has $S = \frac{20}{20}$, with $\frac{1}{36}$ more easily still $S = \frac{20}{20}$, and therefore $Hm = \frac{1}{36}$. She will derive benefit from glasses of $\frac{1}{36}$. "Must I then use spectacles?" "It is desirable, indeed necessary, even by day, particularly if you wish to be free from your nervous headach. Besides, by the proper use of spectacles, when you are alone, you avoid fatigue, and you will now and then be able in company to work at intervals without glasses." "Is it not the case that I have spoiled my eyes?" "Not in the least ; the form of your eye is the original cause of your requiring spectacles at a comparatively early age. Perhaps other instances of the same are to be met with in your family?"

"It is possible, but I had always such good eyes, and can see so far. Can I do nothing to strengthen them?" "Often rest is the chief thing. Cool them now and then. Rub, if you choose, a little eau de Cologne over the eyebrows, but put nothing into the eyes, and depend upon it, the spectacles will cure your nervous headach."

6. *Pr, with M; reading at more than the usual distance.*—Madame U., aged 65, can in clear daylight still easily read good print. M is suspected and found $= \frac{1}{32}$, $S = \frac{18}{20}$. She has spectacles of $\frac{1}{24}$, but these tire her, and the letters are not black. R_2 is at the same time $= 13''$, P_2 not much less. Somewhat surprised at her statement, I request her to hold the book in her usual way. She lays it flat on the table, holds herself quite straight on her chair, and is thus at a distance of nearly 16''. Evidently for such use the spectacles were too strong; she required $\frac{1}{36}$, which gave her a space of from 17'' to 15''. For very small type she would do well to use the stronger glasses. "I never read small print," was her answer.

7. *Rapidly decreasing accommodation, with incipient cataract.*—Heer B., aged 45. His vision has for some time been less accurate than it was, particularly for near objects, and he has used spectacles only at his work. I suspect the existence of slight H. It appears, however, that the eyes are emmetropic, with $S = \frac{14}{20}$. Without spectacles he cannot read even III, for which, with perfect accommodation for 1' distance, only $S = \frac{1}{3}$ would be necessary. There is, therefore, evidently a very slight power of accommodation. The ophthalmoscope and focal illumination reveal radiating opacity of the lens, particularly inferiorly, with extremely slight granular turbidity. Thus the diminution of S and of $\frac{1}{A}$ is explained. The papilla nervi optici is redder (capillary hyperæmia) than is proper to the time of life; the fundus is otherwise normal. With $\frac{1}{20}$ III is easily read at 13''; r_2 lies at the same time at about 18''; p_2 at 10''. He must make only moderate use of these glasses, avoid too much laterally incident light, beware of a bent position, and to this end write at an inclined desk, take care to keep his feet warm, avoid whatever can cause congestion of the head, cool his eyes often with cold water, frequently rub a spirituous fluid strongly over his eyebrows, report himself again at the end of six months, or sooner if anything particular should occur. I say nothing of cataract; "his eyes are in a congested state."

8. *Rapidly increasing presbyopia with H acquisita, with glaucoma simplex.* —Madame K, aged 54, saw perfectly well until her 47th year; in her 48th year she began to use weak spectacles for fine work in the evening; these answered her purpose up to her 52nd year, she then got stronger glasses, but now constantly requires still stronger, and even with them she does not see with facility. She complains of weariness and a feeling of pressure.

At present she uses $\frac{1}{12}$, and with them sees at 14″, not much closer. This great distance is explained by $H\frac{1}{36}$, which, in connexion with her accurate vision at 47, is looked upon as acquisita. In any case, $\frac{1}{A}$ seems to be very limited. However, S is $=\frac{21}{20}$, and is therefore very satisfactory. On handling the eyeball, it feels too hard (T_1 on the right and T_2 on the left eye, according to Bowman). This indicates *glaucoma simplex*. With the ophthalmoscope commencing excavation of the optic nerve is recognised, and on slight pressure with the little finger arterial pulsation; there is no restriction, but in feeble light there is less certain distinguishing of the fingers in the inner part of the field of vision. The iris, the size and mobility of the pupil, the depth of the chamber of the eye, and the sensibility of the organ, are still normal; there are no coloured rings about the candles; the subconjunctival vessels are perhaps somewhat dilated. I speak seriously to her: "There is the commencement of a disease of much consequence, which is sometimes rapidly, sometimes slowly developed. Art can, however, prevent it, for this I can answer. I shall expect to see you again in a month. If redness or pain come on, come to me immediately, even if you are indisposed, for by neglect, but by neglect alone, irretrievable blindness might be the result. I shall give you a few lines for your medical attendant. Meanwhile you must spare your eyes. Reading I will not absolutely forbid, but use a large print, stop often, and immediately whenever you have any feeling of uneasiness." These words are the introduction to the proposal of iridectomy, which at the following visit she has to expect. Humanity urgently requires, that prejudice and ignorance should no longer oppose the use of iridectomy in glaucoma.

CHAPTER VI.

HYPERMETROPIA. H.

§ 19. Dioptric Definition of the different Degrees and Forms of Hypermetropia.

The refracting system of the emmetropic eye has, as we have seen, in the state of rest of accommodation, its focus on the layer of rods and bulbs of the retina: parallel rays, derived from infinitely remote objects, refracted by the media of such an eye, there unite in a focus (Fig. 112 ϕ''). The farthest point of distinct vision r therefore lies at an infinite distance, that is, at the limit of our necessities.

Fig. 112.

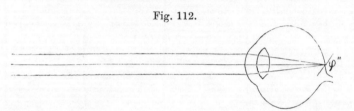

From this ideal state the eye may deviate in two respects and become *ametropic*. The focus of the dioptric system may be situated *in front of*, or *behind* the layer of rods and bulbs. In the first case the eye is *myopic* (Fig. 113), in the latter it is *hypermetropic* (Fig. 114).

Fig. 113.

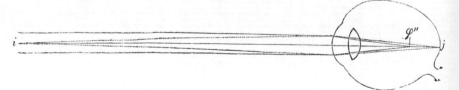

Myopia is a condition which has been long observed, and has been much studied. Hypermetropia, generally as it occurs, was, on the contrary, until quite recently (though mentioned by Ware), almost entirely overlooked, at least its nature and its results were not recog-

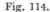

Fig. 114.

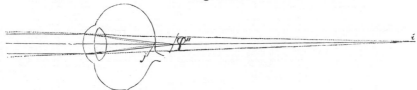

nised. But once discovered and understood, it speedily revealed all
its mysteries, and gave us the key to a number of phenomena, whose
origin had, until then, continued enigmatical : thus the source of
asthenopia and of strabismus convergens was found in this anomaly.
We have, in the first place, here to treat of it in this section, particularly from the dioptric point of view. From this point of view the
definition of H was given. It is also included in Fig. 114. Parallel
rays unite not on the retina, but in φ'', that is, behind the retina. In
order to unite in the retina, for example in j, the rays falling upon the
cornea must already have a converging direction, as the dotted lines in
Fig. 114, which converge towards i. The point which has its image
on the retina, is therefore not a true point, but an ideal or virtual point,
situated behind the retina (for example in i). Such points we do not
see in nature.* From each point of an object the rays always proceed
in a diverging, or at most in a parallel direction (when, namely, the
objects lie at an infinite distance), *never* in a converging direction.
The eye therefore has no need to be able to adapt itself for converging rays. All requirements are fulfilled, when it can bring tolerably
diverging rays to a focus on the retina, and at the same time can relax
itself to accommodation for parallel rays. If it can go farther than
this, it oversteps the measure, and is hypermetropic. It possesses
something useless, and has thereby lost on the other side in what is
useful. In order to see remote objects, it must be actively accommodated ; and in bringing to a focus it yields, for equal range of
accommodation, to the emmetropic eye.

* Converging rays can fall upon our eye only when dioptric surfaces, for
example, those of a lens, stand between the point and the eye. Moreover,
the rays proceeding from the fundus of a myopic eye, or of an eye accommodated for finite distance, when arrived without the eye, acquire a converging
direction. Therefore a hypermetropic person can see with the ophthalmoscope
the fundus of such eyes accurately, and an emmetropic individual, in order to
do the same, must make himself hypermetropic by means of a concave glass.

The degree of H is easily expressed. It is equal to the quantity, by which the relaxation of the eye can overstep the measure, and this is found in the strongest positive glass, with which infinitely remote objects can be accurately seen. If this glass amounts to $\frac{1}{20}$, $\frac{1}{10}, \frac{1}{8}$, H is also $\frac{1}{20}, \frac{1}{10}, \frac{1}{8}$, or, more exactly still, $\frac{1}{19}, \frac{1}{9}, \frac{1}{7}$, since the glass was removed 1″ from the nodal point.

H may be divided into *acquired* and *original*. Of the acquired we have spoken so far (§ 17) as it is developed by the senile changes, in the emmetropic eye. As in the latter, it begins after the 50th year, the original hypermetropia must also, after that period, gradually increase; but only in the same slight degree in which it occurs in the emmetropic eye. Under the head of 'acquired H,' we must here provisionally include aphakia, that is, the condition in which the lens has disappeared from the eye, or at least from the plane of the pupil. That with such a state a high degree of H must, in the ordinary form of the eye, be combined, needs no proof. To this subject I must devote a separate section of the present chapter.

Original H we divide into *manifest* Hm, and *latent* Hl. In my first investigations respecting H, I encountered the difficulty of accurately determining the degree of this anomaly. Thus an eye sometimes at first refused every glass stronger than $\frac{1}{12}$, while it soon afterwards gave the preference to $\frac{1}{8}$, and subsequently again chose $\frac{1}{10}$ or even $\frac{1}{14}$. I assumed that hypermetropic eyes, obliged to put their power of accommodation upon the stretch in order to see remote objects, sometimes involuntarily to a certain degree kept up the tension, even when the proper glasses rendered this not only superfluous, but undesirable for accurate vision. Therefore, from the strongest glasses, with which the eye had, in different trials, still seen accurately at a distance, the degree of H was deduced. These should, as I supposed, completely neutralise the H. But when shortly afterwards, still stronger glasses were sometimes found adapted to the same persons, I discovered my error, and comprehended that those first given had not completely neutralised the H, but that in using them the accommodation to a certain degree continued in operation. This led me to inquire, what the refractive condition of such hypermetropic eyes should be, when by the instillation of a solution of sulphate of atropia, the power of accommodation should be paralysed; and to my surprise, it appeared that not unfrequently in the trials with glasses, the greater part of the H had been suppressed. In slightly myopic, and equally in truly emmetropic eyes, on the contrary, R continues, after artificial mydriasis, nearly unaltered: the power of accommodation here becomes, when the eye is accommodated for r, actually almost wholly relaxed; at most only $\frac{1}{40}$ remains. Evidently, therefore, it is a peculiarity of H, that with the act of vision tension of accommodation is associated, and thus the H is in part concealed. Hence it appeared that in H a manifest and a latent part are often to be distinguished. But it was then also to be suspected, that slight degrees of H, in youthful accommodation, might be wholly suppressed, and in confirmation of this suspicion, experience showed me that where, as in cases of asthenopia and of strabismus, H was with some reason suspected, without being capable of immediate demonstration, a not inconsiderable degree almost always in fact appeared, on paralysing the accommodation.

The conclusion is: that H may be wholly latent, $=$ Hl, and that, where it occurs in the manifest form, as Hm, a latent part Hl may still be supposed to exist. Therefore $H = Hm + Hl$, and if $Hm = 0$, then $Hl = H$. Now, is it also possible that $Hl = 0$, and that therefore H should be entirely manifest $= Hm$? This is actually the case, when in advanced age the power of accommodation is wholly absent, either through paralysis or artificial mydriasis. But even already, while it diminishes, Hm must increase in reference to Hl, and experience actually shows, that even in the 40th year Hl, in reference to Hm, is very slight, and that in the 55th, it may be wholly neglected. Hence it follows, that an originally latent H becomes gradually more and more, and finally, just as the higher degrees, altogether manifest. I have seen cases of Hl in children of ten or twelve years of age, where, in consequence of paralysis produced by atropia, H appeared $= \frac{1}{6}$; others, in which $Hm = $ from $\frac{1}{16}$ to $\frac{1}{20}$, gave place to $H = \frac{1}{5}$. At twenty years of age about one-half of this, at forty more than three-fourths will have become manifest, and at seventy we have to expect simple Hm, in a still higher degree (on account of the supervening diminution of refraction, as H acquisita) than H was originally present (compare, moreover, Fig. 117).

A further division of Hm is that into *absolute, relative,* and *facultative.*

The *absolute* exists, when even with the strongest convergence of the visual lines, accommodation for parallel or converging rays is not to be attained: of this Fig. 115 gives an example. It shows

Fig. 115.

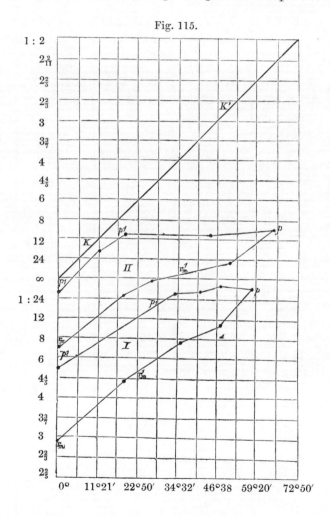

us the boundaries of accommodation of Dr. de Haas,[*] one of the strongest hypermetropics I have met with. It appears that Hm amounts to very nearly $\frac{1}{3}$, and, nevertheless, with strong convergence, Dr. de Haas still attains to nearly the accommodation for parallel rays. He has, in fact, the, for his time of life, very considerable range of accommodation of nearly $\frac{1}{3}$. Some years ago, we may safely infer, while $\frac{1}{A}$ was still greater than it is now, his Hm was not yet absolute. Hence we see that in youth absolute Hm is of rare occurrence. *Relative Hm*, however, even then rather frequently presents itself. Fig. 115, II., represents a case of it in a girl of 17. The manifest farthest point r_m lies about 7″ behind the eye, the absolute nearest point p lies 10″ before the eye, so that, calculated from r_m, $\frac{1}{A}$ is $= \frac{1}{4 \cdot 12}$,—and yet the line $p_1\ p_1\ p$ nowhere passes over the line of convergence K K′. This young person can accommodate for a real point i, but only upon condition of convergence of the visual lines to a point, situated nearer than i to the eye. The H is therefore not absolute, but still it exists in relation to the convergence. For example, in order to see accurately at a distance of 16″, there must be convergence to a distance of 12″, that is, under an angle of 11° 21′. But of this the person in question makes no use. She does not do so even by covering one eye; consequently she now never sees accurately, even monocularily, except with the aid of spectacles, but has, perhaps, when at ten or twelve years of age $\frac{1}{A}$ was still greater, seen accurately even binocularily. When with increasing years $\frac{1}{A}$ shall be reduced to $\frac{1}{7}$, this relative Hm will have given place to the absolute form.

Facultative Hm I have assumed, when objects can be accurately seen at ∞ both with and without convex glasses. A case of this kind is represented in Fig. 116. It is that of a man aged 28, in whom r_m lies 30″ behind the eye, and p, with parallel visual lines, 20″ before the eye; he sees still accurately at a distance as well

---

[*] Author of the Inaugural Dissertation, *Over de Hypermetropie en hare gevolgen*, Utrecht, 1862.

with glasses of $\frac{1}{30}$ as of $-\frac{1}{20}$. His relative range of accommoda-

tion with parallel visual lines therefore amounts to $\frac{1}{20} + \frac{1}{30} = \frac{1}{12}$.

At the distance of 10·5, he can for a short time still see binocularly.

Fig. 116.

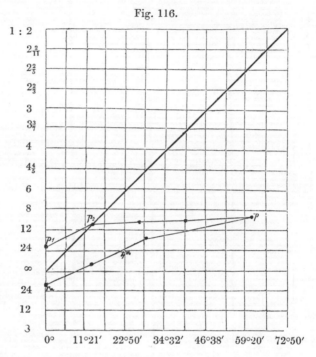

Even before his 38th year this facultative H will have given place
to relative, and about his 45th year, to absolute H.   Does not even
the originally emmetropic eye end by becoming absolutely hypermetropic?

The distinction here made is in all respects justified.   The distinctive character of H is: position of the focus $\phi_{\prime}$ behind the retina
in rest of accommodation.   If, moreover, with the most powerful
tension, $\phi_{\prime}$ remains behind the retina, Hm is *absolute;* if $\phi_{\prime}$ can
reach the retina only with convergence of the visual lines, Hm is
relative; it is, on the contrary, *facultative,* when also with parallel
visual lines $\phi_{\prime}$ can be brought into the retina.   The definitions give
accurate boundaries.   In reference to vision the distinction has, too,

its important aspect, for with absolute Hm vision can never be acute; with relative only monocular vision can be so (and indeed exceptionally); with facultative, on the contrary, binocular vision may also be acute. But the distinction loses much of its importance, inasmuch as in fatigue and weakness, and also regularly with the increase of years, the facultative passes into relative, and the latter into absolute H. To this attention was already directed in the description of the forms enumerated. A diagram (Fig. 117) may

Fig. 117.

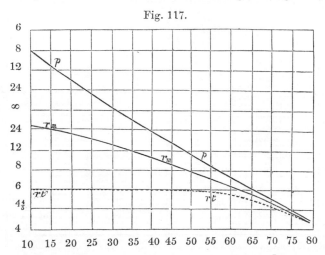

further illustrate it. In the 10th year, with $H = \frac{1}{6}$, Hm is here $= \frac{1}{30}$, but with tension there is still, even without convex glasses, acute vision to some distance from the eye (facultative Hm). With the 25th year, Hm has, with unaltered $H = \frac{1}{6}$, become $= \frac{1}{16}$, and while the absolute nearest point p lies at 30″, a binocular nearest point is no longer present: relative H has supervened. Even in the 31st year p here passes the line ∞, that of the infinite distance, and therewith absolute H is given. Further, while $\frac{1}{A}$ gradually diminishes and finally at 80 years of age becomes $= 0$, the latent part of H, the distance between $r \; r'_m$ and $r_t \; r'^t$ becomes less and less, and at length entirely disappears, where the lines

2

r_m r'_m and r_t r_t meet one another: at the same time the total H has risen from $\dfrac{1}{6}$ to $\dfrac{1}{4\cdot5}$.

§ 20. Form, Position, and Movements of the Hypermetropic Eye.—Apparent Strabismus.

In the preceding section we defined H, from the dioptric point of view. The question now is, on what anatomical deviation this refractive anomaly depends.

A great variety of circumstances may, exceptionally, in this respect, come into play. In the first place, absence of the crystalline lens (aphakia), by whatever cause produced—an important condition, to which we shall devote a separate section. Moreover, diseases of the cornea, attended with flattening, whether of the cornea at large, or of its central portion. Thus, I have sometimes found, with central ulcer of the cornea, a high degree of H, which gave way to E, or even to M, combined with irregular astigmatism, when by mydriasis the lateral parts of the cornea also came into play in direct vision. In commencing glaucoma, too, the eye appears to incline to H, which may be dependent on flattening of the crystalline lens through tension of the zonula Zinnii, if not on a higher cöefficient of refraction of the aqueous, or especially of the vitreous humour: at least the cornea, according to my measurements, does not become flatter, as might have been supposed, from the increased pressure, which appeared necessarily to make the whole eyeball more spherical. Finally, protrusion of the retina through firm chorioideal exudation, may give rise to some H, and by detachment of the retina it may produce even a high degree of the same, which, in that case, soon gives way to blindness.*

The rule is, however, that H depends on a peculiar typical structure of the eye, which may be called the *hypermetropic structure*. The hypermetropically-formed eye is a *small eye;* in all its

---

* According to Ed. v. Jaeger (*Ueber die Einstellungen des dioptr. Apparates*, etc., Wien, 1861, p. 96) H is very characteristic and important as a diagnostic symptom in many affections of the central nervous system and of the optic nerve (bluish coloration combined or not with phenomena of irritation). H is said in such cases often to intermit, not unfrequently simultaneously with the symptoms of irritation. Increased tension would, under these circumstances, be present.

dimensions less than the emmetropic, but especially in that of the visual axis. Immediately around the cornea, the sclerotic has a flat, slightly-curved appearance : the meridians have here a slight curvature; at the equator, on the contrary, the curvature is much greater in the direction of the meridians than in that of the equator itself. A section through the visual axis has the form of an ellipse, of which the visual axis is the short axis (Fig. 118); on the contrary, a section perpendicular to the visual axis, carried through the equator, is almost a circle. The hypermetropic eye is in general an *imperfectly developed eye*. If the dimensions of all the axes are less, the expansion of the retina also is less, to which, moreover, a slighter optic nerve, and a less number of its fibres correspond. Further, the asymmetry in the several meridians (astigmatism) is, in this eye, on an average, greater than in the emmetropic. Both these circumstances explain the fact, at least in part, that in high degrees of H the acuteness of vision is usually below the normal. If, in addition, the development of the cornea has been imperfect, which is comparatively rare, the hypermetropic structure passes into true microphthalmos.—The hypermetropic structure is *hereditary :* if one of the parents suffers from H, we find the same anomaly usually in one or more of the children; sometimes, too, several brothers and sisters are hypermetropic, without the anomaly being observable in either of the parents. How far the structure in question is also *congenital,* I have not inquired. According to von Jaeger's ophthalmoscopic investigations,* the eyes of most newly-born children are, on paralysis of accommodation, moderately myopic; but soon, on further development, these lose M, and in the first years of life mostly become emmetropic. The great difference in the form of the eyes does not occur until a later period. However, von Jaeger did not find even in the first days of life exclusively (78%) myopic, but in 5% emmetropic, in 17% hypermetropic eyes. It may probably be said, that among these last especially the hypermetropics of more advanced age are to be found. At least I have in the fifth and sixth, and sometimes even in the fourth year, demonstrated considerable degrees of H, and have never seen these disappear at a later period.

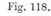

Fig. 118.

* *l. c.,* p. 20.

The shorter visual axis of the hypermetropically-formed eye, which is demonstrable even in life, satisfactorily explains, the form and position of the refracting surfaces being the same, the existence of H. The question, however, is, whether we are right in assuming this similarity in position and form. *A priori* it might be supposed, and it has been not only supposed, but also asserted, that less convexity of the cornea and of the crystalline lens is peculiar to the hypermetropic eye. So far as the cornea is concerned, I am justified by the results of numerous accurate determinations, in denying the assertion. Even in high degrees of H, the radius in the visual line (compare p. 89) is nearly equal to that in the emmetropic eye, and in the highest degrees, when the circumference of the cornea is somewhat less than usual, I found the radius even less. And if this be true for ρ°, still more must it hold good for $\rho_{,}$, the radius in the apex of the cornea (which alone is here concerned); for the angle a between the axis of the cornea and the visual line is greater in H than in E. However, it has really the appearance as if the cornea of the hypermetropic eye were less convex, which, just as in presbyopia, is to be ascribed solely to the diminished depth of the anterior chamber of the eye, and to the relative smallness of the pupil: a more anterior position of the iris and crystalline lens is part of the peculiarity of the hypermetropic structure. The influence of the cornea is thus excluded.—Whether a flatter crystalline lens belongs to the hypermetropic structure of the eye, is quite unknown. It is true that in some eyes the lens is thicker, in others thinner; but, even if we admit that a shorter and longer focal distance correspond thereto (which is not proved), we have no right to place this difference in connexion with H. We know that the cornea has sometimes a particularly long radius, but this is peculiar rather to the highest degrees of M than to H; and accidentally, too, the lens, which in the measurements of Knapp* had a particularly great focal distance, belongs to a myopic eye. Indeed, it is evident that in order to be justified in connecting a flat lens with the hypermetropic structure, we must distinctly demonstrate the presence of the same in hypermetropic eyes. I have tried an indirect method. I have endeavoured to measure the length of the visual axis of superficially-situated hypermetropic eyes, turned strongly inwards, and thence, in connexion with the simultaneously deter-

* *Archiv f. Ophthalmologie*, B. vii., p. 1.

mined radius of the cornea and the degree of hypermetropia, to calculate the focal distance of the lens. But the measurement of the visual axis appeared to be not sufficiently accurate.

Now, in the absence of decisive determinations, we assume that the cardinal points of the dioptric system in the hypermetropic eye have the same position as in the emmetropic. That the crystalline lens in the hypermetropic eye is placed somewhat more anteriorly, we leave out of account, partly for the sake of simplicity, because the influence thereof is slight,—partly in order so far to meet those who feel bound to contend for a flatter crystalline lens in the hypermetropic eye. Now, the position of the cardinal points being the same, we can apply those of the reduced eye, in order to calculate what degrees of H are connected with a given diminution in length of the visual axis. Thus we find :—

With a diminution in length of 0·5 mm., H = 1 : 21·43.

    ,,   ,,   1 mm., H = 1 : 10·34.

    ,,   ,,   1·5 mm., H = 1 : 6·649.

    ,,   ,,   2 mm., H = 1 : 4·302.

    ,,   ,,   3 mm., H = 1 : 2·955.*

In a similar manner we can from the degree of the hypermetropia calculate the diminution in length of the visual axis, and thus the actual length. This has been done in the subjoined table, in which also the position of the centre of motion (compare the method of the determination pp. 185 *et seq.*), and the angle *a* are included. As the basis of the calculation, the values of the reduced eye are taken, and the ascertained diminution in length is deducted from the length of the visual axis (= 22·231 mm., according to the diagrammatic eye of Helmholtz).

* At p. 178 we found

$$f'' - F'' = \frac{F'' \, F'}{f'' - F'}, \text{ or } y = \frac{F'' \, F'}{\zeta} \, ;$$

consequently :

$$\zeta = \frac{F'' \, F'}{y}.$$

If the focus *j* (the retina) lies in front of ϕ'', as is the case in hypermetropia, *y* and ζ are both negative, because $F'' > f''$ and $F' > f'$: even f' becomes negative, so soon as *i* comes to lie behind *h*. As ζ, we find the distance of *i* behind ϕ'; we need that of *i* behind *k*, and $\zeta - G'$ is therefore the distance which we seek. We thus find

$$H = \frac{1}{\zeta - G'}$$

n which $\zeta - G'$ must be expressed in Parisian inches.

No. of the Persons.	Age.	Eye.	H.	Length of the Visual Axis		Position of the Centre of Motion behind the Cornea.	Angle a.
				to the Retina.	to the Posterior Surface of the Sclerotic.		
1	23	D	1 : 16	21·57	22·87	14·67	7
		S	1 : 16	21·57	22·87	13·90	7
2	21	D	1 : 8·75	21·06	22·36	12·95	8·5
		S	1 : 8·75	21·06	22·36	13·12	7
3	22	D	1 : 7·75	20·93	22·23	12·32	8·5
		S	1 : 7·75	20·93	22·23	12·40	9
4	34	D	1 : 6·75	20·75	22·05	12·58	7
		S	1 : 6·75	20·75	22·05	12·85	7
5	26	D	1 : 6·75	20·75	22·05	13·81	8·5
		S	1 : 6·75	20·75	22·05	13·40	8
6	24	D	1 : 3·75	19·77	21·07	13·24	7
		S	1 : 3·75	19·77	21·07	13·39	6
Average				13·22	22·105	13·22	7°·55

To the length of the visual axis to the retina, found by calculation, 1·3 mm. are added for the thickness of the membranes, in
order to obtain the length measured to the outside of the eyeball.
Now this, on an average, amounts in these hypermetropics to
22·105 mm.; and the centre of motion, which is situated 13·22
mm. behind the anterior surface of the cornea, is therefore 8·885
mm. before the posterior surface of the sclerotic: these distances,
13·22 and 8·885, are to one another as 59·8 : 40·2, that is, nearly
as 3 : 2. Thus, as we have already observed, the centre of motion
therefore lies in hypermetropic eyes, although absolutely somewhat
less, relatively more posteriorly than in emmetropic eyes. This
position of the centre of motion, as already the shortness of the axis
in itself, requires in movement little displacement of the optic nerve,
and it is consequently not surprising, that the excursions in hypermetropic eyes are usually a little more: only in No. 6 did any
limitation exist.

In the table the angle a is also stated. Without exception, in
hypermetropics, the cornea is cut to the inside of its axis, by the
visual line, and, as we see, the angle in this horizontal plane amounts,
on an average, to not less than 7°55. The maximum is here
stated as 9°, the minimum as 6°; but in some eyes I have found
still greater deviation, even up to 11°3· In the emmetropic eye
this angle amounts on an average to only 5°082, and in the myopic,

where it may even lie to the outside of the axis of the cornea, and thus become negative, we found it in general somewhat less than 2°. How intimately this angle is connected with M and H, appears especially from the fact, that the maximum in M is exceeded by the minimum in H.   Of this, as we have already remarked, the result is, in myopics apparent strabismus convergens, in hypermetropics apparent strabismus divergens. Our judgment respecting the position of the eyes is determined by the direction of the axes of the cornea, and these are, with a parallel position of the visual lines, in hypermetropics more diverging than in emmetropics; in myopics on the contrary they are less diverging or even converging.   If we consider that between the angle of the axes of the cornea, with parallel visual lines, in the most extreme cases of M and H, a difference of 25° may exist, we shall conceive that this angle is very characteristic of the physiognomy of myopics and hypermetropics, and may indeed suggest the idea of strabismus.   We shall hereafter see what an important part apparent strabismus plays in the production of the true, how the apparent diverging promotes the development of true converging strabismus, and *vice versâ;* and the importance of the angle *a* will thus become still more evident.   Here it remains only to treat of the question, on what the different values of this angle depend.   Fig. 119 distinctly shows, that in the first place the position of the yellow spot *l* in reference to the axis of the cornea determines this angle.   But in the second place, the distance *k g,* from the nodal point to the retina, is to be taken into account.   It is evident that, if in the hypermetropic eye, where this distance is particularly short, the yellow spot *l* is only at the ordinary distance from *g* (a point of the prolonged axis of the cornea), the angle *a,* under which *l l'* and *g a* intersect one another in *k,*

Fig. 119.

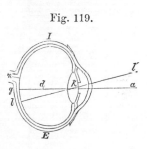

becomes greater. In this, therefore, really lies in part the cause of the greater value of *a* in hypermetropic eyes; but for the most part this greater value must still be explained by the more external position of the yellow spot. This position is connected with the arrested development, especially of the external portion of the hypermetropic eye.   It is, on the other hand, as shall further appear, precisely the extraordinary development and morbid distention of the outer parts

in myopics, which make the yellow spot in them approach the axis
of the cornea, and sometimes even to pass it.

NOTE TO § 20.

It appears to me that the so-called *strabismus incongruus* of Johannes
Müller (*Zur vergleichenden Physiologie des Gesichtssinnes*, Leipzig, 1826,
p. 230), which has sometimes been rather lightly disregarded, is nothing
else than the above-described *apparent strabismus*. It is true, Mueller has
not recognised the relation of this deviation to the anomalies of refraction,
nor has he expressly connected it with the position of the yellow spot. But
what else can he have in view when he says : "Moreover, this species of
strabismus is *not rare*, though in general it is *but slight*, so that *the look being
otherwise steady and the integrity of both eyes being equal*, there is little
striking with regard to internal changes ?" He states that in these cases the
muscles of the eyes are quite sound. His definition, too, is applicable to
our apparent strabismus. "The kind of strabismus I refer to is," he says,
"congenital" (which is correct, at least for the apparent diverging strabismus of hypermetropics) "and incurable; it depends on a difference in the
position of the identical points of the retinas of both eyes; so that these are
indeed perfectly identical in a subjective respect, but in the two eyes the
identity belongs to different meridians, that, for example, the central point
of the retina in the one eye corresponds to an identical point of the
other eye, which is removed from the central point of that eye."
He illustrates his meaning with a figure, from which it might be inferred that, in his opinion, only in one of the eyes the visual line
(by him called "visual axis") and the axis of the cornea (his "axis
of the eye") would not coincide. —A particularly well-marked case
of this kind is described by von Graefe, under the name of "apparent
incongruence of the retina, through anomalous entrance of the
optic nerve" (*Archiv f. Ophthalmologie*, Band I., Abth. 1, p. 435),
where the yellow spot, together with the optic nerve, was in one eye
strongly displaced inwards. The writer contrasts this case with another of
"*true* incongruence of the retinas" (Ibid., p. 105), in which the yellow-
spot is said to have occurred in one eye at the nasal side of the optic nerve.
I must observe that this last case appears to me somewhat problematical; nor
have the cases recorded by Alfred Graefe, in his clear and able paper
(*Klinische Analyse der Motilitätsstörungen des Auges*, Berlin, 1858, pp. 228
et seq.), convinced me. I see that Artl likewise still doubts the existence
of the true strabismus incongruus (*Die Krankheiten des Auges*, B. III., p.
320). If we consider the imperfect acuteness of vision of the part of the
retina used in fixation, another explanation, which has occurred also to von
Graefe himself, may very well be given. If I cannot therefore consider it
proved, that other forms of incongruence occur than those here described

under the name of apparent strabismus, I willingly apply to these the words of von Graefe: "I would certainly attribute these not to incongruence of the retinas, but to *asymmetrical development* of the two halves of the bulb."

The development of the hypermetropic eye deserves to be more closely examined. With it important questions are connected. It is certain, that in the lower orders of society H is more common, as in the higher M is more frequently met with. Now, hereditarily thus transmitted, these anomalies must nevertheless undoubtedly have in the first instance been produced, and must still be promoted, by special practice. With respect to M this seems to me indeed explicable: the stooping position, probably also the increased pressure in accommodation for near objects, may promote the distention of the eyeball. But the same holds good also for H: there are comparatively more hypermetropics among the lower orders, and these want all tendency to become myopic. Now, if H were based upon a flatter lens, it would be comprehensible, that during the development of the lens want of accommodation for near objects should make it remain flatter, just as, by being subject in a more convex condition to the nutritive changes, it might at last retain a more convex form. But just as little as a more convex lens is demonstrated in M, is a flatter one in H. Nevertheless, I have asked myself whether in the promotion of H, by want of accommodation for near objects in childhood, there was not an indication that the crystalline lens in H should be somewhat flatter. But I must say that the indication is too slight. Moreover other hypotheses present themselves. For instance, if in accommodation for near objects, the fluids of the eye are brought under higher pressure, it can be understood how want of this pressure might retard the development of the circumference of the eyeball, and thus favour the hypermetropic form.

These remarks may tend to direct attention to the investigation of the development of eyes, especially of such as are hypermetropic, even in the first years after birth; the merit of having made a beginning in this direction must be awarded to Ed. von Jaeger.

§ 21. PHENOMENA. — DIAGNOSIS. — THE VISION OF HYPER-METROPICS.

The diagnosis of H is attended with little difficulty. I have already laid it down as our duty, systematically to examine the refractive condition of every ophthalmic patient, and no case of H will easily escape him who does so. But before this examination has been begun, before we have even tested the power of vision, the external appearance will often have made us already suspect the presence of H. In the first place, we find an indication in the

anatomical peculiarities, spoken of in the preceding section. The
flat anterior surface of the sclerotic, the strong curvation of its
meridians in the region of the equator, the shallow position of the
iris, the relatively small pupil, the apparent diverging strabismus,
all these give a peculiar physiognomy to the eye. But there is
still more. In the form of the face, too, the existence of H is not
unfrequently expressed. If I am not mistaken, the peculiarity
which here prevails, depends chiefly on the shallowness of the orbit.
The margins of the sockets are flatter, less curved, the whole face is
flattened, with little relief; there is little rounding in the cheeks,
because the anterior surface of the face quickly passes into the lateral
flatness. Often, too, the nose is but slightly prominent, and the
upper part of its dorsum is so little marked that it can scarcely give
support to ordinary spectacles. The eyelids are flat and broad, the
eyes are far from one another; the same is true of the orbits, at least
of their outer margins, whose mutual distance is easily measured.
Otherwise, so far as the position of the hypermetropic eyes is concerned,
it is sometimes very deep, sometimes superficial, so that nothing is
to be inferred from it.—It must be observed, however, that the form
here described is far from being constant. But that a connexion
does exist between the refraction of the eye and the form of the face,
appears most distinctly from the asymmetry of the bones of the latter,
including the frontal bone, which almost without exception accompanies a great difference of refraction in the two eyes. In general, we
find in such cases the eye on the hypermetropic side placed farther from
the root of the nose, and together with the whole side of the face
sloping backward. It is as if the bones of the face on this side are
in general less developed. Thus the orbit also is less deep, and to
this corresponds a smaller eye, with a shorter axis of vision, which
again in its turn is connected with a shallower socket. We shall
subsequently have to devote a separate chapter to difference in
refraction between the two eyes, and we shall then revert to this
subject of the asymmetry of the skull and face.

If we find the physiognomy here described in a young person,
who presents himself as a patient, without the external appearance
of the eyes betraying any disease, we may with the greatest probability infer the existence of hypermetropia. To the question: "Can
you continue to work long?" we obtain almost without exception
a negative answer. This rapidly supervening fatigue, the most

usual phenomenon of certain degrees of H, we shall study more fully, in the following Section, under the name of *asthenopia*.

We have now in these cases, as well as in those where all indication is wanting, with the aid of glasses to ascertain more exactly the true state of things. It has already been stated that hypermetropia is perfectly characterised, when with the aid of positive glasses the vision of distant objects is acute; the strongest glasses, with which the acuteness of vision still continues perfect, show us, in the manner before described, the position of the farthest point, and with it the degree of the hypermetropia. Nevertheless, even with such assistance we are still liable to error. In the first place, as has already been stated, the hypermetropia may be *latent*. After the twenty-fifth year, a part even of very moderate degrees of H is usually manifest; but at a very early period of life the strong power of accommodation may completely suppress comparatively high degrees, and such may therefore exist, even when weak positive glasses already diminish the distinctness of vision at a distance. I formerly supposed that when even with weak negative glasses, for example, of $-\frac{1}{40}$ or $-\frac{1}{30}$, the patients asserted that they could see as well or even better than without glasses, we might infer, if not the presence of myopia, at least the absence of hypermetropia; but this opinion, too, has been corrected by experience. I have found that young patients sometimes involuntarily suppress even the hypermetropia increased by the negative glass, and that they have such a fancy for the smaller forms of letters and of other objects, that they imagine that they distinguish them as well, if not better, than with the naked eye. That they are mistaken in this, is evident, but it is not always easy to prove this; for hypermetropic persons, with good accommodating power, lose very little with negative glasses, at all events very much less than myopic individuals gain by them. If the phenomena in other respects justify us in suspecting the presence of hypermetropia, but do not fully demonstrate it, we must have recourse to a mydriatic, whereby the power of accommodation is paralysed, and the hypermetropia, so far as it exists, is rendered entirely manifest. Sometimes, in such cases, examination with the ophthalmoscope is sufficient, without the employment of the mydriatic, to establish the existence of hypermetropia. In the passive condition of the eye thus examined, in fact, the power of accommodation not unfrequently becomes more relaxed than when the organ is fixed even with parallel visual lines.

In the second place, we must be especially upon our guard, if the acuteness of vision S is very much diminished. In this case the recognition of objects depends less on the sharpness of the retinal images, which, nevertheless, are not acutely seen, than on the magnitude of the images. We may imagine the retina in amblyopic persons to be a very coarse canvass, on which very small objects, even though accurately drawn, are not so well distinguished as larger objects, though bounded by less sharply-defined contours. Or we may suppose very small images to be less accurately drawn on a finer texture, whereby the advantage obtained by increased magnitude readily counterbalances the disturbance, caused by a further loss of sharpness, —in like manner as the strongest eye-pieces in microscopic examination, although they render the images more diffuse, often place us in a position to recognise with greater certainty the form of the smallest visible objects, than was possible with weaker eye-pieces (with the same object-glass). We thus readily understand why amblyopic patients, even when they are not hypermetropic, often choose positive glasses : the greater size of the images is particularly serviceable to them. Where there is any doubt, in this case also ophthalmoscopic examination seldom fails us. In mydriasis, too, positive glasses, on account of the now so much more rapid increase in magnitude of the circles of diffusion, will not readily be chosen, unless hypermetropia actually exists. In general, we must in such cases attend to the magnitude of the pupil. I have seen some instances of extraordinarily small, whether natural or artificial, pupils, which, connected with a certain degree of amblyopia, on account of the improved power of vision at a distance caused by strong positive glasses, incorrectly led the observer to infer the existence of a high degree of hypermetropia. In very rare cases, too, diseases of the cornea may lead us into error. A slight flattening, and especially transparent ulcers opposite the pupil, cause myopia to disappear, or render the person hypermetropic, which altered refraction is removed when the ulceration is healed, and often even on dilatation of the pupil. Lastly, I must caution the reader against making an examination with dirty or dull glasses. Of course, if the glass is dirty or grows dull before the eye, which very readily happens with cold glasses, it will, although it corrects the existing anomaly of refraction, be rejected. If we doubt whether this influence is in operation, we should hold glasses of equal negative focal distance before the positive glasses placed in the frame, in which case the patient ought to see as well as without glasses. If care has been taken to have the glasses clean, this method is very much to be recommended, if we obtain confused answers, especially if we think the credibility of the patient is to be doubted.

As to the functions of the hypermetropic eye, we, in the first place, often find the acuteness of vision diminished. In the slight degrees there is in this respect seldom any difference to be observed, but in high degrees it is almost exceptional to find $S = 1$. It is evident that with glasses which neutralise the hypermetropia, the acuteness of vision becomes greater, than it was without glasses: in fact by the use of these, the nodal point is moved more forwards than when the convexity of the crystalline lens, increased by extraordinary tension of accommodation, brings the focus into the retina, and the retinal images therefore become greater (compare p. 152). Even then, however, in high degrees of H, S often remains below the normal. The cause of this diminished acuteness of vision is to be explained partly from the structure of the eye. On account of the shorter distance between the nodal point and the retina, the retinal images are smaller than in the emmetropic eye, and this will in general continue also with the use of convex glasses, unless strong glasses are required and these are held comparatively far from the eye. It is only if the slighter optic nerve should possess an equal number of nerve-fibres, and the smaller surface of the retina should contain an equal number of percipient elements as in the emmetropic eye, that the smaller magnitude of the retinal images would be wholly, or at least partially compensated; but we have no right to assume such a relation. Moreover, as I have already remarked, the hypermetropic eye is, more than other eyes, liable to asymmetry. In the Chapter on Astigmatism, it will be more fully explained in what manner the acuteness of vision diminishes in consequence thereof. Here I shall remark only, that even after the correction of the astigmatism and of the hypermetropia, the acuteness of vision usually remains rather considerably below the normal. In general it may even be said, that when in high degrees of H, the glasses are also so placed before the eye, that the retinal images may be considered to attain the normal magnitude, the acuteness of vision, nevertheless, in many cases, does not reach the normal. The cause of this we know not. Probably an accurate microscopical examination of the yellow spot would enable us to account for it.—In addition to this diminution of the acuteness of vision depending on congenital deviation, an acquired one frequently occurs in hypermetropia. Thus when only one of the eyes is in a high degree hypermetropic, this eye is usually but little used, and this exclusion, with psychical suppression of the images, leads to amblyopia. Chiefly, however, when strabismus is developed in one eye, to which precisely in hypermetropia a special tendency exists (compare § 24), the acuteness of vision rapidly diminishes considerably, and indeed particularly in the region of the yellow spot. In this last case, when the eye, moreover, on closing the other, no longer fixes, no improvement of the acuteness of vision is to be expected. But if there be no strabismus, or if the deviated eye, on closing the other, still looks at least by preference directly, that is with the yellow-spot, systematic practice with a strong positive glass is almost always capable of considerably improving the sight. It is then sufficient to practise the weak eye for eight or ten minutes three times a-day, while the other eye is closed, and with the aid of the glass just mentioned, in deciphering or reading a large type. A great number of cases justifies me in asserting that the practitioner will seldom find this plan to disappoint him.

What properly characterises the vision of hypermetropics, is not the diminished S, but the abnormal refractive condition, which requires another use of the power of accommodation. After all that has been already stated, I have but little to say in reference to this point. It is understood that the hypermetropic person begins his accommodation with a *deficit*. The emmetropic relaxes that power as much as possible, and then sees acutely at an infinite distance; he converges and accommodates as of his own accord for the distance of the convergence, in youth up to six, five, and four inches and less; everywhere he moves about in the middle of the relative range of the accommodation, which belongs to the given convergence. On the contrary, the hypermetropic individual, in order to see at a distance, must already bring his power of accommodation into action: that is his *deficit*. Commencing with this, he has still for each convergence to add as much range of accommodation as the emmetropic person. It is true we may say, that his accommodation adapts itself to the refractive condition: he learns, forced by necessity to practise, with relatively little convergence to bring a relatively great part of his accommodation into action, and can, finally, even no longer omit the increased tension; but constantly, at each convergence, he finds himself still nearer to the maximum of the corresponding possible tension, and both his absolute and his binocular nearest point lie farther from the eye than they do in the emmetropic subject.   Moreover all this holds good for the facultative hypermetropia in youth : the actual disturbance may here still be absent; the eyes may fulfil their daily requirements; not a complaint may be heard.   But with the advance of years, while the absolute range of accommodation diminishes, the relative, for a definite convergence, falls too short : fatigue now rapidly supervenes, and thus even in the slightest degrees of hypermetropia premature presbyopia occurs, which has more of the character of asthenopia, the higher the degree of the facultative hypermetropia is, and the earlier the age at which difficulty in working at near objects sets in.—The case is much worse in relative hypermetropia.   In it, as we have seen, there may still be accommodation for parallel and even for diverging rays, but only on condition that the eyes converge to a point, situated nearer than that from which the rays proceed.   Binocular vision and acute vision thereby exclude each other.   With one eye, under excessive convergence, there might be acute vision; but generally speaking, no use is made thereof, and if this takes place, there is periodical, to be followed by persistent, strabismus.   In very young subjects relative hypermetropia is rather unusual.   It must be a very considerable degree of that affection which, with $\frac{1}{A} = \frac{1}{3}$ or $\frac{1}{4}$, might not for a short time be overcome, and which even at a certain convergence should not admit of sufficient binocular accommodation.   But at a somewhat more advanced time of life, even so early as in the twenty-fifth year, many cases of H already belong to this category.   Vision is in these cases unfortunately circumstanced.   Properly speaking it is never accurate either for distant or for near objects, and every effort to distinguish anything, to which is united great knitting of the brow, is rapidly followed by fatigue.   Persons with such hypermetropia are always seeking the distance at which they distinguish relatively well.   They hold the book now farther off, then again closer, sometimes at only two or three inches from the eye; but even if the print is large and distinct, they quickly end by throwing the volume away.   Very bright light is a great advantage to them, because with a small pupil the circles of diffusion become less.   They therefore endeavour, although less generally than myopic persons, to diminish the latter by other means, for example, by narrowing the space between the eyelids.   I have seen a boy of eight years, very weak and delicate, with

17

amblyopia of the left eye, and with $H = \frac{1}{7}$, and very little range of accommodation of the right eye, who used his nose to diminish his pupil. When he wished to distinguish anything, particularly in looking at a distance, he turned his head to the right, and looked with the right eye directly along the nose, which thus covered a portion of the pupil.—How inconceivably happy we make such persons with proper spectacles, which are a natural complement of their eyes, and have been so long withheld from them, I need not say.—Absolute hypermetropia we scarcely ever find with the normal accommodating power of youth. Only a couple of cases of this kind have occurred to me : in the one the hypermetropia amounted to $\frac{1}{2\cdot97}$, in the other to $\frac{1}{3\cdot5}$. My friend William Bowman has enabled me to communicate a case (see p. 290), in which glasses of $\frac{1}{1\frac{7}{8}}$ being employed for distant vision, the degree of H was $= 1 : 1\cdot7$, in fact, more than enough to make it necessarily absolute. The cases of absolute, as well as those of the higher degrees of relative H, present almost exactly the image of myopia, complicated with amblyopia, with which they are therefore confounded. Small print such hypermetropics cannot read—they appear, therefore, to be amblyopic,—and larger type they can read only when it is very close to the eye—just like myopic persons. From the latter they are distinguished by the fact, that at a greater distance they see objects comparatively as well, that is under equal angles, as near ones ; and moreover by this, that with positive spectacles they can read the same print at a greater distance than without spectacles. The enigma, why, while the eye is hypermetropic, small objects are distinguished near the eye more easily than at some distance, for example, at that of one foot, has been partly solved by von Graefe* by a simple calculation, whence it appears, that in such eyes, on the approach of the object, the retinal image increases more in magnitude than the circles of diffusion, (partly also because we have to do more with polyopia than with simple circles of diffusion), so that the form of the object can be better distinguished. Of the correctness of this, we can easily be satisfied, by making ourselves strongly hypermetropic with negative glasses, and then, without altering the accommodation, bringing large letters

* *Archiv f. Ophthalm.*, B. ii. H 1, p. 181.

at different distances before the eye. We shall thus distinguish more easily near the eye, than at the distance, for example, of one foot. We will, however, at the same time find, that in recognising objects we are far behind such hypermetropics, whose anomaly of refraction has the same degree as that which we produce in ourselves. For this there are different reasons. In the first place the hypermetropic in this case accommodates as strongly as possible, in which he succeeds admirably by convergence upon a proximate point; consequently, too, his pupil becomes narrower; moreover, by approximating the eyelids he diminishes still further the effect of the circles of diffusion, and thus probably makes a single image come forth more strongly from their polyopic surface; in some cases also regular astigmatism plays a part therein, and, finally, he has by practice learned from imperfect retinal images to deduce the true forms of the objects. In this manner I believe we can explain the comparatively great degree of power of distinguishing very near objects possessed by persons strongly hypermetropic, without being obliged to take refuge in a somewhat mysterious faculty of suppressing the circles of diffusion.

From the above it follows that the indication of the existence of slighter degrees of H is derived chiefly from the phenomena of asthenopia, the most important result of hypermetropia, to the consideration of which we now proceed.

§ 22. ASTHENOPIA.

A peculiar morbid condition of the eyes has long attracted the attention of ophthalmologists. The phenomena of which it is composed are highly characteristic. The eye has a perfectly normal appearance, its movements are undisturbed, the convergence of the visual lines presents no difficulty, the power of vision is usually acute,— and nevertheless in reading, writing, and other close work, especially by artificial light, or in a gloomy place, the objects, after a short time, become indistinct and confused, and a feeling of fatigue and tension comes on in, and especially above, the eyes, necessitating a suspension of work. The person so affected now often involuntarily closes his eyes, and rubs his hand over the forehead and eyelids. After some moments' rest, he once more sees distinctly, but the same phenomena are again developed more rapidly than before. The longer the rest has lasted, the longer can he now continue his work. Thus, after the rest of Sunday, he begins the new week with fresh ardour and fresh power, followed, however, by new disappointment.

2

If he is not occupied with looking at near objects, the power of vision appears to be normal, and every unpleasant feeling is entirely absent. If, on the contrary, he endeavours, notwithstanding the inconvenience which arises, by powerful exertion to continue close work, the symptoms progressively increase: the tension above the eyes gives place to actual pain, sometimes even slight redness and a flow of tears ensue, everything is diffused before the eyes, and the patient now no longer sees at first well, even at a distance. After too long-continued tension, he is obliged to refrain for a long time from any close work. It is remarkable that pain in the eyes themselves, even after continued exertion, is of rare occurrence.

At first this condition was considered as a sort of amblyopia. It was called *hebetudo visus, amblyopie presbytique*, or *amblyopie par presbytie*. By degrees the cause was sought more and more in the organs of accommodation, at first in the action of the external muscles, subsequently in that of the internal muscular elements; and in the same measure was the importance of the retina thrown into the shade. Excessive tension of accommodation was looked upon as a satisfactory cause of the troublesome symptoms which, it was hoped, might be overcome by rest.

Evidently, however, when it was supposed that the origin of asthenopia was thus explained, the facts were overlooked that thousands in like manner, sometimes in a still higher degree, put their power of vision upon the stretch, without being visited by the troublesome phenomena of asthenopia or impaired vision, and that, on the other hand, these phenomena not unfrequently occur in men, nay, even in children, who had exacted but little from their power of vision.

Since the same cause does not produce in every one the same deviation, writers are accustomed to take refuge in a *peculiar predisposition*. Thus the difficulty is set aside. But if the foundation of this peculiar predisposition be dark and obscure, pathogeny has gained but little from the adoption of this course. I therefore felt called upon to propose to myself the question, on what the so-called predisposition to *asthenopia* (so the condition was now more generally called) might depend, and I soon became convinced, that a congenital deviation, namely, a moderate degree of hypermetropia, is at the bottom of it. The hypermetropia is here, however, more than predisposition. The asthenopia—I mean the *tendency* to fatigue in looking at near objects—is already wholly included therein.   Every hypermetropia which, with reference to the range of accommodation, has attained a certain degree, is at the same time asthenopia.   If the symptoms sometimes do not manifest themselves until twenty-five years of age, or even later, this is to be ascribed merely to the fact, that previously the range of accommodation was sufficiently great, easily to overcome the existing degree of hypermetropia.   We should beware of confounding the exciting circumstance with the cause of the affection.   The exciting circumstance of the phenomena consists in continued tension in looking at near objects; the cause, on the contrary, is the hypermetropic structure of the eye.   In fact, asthenopia is not the fatigue itself, but the want of power, through which the fatigue occurs.   The distinction made here is applicable to other conditions.   When a person going up hill is soon exhausted, the exertion is indeed the exciting circumstance of the weariness, but the cause is to be sought in the slight energy of the muscles with reference to the weight of the body.   This disproportion exists at all times, although the person ascends no hills.   By practice it will even be partly overcome, and only after repeated excessive exertion, without sufficient intermission, does the fatigue occur still earlier than before.   Just so is the relation of hypermetropia to asthenopia: after each excessive exertion longer rest is required; but total want of practice makes, on the first effort, the phenomena follow still more quickly.   The analogy is perfect.

I have already asserted that hypermetropia is usually at the bottom of asthenopia.   The truth of this assertion has been doubted.   I now, however, go a step further, and venture to maintain, that in the pure form of asthenopia hypermetropia is scarcely ever wanting.

The doubts which were expressed are to be ascribed, on the one hand, to insufficient investigation,— observers sometimes found no Hm, and neglected to examine whether the H was suppressed by accommodation; on the other hand, to confusion with other morbid forms.   I readily admit, that many different conditions were included under the name of hebetudo or asthenopia.   When inconvenience was felt on continued exertion, this appeared to some sufficient to justify the inference that asthenopia existed.   On this account different forms of irritation, congestion in myopic eyes, hyperæsthesia of the eye, with increasing pain on exertion, different affections of the retina and of the choroid, nay even the beginning of trachoma, and foreign bodies in the sac of the conjunctiva, might all be united under one denomination.   But I cannot concur in the adoption of such a primitive semeiotic method. It leads inevitably to confusion of ideas and of conditions. When I asserted that asthenopia is the result of the hypermetropic structure of the eye, I was thinking, not of a symptom, but of a portrait of disease, such as has been drawn above, and in this sense I can fully maintain my assertion. In general, if the portrait be faithfully and perfectly copied from nature, we run little risk of find- more than one condition, to which it applies.

Now that it has actually been shown, that asthenopia depends on H, it appears to be so natural a result of the latter, that the in- ference evidently suggested itself *à priori*. Extraordinary tension of accommodation is required by the ordinary employments of young eyes. From youth the eye adapts itself to these requisites, so far as it is able to do, so that the range of accommodation alters its margin and the H becomes in part even latent. But, in spite of all this, it finally falls too short. The diminution of the range of accommodation with the time of life explains it satis- factorily. The asthenopia then gradually sets in, at first only under less favourable conditions of illumination, and extraordinary exertion or headache, subsequently on all occasions and without exception when close work is performed even for only a comparatively short time. In general the symptoms of asthenopia show themselves the earlier, the higher the degree of H is, on which they depend. I found the year of life at which the asthenopia begins to be about equal to the denominator of the fraction by which the degree of H is expressed: with $H = \dfrac{1}{10}$ we may expect the commencement of asthenopia in the tenth year, with $H = \dfrac{1}{25}$ not until the 25th year. With $H = \dfrac{1}{40}$ it in the fortieth year nearly coalesces with the presbyopia, and the symptoms are then less characteristic. Finally where H is absent, presbyopia is developed, as we have above seen (p. 215), not with the complaint of fatigue, but with that of defective vision for near objects. The cause of this is evident. Asthenopia, namely, depends upon the fact, that not only at a distance of 6, 8, and 10 inches, but likewise at that of 12″, 16″, and 20″, and even at an infinite distance, acute vision takes place only with special effort of the power of accommodation. In the commencement of presbyopia in a normal eye on the contrary, vision at 8″ is absolutely impossible, but at 12″, or at least at 16″, it takes place without special exertion, and at a great distance the weakest positive glass has even an injurious effect. The hypermetropic eye is therefore little or not at all benefited, by removing the object some inches further; the presbyopic, on the contrary, is thereby relieved of all extraordinary exertion. The former is obliged to cease working; the latter continues to work without trouble, provided the visual angle at the distance of 16″ is not too small. While, even at the commencement of the exertion, the presbyopic eye sees distinctly only at a greater distance, the need of spectacles, to make vision at a *shorter* distance *possible*, is evident. In the hypermetropic eye, on the contrary, there may at first be very acute vision for near objects : the need of spectacles, which would in this case serve to make vision at *any* distance *easier*, was therefore often overlooked.

For this difference between presbyopia and hypermetropia, the relative range of accommodation of the normal eye, in incipient presbyopia, sufficiently accounts. Beyond the binocular nearest point, in incipient presbyopia, the positive part of the range in question rapidly increases rather considerably, while in the hypermetropic individual it increases only slowly, and at each convergence remains a very subordinate part. But neither in this also is everything included. I started provisionally from the supposition, that in the same eye, for traversing equal parts of the range of accommodation, equal exertion of the muscular system is required. But this is, however, far from being perfectly true. Both the complicated mechanism and the mode of action of the effect obtained render it almost inconceivable, that this exact proportion should ever exist. But particularly in presbyopic persons, whose crystalline lens has become firmer and has gradually shifted forwards, this proportion is by no means to be expected. The result thereof is this : that in comparison to its magnitude, the positive part of the relative range of accommodation in the presbyopic individual represents more muscular tension than the negative part, and that therefore in the latter the relation between these two parts may be more unfavourable than in the youthful eye, and may yet not produce fatigue so early.

The condition for the occurrence of asthenopia may now be still more generally formulized : it is the presence of a rather considerable, but at the same time insufficient, range of accommodation. Now

in general this insufficiency is attributable to H, as has been fully
explained. But it may proceed also from want of energy. This
last occurs exceptionally, especially in general weakness, from loss
of blood or otherwise, and in paresis. In both these conditions
there is this peculiarity, that a brief but rather powerful muscular
exertion is possible, but that the energy employed is almost immediately lost. We observe this in all muscles, and it is true also of
those of the eye. A half-paralyzed arm is still raised with force, but
it immediately falls powerless : a single almost spasmodic contraction
has, as it were, exhausted the muscular power. In like manner the
eye is accommodated, for a moment, to a rather near point, but relaxation forthwith ensues, and persistent tension is impossible. We
now easily understand, how under weakening influences, for example,
after exhausting diseases, after loss of blood, phenomena manifest
themselves, which have the greatest resemblance to those of asthenopia in consequence of H. These phenomena occur with
especial rapidity and characteristically, when a slight degree of H
exists, which on-an energetic accommodation was hitherto still easily
overcome. The same is true of paresis of accommodation, as will
hereafter be explained. If in these cases the H be entirely absent,
the condition is distinguished, among other things, from ordinary
asthenopia, by the fact, that now at least vision at a distance is
possible without tension of accommodation, and therefore persistently. In H this is not the case. Of course, the phenomena are
developed the more rapidly, the closer to the eye the objects
must be seen, (for its proximate binocular point even the powerfully accommodating emmetropic eye is asthenopic) ; but even in
looking at a distance, the phenomena of asthenopia would in the
hypermetropic not be absent, if there were necessity to accommodate accurately for a long time uninterruptedly for distant objects.
I am convinced that the asthenopic person, who states that he
experiences no trouble in ordinary life, and that he sees well at a
distance, in turns relaxes his accommodation, and is only thus preserved from fatigue. Accordingly some, as even Mackenzie remarked,
state too, that remote objects also on being fixed, sometimes become
indistinct. Now this, I repeat, is inconsistent in emmetropia, even
when the power of accommodation has quite lost its energy.

There are still other morbid states, whose symptoms have some
resemblance to those of asthenopia. To these belong especially
insufficiency of the internal recti muscles, which von Graefe* has

* *Archiv f. Ophthalmologie*, B. iii. 1, p. 308, and B. viii. 2, p. 314.

studied with such excellent results, and to which I shall revert in speaking of the movements of the myopic eye, where this insufficiency is more particularly apt to occur. This form was distinguished by von Graefe, under the name of asthenopia muscularis, from that here described, which may be called the accommodative asthenopia. —In astigmatism too, we shall find phenomena, resembling those of asthenopia. I shall endeavour, in the proper place, to examine how far special peculiarities characterise each of these morbid forms.

An emmetropic person can easily form an idea of the vision of the hypermetropic, and of the conditions and phenomena of asthenopia, by making his own eyes hypermetropic by means of the negative glasses required for that purpose. The only condition necessary is, that he have a tolerably good accommodating power. The tendency to bring this into action takes place immediately, and, as it were, involuntarily. At a certain strength of the negative glass he sees distinctly and acutely by, at each angle of convergence, increasing his accommodation with the degree of the produced H. But fatigue will ensue, and he will easily satisfy himself of the difficulty of continuing to see accurately also at a distance.—The young myopic individual needs only to take too strong negative glasses, in order to bring himself into the same state. If the myopic person have somewhat exceeded his fiftieth year, he needs only to neutralise his myopia in order to observe in himself the phenomena of presbyopia: for those of asthenopia he has then lost the capacity.

It will have been evident to the reader, that the phenomena of asthenopia proceed from nothing else than from fatigue of the muscular system of accommodation. In what this fatigue consists deserves to be more closely examined.

In my investigations[*] respecting the elasticity of muscles, I have distinguished two forms of fatigue.

One form proceeds from the actual energy,[†] produced by the muscle. The work consists in the moving of a load. The load may be the body itself or some part of the body, which is moved, or, in addition thereto, an object external to the body.

Distinguished from this is the fatigue, which is the result of the simple extension of an elastic muscle in a state of contraction.

* See the preliminary communication in *Verslagen en mededeelingen der Koninklijke Akademie van Wetenschappen*, 1859, D. ix., p. 113.

† I use the terms of Mr. Rankine, adopted also by Mr John Tyndall (*Heat considered as a mode of motion*. London, 1863, p. 137.)

This takes place when a burden is held, without being moved, as, for example, when, with the arm bent at a right angle at the elbow-joint, the hand is loaded with a weight : the arm and the weight remain in the same place, and yet fatigue soon occurs. At the moment when the weight was placed in the hand, some actual energy (chemical action in the muscle) was indeed required to make the arm continue in the same position : the muscles (mm. biceps et brachialis internus) had to contract more strongly, in order in the state of extension induced by the weight, to remain as short as before, and the actual energy (the chemical action) was thus converted into a potential energy (elastic tension). Moreover, the muscular contraction gradually increases as much as the greater extensibility, accompanying the increasing fatigue of the muscles, requires. It has, in fact, been proved that, accordingly as the muscle becomes more fatigued, its extensibility increases, and this increasing extensibility gradually requires augmenting contraction, in order, under the extending action of the same load, to keep the muscle as short as it was. This is evident from the fact, that on the unexpected removal of the load, the arm bends involuntarily, as a result simply of the previous extension of the elastic contracted muscle,—the more strongly, the longer the weight has rested on the hand ; and in that involuntary motion of the arm the potential energy of the extended muscle again becomes actual. Finally, also, there was continually some actual energy in the oscillations of the electric currents, composing the negative deflection of the tetanized (contracted) muscles and nerves, and most likely converted into heat. It was therefore under more than one mode that, without external phenomena having been visible, some energy was actual, while arm and weight, unaltered, occupied the same place. But that energy, in its different modes, seems to be very small in comparison to the often repeated lifting of the same weight. I therefore think the fatigue proceeding from the performance of labour, must be distinguished from that arising from simple extension. According to the law of the conservation of energy, we may, in the first case, expect more metamorphosis of matter in the organism. The acceleration of the heart's action appeared to me to be the measure thereof. I found, in fact, that when a weight is held during some minutes resting on the hand of the bent arm, the pulsation of the heart is much less accelerated than when, during an equal space of time, the weight is alternately taken off by another, and with extended arm placed again upon the hand, and now by flexion raised once more to the original height. The feeling of fatigue in the muscle is, however, in the latter case not greater than in the former.

In explanation of the fatigue, which is the result of the performance of labour, we may take refuge in an accumulation of products of metamorphosis of matter in the muscular tissue, which really goes hand-in-hand with it. The fatigue, proceeding from extension, under the influence of a load not further moved, may, partly at least, have another source. Thus the extension might give rise to pressure on the nerve-filaments in the muscle : in fact, without the extension by a load, fatigue does not arise in the muscle, though contracted in an equal degree. Probably, however, it depends partly also on an increase of the products of the metamorphosis of matter in the muscular tissue, produced not so much by an accelerated formation, as by retarded elimination. Indeed, in uninterrupted contraction the vessels are compressed and the circulation is impeded, while in motion from muscular action the latter is excited and accelerated. That accumulation of products of metamorphosis is co-operative, is, moreover, admissible, because in both cases the coefficient of elasticity of the muscle decreases,—which coefficient may, I think, be connected with the presence of some products of metamorphosis in the nutritive fluid of the muscle. But this is not the place to enter more fully into this question. It is sufficient to have directed attention to the distinction to be made.

Now, to which form of fatigue does that belong, which arises from persistent accommodation for accurate vision in the hypermetropic eye ?

Evidently we have here to do with persistent extension of the muscle in a state of contraction. The extension is the result of the resistance exercised by the parts involved in the accommodation, while their form and position undergo a change. By virtue of elasticity they resume their original form and position, so soon as the contraction of the internal muscular system of accommodation ceases. The latter must, therefore, in order to produce persistent accommodation, be in a state of permanent contraction. This permanent contraction causes fatigue, and the fatigue, promoted by extension, increases, as was above remarked, the extensibility : in consequence of this law, the contraction must be always increasing, in order to keep the muscle equally short and to make it permanently exercise the same force (in equilibrium with the resistance). Sooner or later therefore the fatigue must pass into powerlessness. A moderate contraction,

such as is required in the normal eye, may be kept up without fatigue
for almost an entire day. A degree of contraction is even possible, at which the recovering power of the muscle removes, *pari passu*,
the fatigue proceeding from contraction : the extensibility in that
case does not increase. This applies particularly to involuntary
muscles, consisting of fibre-cells, to which (at least in mammalia) the
internal muscles of the eye belong. But where hypermetropia exists,
such a degree of contraction is required, that increasing fatigue, at
length proceeding to complete loss of energy, cannot long be absent.
Thus all the phenomena of asthenopia are readily explained. It
seems to me that there is therefore no reason for resorting in addition either to the condition and the function of the retina, or to
pressure of the fluids, or to obstruction to the circulation.

To fatigue through work, as has been above said, the same law
is applicable : here, too, the coefficient of elasticity diminishes; here,
too, the extensibility is therefore increased. Actual work is done by
the muscular system of accommodation, when the eye is accommodated alternately for different distances. This, however, need scarcely
ever take place to such a degree as to give rise to fatigue.

What are the results of continued excessive tension of accommodation in asthenopia?

In former years, especially, the most fearful consequences were predicted from it. Asthenopia was considered to be the first stage of, or at
least to be intimately related to, amblyopia, and the latter, it was supposed, threatened the destruction of the asthenopic eye, if it was not
condemned to almost absolute rest. Precisely the mode of treatment of
oculists, in giving asthenopics no spectacles or insufficient spectacles,
has placed me fairly in a position to satisfy myself of the unfounded
nature of their fears. I have seen hundreds of asthenopic patients,
who from youth up to their 30th or 40th year, some to an advanced
period of life, had every day anew, without spectacles, or with too
weak spectacles, obstinately pushed the tension of accommodation
to the uttermost, and I have never seen a diminution of the acuteness of vision arise from such a course. It appears also, that in H
a certain immunity against many kinds of diseases, which threaten
the power of vision, actually exists ; it is certain, that by excessive
tension of accommodation the retina is not brought into danger.—
In rare cases, perhaps in one in a thousand, I have observed that
on every effort to see near objects, almost immediately violent pain
arose in the eye, evidently connected with the contraction of the
muscles of accommodation. This painful spasm made it necessary

for the patient directly to refrain from work.   Nor did the use of spectacles avail him, for in each case near objects were seen with convergence, and the tension of accommodation connected with this convergence, was sufficient to excite the pains.   These remarkable cases, the cure of which was obtained by the regular instillation of sulphate of atropia, which completely excluded the accommodation, while strong glasses meanwhile rendered work possible, I shall have to describe more fully in speaking of the anomalies of accommodation.

An evident proof, that neither the nature nor the causes of the phenomena of asthenopia had been fully ascertained, notwithstanding many endeavours to investigate them, is to be found in the host of names by which this condition has been designated by different writers. They are almost innumerable : *debilitas visus* of Taylor, *amblyopia a topica retinæ atonia* of Plenck, *affaiblissement de la vue* of Wenzel, *Gesichtsschwäche* or *hebetudo visus* of Jüngken, *dulness of sight* of Stevenson, *debollezza di vista per stanchezza di nervi* of Scarpa, *dimness of vision* of Middlemore, *visus evanidus* of Walther, *impaired vision* of Tyrrel, *amaurosis muscularis* of J. J. Adams, *affection of the retina from excessive employment* of Lawrence, *lassitudo ocularis* or *disposition à la fatigue des yeux* of Bonnet, *kopiopie* or *ophthalmokopie* of Pétrequin, *Schwäche der Augen* of Chelius, *amblyopie par presbytie ou presbytique* of Sichel, *languor oculi* of Arlt, *slowly adjusting sight* of Smee, *impaired vision from overwork* of Cooper, and perhaps many others still.

Our knowledge of asthenopia commenced with that of the phenomena of the affection. By degrees the description thereof became more true and more accurate, and what did not belong to it was separated from it. It is evident that in a condition such as this, constituting a part of the floating idea of weakness of vision, occurring with many complications, and presenting numerous varieties, according to the time of life and the use made of the eyes, there was great difficulty in sketching a typical picture, so long as the cause of the leading feature of the affection, and therefore its nature, were unknown. So it was possible that although even Taylor* had given a good sketch in the following words :—"dantur exempla, ubi statim ab initio lectionis, et post eam, litteræ confuse permixtæ videantur, et hinc legentes a lectione prohibeantur, quod etiam acu subtili nentibus, vel aliud quodcunque negotium, ejusmodi longam axeos directionem certum versus objectum quoddam requirens, tractantibus, accidere solet," the well-defined lineaments of the picture were again obliterated by unessential phenomena and mixed up with those of amblyopia. According to this the cause of the affection was now generally sought in the retina or in the chorioidea. That Plenck† was inclined to this opinion, is at once evident from the name he

---

* Taylor, *Nova Nosographia Ophthalmica*, § 189, p. 151.   Hamburgi et Lipsiæ, 1766.

† Plenk, *Doctrina de morbis oculorum*, p. 188.   Viennæ, 1792.

gave it of *amblyopia a topica retinæ atonia*. Scarpa* sees in the affection fatigue of the nerves, especially of those which have direct reference to vision ; and if the picture, sketched by Beer†, was to be considered as sufficiently characteristic, we might say also of him, that he ascribes the disturbance to a weakness of the retina, or to a change in its structure. Without determining the nature of the affection, Lawrence ‡ also states, that this is to be sought in the retina, perhaps primarily in the chorioidea, but still he clearly shows that, while the acuteness of vision is perfect, it has been incorrectly classed together with amblyopia, and Tyrrel § endeavours, rather by number than by force of arguments, to prove that a preceding congestion of the chorioidea is the primary cause of asthenopia, which congestion might even pass into chorioiditis. At first Sichel ‖ is yet farther from the truth : he looks upon the affection as the beginning of amblyopia, " le premier degré d'amblyopie où le malade voit parfaitement ou *presque* parfaitement bien, mais où la vue ne supporte pas la moindre fatigue et se trouble, dès que le malade applique les yeux pendant quelque temps ou même pendant quelques minutes." Jüngken¶ still distinguishes his *hebetudo visus*, of which he assumes not less than ten varieties, from the proper amblyopia, and remarks very justly, that it is distinguished from the amblyopias by the fact, that in the latter "the power of vision has already suffered, that the patient in general can no longer distinctly recognise objects, which in weakness of sight (asthenopia) is by no means the case ;" but he adds : "this latter may, however, pass into amblyopia, and this is usually the case, if its causes are not removed."

It is by Bonnet (*Gazette médicale de Paris*, 4th September, 1841), and particularly by Pétrequin (*Ann. d'Oculist.*, v. p. 250, and vi. p. 72, 1841 and 1842), that we first find the retina excluded, and the primary cause of asthenopia sought in the muscular organs of the eye, especially in those of accommodation. The external muscles were by them put most prominently forward, and being too much preoccupied with the idea of tenotomy, in order to cure the asthenopia, they thought more of an injurious pressure of the muscles than of fatigue. Mackenzie,** too, comes, in his remarkable treatise, to the conclusion, "que ce sont les organes ou l'organe d'ajustement, qui sont affectés dans cette maladie, et qui en sont probablement le siége principal." Perhaps he would have ventured to exclude the retina ; but he thought he had observed, that myopics also are subject to asthenopia,

---

* Scarpa, *Trattato delle principale Malattie degli Occhi*, Vol. ii. p. 241. Pavia, 1816.

† J. G. Beer, *Lehre von den Augenkrankheiten*, Theil ii. p. 17. Wien, 1817.

‡ Lawrence, *Treatise on the Diseases of the Eye*, p. 566. London, 1841.

§ Tyrrel, *Practical Work on the Diseases of the Eye*, Vol. ii. p. 25. London, 1840.

‖ Sichel, *Traité de l'ophthalmie, la cataracte et l'amaurose*, p. 646. Paris, 1837.

¶ Jüngken, *Die Lehre von den Augenkrankheiten*, p. 780. Berlin, 1832.

** *Mémoire sur l'asthenopie ou affaiblissement de la vue. Annales d'Ocul.*, Tome x. pp. 97, 155.

and that convex glasses do not protect the wearer against attacks of that affection. Elsewhere (*Practical Treatise*, 1854, p. 984, 4th edition), we read again: "Were it entirely a disease of the apparatus of accommodation, looking through a small aperture, by making the use of the accommodating power unnecessary for the time, would make vision distinct." It hence appeared perfectly logical, not to seek the seat of the affection simply in the accommodation. The observation was, however, incorrect. The difficulties which myopics sometimes experience, represent another form of disease, and moreover we have reason to believe that Mackenzie has incorrectly supposed the existence of myopia in some of his patients. As to the attacks during the use of convex glasses, we shall see that Mackenzie was too timid to give glasses of sufficient strength, and asthenopia is, of course, not to be removed by the use of too weak glasses, and lastly, asthenopics really see, when they are tired, comparatively well and easily through a small opening.

From this time we find fatigue of accommodation mentioned by different writers, as at least a coöperative cause of asthenopia. Sichel* had not yet a just idea of accommodation, but he had nevertheless arrived at the conviction that his *amaurose presbytique*, which he now himself identified with asthenopia, occurred only in presbyopic eyes, and this point he correctly maintains against Mackenzie. But, on the other hand, he keeps up the connexion with amblyopia, and still thinks that this affection may very easily pass into incurable amaurosis.

With good result, the implication of the retina in asthenopia was by Böhm† set still further aside. He shows especially, that nerves of motion are much more liable to be affected with fatigue than nerves of sense, and he consequently seeks the primary cause of the affection in the motor nerves of the eye. It is true that Böhm's theory remains somewhat obscure and indefinite, in consequence of the part he ascribes to the external muscles of the eye, and of his not very clear ideas of near- and farsightedness; but in non-squinting asthenopics he recognises as the cause of the affection, the want of permanent power of accommodation for near objects, and with great satisfaction he mentions that he has, by means of convex glasses, delivered many asthenopic patients from their troubles. Böhm is, in truth, the first who unconditionally recommended the use of convex glasses in asthenopia. As, however, he did not hit upon the principle for the determination of the required strength of these glasses, those he prescribed were in general far too weak $\left(\frac{1}{80} \text{ to } \frac{1}{40} \right)$. from which, indeed, much could not be expected, and, moreover, supposing that he had to do with an anomaly of accommodation, he still adhered to the hope of being able to cure the asthenopia. Böhm's theory was almost unconditionally adopted by Ruete.‡ This sagacious author expressly states that the exciting causes are not known, and

* *Leçons cliniques des lunettes et des états pathologiques, consécutifs à leur usage irrationnel.* Bruxelles, 1848.

† L. Böhm, *Das Schielen*, p. 117.

‡ Ruete, *Leerboek der ophthalmologie in het Nederduitsch bewerkt en met aanteekeningen voorzien door* Professor Donders, p. 713. Utrecht, 1847.

that the disease may be congenital and sometimes hereditary : thus he appears to be upon the point of asking what may be the organic basis of the affection, but he finally contents himself with the conclusion, that "the proximate cause, as Böhm has proved, is a weakness of the motor nerves of the eye." Thence also his hope of curing the disease.

Others have been less circumspect in the assumption of exciting causes. The majority of these observers believed the causes they assigned to be alone sufficient to produce asthenopia. Among these causes, excessive tension of accommodation for near objects was especially mentioned. The very names given by some to asthenopia, "Affection of the Retina from excessive employment" of Lawrence, "Impaired Vision from overwork" of Cooper,* show how much importance was attributed thereto. By Carron du Villards† we find asthenopia even described as a *peculiar* form of disease, from which the embroiderers of Nancy were said to have particularly suffered, and soon after the same affection was found among the lacemakers of Brussels. Sichel, too, thinks that particular callings develop this condition. Thus the circumstance under which the existing anomaly might manifest itself by peculiar morbid phenomena, was considered to be the cause of the anomaly itself. This cannot cause surprise. Up to the 16th, the 20th, nay, even to the 25th year, the power of vision had continued normal; no complaints were made; but gradually, precisely in persons who were almost incessantly occupied with close work, the continuance of the latter had become more and more difficult, and if the work was for some time suspended, improvement took place. Could it be otherwise than that the affection should be considered as a purely acquired condition, and that the cause of it should be sought in excessive tension ?—In addition, a long train of causes has been drawn up by Mackenzie and others from circumstances which accidentally coincided with the development of the phenomena.

If we glance back at what has been above stated, we find that asthenopia at first lay concealed in amblyopia, that it gradually—although still referred to amblyopia, whether as predisposition, whether as the commencement, or, finally, as a peculiar form of that affection—emerged from its obscurity, that afterwards, without the participation of the retina being as yet denied, its seat was sought more and more in the organs of accommodation, until at last the retina was almost completely excluded, and the condition was looked upon as a disease of the motor nerves and of the organs of motion of the eye.

At this time the source of the power of accommodation had not yet been discovered, much less had its mechanism been demonstrated. There was almost as much reason to assign the principal part in that function to the external muscles of the eye, as to the muscular system situated in the eye. This led to the supposition that asthenopia was to be sought in a spasmodic contraction of some external muscles of the eye, and there were practitioners who had the courage to cut through these muscles. This is a melancholy page in the history of operative ophthalmic surgery. It is

---

* White Cooper, *On Near Sight*, etc. p. 124.

† *Annales d'Oculistique*, Tome iii., Supplém. p. 256.

the more sad, because thereby in general ignorance is exposed, so great, that myopia, presbyopia, and asthenopia were not even distinguished, and because, on the other hand, we find results communicated to which, to use no harder expression, we will, with Mackenzie, apply only the words of Scarpa: "Istorie di guarigioni sorprendenti, e poco dissimili dai prodigi."

Much may, however, be alleged in exculpation. In the first place, history shows that every discovery, and certainly also every new operation, usually leads to exaggeration. This is the result of an enthusiasm deeply rooted in human nature, and which has also its good side. Without it truth appears to gain no victory in the domain of science. Moreover, in the operation for strabismus, improvement of the power of vision was actually obtained, and many now thought that this improvement was the result of a change of refraction: in the then position of science this was certainly rather to be expected than an even now unexplained improvement of the acuteness of vision. We may also assume that, even when asthenopia existed without strabismus, the rest which the patients had to observe for some time after the operation caused the fatigue, on an endeavour to read, to occur less quickly. Besides, it is easy to understand, that when the musculus rectus internus was cut through, stronger tension of accommodation, with convergence of the visual lines to a certain point, became possible, just as may be effected by means of a prismatic glass with the refracting angle directed inwards. In any case, we will not judge harshly of the operators of that season of rage for operating. It is enough that for a time the cause of asthenopia was sought in the external muscles of the eye, and that the results obtained on division of the latter were supposed to furnish a fresh proof of the correctness of the views of those who referred it to them. Asthenopia was in these cases really the subject of discussion. Although here Bonnet,* for whom the priority of the application of the division of the muscles in these cases is claimed by Phillips and Guérin,† as well as Cunier,‡ is speaking of myopia, the cases communicated by these writers leave no doubt respecting the nature of the affection. They supposed that myopia existed, whenever anyone could decipher a certain print better near the eye than at the distance of a foot, and they thought that the myopia had given way, or was diminished, when such a person could subsequently distinguish the same print at a greater distance, or could continue his work longer.

From this error even Ludwig Böhm was not completely free. After the discovery of the principle of accommodation, nothing more was said of abnormal pressure of the muscles of the eye, nor of dividing the latter as a remedy for asthenopia. Stellwag von Carion § refers asthenopia exclusively to a diminution of accommodation, and, indeed, in particular to

---

* *Annales d'Ocul.*, Tome vi., p. 73.

† *Ibid.*, Tome v., p. 31.

‡ *Ibid.*, Tome v., pp. 139, 173.

§ Stellwag von Carion, *Die Ophthalmologie vom naturwissenschaftlichen Standpunkte aus.* Bd. ii. Erlangen, 1855.

18

presbyopia. " In the majority of cases,"—thus he expresses his opinion,—
" normal vision passes under the phenomena of asthenopia into presbyopia, and kopiopia never comes so remarkably under observation as in the
eyes of elderly people. It belongs quite especially to the later epochs of life ;
and if it is sometimes observed in youth as the precursor of presbyopia,
the attending circumstances are in general of such a nature, that a condition
of the muscle analogous to involution is highly probable." He could not
say more plainly that he considers asthenopia to be a lesion of accommodation. Von Graefe* puts the question on as broad a basis as possible, by here
assigning to asthenopia only a symptomatic signification. Thus he demon-
strates the existence of asthenopia muscularis, proceeding from insufficiency
of the musculi recti interni. Moreover, he brings asthenopia into connexion
with slight degrees of presbyopia. And when he further sees asthenopia
arise, " where the nearest point is but little removed, but where still the
region of permanent accommodation lies considerably farther from the eye
than is normally the case," he seems really on the point of thinking of hypermetropia. In other respects, von Graefe attaches more importance to the
influence of the retina than I think ought to be assigned to it. Finally,
he observed asthenopia in consequence of " actual paresis of accommodation," and in truth the description of the latter may almost completely
apply to asthenopia, the result of hypermetropia.

Our knowledge had reached this point, when I† discovered the cause of
asthenopia in the hypermetropic structure of the eye. The supposed anomaly
of accommodation then became an anomaly of refraction, the connexion of
asthenopia with the circumstances under which fatigue is manifested was
made most clear, the necessity of complete relief by spectacles was proven,
while at the same time the hope of a radical cure of asthenopia was extinguished for ever.

---

§ 23. Treatment of Hypermetropia, with Special Reference to Asthenopia.

The treatment of asthenopia has always been called "rational."
I remember the time when this qualification was considered to be an
honour, and when he who in medicine stood upon mere empirical ground, was regarded with disdain. Fortunately, a change has
taken place in this respect. It has become more and more evident that,
even with perfect knowledge of the nature of an anomaly, the final
decision must remain with empiricism, and that, with our defective

* *Archiv für Ophthalm.*, Bd. ii., Abth. i., p. 169.
† *Nederlandsch Tijdschrift voor Geneesk.* Jaarg., 1858, p. 473.

and imperfect notions, science can, with respect to therapeutics, at the most, occasionally suggest what deserves, by preference, to be submitted to investigation, and that her further duty is to endeavour to explain what has been ascertained.

Asthenopia has been looked upon as the result of an enfeebled power of accommodation. Hence its " rational" treatment was directed against the causes of debility, and demanded, above all things, rest of accommodation. With this view, Tyrrell prescribed a systematic treatment. Now, rest was certainly most perfectly attainable by avoiding all work in which looking at near objects was necessary, and where the latter could not be wholly dispensed with, it was thought that the same object might be attained by the use of convex glasses, although, on account of the tension of accommodation connected with convergence, this plan would necessarily be less successful. This constituted the first period of the treatment, in which the organs of accommodation should by rest be relieved from their morbid state. Again on rational grounds, the second period must follow—that of practice : the spectacles were gradually weakened, and close work was permitted for longer and longer intervals, though with the strict injunction to suspend the work on the occurrence of the least fatigue. Thus it was hoped that the asthenopia might be permanently overcome. Many also actually asserted—and in good faith—that they succeeded in this. But were the patients not desired always to take care of themselves ? Did not the prescribed spectacles remain in their hands ?—and would not many, desiring to be relieved from a long-continued treatment, have represented their state too favourably, and when they got worse, have simply stayed at home ? I am convinced that the great majority, if they used their eyes as formerly, would be equally affected by the same troublesome symptoms.—On the supposition that the retina was in some measure implicated in the affection, Böhm and Ruete thought it " rational " to recommend that the convex glasses should be blue. And, indeed, this might, if, as usual, the glasses allowed were too weak, on account of the greater refrangibility of the blue rays, even if the retina was not over-sensitive, be attended with some advantage, which cannot be said of the London *smoked glass* recommended by Fronmüller, by the simply light-diminishing action of which it is certain that few asthenopics would be benefited.

All ophthalmologists did not, however, boast so much of the ex-

2

cellence of their results. " In many cases," says Mackenzie, treating
of the prognosis of asthenopia, "it is our duty to declare the
disease incurable. If the patient is a young lad, bound apprentice
to a sedentary trade, and the disease, from its duration and its
mode of origin, not likely to yield to treatment, we may advise
him to turn shopkeeper, to apply himself to country work, or to
go to sea : if a female, occupied constantly in sewing, to engage in
household affairs, or any other healthy, active employment. Many
a poor man have I told to give up his sedentary trade, and drive a
horse and cart; while to those in better circumstances, and not far
advanced in life, I have recommended emigration, telling them that
though they never could employ their eyes advantageously where
much reading or writing was required, they might see sufficiently
to follow the pastoral pursuits of an Australian colonist."

What is the reason that, before taking so decided a step in the
destination for life of a man, it has not been without prejudice investigated, what the effect would be of the constant use of stronger
convex glasses ? Is it prejudice, in general, against the use of the
latter by young persons ? Or had the old apprehension that asthenopia might lead to amblyopia found fresh support in the experience that, after the use of sufficient convex glasses, the eyes (as we
now know, in consequence of displacement of the relative region
of accommodation) soon act in close work still less perfectly than
before ? Certainly the prejudice must be deeply rooted; for there
lay a very significant hint in the observation drawn by Mackenzie
from life : " A child, the subject of asthenopia, engaged in learning
his lesson, complains he cannot see, and repeats the complaint so
frequently, especially by candlelight, that his father or grandfather
at last says, ' Try my glasses.' *The child now sees perfectly*, and
night after night the loan of the glasses is required before his task
can be finished." And yet he adds, "It would have been better
had glasses been selected of the longest focus, which would have
enabled the child to read, or, better still, he had been put to bed,
and the lesson left till daylight." There is no doubt that
Mackenzie gave far too weak glasses, and therefore he concludes with
the unsatisfactory words : " In some instances the state of asthenopia
is so very easily excited, that the patient is never able to apply
himself to any trade requiring the ordinary use of sight. These
facts are sufficient to show the serious nature of asthenopia. It is
an infirmity much more to be dreaded than many disorders of the

eye which, to superficial observation, present a far more formidable appearance."

It is a great satisfaction to be able to say that asthenopia need now no longer be an inconvenience to any one. In this we have an example, by what trifling means science sometimes obtains a triumph, blessing thousands in its results. The discovery of the simple fact that asthenopia is dependent on the hypermetropic structure of the eye, pointed out the way in which it was to be obviated. Could it be otherwise than that, with the correction of the hypermetropia by means of convex glasses, its resulting asthenopia must also disappear? But here, too, science might mislead one. For it might appear rational to determine the degree of the total hypermetropia, and to neutralise this entirely, and at first I proposed this method. But I had overlooked the fact, as experience soon taught me, that even in the use of completely neutralising convex glasses, the hypermetropia remained in part latent, in consequence of which not only was the vision of distant objects with these glasses indistinct, but also, with moderate convergence, the eye was still always accommodated for a too near point. The unpleasant sensation connected with the relaxation to the minimum of the relative range of accommodation, whereby in this case also vision at an ordinary distance was not yet acute, caused the object to be brought closer and closer to the eye, and thus we saw the patient fall from Scylla into Charybdis— that is, from accommodative into muscular asthenopia. My error lay in supposing a neutralised hypermetropic to be equal to an emmetropic eye, which, as I have above (p. 123) shown, is by no means the case. Thus it is in general : science theorises ; practice tests and rectifies her hypotheses, and of this rectification science has, in order to restore herself, again to give account.

In the establishment of the rules to which experience led me, I must distinguish between two series of cases: a, those which, with normal range of accommodation, are exclusively dependent on H ; b, those where diminution of the range of accommodation, or want of energy, plays a more or less important part.

The great majority of the cases belong to the *first* category : hypermetropia is the cause, and, indeed, the only cause, why close vision cannot be maintained. It is self-evident that this form occurs only in youth, when, if the eye were emmetropic, the idea of the existence of presbyopia could not yet be entertained. Indeed, as I have already explained, a certain range of accommodation belongs to the conditions of asthenopia. Many announce themselves as asthenopics at from the eighteenth to the twenty-sixth year of life, when $\frac{1}{A}$ has descended to $\frac{1}{5}$ or $\frac{1}{6}$. The majority of these are females. The cause of this appears to me to consist exclusively in the occupation. He who is not constantly occupied with close work acquires, even with a moderate degree of H, no symptoms of asthenopia. Now, in most female occupations, continued close vision is undoubtedly more required than in those of males; and in certain ranks of society, where the man is almost wholly exempt from special tension of accommodation, sewing and darning in the evening, and often by bad light, fall, in addition to her household work, to the lot of the woman. In this alone, and by no means in the more frequent occurrence of H, I think we must seek the cause why the complaint of asthenopia is oftener heard from women than from men.

The first thing we have to do in asthenopia is to determine the degree of the manifest hypermetropia—in other words, to examine what is the strongest convex glass with which the vision of distant objects becomes acute. This glass is, however, seldom sufficient completely to guard against fatigue in close work. The patient may, nevertheless, be allowed to read with it at our consultation; but it is only when he can do this without any inconvenience, and when, moreover, with these glasses the binocular nearest point p_2 lies but a little farther from the eye than in the emmetropic organ at the same age, we can determine in favour of commencing their use. But we often find immediate indication to give him somewhat stronger glasses, for example, of $\frac{1}{16}$ with $Hm = \frac{1}{20}$: in very young persons, in whom we may expect much Hl, and, moreover, in those who are somewhat more advanced, for example, at thirty years of age, when the range of accommodation has undergone much diminution, glasses which correct only the Hm are scarcely ever sufficient. If the patient can easily return, the glasses thought suitable are given him, without any further direction than never to work without the spectacles, every half hour to interrupt his work for some minutes, to avoid excessive fatigue, and in about eight days to bring a report of how he finds himself. Almost invariably he returns with expressions of satisfaction and gratitude. He now obtains permission to use his eyes at his own discretion, and is requested to return, if he feels any inconvenience—in any case after the lapse of a year or two, when probably the Hm shall have somewhat increased, and the use of stronger spectacles shall have become advisable. But it may also appear that the glasses were either too weak or too strong. If too weak, the asthenopia has not been entirely removed; and we now often find, especially on some fatigue, a rather higher degree of Hm than before : we also find that p_2, defined with the glasses, is further from the eye than it ought to be; —of course, we must then go up, often even above the Hm now ascertained, and bring the p_2 nearly to the normal distance. If the glasses were too strong, the work had to be held too near the eye ; acute vision was, indeed, thus attained, but a peculiar sensation of fatigue ensued (muscular asthenopia). This complaint, although rare, occurs sometimes, even when only the Hm has been neutralised: the explanation of this is found in the too powerful tension of accommodation excited each time, and depending upon habit, precisely at a convergence of from $10''$ to $14''$. Under such circumstances, we must really begin with weaker glasses, and pass over to stronger ones in proportion as the extraordinary tension ceases. In the other cases, the holding the book too near is combined with the complaint, that with the spectacles distant vision is so particularly bad. I may say that of late years it has seldom occurred to me, that the glasses chosen with attention to the above rules have not completely answered their purpose. I very seldom, also, find it necessary in asthenopia to have recourse to the employment of mydriatics for the determination of H. It is only in those cases where the asthenopia justifies us in supposing the existence of H, and where, nevertheless, no Hm is observed, not even on moderate fatigue,—further, when the spectacles fixed on and modified on good principles, do not answer,—perhaps, also, when we can see the patient only once, that the employment of a mydriatic is required in the interest of the patient. But it is, however, perfectly justifiable for the sake of the more accurate study of the connexion between Hm and Hl, the more so because, during mydriasis, if necessary, close work may be very well performed with stronger spectacles. If we now know Hm and Hl, we give glasses which neutralise Hm and about $\frac{1}{4}$ of Hl : in general they will answer the purpose either immediately, or after a few weeks.

Hitherto, as we have seen, ophthalmologists endeavoured, by the use of progressively weaker glasses to obtain a radical cure of asthenopia. With the knowledge of the cause of asthenopia this endeavour is completely reversed. We wish gradually to give stronger glasses, and therefore we investigate from time to time in our asthenopic patients, the position of the relative region of accommodation, or perhaps only the Hm, and if the latter appears to be increased, we give according to the rules laid down, other and stronger glasses. It is not until the H has almost completely given way to Hm, and the relative region of accommodation has on the whole acquired a normal position, that we have, in the use of the glasses so indicated, a decided guarantee against the return of the asthenopia, and in young persons the same glasses are now adapted for distance and for near objects. With this strengthening of the glasses laymen have sometimes made known their fears to me that, at last, no spectacles should be found strong enough to accommodate their eyes. To persons in their situation this fear would certainly appear to be justified. We may, however, quite set them at ease on this point. I usually take the trouble to explain to them, that if once the deficient power of the eye shall be entirely made good, the limit for the strength of the glasses is provisionally attained, and that what the senile changes at a more advanced period of life in general demand, can still very easily be added. It is evident that even under the most unfavourable circumstances, we cannot easily be obliged to rise to such strong glasses as are necessary in aphakia. To these unfavourable circumstances belong amblyopia, and especially deficient range of accommodation. What has already been said on these points in speaking of Pr, may be here also the guide of our treatment. Rules for the management of the combination of H with Pr are there given. I have in this place only to mention, that in amblyopia of one eye, in consequence of exclusion, separate practice of this eye with a reading or magnifying glass several times daily, for some minutes at a time, is indicated.

So much for the use of spectacles for near objects. It is now an important question, whether asthenopics should also in ordinary life wear glasses for distant objects. On a superficial view there appears to be no objection to such a plan. Why should a person not remove the Hm, and thus make the acute vision of distant objects, without extraordinary tension, possible? Undoubtedly, if we could make the glass an integral part of the eye, we should have no reason to hesitate. We should then even be justified in neutralising almost the whole H, convinced that the relative region of accommodation would soon adapt itself to the new refractive condition. But this is not the case : the glasses do not stand *in* the eye, but *before* the eye, and are sometimes not even at hand. Hence it is of great consequence, that the patient should be able to distinguish tolerably well also without glasses, and it is certain that if the hypermetropic individual accustoms himself to wear correcting spectacles, he will gradually lose the power of distinguishing without glasses. That is the unfavourable side of the question of wearing spectacles. Even in employing spectacles for near objects he loses in part the advantageous use of his accommodation : but in this case an actual necessity is in question, and he has, therefore, no choice. Not so with respect to looking at distant objects. With repeated strong tension of accommodation the power of vision, as we have seen, remains undisturbed in hypermetropic individuals. From the tension necessary to see distinctly without spectacles at a distance, which is each time required only as for a moment, no injurious effect is certainly to be expected. Therefore this may safely be required of the accommodation. Consequently, when H is still wholly facultative, when the persons can even say to us : " in ordinary life, I have no inconvenience, and at a distance I see excellently,"—we should not press spectacles on them to be worn constantly. At most we may say to them, that, when they have become somewhat older (when the facultative H shall have given place to relatively absolute) they will derive great advantage from the use of spectacles for distance also ; they can then apply to the oculist, so soon as they observe that they no longer distinguish satisfactorily at a distance.* But it is quite ano-

---

* Last year I had the good fortune to meet an English gentleman, eminent in the scientific world. I observed that he saw with spectacles of $\frac{1}{8}$ at 11″ distance, and concluded therefore that he was hypermetropic. "You do not see well at a distance," I remarked to him. " O no ! " replied the able and vigorous veteran, " I no longer recognise the characters of minerals, as I formerly did, at a great distance, and if I wish to look at them before my feet through my spectacles, I stumble over them." " Go," I rejoined, " and ask the optician for glasses of $\frac{1}{30}$." On the following day he wrote to me: " I cannot tell you how grateful I am for the *new* sense you have given me. I now see the eyes of the handsome girls, and the wrinkles of the old ladies as well as when I was a young soldier."

ther matter, when, even in youth, relative or absolute H exists; then, notwithstanding every effort of accommodation, distant vision is not acute, and we need not now hesitate to assist it with glasses. The best result attainable, under such circumstances, consists in this: that the same spectacles, which are not too strong for distance, should be sufficient for ordinary close work. With the usual range of accommodation this result is obtained in spite of the disadvantages connected with the use of convex glasses (compare p. 145), so soon as the relative region of accommodation has sufficiently shifted, and therefore the indication here is, by causing the patient always to wear spectacles (at first weaker ones) to promote this change of place.

With respect to the second category of asthenopia, I have here but little to say. The cases contained in it are characterised by the fact, that the accommodation itself is disturbed or morbidly diminished, and the proper place to consider them is therefore where in the Second Part I shall have to speak of the anomalies of accommodation. Here it may be in general remarked, that, when in asthenopia either no, or comparatively very slight, H exists, and where, moreover, muscular asthenopia is excluded, we may suspect the presence of disturbed or morbidly diminished accommodation. To this point our investigation must then be directed. If general weakness is exclusively the cause, recovery from the asthenopia is to be expected, if we succeed in restoring the strength. If paresis of accommodation exists, without H, the asthenopia of course gives way when the paresis is removed. In either case convex glasses are meanwhile useful. Where painful accommodation exists a special treatment is required.

What I have to say with respect to the treatment of H in general, apart from asthenopia, is included in the foregoing. As to the slightest degrees of H, which scarcely produce asthenopia, they require merely, as has been mentioned while on the subject of presbyopia, that the use of spectacles be permitted some years earlier than usual. The most extreme degrees are in their symptoms characterised by the fact, that very near the eye, the same type is read comparatively better than at a distance. The explanation of this apparent paradox has already been given. Since at a distance also vision is not acute, the suspicion of a complication of myopia with amblyopia readily suggests itself. Moreover, the aggregate of the symptoms of asthenopia does not appear distinct: from the beginning the difficulty is there, and results of fatigue do not so readily present themselves. And yet in this case relief is also above all to be sought specially in the use of convex glasses. They are necessary not only for the easy performance of close work, they are desirable also for seeing at a distance. Here we need not be afraid of obtaining, by their means, a less desirable⁻ displacement of the relative range of accommodation (compare p. 125). The strength of the requisite glasses is deduced from the degree of Hm and H. For ordinary wear the glasses must completely neutralise Hm. In reading the spectacles fall somewhat on the nose, and frequently the same glasses are now also sufficient for that purpose; if they are not, we give some a little stronger, so that p_2 comes to lie within the desired distance of distinct vision. Accordingly as Hm increases, we strengthen the glasses. Where complication with presbyopia exists, the use of two pairs of spectacles, one to wear generally, the other for close work, is indispensable. When strong glasses are necessary, the preference is to be given, among other reasons, for the more advantageous position of the principal points, to periscopic glasses, whose concave surface must be turned towards the eye.

Are we in H to hope for a radical cure? The answer must be in the negative. *A priori*, we should think, that, as the emmetropic eye may become myopic, and as myopia may be progressive, H might give place to E and even to M. In fact it appears possible that H of the as yet undeveloped eye might disappear during the years of development. But if the development have once taken place, I have never seen H give way, in the healthy state I have never seen it pass into E or M: this occurs only where there is increasing convexity from disease of the cornea. On superficial examination one may be deceived in this respect. A gentleman, aged 54, had been obliged to use convex glasses so early as in his 36th year, and now he preferred working without spectacles. With $S = 1$ he had $M = \frac{1}{15}$. Had H in this case not given way to M?

I found that his power of accommodation was completely paralysed, and that it had been so from his 36th year, and ophthalmoscopic investigation indicated progressive M. It therefore readily suggested itself that at the age of 36 the paralysis of accommodation, with $M = \frac{1}{20}$ or $\frac{1}{30}$, had rendered convex glasses necessary, which through the progress of M had become superfluous, and indeed inapplicable. Hence it is evident that the eye, when of hypermetropic structure, has no tendency to M. And if a modification in this direction does not sometimes spontaneously occur, it is not to be expected that art should in such a case be able to do anything. How could we, without bringing the eye into danger, endeavour with any force to make the cornea more convex or the visual axis longer? The cure of ordinary asthenopia by division of the muscles belongs to the fables of the period of operative mania, to which I have in the course of my historical remarks more than once alluded. We understand that tenotomy of the mm. recti interni interferes with the convergence, and that therefore with certain degrees of the latter in binocular vision more tension of accommodation can be associated. This tenotomy acts in the same manner as prismatic glasses with the refracting angles turned inwards, from which asthenopic persons in fact derive some advantage. In two instances, where the action of the recti externi was evidently very weak, von Graefe has* also actually put in practice tenotomy of the interni. He adds, however, correctly, that this method, contrasted with the simple choice of spectacles, is more interesting than practical. And in truth the hypermetropia cannot be diminished either by this or by any other operative method, and the asthenopia will not be permanently removed. I may add that when in developed strabismus convergens correcting tenotomy is performed, the use of the convex glasses is still often necessary, to prevent asthenopia and relapse of the strabismus. It is only where the asthenopia depends on insufficiency of muscles, that the operative method can have its triumphs.

Some cases, which I shall now in conclusion relate, will afford me the opportunity of introducing a few additional practical hints.

H does not always cause disturbance, and correction is then unnecessary.

I. An elegant lady, aged 22, is under treatment for slight granulations. At a distance her vision is acute, with negative glasses it is not so good, with $\frac{1}{40}$ and indeed with $\frac{1}{24}$, it is as acute as without glasses, but unpleasantly large: "men are like giants." There was consequently $Hm = \frac{1}{24}$, and we may probably infer $Ht = \frac{1}{14}$. Nevertheless she had experienced no

---

* *Archiv f. Ophthalmologie*, B. viii. Abth. 2, p. 321.

kind of inconvenience. But read "she did not much," and of work she "did nothing." Had she been obliged to do much close work, asthenopia would not have been absent. Indeed, she now remembered that she could not see the finest things so accurately as other ladies of her age, and that she had even, in gazing at distant objects, sometimes observed a dimness. She had a horror of spectacles. Perhaps, being well able to comprehend this, I ought not to have predicted, that with her 30th year she would have need of them ; the recommendation to call in advice, whenever she should not see near objects well, would have been sufficient. Indeed for the moment there was no indication for spectacles, which would only have produced an, as yet, undesirable displacement of the relative range of accommodation. On account of the existing H, stricter rest had to be enjoined, so long as the granulations lasted, than is otherwise necessary.

We learn to distinguish, at first sight, an ordinary case of asthenopia, the result of H.

II. Miss H., aged 19, is announced. She has a florid look, has clear eyes, without a trace of disease, blue iris, mobile pupil, not a very deep globe, flat margins to the socket, the visual axes appear to diverge. I suspect asthenopia. I make her read and bring the book to 6″: reading becomes difficult ; at 5″ it is impossible. There is either H or diminished $\frac{1}{A.}$ My eye falls on those about her, I see a brother with converging strabismus. This was decisive in favour of H. "You cannot persevere with your work." She answers : "No." "On exertion you get a feeling of tension over the eyes, press upon the part with the hand, rub over the closed eyes, and then it passes off, but only for a short time ?" "Precisely," is the answer. Confidence is gained. "You have no pain in the eyes ?" "At a distance you see well ?" "Yes." "After a long rest you can continue your work better ?" "Yes, yes."—With $\frac{1}{18}$ she distinguishes well at a distance, and moving the glasses at the first moment not so well ; with $\frac{1}{16}$ not so acutely as with $\frac{1}{18}$, with $\frac{1}{24}$ not more acutely ; between the two eyes there is little difference. Ophthalmoscopically all is well. I learn further, that for some years the inconvenience felt in working has been always increasing ; that formerly when weakened by fever, she could for a time neither read nor sew ; that she once tried a pair of spectacles, but was strongly cautioned against wearing them, &c., &c. She gets spectacles of $\frac{1}{16}$ to work with, with a recommendation now and then to pause for a little, and at first not to do much in the evening. At the end of a week she has forgotten her ailment. She now works too with less trouble occasionally for a short time without spectacles, which I advise her to do, though with the recommendation to return to the use of the spectacles on the least trace, or rather before the occurrence of fatigue.

Asthenopics have sometimes a sad past, and live in a gloomy future.

III. The Rev. G. D., aged 52, looks dejected. " My good Professor," he says, " I come to you, for I feel that I am getting blind ! " For the last twenty years he has thought that within a year he should be blind; and, singularly enough, although he still sees, he continues to look upon every year as the last ! Such is the man ! His life has been a struggle with his eyes. Even as a child he read with difficulty. When a student, the least exertion fatigued him, and he was compelled to learn more by hearing than by his own study. As a preacher, he has been obliged to write his sermons in a rather large hand, and still to get them off by heart. And, what was the worst part of it, he never read nor worked without the idea that he was thus hastening his blindness—interfering with the concentration of his mind upon any definite object. The same fear of blindness had restrained him from a matrimonial alliance with which he believed his happiness for life to be connected. He trusted in art. He had faith in a person he consulted in Germany ; and if the optician had sometimes given him spectacles which had brought him relief, these were mercilessly taken from him again by the oculist on the first consultation, as a treacherous instrument which must, in the end, inflict upon him the total loss of his sight. At last he had in his fortieth year, got convex glasses of $\frac{1}{40}$, and he now uses $\frac{1}{20}$. " Do you see with these spectacles at a distance ? " was my first inquiry. " Something better," he replied, " but still very imperfectly." I tried $\frac{1}{10}$: "Much better" was his verdict ;—subsequently I gave him $\frac{1}{8}$: "Still better." In a word, there was H $= \frac{1}{7}$ with S $= \frac{17}{20}$, and, with his slight range of accommodation, he needed glasses of $\frac{1}{5\cdot5}$, in order to make reading at the distance of a foot easy. He got $\frac{1}{7}$ to wear. The man was grateful as a child. He left me as one saved from destruction.—Such victims of the prejudice against the use of convex glasses are not uncommon.

Where H exists, paralysis of accommodation may give rise to disquieting symptoms.

IV. E. K., a boy of ten years, son of Dr. K., remarks in the morning that he is not in a condition to read. His father sees that the pupils are rather large and are immovable. Paralysis of accommodation occurs to him ; but at a distance also, the boy cannot properly distinguish objects: "there must consequently be a lurking affection of the optic nerve or of the brain." He brings his son to me. I establish the fact of paralysis of the sphincter of the pupil in both eyes. Neither on convergence, nor on the incidence of strong light, does contraction of the pupil arise: accommodative and reflex movements are both absent. The inference that there is paralysis of accommodation is thus justified. Why cannot the boy see even at a distance? A glance with the ophthalmoscope clears all up: it appears I must accommodate about $\frac{1}{12}$ in order to see in the uninverted image the fundus oculi; and, as I am emmetropic, our boy has therefore H of about $\frac{1}{12}$. With $\frac{1}{12}$ he then saw admirably at a distance; with $\frac{1}{6}$ he read at the distance of a foot. All fear of an affection of the system of the optic nerve was gone. In speaking of the anomalies of accommodation, I shall revert to such cases. Here it may suffice to observe that within four weeks the paralysis had given way, the H had again gradually become for the most part latent, and that in what the boy had to do or to read, he now no longer complained even of fatigue. In a few years asthenopia may be expected, and the use of the convex spectacles while working will then be indicated.

Paresis of accommodation in young persons is scarcely distinguishable from asthenopia through H.

v. H. J., a boy aged 14, is brought to me, complaining that for some time he has been unable to read. He looks pale and weakly. I suspect asthenopia, whether in consequence of a slight degree of H, with peculiarly debilitating causes, or in consequence of paresis of accommodation. The pupils move well. " Do you feel weak ? " " Yes, I have not yet recovered my strength after an attack of sore-throat." The articulation of words is imperfect, he speaks through his nose, and the soft explosive consonants (b, d, and g) are, especially at the end of the words, pronounced as corresponding nasals (m, n, ng) (paresis of the palate). These symptoms are characteristic as the result of angina *diphtheritica* (better, *diphtherina*). I therefore infer the existence of paresis, notwithstanding the movable pupils. At a distance S is $= 1$, and neither convex nor concave glasses are borne: consequently we have to deal with E. The nearest point lies, instead of at 3″, at 9″, and can be maintained there only for a moment, as by spasmodic tension. The statement of the case is more accurately formulated as: Reading can be maintained only for a moment, vision at a distance is excellent. From ordinary asthenopia, in consequence of H, the condition is distinguished by its rapid appearance (*N.B.*, about a fortnight after the symptoms of angina had given way), by the easy *permanent* vision at a distance (this was not observed by the patient, but was found on examination), and by the almost immediate occurrence of fatigue and of absolute impossibility of seeing near objects.

Muscular asthenopia may be connected with H.

vi. P. C., aged 20 years, comes with the ordinary complaint of asthenopia, which has existed from youth. $Hm\frac{1}{60}$ is established, and $H\frac{1}{24}$ given to read, wherewith p comes to lie at 6″. At the end of a week the patient comes again; he can persevere somewhat, but not much, longer. Paralysis by atropia discloses $H = \frac{1}{12}$. Glasses of $\frac{1}{16}$ are permitted, with which, after the paralysis of accommodation has ceased, every distant object is in a mist, and the patient reads by preference at only 8″ distance, notwithstanding that $S = 1$: moreover, the unpleasant tension in the eyes and in the forehead becomes greater than before. Insufficiency of the muscles now suggests itself. The movements are free in every direction; the convergence, on the contrary, is, on the approach of the object, maintained only at 5″, and behind the hand, the one eye deviates much more rapidly outwards; on the contrary, there is at a distance single vision, when a prism of 10° is held before the eye with the angle outwards, for which a divergence of the visual lines of about 5° is required (compare p. 132.) Evidently, therefore, the mm. recti interni are insufficient. Glasses of $\frac{1}{16}$, placed very close to one another, make the convergence required somewhat less, but render no assistance. Permanent help is derived only from spherico-prismatic glasses $\left(\frac{1}{16}\right.$ with a prism of 5°$\left.\right)$. In this case we should have been justified in cutting through, in one of the eyes at least, the tendon of the m. rectus externus; the convergence would have become easier, and yet even at a distance there would not have been double vision. " Shall I then be able to read without spectacles? " I was obliged to give a negative answer. Indeed, when the convergence became easier, less tension of accommodation could be associated therewith, and the existing H would therefore, still more than before, give rise to asthenopia. Therefore, too, in the combination with a prism, the convex glass must be rather strong $\left(\frac{1}{16}\right)$. My answer made the patient shrink from the operation. The almost perfectly latent existence of the H was connected with the insufficiency of the mm. interni; the prism alone, without combination with a spherical glass, made a greater portion manifest.

Strong H in a child has hitherto been almost invariably regarded as M.

VII. A girl, aged six years, is said to have very weak eyes. If she wishes to see anything, she runs to a bright light, and holds the object directly before her eyes. Her anxious parents had taken much advice respecting her; the child was generally considered to be near-sighted. The fact that she so particularly looks for bright light, in order to see anything well, makes me doubt the correctness of this opinion: in that case considerable amblyopia would necessarily be combined with the myopia.

From the external appearance, I had scarcely a doubt of the existence of H. At the distance of 3″ the child saw, with her head aslant and her eyelids nearly closed, No. III of Snellen; smaller letters she did not see; with $\frac{1}{6}$, on the contrary, she saw II at 8″: so the proof was supplied. S was $= \frac{1}{2}$. Probably astigmatism exists, to be more fully investigated at a somewhat later period, when the patient shall be able to give a more accurate account of herself. Meanwhile, she may provisionally use $\frac{1}{6}$ in learning,—if she chooses she may also wear them habitually. "This she would rather not do."

Even with a slight degree of H, tension of accommodation may be painful.

VIII. Mr. X., a lithographer, aged twenty-one, has, until some months ago, been able without trouble to perform even his work. Now and then, it is true, he got a pain in his eyes, but that he attributed to excessive exertion. Of late, however, the pains are so frequent, and rapidly become so violent, that he is obliged to forego his work. Above the eyes he feels at most a slight pressure; in the eyes themselves the pain settles, and is at the same time stinging and oppressive. Soon after leaving off work the pain always ceases, and if he refrains from exertion, and from fixing his sight strongly, it does not return. Objectively no morbid change is perceptible in the eyes. The movements, too, are normal; divergence with prisms held before the eyes is impossible. Examination indicates only Hm $= \frac{1}{36}$. After artificial mydriasis we obtain Hm $= \frac{1}{24}$. Glasses of $\frac{1}{36}$ and of $\frac{1}{24}$ are of no use. Indeed, at the patient's time of life, and with his range of accommodation $= 1 : 4\cdot3$, he would easily have overcome the existing H. Former cases had taught me, that all medication in this instance would be useless, except daily repeated paralysis by atropia. To this I had in the present case immediate recourse, at the same time prescribing glasses of $\frac{1}{24}$ for distant, and of $\frac{1}{8}$ for near objects. The pain forthwith ceased.—This case belongs properly to the anomalies of accommodation, to which I shall revert more at length. I have communicated it here, because I have observed such instances of painful spasm, on every tension of accommodation, only where H exists. It is true they are rare: altogether I have seen but three.

We must beware of mistaking apparent for true asthenopia.

IX. Mrs. N., aged thirty-three years, a nervous, weak little person, complains that she cannot continue her work. She soon becomes tired and suffers pain,

19

the eye begins to weep, and she cannot resume her occupation during the entire day. In the evening especially she is obliged strictly to avoid all exertion; occasionally, too, some photophobia is present. I make her read : she holds the book at about 10″, and says she can still distinguish accurately when I bring it 5″ nearer. Already I suspect that no H exists. At a distance S appeared only $= \frac{1}{2}$; but while positive glasses diminish still more the acuteness of vision, S becomes $= 1$, with the use of $- \frac{1}{36}$: there is consequently $M = \frac{1}{36}$. Closer investigation of her case shows, that it differs in many respects from asthenopia by H. She has pain in the eyes themselves, which, properly speaking, always continues, and only increases on exertion; the characteristic tension above the eyebrows is, on the contrary, absent; moreover, to the last moment she sees acutely, and it is only the pain which makes her give up work. With these symptoms there is now a slight irritation of the eyes persistently present. Ophthalmoscopic investigation reveals capillary hyperæmia of the optic nerve. Nothing more is to be seen. Such cases are not uncommon; they occur mostly with myopia, but they are also met with in other eyes. It is a not well explained form of hyperæsthesia, in connexion with symptoms of congestion. Blue glasses, resting the eyes, stimulating derivatives, &c., are only too often tried in vain. To refer such cases to asthenopia is to call two conditions widely different both in essence and in symptoms, by the same name.

Absolute H of the highest degree simulating M with amblyopia.

(Case kindly communicated by Mr. Bowman to the author, compare p. 258.)

Mr. T., twenty-five years of age, has very small globes—as far as can be judged they would appear of this size on a horizontal section (Fig. 121 a).

Fig. 120.

Fig. 121.

Fig. 120 represents about the size of cornea and pupil. The antero-posterior diameter is too short, but so also are the transverse and vertical, so that the eye does not look too *flat* on a lateral view. The anterior chamber is shallow (the iris near the cornea)—the pupil has this range under varying light ◎. As to the presence of the lens, the patient was unwilling to have the pupil expanded by atropia; but I perfectly satisfied myself by the catoptric test that the lenses are present—the reflexion from the front being very distinct. The convex form of the iris and the prominence of the pupil are also evidently due to the iris being thrown forwards by the lens.

When I first saw Mr. T., in 1856, he was at College, and had distinguished himself by scholarship, but his sight had become much fatigued, and he accordingly consulted me. He was using for the right eye a convex glass of $\frac{1}{7}$ for distant vision, and when he held this glass at 2 or 3 inches in front of the eye, he could read a book held two feet off. Without a glass he could read the smallest print (diamond = Jaeger No. 1) at about $\frac{3}{4}$ of an inch from the eye.

He had up to this time always used the right eye, and attempts were made to bring the left eye into use, but without success as regards comfort, though the vision of that eye improved under them.

In the summer of 1857 he had come to use the right eye in reading, without a glass, and holding the print very close. He could thus read with tolerable comfort.

In May, 1862, he had been some time in the habit of employing strong convex glasses, viz., $\frac{1}{1\frac{5}{8}}$ for distant vision, being then able to see Jaeger, No. 18, at eight feet; and $\frac{1}{1\frac{1}{4}}$ for reading, being then able to see Jaeger, No. 2, at 4″, with comfort, unless in a strong light.

---

§ 24. Strabismus convergens, the Result of H.

Strabismus is a deviation in the direction of the eyes, in consequence of which the two yellow spots receive images from different objects. In strabismus the visual lines do not cross one another in the point it is desired to observe; only one of the two, that of the undeviating eye, is directed to that point. Under this deviation not only does the expression of the face suffer from the want of symmetry in its most eloquent parts, but the power of vision, at least in one of the eyes, is usually disturbed, and the squinter always loses the advantage of binocular vision.

Strabismus is not an independent morbid condition; as is comprised in the definition given, it is only a symptom. We may add, that it is a symptom, dependent on very different conditions, and as such connected with other very different phenomena. He who proposes to write a manual, and in it to treat systematically of all defects of the eye, will more than once meet with strabismus, as a more or less constant result of definite conditions. It will repeatedly occur as a constituent of a compound anomaly, in which it is connected with the cause on which it depended, and with all the results of that cause. But there will be no room for it as an independent

2

form of disease.   It is only in a book on semeiotics that we have to
treat of strabismus in general.

If this view has been long received, writers have not been faithful
to it.   To ascertain this, it is sufficient to consult the manuals.   A
special chapter is devoted to strabismus.   In this everything which
has reference to this deviation is treated of; elsewhere strabismus is
only incidentally mentioned. Even in the investigation of its causes, all
forms, different as they may fundamentally be, are treated of alike.   In
the monographs the case is sometimes no better.   Is it, then, strange
that the pathogeny of strabismus is still so very obscure?   It is an
attribute of human nature to suppose for each phenomenon which
occurs an external cause, and readily to assume as such the first which
presents itself.   From this rashness and credulity pathology has not
entirely freed itself.   With respect to strabismus, the cause is, on
the authority of mothers and nurses, often sought in all kinds
of accidental circumstances, and thus the source of the abnormity, which originally consisted in the form of the eye, is overlooked.

We now know that by far the greater number of cases of strabismus are connected with anomalies of refraction.

According to the direction of the deviation, two forms of oblique
vision are specially to be distinguished : strabismus convergens and
strabismus divergens.   The main result of our investigation may be
expressed in these two propositions .—

1. *Strabismus convergens almost always depends upon hypermetropia.*

2. *Strabismus divergens is usually the result of myopia.*

We have here to treat only of strabismus convergens.

Experience, in the first place, shows, that strabismus convergens
is, in the great majority of cases, combined with H.   In 172 cases
investigated by us, H was 133 times proved to exist in the undevi-
ated eye.   In nine cases myopia existed, five times to such a great
degree that the form of the distended, but little movable, eyeball,
admitted of no other condition ; in thirteen cases difference of refraction of the two eyes was recorded ; five times inflammation was the
cause ; at least five times paralysis had gone before ; three times
there was complication with congenital cataract, twice with
nystagmus.—It is evident how greatly H preponderates : it occurs
in about 77 per cent. of the cases.   And yet I am convinced, that
if we could investigate without distinction all cases of strabismus con-

vergens which occur in a given population, H would be met with relatively still more frequently. In the first place, ordinary cases of strabismus convergens are seldom brought to the oculist, and these are precisely the cases in which H is the only cause : if inflammation, paralysis, or any special complications be present, the patients do not delay to call in help ; and thus, in proportion to the whole, a greater number of these exceptional cases comes to be seen. Moreover, cases are included, which it is not usual to refer to the head of strabismus convergens, as tolerably recent instances of paralysis of the abducent muscle; too strongly convergent, nearly immovable myopic eyes, &c. And, finally, some ordinary certainly rather than extraordinary cases, whose pathogeny was not wholly cleared up, have been neglected.—I therefore do not hesitate to declare, that it is exceptional, to find strabismus convergens without hypermetropia.

In general, it is not the highest degrees of H with which strabismus is combined. Often even, at least in young persons, the hypermetropia is completely latent : it was involuntarily neutralised by tension of the power of accommodation, and appeared first on artificial paralysis of the accommodation. Where it was manifest, it amounted to from $\frac{1}{30}$ to $\frac{1}{10}$, rarely to $\frac{1}{7}$ or more. The total hypermetropia was, so soon as it was manifest, usually not examined, but of course attained, especially in young subjects, a considerably higher degree. With $\frac{1}{30}$ manifest H more than $\frac{1}{15}$ total H may in general be assumed; for where, with complete want of manifest, the total was defined under the influence of paralysis of accommodation, the latter was seldom under $\frac{1}{15}$.

Since in strabismus convergens H in general exists, no other connexion is conceivable than that H is the cause of the deviation. H is, indeed, the primary anomaly, to be sought in the structure of the eye, and originally proper to the organ; strabismus is the secondary condition, which does not arise until some years after birth. In the first period, in the commencement of the so-called periodical oblique vision, it can be proved that H already exists : unquestionably, therefore, it precedes the squinting. And if we add, that the incipient strabismus again gives way, when the hypermetropia is neutralised by a convex glass, we readily infer that H may produce strabismus. The only question, therefore, is, how it can do this, and the answer is evident.

The hypermetropic individual must, in order to see distinctly, accommodate comparatively strongly. This holds good for all distances. Even in looking at remote objects he must endeavour to overcome his hypermetropia by tension of accommodation, and in proportion as the object draws near, he must still add so much accommodation, as the normal emmetropic eye should need on the whole. The vision of near objects therefore especially requires extraordinary tension. Now, as we have seen (compare p. 110), there exists a certain connexion between accommodation and convergence of the visual lines : the more strongly we converge, the more powerfully can we bring our faculty of accommodation into action. A certain tendency to increased convergence, so soon as a person wishes to put his power of accommodation upon the stretch, is therefore unavoidable. This tendency exists in every hypermetropic person. An emmetropic person may also convince himself of this by holding negative glasses before his eyes, and thus bringing the latter temporarily into a condition of hypermetropia. He will distinctly remark, that on the endeavour to see accurately, double images every time threaten to appear as the result of increased convergence, and that he soon has a choice only between indistinct vision and squint. Probably this conflict exists unconsciously in the case of all hypermetropic persons.

Hypermetropia is a very widely spread anomaly. I am convinced that it occurs still more frequently than myopia. Now, if strabismus convergens is in general the result of hypermetropia, the latter evidently is very often met with without strabismus; we may even say, that only in a comparatively small number of cases of hypermetropia is strabismus developed. This, however, need not by any means surprise us. In general, in fact, the necessity of seeing an object *single* with both eyes together, is deeply felt. The direction of the visual lines is thereby forcibly determined. Of this I convinced myself, many years ago, in my experiments on the action of prismatic glasses.* If we bring a weakly prismatic glass, with the refracting edge turned inwards, before one of the eyes, the fixed object is directly seen double, but increased convergence is immediately involuntarily produced, which makes the double images

* *Nederlandsche Lancet*, 2ᵉ Ser., D. iii. p. 233. 1845.

coalesce; and if, some moments later, we again remove the glass, double images for an instant reappear, which, however, equally rapidly disappear, in consequence of lessening the convergence. Now, it is as if the double images, of their own accord, again coalesce: the movement made takes place so spontaneously, that the person is not even conscious of it. This abhorrence of double images, or rather the instinctive adherence to binocular vision, preserves most hypermetropic individuals from strabismus. They sacrifice the advantage of seeing accurately, rather than to allow that on the two yellow spots different objects should form their images. In this, therefore, we find the reason, why not nearly all hypermetropics squint. If one eye be covered with the hand, while it, as well as the other, is open, the visual line will, in *most* hypermetropics, rapidly deviate inwards. The same thing takes place when an emmetropic person holds a negative glass before the uncovered eye.

The question which now suggests itself is : What circumstances must coöperate to give rise to strabismus in hypermetropic individuals?

These circumstances are of a twofold nature : *a,* those which diminish the value of the binocular vision; *b,* those which render the convergence easier.

To the first class belong :

1°. *Congenital difference in the accuracy of vision, or in the refractive condition of the two eyes.*—In hypermetropia the accuracy of vision is often imperfect, whether in one or in both eyes. This is in part attributable to astigmatism, in part to a still unknown imperfection of the retina. If the diminished accuracy of vision affects only *one* eye, then, on too great convergence, the image of this eye will not so much disturb vision. The same is the case when the degree of H in the deviating eye is greater, and the image in this eye is therefore less accurate. In either case, consequently, strabismus will more easily arise. But the tendency doubly increases when both circumstances, a higher degree of H and diminished accuracy of vision, as is often the case, occur combined in the same eye. If the eye has long been deviated, there arises a secondary diminution of the accuracy of vision, as a result of strabismus, to which I shall subsequently revert. In that case, however, we can, with the aid of the ophthalmoscope, often demonstrate a still higher degree of H of this eye.

2°. *Spots on the cornea.*—It is often remarked, that in oblique vision the deviated eye, or, indeed, both eyes, exhibit opacity, or spots on the cornea. Pagenstecher and Saemisch have recently called attention to the frequent occurrence of corneal spots in strabismus. It does not appear to me, however, that spots on the cornea should, in themselves, be capable of exciting strabismus. Although the image of the second eye is less perfect, experience shows that even then the preference is given to binocular vision ; nor is it explicable that one of the eyes should be inclined to deviate, merely for the purpose of making a quite different, rather than, it is true, an unequal, but still corresponding, image fall upon the yellow spot. Ruete* has, upon good grounds, in this way decided the contest between Beer and Joh. Mueller. But it is quite a different question whether, where hypermetropia exists, specks on the cornea and other obscurities might not increase the tendency to strabismus ; whether the less accurate image in the visual axis might not make the image less disturbing, and diminish the abhorrence of an accessory second image. I am very much inclined to assume this. At least, I find specks on the cornea much more common in hypermetropia with strabismus, than in hypermetropia without strabismus. It is true, there may be still another connexion between specks on the cornea and strabismus, to which Ruete† has already directed attention : an inflammation, namely, which produces these specks on the cornea, may extend beneath the conjunctiva to some of the muscles or their envelopes, and produce, first, a spasmodic, and afterwards a nutritive, contraction. Such cases I have already above mentioned. They are, however, comparatively rare ; but they may in part explain the preponderance of specks on the cornea in hypermetropia with strabismus.

In the second place, as I have remarked, the origin of strabismus is promoted by circumstances which render convergence easier. Under this head are to be noted :

1°. *Peculiar structure or innervation of the muscles ; easy mobility of the eyeballs inwards.*—Not unfrequently a congenital insufficiency of the musculi recti interni occurs. It may readily be assumed that the opposite also may be the case ; and, in fact, some eyes converge without any particular tension up to 3″, nay, even up to 2″, and

---

* *Lehrb. der Ophthalmologie f. Aerzte und Studirende.* B. ii. p. 520. Braunschweig, 1854.   † *l. c.* p. 537.

less, from the eye. We may assume that form and position of the eye-ball exercise as much influence in this respect as the structure or innervation of the muscles.

Now, while in insufficiency of movement inwards we have a guarantee against strabismus convergens, free motion in this direction will increase the tendency to this form of oblique vision. By many the latter can, in a high degree, be easily produced at will—by others, not at all, or only with great difficulty; and when it is stated that such voluntary squinting, often produced for the sake of imitation, or of mockery, has, with some, given rise to permanent strabismus, I readily admit it, but on condition that hypermetropia at the same time existed. Moreover, I have not been able to satisfy myself that a special tendency to strabismus may be hereditary. Let me be understood. In a very high degree hypermetropia is hereditary. It is a rare thing, with hypermetropic structure of the eyes in one of the parents, not to find hypermetropia also in some of the children. But whether this hypermetropia in the parents was combined with strabismus or not, has, if any, certainly only slight influence in the development of strabismus in the hypermetropic children born of them. If in a family one or two labour under strabismus convergens, we may be nearly sure that in some other members hypermetropia will occur; but that in the same family most of the hypermetropics should be affected with strabismus, has very rarely occurred to me.

2°. *Relation between the visual line and the axis of the cornea.*— We have above seen (p. 182) that in general in hypermetropic individuals, in order to give a parallel direction to the visual lines, a more than ordinary divergence of the visual axes is required. Thence we have in so many hypermetropic persons apparent strabismus divergens. On the other hand, we know that most eyes can with difficulty be brought to a state of divergence: a weak prism, with the refracting edge held outwards before the eye, produces double images, which most people are not able, by divergence of the visual lines, to overcome. Even for the sake of single vision, many do not succeed in diverging some degrees more. It is therefore natural to assume, that when for single vision more than ordinary divergence of the corneal or visual axes is required, the divergence may very easily be insufficient, and that, accordingly, as a matter of course, for seeing at a shorter distance also, there may readily be too great convergence. What was treated of under 1°

facilitates convergence in an absolute manner. Comparatively, the relation between the visual line and the axis of the cornea has, in hypermetropics, the same result. Now, if, in looking at a distance, the requisite divergence of the axes of the cornea easily falls short, the convergence will likewise, under the influence of the hypermetropia, in looking at near objects, be relatively too great. The condition for the development of strabismus is thus given. In fact, it often seemed to me that in squinters, after tenotomy, a considerable degree of divergence of the axes of the cornea was required to make the visual lines assume a parallel position;—often the eyes are apparently quite properly directed, and yet when, on fixing a remote point, one and the other eye are alternately covered with the hand, we observe that the eye just opened has each time to make an extensive movement outwards, to fix the remote point. Sometimes this is to so great a degree the case, that for binocular vision, at a distance, a deformity by divergence would be required. This leads me to suspect that while in general the great angle a promotes the occurrence of strabismus convergens with H, an extraordinary magnitude of this angle predisposes more particularly to this form of strabismus. In order to test this suspicion, the angle a was measured in ten cases of strabismus convergens. The measurements were in great part made by Mr. Hamer, now house-surgeon in our Ophthalmic Hospital, according to the method already described, with his usual accuracy. The results are presented in the subjoined Table I.

TABLE I.

Persons.	Sex.	Age.	Deviation.	Eye.	Refraction. Hm.	H.	a	S.	Observations.
1	m.	23	Str. C. Od.	Od.	$\frac{1}{10}$?	$\frac{1}{8}$	5°.8	0.2	
				Os.	$\frac{1}{28}$	?	6°.5	0.67	
2	m.	15	Str. C. Os.	Od.	$\frac{1}{12}$	?	6°	1.	
				Os.	$\frac{1}{12}$	?	7°	0.28	
3	f.	25	Str. C. Od.	Od.	?	?	6°.75	0.1	
				Os.	$\frac{1}{40}$	?	6°.5	0.85	
4	m.	16	Str. C. Od.	Od.	?	?	?	0.01	Does not fix.
				Os.	in H $\frac{1}{28}$? in V $\frac{1}{8}$	in H $\frac{1}{12}$ in V $\frac{1}{24}$	7°	0.45	
5	f.	23	Str. C. Od.	Od.	in H? in V ?	in H $\frac{1}{24}$? in V $\frac{1}{40}$?	8°	0.2	As ?
				Os.	$\frac{1}{20}$?	in H $\frac{1}{11}$ in V $\frac{1}{16}$	7°	0.5	As $= \frac{1}{35}$
6	m.	12	Str. C. Alt.	Od.	? ?	in H $\frac{1}{16}$ in V $\frac{1}{8}$	7°.5	0.4	As $= \frac{1}{16}$
				Os.	? ?	in H $\frac{1}{10}$ in V $\frac{1}{20}$	8°	0.25	As $= \frac{1}{20}$
7	m.	19	Str. C. Alt.	Od.	1	$\frac{1}{6}$	8°.5	0.66	
				Os.	$\frac{1}{12}$	?	7°	1.	
8	m.	22	Str. C. Os.	Od.	$\frac{1}{16}$	$\frac{1}{6}$	9°	1.	Strabismus, yielding on mydriasis Od.
				Os.	$\frac{1}{11}$	?	7°.5	0.41	
9	f.	18	Str. C. Od.	Od.	$\frac{1}{20}$?	?	?	0.025	Does not fix.
				Os.	$\frac{1}{24}$	?	9°	0.4	
10	f.	16	Str. C. Alt.	Od.	$\frac{1}{18}$	?	10°.1	1	
				Os.	$\frac{1}{16}$	?	9°	1	

Hm.	signifies	Hypermetropia manifesta.
H.	,,	,, totalis, after mydriasis.
a.	,,	the angle between the axis of the cornea and the visual line.
S.	,,	the sharpness or accuracy of vision.
Str. C. Od.	,,	Strabismus convergens oculi dextri.
Str. C. Os.	,,	,, ,, ,, ,, sinistri.
Str. C. Alt.	,,	,, ,, ,, alternans.
As.	,,	Astigmatism.
In H.	,,	in the meridian of minimum of curvature (usually the horizontal).
In V.	,,	in the meridian of maximum of curvature (usually the vertical).
?.	,,	value not determined, or not accurately determined, or not to be determined.

In No. 8, permanent strabismus was demonstrated, which, singularly enough, on artificial mydriasis of the sharp-sighted right eye, temporarily disappeared : the left eye was now properly directed, without the right deviating in its turn.

This Table again shows what has already been seen, that the angle a for both eyes of the same person is in general nearly similar. Therefore for No. 4 Od. and No. 9 Od., which on account of diminished S did not fix, a was, on calculation of the average, assumed $= a$ of the left eye. As an average we now obtained $a = 7°.63$. This but slightly exceeds $a = 7°.3$, previously found as the average in non-squinting hypermetropics ; but in order to make the influence on the position of the centre of motion appear strongly, particularly high degrees of H were designedly selected, in consequence of which a also increases. In order to have a better ground of comparison, the angle a was therefore determined also in some cases of H, in degree about equal to H of squinters. The results are comprised in the annexed Table II.

TABLE II.

Persons.	Sex.	Age.	Eye.	Refraction.			a	S.	Observations.
				Hm.	H.	H.?			
1	m.	19	Od.	$\frac{1}{26}$	?	$\frac{1}{14}$	$4°.5$	0.85	As. ?
			Os.	$\frac{1}{28}$	$\frac{1}{16}$	$\frac{1}{16}$	$3°.6$	0.85	As. ?
2	f.	50	Od.	$\frac{1}{12}$	?	$\frac{1}{13}$	$5°$	?	
			Os.	$\frac{1}{12}$	?	$\frac{1}{12}$	$5°$	?	
3	m.	55	Od.	$\frac{1}{12}$	?	$\frac{1}{12}$	$5°$	?	
			Os.	$\frac{1}{13}$	?	$\frac{1}{12}$	$5°$	?	
4	m.	60	Od.	$\frac{1}{28}$	?	$\frac{1}{60}$	$5°.75$	1	
			Os.	$\frac{1}{26}$	?	$\frac{1}{55}$	$5°.5$	0.95	
5	f.	21	Od.	$\frac{1}{36}$	?	$\frac{1}{12}$	$6°.25$	1	
			Os.	$\frac{1}{36}$	?	$\frac{1}{12}$	$5°.9$	1	
6	m.	9	Od.	$\frac{1}{12}$	?	$\frac{1}{6}$	$6°.5$	?	
			Os.	$\frac{1}{12}$	?	$\frac{1}{6}$	$6°$	?	
7	m.	14	Od.	$\frac{1}{16}$	$\frac{1}{6}$	$\frac{1}{8}$	$7°$	0.4	As.
			Os.	$\frac{1}{20}$	$\frac{1}{6}$	$\frac{1}{6}$	$6°$	0.32	As.
8	m.	62	Od.	$\frac{1}{6}$	?	$\frac{1}{7}$	$7°$	0.25	
			Os.	$\frac{1}{6}$	?	$\frac{1}{7}$	$7°$	0.25	
9	f.	13	Od.	$\frac{1}{24}$	?	$\frac{1}{7}$	$8°.5$	1	
			Os.	$\frac{1}{20}$	?	$\frac{1}{6}$	$8°.75$	1	
10	m.	36	Od.	$\frac{1}{24}$	?	$\frac{1}{11}$	$8°.8$	1	
			Os.	$\frac{1}{24}$	?	$\frac{1}{11}$	$9°.2$	1	
11	m.	21	Od.	$\frac{1}{10}$	?	$\frac{1}{6}$	$9°$	0.9	
			Os.	$\frac{1}{10}$	?	$\frac{1}{6}$	$9°$	0.9	

Column H ? gives the total Hypermetropia, reduced by calculation to the period of youth.

Now, in the first place, we find among these non-squinting hyper-metropics a on an average $= 6°.56$, that is, $1°.07$ less than in squinters. In the second place, it appears further, that the degree of H has an influence upon a. Comparison with the average $a = 7°.3$, found in higher degrees of H, at once indicates this. But still more distinctly does it appear in Table II., in which the persons are arranged according to the magnitude of a, and the suspected degree of the total H, at 14 years of age, was calculated under H? It immediately strikes the eye, that the latter keeps about equal pace with a. In estimating H?, the ascertained Hm, and sometimes also H, were made use of, the time of life being borne in mind ; the estimate certainly deviates little from the truth. The result, therefore is, that, with equal degrees of H, high values of a especially predispose to strabismus convergens. To this result I attach the more importance, because it *in general* proves, that the greater angle a, proper to H, is not indifferent in its bearing on the connexion between H and strabismus convergens.

In the highest degrees of H, strabismus is rarely observed. This need not surprise us. In such cases the power of accommodation is, even under abnormally increased convergence, not sufficient to produce accurate images, and such hypermetropics are thus led rather to the practice of forming correct ideas from imperfect retinal images than of, by a maximum of tension, improving the retinal images as much as possible. We have already seen, that strabismus is met with chiefly in mean degrees of H. These belong to facultative and relative hypermetropia : the eye can adapt itself for parallel and even for diverging rays, and can moreover maintain this accommodation for some time, yet often only with convergence of the visual lines to a point, situated closer to the eye than the point whence the rays proceed. The minimum of H, at which strabismus occurs, depends undoubtedly on the angle a, and on the range of accommodation : the less the latter, and the greater a is, the less degree of H will be sufficient. But diminished energy or paresis of accommodation by itself is as little liable to produce strabismus, as is the diminution of the range of accommodation connected with the increase of years.

As to *external causes*, we often find mention made of the fixing of near, and particularly of laterally placed objects, as a feather of the cap, the flame of a candle, a toy or such like. From what has been said, it will have been seen that I attach but little influence to these things. At least, I am convinced that the *emmetropic* eye will not in this way

be led to squint.   But I would not venture so unconditionally to
assert, that, for the hypermetropic eye, no cause of strabismus might
be found therein.   Particularly the fixing of laterally placed objects,
might have influence in this way.   For under these circumstances
the fixed point can be seen only by one eye, since the field of vision
of the other is limited by the nose; and if only the one eye sees
the object, the second eye wants the guide which directs its movements, and there is nothing to prevent too strong convergence, for
the sake of distinct vision.   It seems to me that there is no ground
for denying, that in this manner the internal muscles of the eye
might acquire a preponderance, which would promote the further
development of strabismus.

I have above remarked, that oblique vision differs in kind and
form, according to its causes and to the nature of the affection,
of which it is the result, and with which it occurs in one and the
same morbid type.   This is quite true of oblique vision, proceeding
from hypermetropia.   But as this is the most usual, the typical
form of strabismus convergens, it is very natural that what is described as strabismus in general, should be applicable precisely to
this form.   I may be permitted to give a short sketch of it.   In
doing so I must advert to some well-known matters, but I shall
thus best find opportunity to add what is still deficient respecting
the nature, the symptoms, and the pathogeny of the affection.

Converging strabismus, in consequence of H, *we see* to arise
mostly about the 5th year, probably because the effort to see accurately then begins to be developed; the range of accommodation is
now also sufficiently great, by means of somewhat increased convergence, easily to overcome the H.   To *reports* of its occurrence
at, or shortly after birth, in consequence of convulsions or of other
diseases, no credit is in general to be given.   Exceptionally it
commences after the 7th, extremely rarely so late as the 18th year,
unless special accessory causes exist.   At first the deviation is
transient, connected with fixing, that is with an effort to see accurately, sometimes only with the fixing of near objects : it passes off
again when the fixing ceases or the eyes are closed.   This is the so-
called periodical squint, by some described as a distinct period.   Even
in this period, and when the strabismus is developed first in the 16th
or 18th year, we very rarely hear a complaint of double vision.   This
is explained, in my opinion, by the fact, that the deviation arises

only on the effort to see a given object accurately. On that object
the attention is fastened. To it the one visual line remains directed.
Now the double image of it lies in the deviating eye at some distance
from the yellow spot, and must therefore appear indistinct, so that
beside the direct fixed one, it is not easily seen as a second image.
And on the yellow spot appears the image of a wholly different object, with which the observer is in general not occupied, and from
which it is therefore easy to abstract. But when the deviation,
before S is much diminished, occurs involuntarily, without a special
effort to see accurately, there is occasionally some transient double
vision. The periodical form of squint on looking at near objects, just
described, sometimes continues as such. Stoeber* and Artl† have
each described a remarkable instance of this nature, the cause of which
was unknown to them. In most cases, however, the squint soon becomes constant. The rule is, that invariably one and the same eye
deviates (strabismus simplex); this held good even when the squint
was still transient: when it occurs under the form of strabismus
alternans, with H, other causes are often in operation. The squint is
usually concomitant; the movements are free; the excursion normal
although with excessive mobility inwards, limited outwards, *in both
eyes*, even when the one constantly deviates, the other being steadily
properly directed; this is found also to be the case when the squint
is still periodical. Both the internal muscles of the eye are therefore
to be considered as shortened. The shortening, at first dynamical,
has in the constant strabismus become organic : it is the result of
excessive action, with relaxation of the antagonistic muscles; morbid
structural change does not exist. That both internal muscles are
shortened, depends upon the habit of keeping the fixed object to the
side of the deviated eye, so that even in the non-deviated eye the
musculus rectus internus is brought into relatively strong contraction. In this position the H of the non-deviated eye is best
overcome. Also when the strabismus has become constant, a comparatively stronger tension of the internal recti muscles is connected
with the fixing of an object, whereby the angle of squinting is increased—of course in a less degree where a great angle of deviation
already exists, because increased tension is then attended with less
motion : after tenotomy the increase of the convergence often again
appears very well marked in these cases on fixing an object. This
increase of convergence on fixing, when a correct position has been

* *Ann. d'Ocul.*, 1855, T. xxxiii. p. 177.　　† *l. c.* T. iii. p. 312.

obtained by tenotomy, is important in a double point of view. In the first place, as it relates to adults, who state that they feel this convergence distinctly, and at the same time perceive that they produce it, as it were involuntarily, in order to see more accurately. More direct proof that H may lead to strabismus, and how it may do so, could certainly not be given. We have here, in a certain sense, a return to the first period, with this difference, that the deviation can now be observed by the person himself in its cause and in its signification, while, just as in the original first stage the *commencement* was to be obviated by means of convex glasses, which should neutralise the H, the *relapse* is now to be prevented on the same principle.—The practical indication, after tenotomy in such cases, to give convex glasses during work, furnishes the second point, in regard to which I called the phenomenon important.

In strabismus simplex the acuteness of vision suffers more and more in the deviated eye. At first, on bringing the hand before the fixing eye, the deviated eye directs itself properly to the object; even when the hand is taken away, the originally deviated eye may continue to fix, soon, however, usually when movement is required or even on the first winking of the lids, giving way to the other. The acuteness of vision in the deviated eye has then already diminished, but it continues still for a considerable time satisfactory, may be recovered by practice, and improves almost always immediately after tenotomy. After some time, however, on closing the fixing eye, the deviated eye usually directs its visual line no longer to the object; the line passes to the inside, so that the retinal image of the object comes to lie also on the inside of the retina. When this takes place, we may infer, that in the visual line and besides in the field of vision common to the two eyes, the acuteness of vision of the deviated eye is much diminished, while, on the contrary, that of the indirect vision, on the innermost part of the retina, in so far as it has its own field of vision and perceives objects, which are not represented on the retina of the other eye, has continued undiminished. It is again von Graefe, who has first accurately investigated this loss of physiological sensibility through psychical exclusion. And this is indeed a remarkable phenomenon! That through attention we can sharpen our senses, is an admitted fact. How rapidly, on the other hand, a nerve may become blunted, from whose impressions we wish mentally to abstract ourselves, the case here described supplies an example important for physiology at large. Although no organic changes of the retina are to be observed, no improvement of any importance is to be obtained, if fixing no longer occurs under any circumstances, either by practice or by tenotomy.

But we must not too rapidly decide this point. There is a period in which the deviated eye will not see large objects otherwise than indirectly, and nevertheless, on using a convex glass, it will quickly look directly, that is, use the yellow spot, to recognise comparatively small objects, for example the letters of No. X and No. XX. In this period we may by practice and by tenotomy sometimes still attain a brilliant success.

A word still as to the practical application of what has been said. I have already above stated, that so long as strabismus occurs only intermittingly with fixing of an object, its development may be prevented by wearing convex glasses, which neutralise the existing H. This I first observed in a young man, who in his 18th year began for the first time to squint in fixing. He had $Hm = \frac{1}{20}$. After he had worn glasses of $\frac{1}{20}$ for two days, he began to be no longer able, for the sake of seeing accurately, to make one eye deviate. He then saw also at a distance indistinctly, and it was not until half-an-hour after putting off the spectacles that he again succeeded in producing the squint, and thereby distinguishing accurately. By continuing to wear the spectacles, the squint ceased to be produced, and the tendency to it was completely lost.—If the squint sets in very early in life, wearing spectacles is of course attended with difficulties, and particularly when the patients are of the female sex, they are unwilling to be condemned to wear glasses during their whole life. In such cases I generally confine myself to advising them to look twice daily for some minutes, with the deviating eye alone,* which practice is sufficient to prevent the diminution of the acuteness and the limitation of the field of vision : at a later period, when the strabismus is confirmed, the operation of tenotomy is performed. Where the patient preferred obviating the strabismus by wearing spectacles, I willingly consented to it, and almost invariably the object was thus attained. Mooren,† too, has recently stated that, where a tolerably high degree of Hm existed, he has, in the first stage of strabismus, with

* Mydriasis, by atropia, of the eye which is usually properly directed immediately causes the other to be used, and is therefore sometimes recommended in the case of young squinting children, on whom it is undesirable as yet to operate.

† *Klinische Monatsblätter f. Augenheilkunde*, B. 1, H. 1, 1863.

20

good result prescribed the use of convex glasses. In comparatively
great degrees of H the prevention of strabismus is, in fact, more
particularly desirable, because subsequently, even after full tenotomy, the tendency to strabismus continues, and, in order to prevent
a relapse, the use of convex glasses, at least for close work, is still
necessary. Moreover, I have observed, that when hypermetropics
with already confirmed strabismus, especially after insufficient tenotomy, regularly wear convex glasses, the degree of strabismus often
diminishes so much, that the deformity is almost entirely removed.

If we now inquire whether the cause of strabismus was ever before sought
in hypermetropia, this question may be answered in the negative. Indeed,
this could scarcely be otherwise. It is only a few years since hypermetropia was properly understood ; and the forms which are wholly or in great
part latent, were overlooked, until I satisfied myself of their existence, and
immediately began to perceive their relation to strabismus. But to this
conclusion, what had been observed and recorded by my predecessors, in a
certain degree contributed. Not to mention some isolated observations,*
which after the discovery of hypermetropia, clearly enough demonstrate the
existence thereof in strabismus, I must, in the first place, refer to Böhm's†
investigations upon squinting, where it is plainly stated, that squinters
can distinguish a certain print with the aid of *convex* glasses at a *greater*
distance than with the unaided eye. In this observation of Böhm there is an
essential value. It might have led to the discovery of hypermetropia, and
particularly of hypermetropia with strabismus, if he, with a thorough
knowledge of dioptrics, had comprehended and properly explained the fact
he had observed. In place, however, of thinking of a condition, in which
the retina lay in front of the focus of the eye, Böhm has recourse to an
enigmatical connexion of "physical presbyopia" with "vital myopia."
And in any case he was far from seeking therein the *cause* of strabismus.
In investigating the origin and causes of the latter, he falls into the same
error as all his predecessors. He tries to find out the causes, not of a
definite form of strabismus, *i.e.* of a true form of disease, but of a symptom :
strabismus in general. Consequently, the causes of wholly different conditions were all investigated and studied together in heterogeneous connexion. That in this way the pathogeny of strabismus would not disclose its mysteries, might indeed have been anticipated. But there is more to be said
against the reasoning. Where Böhm treats of the "origin of squinting from the
condition of the eye " (p. 5), and further speaks of "the etiology of strabismus,
originating from the eye" (p. 16), the state of the *deviating* eye is and remains for
him the principal point. He speaks here of " shortsightedness of the *one* eye,
with normal behaviour of the other," of " Hebetudo of the *one* eye," of " weakness

---

* Conf. de Haas, *Geschiedkundig onderzoek omtrent de hypermetropie en
hare gevolgen*, 1862. Diss. inaug., p. 61.

† Böhm, *Das Schielen*, Berlin, 1845.

of vision of *one* eye," and always makes the eye affected with the anomaly deviate. In this deviation he sees the endeavour to exclude this eye, but by no means an effort to improve the accuracy of the retinal images in the non-deviating eye. What we have above assumed as one of the circumstances, under which the eye more easily allows itself to be withdrawn from the binocular vision, is for him the all-decisive cause. Böhm was, therefore, as far as any one else from comprehending the origin of converging strabismus.

Subsequently, von Graefe* was certainly on the point of recognising the cause in hypermetropia. He, however, did not treat definitely of the pathogeny of strabismus. He even asks pardon, when, in passing, some observations on the subject fall from his pen. But we value these observations as so many useful hints, although, as it did not occur to him to include hypermetropia as an element therein, his efforts necessarily remained in great part fruitless.

Von Graefe puts it prominently forward as a well-known fact, that persistent strabismus is very often, indeed generally, preceded by an "intercurrent or periodical squint." Subsequently he remarks, that all cases of intercurrent strabismus do not run into the persistently concomitant variety. So long as this has not taken place, these cases must, with respect to the question of operative aid, give rise to special observations. Therefore, von Graefe proceeds to speak of them. But evidently he felt that the phenomena, peculiar to these cases, had a particular value for the investigation of the pathogeny of the affection; for from the pathogenetic point of view, he specially considers the three categories, distinguished by him:—

1. Patients who, with a careless glance, do not accurately fix any definite object, whether near or distant. Von Graefe considers that a disturbance of binocular vision might proceed from the squinting eye, and that therefore this image should be voluntarily set aside. That permanent strabismus might be thus produced is evident. But he does not think that everything is thus explained. "When under particular circumstances of the act of vision, namely, in acute perception of the retinal images," (thus we read, *l. c.* p. 281), "a deviation takes place, but not otherwise, an active connecting link must each time be sought between the act of vision and the muscles of the eye." Further: "if it [the link] is not the disturbance of the stereoscopic retinal images, the conditions of the accommodation next present themselves." In reference to the first quotation, von Graefe, however, remarks, that at every distance, even behind the covering hand, on fixing an object the one eye deviates, and while, with respect to the latter quotation, he did not understand that hypermetropia might be the cause of it, he could give no other than this somewhat obscure explanation: "Every action of the organ tending to the elaboration of visual perception, reflects the stimulus to the irregular contraction upon the affected muscle."

2. Cases in which the visual axes are directed with precision to a definite distance (eight inches, one foot, four feet), but where, at a greater distance,

---

* *Archiv f. Ophthalmologie*, B. I., Abth. I., p. 17.

2

a deviation arises.   These are almost invariably connected with near-sightedness.

3. Cases of which he says: " The pathological convergence occurs only with accommodation for near objects."   The phenomenon appears equally on covering the squinting eye, and must, consequently, says von Graefe, depend on the condition of accommodation, "probably on increase of the muscular resistance with the augmenting refraction of the eye."   " The increase of the muscular tension," he continues, " arouses in the affected muscle the slumbering impulse to the irregular contraction."   He refers further to the singular cases, in which, in looking at both near and distant objects, strabismus convergens arises, but where, at a medium distance, the vision is binocular.   He explains this partly from myopia, but he adds that often hyperpresbyopics and presbyopics are met with in this group ; sometimes myopia appeared to exist in distance, etc.. etc.   He, at last, formulises his views in the following manner : " For all distances of the visual object there exists, according to the natural inclination to tension, a slight degree of pathological convergence.   If a higher refractive condition be taken, whether through approximation of the visual object, or by holding a concave glass before the eye, the morbidly increased contraction arises; in a medium or low state of accommodation, and with proportionally large retinal images, the prevailing muscular tendency is, in the interest of single vision, counteracted; for a greater distance, with diminishing magnitude of the retinal images, this can no longer take place, double images arise, which are again removed from one another by a morbid muscular contraction."

Finally, Alfred Graefe[*] proposes to himself the question, in a case of intermittent strabismus, not quite correctly called spasmodic, whether it is the "conditions of accommodation," which "cause the deviation of the right eye?"   And when he answers: " Certainly not, for it has been expressly shown in the commencement of this chapter, that the deviation always occurs so soon as an object is fixed, and that it is therefore completely independent of the actual state of the accommodation," it clearly appears, that he did not think of hypermetropia, which required a tension of accommodation even for distant objects.

From all this it will be seen, that in literature hints were not altogether wanting, which might lead us, after the recognition of the slighter degrees of H, to bring strabismus into connexion with the same.

Of H, as the cause of strabismus convergens, I have only cursorily treated,[†] but I have long since, on different occasions, described the results I have obtained.   The subject I had not lost sight of.   But I wished to take it up somewhat more fully, and to inquire in general, with what anomalies of the eye the different forms of strabismus are connected.   It occurred to me, that

---

[*] Alfred Graefe, *Klinische Analyse der Motilitätstörungen des Auges.* Berlin, 1858, p. 214.

[†] *Ametropie*, 1860, p. 45, and *Archiv f. Ophthalmologie*, B. VI. Abth. 1, p. 92.

such an investigation might tend to clear up the pathogeny of strabismus. The investigation required the statistical method. In a great number of squinters, therefore, everything was determined for both eyes, which appeared possibly to be the cause or the result of this anomaly, or to be capable of in any way explaining its origin : sex, age, and ordinary occupation were noted ; of each eye in particular were determined the refractive condition, the range of accommodation, the acuteness of vision, the extent of the movements, these last in connexion with the variable or unvariable angle of squinting ; to these points were added the time and mode of origin, the hereditary causes; finally, complications of various kinds and peculiar disturbances in vision (limitation of the field of vision, double vision, etc.). In this inquiry, several of my pupils, and in particular Dr. Haffmans, ably and zealously assisted me. The registers relating to this subject embrace 280 cases. It is true that in very many instances not all the determinations just mentioned were made, and the accuracy of other cases leaves something to be desired : he who knows by experience, how much time and trouble are necessary, especially in children, or in unintelligent persons, satisfactorily to investigate both eyes with respect to their function, will very easily understand this. But this will not prevent many a question respecting strabismus from finding its answer in the facts collected. Here I have been obliged to confine myself chiefly to the pathogeny, and indeed, in particular to that of strabismus convergens. In the following chapter, treating of myopia, I shall have to speak of strabismus divergens.

After my preliminary communication, the fact that H often exists in strabismus convergens, was confirmed in different quarters. Special communications on this subject we have received from Pagenstecher and Saemisch (*Klinische Beobachtungen aus der Augenheilanstalt zu Wiesbaden*, 1 ste Heft, 1861, and 2e Heft, 1862), and from Mooren (*Klinische Monatsblätter f. Augenheilkunde*, herausgegeben von Dr. W. Zehender. Jahrg. 1863, pp. 37 *et seq.*), who, however, confined themselves to the determination of the *manifest* hypermetropia, and therefore found the proportion of H in strabismus convergens less than I did.

---

§ 25. APHAKIA.

The absence of the lens in the dioptric system of the eye is in many respects an important condition. It must, therefore, be considered strange, that writers had neglected to give it a name. I have proposed to designate it by the term aphakia, and this word is beginning gradually to find acceptance.

Aphakia may be produced by different causes. It occurs most frequently as the result of operation for cataract or of a wound, which has given rise to gradual solution of the lens. When the lens has by luxation or depression of cataract disappeared from the plane of the pupil, though it may still be present in the eye, it no longer belongs to the dioptric system, and we are therefore most fully justified, in speaking of anomalies of refraction, in calling the condition, in this case also, by the name aphakia. Luxation of the lens is usually the result of a wound. Very remarkable cases of spontaneous luxation of the lens are communicated by Bowman.* In the writings of von Graefe I have seen it mentioned that he has observed congenital aphakia in many members of the same family. Such cases have not occurred to me. Partial luxation of the lens, causing the equator of the lens to correspond to the plane of the pupil, is, on the contrary, very frequently met with, and is not uncommonly found in several children of the same parents. This state cannot, however, be considered as aphakia; it belongs rather to irregular astigmatism.

In the condition of aphakia the eye is, complicated as it is in its normal state, the simplest imaginable dioptric system. In consequence of the slight thickness, in fact, and the nearly equally curved surfaces of the cornea, we may safely neglect the slight difference in the coefficient of refraction between the cornea and the aqueous humour, and therefore suppose that the aqueous humour extends to the anterior surface of the cornea; and as, moreover, the coefficients of refraction of the vitreous and aqueous humours are equal, we have in the aphakial eye only one refracting surface to take into account, namely, the anterior surface of the cornea. Hence it follows that, in order to find the cardinal points, we need know only the radius of the cornea and the coefficient of refraction of the aqueous humour. Now as the coefficient we have, with Helmholtz, assumed $1\cdot3365$; as the radius of curvature, in the apex of the cornea,† we may, according to our measurements, take as the average $7\cdot7$ mm. We thus obtain the subjoined system (*Fig.* 122. Compare pp. 40 and 44).

$$\text{F}' = h \, \phi' \, (= 7\cdot7 : (1\cdot3365 - 1) = 22\cdot88.$$
$$\text{F}'' = h \, \phi'' \, (= 7\cdot7 \times 1\cdot3365 : (1\cdot3365 - 1) = 30\cdot58.$$
$$h \, k' = \text{F}'' - \text{F}' = 7\cdot7.$$

Hence it appears, that the visual axis, with normal curvature of

* *Lectures on the parts concerned in the operations on the eye.* London, 1849, pp. 131 *et seq.*

† The cornea is not spherical, but somewhat ellipsoidal, and, in fact, with such eccentricity, that the spherical aberration is partially removed. In the calculation the radius in the apex must form the basis.

the cornea, should have a length $h \, \phi'' = 30{\cdot}58$ mm., in order, in the

Fig. 122.

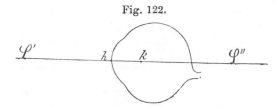

absence of the lens, to bring parallel rays to a focus on the retina. Now, since this axis is, almost without exception, much shorter, the aphakial eye must in general be in a high degree hypermetropic. In order to find the degree of this H, with a given length of the visual axis, we need only calculate to what point behind the cornea the incidental rays must converge, in order, after refraction by the cornea, to unite on the retina. This is done according to the formula (see p. 44)

$$f' = \frac{F' f''}{F'' - f''}$$

in which f'' is the length of the visual axis, and f' the point sought behind the cornea. We find

$f'' =$ mm.	$f' =$ mm.	$f' =$ Par. inches.	H
30·58	∞	∞	$\dfrac{1}{\infty}$
29	420	15·5	$\dfrac{1}{15{\cdot}5}$
28	248·3	9·2	$\dfrac{1}{9{\cdot}2}$
27	172·5	6·3	$\dfrac{1}{6{\cdot}3}$
26	129·8	4·75	$\dfrac{1}{4{\cdot}75}$
25	102·5	3·75	$\dfrac{1}{3{\cdot}75}$
24	83·4	3·1	$\dfrac{1}{3{\cdot}1}$
23	69·4	2·6	$\dfrac{1}{2{\cdot}6}$
22	58·6	2·2	$\dfrac{1}{2{\cdot}2}$

Hence it directly follows, what glasses the aphakial eye requires, with different lengths of the visual axis, for acute vision at a distance. We need, indeed, to the ascertained distance f', to add only the distance x between the glass and the eye (compare p. 144), in order to find the focal distance of the glass required. If we establish $x = 0\cdot5''$, we therefore need, with $f'' = 29$ mm., glasses ($15\cdot5 + 0\cdot5$ $= 16$) of $\dfrac{1}{16}$; with $f' = 24$ mm. ($3\cdot1 + 0\cdot5 = 3\cdot6$) of $\dfrac{1}{3\cdot6}$, etc.

On the other hand, we can further calculate the length of the visual axis, when the focal distance of the required glass is known. If x be assumed $= 0\cdot''5$, glasses of

1 : 2·5 correspond to a length of the visual axis $f'' = 21\cdot5$ mm.

1 : 3	,,	,,	,,	,,	$f'' = 22\cdot9$,,
1 : 3·5	,,	,,	,,	,,	$f'' = 23\cdot9$,,
1 : 4	,,	,,	,,	,,	$f'' = 24\cdot6$,,
1 : 5	,,	,,	,,	,,	$f'' = 25\cdot7$,,
1 : 6	,,	,,	,,	,,	$f'' = 26\cdot5$,,
1 : 10	,,	,,	,,	,,	$f'' = 28\cdot1$,,
1 : ∞	,,	,,	,,	,,	$f'' = 30\cdot58$,,

Experience has shown, that in the majority of cases glasses are required of from 1 : 3 to 1 : 3·5, placed at 6''' from the eye. This corresponds to a length of the visual axis of from 22·9 to 23·9. This length coincides nearly with that of the emmetropic eye. But if the eye was myopic before the development of cataract, weaker glasses are, after the operation, sufficient. A case even occurred to me, in which the accuracy of vision of distant objects was incapable of improvement by either positive or negative glasses. In this instance the visual axis of the eye, emmetropic with aphakia, had actually a length of rather more than 30 mm., and we may assume that so long as the crystalline lens was still present, myopia of about $\dfrac{1}{3}$ had existed. In a second case, in a woman, aged 36, glasses of 1 : 133 were sufficient; in a man, aged 73, glasses of $\dfrac{1}{8}$. In this instance there must have existed, before the occurrence of the cataract, a myopia of rather more than $\dfrac{1}{5}$, which had now given way to H $= 1 : 7\cdot5$. The patient now declares that he can see without spectacles better at a distance than he could in his youth before the occurrence of the cataract; as the pupil is now smaller than it formerly was, this is not surprising. In the two other cases mentioned, the difference must have been still greater. The woman, aged 36, had only one eye (the other was atrophic); and in that operated on by me there had remained from youth, after perforation of the cornea, a lateral leucoma with synechia anterior. Notwithstanding, she declared that with this one eye she now saw better for ordinary purposes than had ever before been possible for her with both eyes. But for near work she now required spectacles of $\frac{1}{8}$, which formerly she had been able to do without.—It is a very common case, that for seeing at a distance in aphakia, glasses of $\frac{1}{6}$ or $\frac{1}{5}$ are sufficient, which, when the form of the cornea is normal, proves that the visual axis is longer than usual. Now, in all these cases myopia has previously existed, and the connexion between M and length of the visual axis is thus in aphakia most clearly brought to light (compare p. 88). Especially in cases of congenital cataract have I been able to satisfy myself of this. It has appeared to me that this condition is usually connected with a myopic structure of the eye. We know that under these circumstances not the entire crystalline lens is obscured, or rather, that ordinarily only some laminæ are obscured, while the nucleus, and especially the peripheric layers, are transparent. Now, if the transparency of these last is tolerably perfect, vision often becomes pretty good on artificial mydriasis. It is then only rarely that positive glasses are required for reading, etc., notwithstanding that the power of accommodation is removed. The degree of the myopia is now also still easily determined. In connexion with this M we shall find, that when the operation has become necessary, and the lens is removed, glasses of from $\frac{1}{4}$ to $\frac{1}{6}$ are in these cases usually sufficient for seeing at a distance. Sometimes I have had the opportunity of determining, in the same eye, the degree of M before, and that of H after, the operation. In the three cases which were most accurately investigated I found:

AMETROPIA.		Radius of Curvature of the Cornea.	Calculated length of the Visual Axis.
Before the Operation.	After the Operation.		
M = 1 : 6	H = 1 : 5·12	7·6	25·96
M = 1 : 8·5	H = 1 : 4·5	7·92	26·36
M = 1 : 24	H = 1 : 3·2	8·04	25·02

It so happens that the radius of curvature of the cornea is in the first case somewhat less, in the last two somewhat greater than usual. Therefore the visual axis proves, in comparison to the degree of M, in the last two cases particularly long: with $M = 1 : 8\cdot5$ it is even somewhat longer still than with $1 : 6$. It would therefore be incorrect to assume, that with $M = \dfrac{1}{24}$ the visual axis is usually 25 mm. long. That from the above observations the focal distance of the original crystalline lens, in a given position, may be calculated, the reader will, no doubt, have already understood. I hope to do this hereafter for a greater number of cases.

Original H, too, makes its influence felt where aphakia has supervened. In one case even of congenital cataract, H was found after operation in the right eye $= 1 : 2\cdot44$, in the left $1 : 2\cdot43$. These eyes were evidently rather small (approaching to microphthalmos), without particularly marked curvature of the cornea, and the hypermetropic structure was in them not to be mistaken. Moreover it is in general rare in aphakia to find $H > 1 : 2\cdot5$. Where I met with $H = 1 : 2\cdot4$ or $1 = 2\cdot3$, I could during life, the eye being strongly turned inwards, very well satisfy myself that the visual axis was shorter than normal, and calculation, after measuring the radius of curvature of the cornea, gave the same result.

The existence of aphakia is, at the first glance, not very easily recognised. Often the anterior chamber of the eye is deep, and we find a certain degree of iridodenosis; but none of these phenomena are characteristic. The search for the reflected images of Purkinje is decisive (compare p. 11): the two reflected images of the lens are absent. Moreover, the sectors and the direction of the fibres of the crystalline lens are easily seen on lateral illumination with light concentrated by a lens, particularly with the aid of a magnifying glass, as Helmholtz first remarked: where these are wanting, we may infer the existence of aphakia. Finally, the degree of H, whether established by experiments with convex glasses, or by ophthalmoscopy, in connexion with the form of the eye, cannot deceive us. When after a blow or knock upon the eye the power of vision has suddenly diminished, without very manifest disturbances in the organ, we should specially bear in mind the possibility of the lens having disappeared from the plane of the pupil, in consequence of luxation, and we should satisfy ourselves upon this point in the manner above described.

The acuteness of vision is in aphakia usually imperfect. The cause of this is almost always to be sought in turbidity of the surface of the pupil. Even after the most successful operations for cataract, where on inspection the pupil appears completely black, we shall, on examination with the ophthalmoscope, and especially with concentrated incident light, usually find some turbidity, depending chiefly on a slight deposit on the inner surface of the capsule of the lens. In consequence of this a portion of the light becomes diffused, and diminishes the sharpness of the retinal images. Slight as this turbidity may be, it has great influence, as appears from the fact that when even only a small part of the plane of the pupil is perfectly clear, vision immediately becomes comparatively very good. The clearest pupils I have obtained in some cases of operation for cataract by solution, where moreover, on account of the larger retinal images produced by the use of convex glasses, S was $>$ 1. In other cases we may be content, when S $= \frac{2}{3}$ or even only $\frac{1}{2}$, which is sufficient for all practical purposes. A change in the curvature of the cornea, which gives rise to tolerable regular astigmatism, is, after extraction, also not unfrequently the cause of diminished S. This may, as will hereafter appear, be in great part corrected by a certain inclination of the glasses.

That, on account of the high degree of H, without convex glasses the power of vision in aphakia leaves much to be desired, needs no proof. Vision will be the more imperfect, the larger the pupil is, to which, for equal degrees of H, the magnitude of the circles of diffusion is proportionate. But even with the use of glasses a large pupil has considerable disadvantages. The power of accommodation is, in fact, as I shall more fully show, in aphakia completely removed, and a glass, therefore, gives a distinct image only for a definite distance. All points, which are either more or less remote from the eye, are now of course seen with circles of diffusion which are larger, the larger the pupil is. With a narrow pupil the smallness of the circles of diffusion even of objects, for whose distance the eye is not accommodated, might lead one to suppose, as has often happened, that the power of accommodation in aphakia is not removed. It is on account of the great advantages for vision of a small pupil in aphakia, that we cannot consider the performance of iridectomy, especially inferiorly, in the operation for cataract, as an indifferent matter. We know that Mooren, Pagenstecher, Jacobson and others, each in his own way, have given their advice in favour of it. That iridectomy, not only when the object is by numerous punctures to cause a soft lens to be absorbed, but also in extraction, much diminishes the dangers of the operation, is fully established. For many years I have observed this. For this reason I have, when there is a tendency to prolapse, or when a portion of the iris has suffered much, advised the performance of iridectomy.* Moreover, following the example of von Graefe, I in general make iridectomy precede operation by puncture. But this iridectomy is performed superiorly. In this case the part which has suffered excision is almost completely covered by the upper eyelid, and the circles of diffusion therefore do not become greater. It is quite a different matter when the iridectomy is performed inferiorly. Hence I cannot, even where there is less danger of losing the eye, so unconditionally adopt the method of Jacobson, who performs every extraction by flap-section inferiorly, and at the same time cuts out a great piece of the iris. If this method with the flap above gives an equally satisfactory result, I should be rather inclined to follow it.

With respect to vision in aphakia, I have further to mention, that the polyopia, dependent on the crystalline lens, the rays proceeding from points of light, and the streaks of light on entoptic investigation are wanting (compare p. 200). On the contrary, regular astigmatism of the cornea, as shall be more fully shown in the chapter upon this anomaly, makes its appearance most distinctly.

In order to prescribe the most suitable glasses in aphakia, we begin by determining what glasses are required for distance: the best object for this purpose is a point of light. We now easily calculate from the result obtained, what focal distance is necessary for near objects.

In order, for example, distinctly to see a point, situated at the distance y from the lens, the rays proceeding from it must, after having passed through the lens with focal distance F^2, converge to the same point as the rays proceeding from ∞, after having been

---

* See *Ametropie en hare gevolgen*. Utrecht, 1859, p. 85.

refracted by the lens with focal distance F_1. Consequently,

$$\frac{1}{y} = \frac{1}{F_2} - \frac{1}{F_1}.$$

With y the distance from the point of distinct vision to the glass lens is found. Let x be the distance between this lens and the anterior surface of the cornea, then in using the lens with the focal distance F_2, the distance from the point of distinct vision to the cornea $f = y + x$.

A few examples may illustrate this.

Let the eye, in order to see distinctly at a great distance, need a glass of $1 : 3\cdot5$ at $\frac{1}{2}''$ from the eye: how far from the eye will the point of distinct vision lie, if this lens be replaced by a lens of $\frac{1}{3}$?

This calculation is:

$$\frac{1}{y} = \frac{1}{3} - \frac{1}{3\frac{1}{2}}$$

$$y = \frac{3 \times 3\frac{1}{2}}{3\frac{1}{2} - 3}$$

$$y = 21$$

$$f' = 21\frac{1}{2}''$$

And if the second lens has only $2\frac{1}{2}''$ focal distance,

$$\frac{1}{y} = \frac{1}{2\frac{1}{2}} - \frac{1}{3\frac{1}{2}}$$

$$y = \frac{2\frac{1}{2} \times 3\frac{1}{2}}{3\frac{1}{2} - 2\frac{1}{2}}$$

$$y = 8\frac{3}{4}$$

$$f' = 9\frac{1}{4}$$

With the lens of $3''$ focal distance vision will therefore be acute at $21\frac{1}{2}''$, with that of $2\frac{1}{2}''$ at $9\frac{1}{4}''$. With a lens of $2''$ this distance lies only at $5\frac{1}{6}''$.

If we wish to know the focal distance F_2 required in order to see acutely at a given distance y, this is found from the formula:

$$\frac{1}{F_2} = \frac{1}{F_1} + \frac{1}{y}.$$

But the question is then, whether we shall have at our command a lens of the calculated focal distance. The object may, however, in case of any difficulty upon that point, be attained, as shall hereafter appear, by modifying the distance of the lens from the eye.

With respect to the choice of glasses in aphakia, we should not forget, that, especially in old people, completely as the operation may have succeeded, the power of vision is seldom perfectly acute, and that, consequently, in order to read a smaller kind of type, the point of distinct vision must be brought rather near the eye. Not unfrequently this distance may amount to not more than 6″. In young subjects, in possession of acute power of vision, it may be considerably greater, the more so because in aphakia the retinal images far exceed in magnitude those of the same eye, before it was deprived of its lens. The dioptric system is altered: instead of a lens *in* the eye, a lens is now placed *in front of* the eye, and consequently the united nodal point is moved forwards. If the lens be farther removed from the eye, the nodal point will come to lie even before the cornea. Hence it appears that the retinal images must be larger, and that they increase still more in magnitude with the removal of the glass from the eye.

This increase of magnitude, which, in using a weak glass held at a great distance, becomes very considerable, is found by comparing the magnitude of the retinal image β_1 of the original eye with β_2, the retinal image of the aphakial eye, combined with a convex lens. The subjoined table gives a view of the increase of magnitude, which we obtained on calculation.*

Focal Distance of the Lens employed.	Distance of this Lens from the Cornea.	$\beta_1 : 1 = \beta_2 :$
3	0·5	1·322
4	1·5	1·763
5	2·5	2·203
6	3·5	2·644
8	5·5	3·525
10	7·5	4·406
16	13·5	7·050

* We should bear in mind, that for remote objects
$$\beta_1 : \beta_2 = G_1'' : G_2'' = F_1' : F_2',$$
$\beta_1 \ G_1''$ and F_1' having reference to the originally emmetropic eye, β_2, G_2'' and F_2' to the aphakial eye, in connexion with a convex lens.

In calculating the increase of magnitude, under the use of different convex lenses, we assumed:
$$F_1' = 0·5734,$$
in an eye, with a radius of the cornea of 7·7 mm. and a length of the

Hence we see, that, when in aphakia, with $H = \frac{1}{3}$ a lens of $\frac{1}{16}$ is held at $13.5''$ from the eye, the patient sees objects rather more than seven times larger than he did with the original eye, furnished with a crystalline lens. This vision is about the same as that of the emmetropic eye using glasses of $\frac{1}{2.5}$ would be, on looking through glasses of $\frac{1}{16}$ at $13''.5$ distance. The combination is, therefore, equal to that of a Dutch or Galilean telescope. In aphakia we find it under the simple form of a lens of from $10''$ to $20''$ focal distance, while the hypermetropic eye plays the part of an eye-piece. Other strongly hypermetropic eyes, without aphakia, can likewise make use of the same.

In the above theory and calculation, we have assumed that in aphakia the power of accommodation does not exist. It is an important question whether we are justified in doing so. For if it can be proved that in aphakia no trace of accommodative power remains, the inference would seem to be legitimate that this power depends exclusively upon a change of form in the lens. Hitherto this question has not been rigidly investigated. It is true that Thomas Young* had already in some cases of aphakia examined the eye with reference to its accommodative power; but the eyes at his disposal were not particularly well adapted for the purpose, and he moreover thought the result only tolerably satisfactory in proving the absence of the accommodating power. Von

visual axis of 22.9 mm., thus having, with aphakia, $H = \frac{1}{2.5}$. Now we found, with the use of different glasses,

$$F_2' = \frac{F' F}{F' + F - x}$$ (compare Helmholtz, *Dioptrik*, p. 58), F being the focal distance of the lens, F' the anterior focal distance of the aphakial eye, and x the distance from the convex lens to the cornea. In this case x must always be $= F - 2.5''$. — We see from the above table, that β is proportionate to F, which may be at once deduced from the formula: the numerator increases proportionately to F. On the contrary $F - x$ (in our case $= 2.5''$), and with it the whole denominator, is an invariable quantity. Consequently if F_2' increases proportionately with F, this holds good likewise for β_2, the value of which is proportionate to F_2'.

* *loc. cit.*, pp. 46 *et seq.*

Graefe,* on the contrary, found that some accommodating power remained. He remarks, however, that those who made the most accurate, and, on repeated investigation, the most uniform, statements, had the least range. Whatever else we find here and there noted respecting the occurrence of considerable range of accommodation in aphakia, proves only that the writers had no idea of the degree of distinctness of vision, even in imperfect accommodation.

My investigations have led me to the conviction, that in aphakia not the slightest trace of accommodative power remains. In old people, and with imperfect acuteness of vision, observers sometimes think they are able to prove the existence of a certain amount of range of accommodation; but in young persons, with perfectly clear pupils and great acuteness of vision, in whom precisely we might still expect to find some accommodative power, it is quite evident that the latter is entirely lost. A young person, of perfect, indeed of extraordinary, acuteness of vision, who was himself interested in the investigation, had suffered from congenital cataract, and had been operated on by me in both eyes with the most complete success. With glasses of $\frac{1}{3}$, placed at 5''' from the eye, he saw, at a great distance, a point of light sufficiently round and perfectly defined. A sight (*vizier*) was placed in the direction between one of the eyes and the point of light, and when he now looked with converging visual lines towards the sight, the point of light remained unchanged or became somewhat smaller and sharper, without changing its form. If the lens was removed only ¼''' more or less from the eye, the distant point of light had ceased to be a defined, round point, and was elongated in one direction, to the form of a line; now even with the most powerful exertion, and convergence in the point of the sight, the line of light became only somewhat shorter, without however a point making its appearance. This shortening, as well as the diminution of the acutely seen point, depended upon narrowing of the pupil, which was, indeed, directly observed. The experiment was repeated separately for each eye, with a like result. Behind the black plate, which in the trial was placed before the one eye, the turning of this eye, in looking towards the sight and towards the remote point of light, could be observed. The force of the experiment, therefore, leaves nothing to be desired. No accommo-

* *Archiv f. Ophthalm.*, B. II. Abth. i. p. 188.

dation whatever existed. Nevertheless in this case also a small margin of distinct vision was, on examination with the optometer, observed,— a proof that we cannot thence infer the existence of accommodative power.

In a second similar case, that of an intelligent young man, the total absence of accommodative power was in like manner proved. In this instance it was, moreover, established, that when a point of light was acutely seen at a distance, through a given lens, the addition of a lens of $\frac{1}{180}$ or $-\frac{1}{180}$ (by the combination of $\frac{1}{30}$ with $-\frac{1}{36}$ or of $\frac{1}{36}$ with $-\frac{1}{30}$) produced the well-known change in the point of light: the patient constantly stated that by $\frac{1}{180}$ the point of light was extended in the vertical, by $-\frac{1}{180}$ in the horizonal direction to a short line. On the other hand, the convergence of the visual lines, with the effort to see near objects, was not followed by the slightest change of form; consequently there was no reason to suppose the existence of accommodative power. I must add, that at the moment when he directed his attention entirely to the sight, an actual change in the sharpness of the point of light was still observed immediately on unexpectedly pushing before him a lens of $\frac{1}{180}$ or $-\frac{1}{180}$.—Subsequently I have, at different times, tried a similar experiment, in which glasses of $\frac{1}{300}$ or of $-\frac{1}{300}$ (a combination of $\frac{1}{50}$ with $-\frac{1}{60}$ or of $\frac{1}{60}$ with $-\frac{1}{50}$) produced an evident change of form in the image of light, while on varying the convergence and endeavouring to accommodate, no change whatever took place. The range of accommodation therefore amounts, in aphakia, even in a youthful eye, certainly to less than $\frac{1}{300}$, and may therefore be considered $= 0$. It may well surprise us, that v. Jaeger, who is aware of these investigations, still speaks of accommodation in aphakia (*l. c.*, p. 111).

The complete want of accommodative power may readily mislead to the idea, that in aphakia glasses of different focus are necessary

21

for each distance. Fortunately this is not the case. An accommodative power remains, the mechanism of which is extremely simple.
The drawback is, that the hand must in it perform the active part.
The power of accommodation to which I have alluded, consists in
the alteration of the distance between the glass and the eye. The
lens placed before the eye has been substituted for the crystalline.
It can also take on itself the part of the accommodation. It cannot
do this by altering its form, like the lens in the eye, but it holds to
the old theory, according to which the power of accommodation was
made to depend upon displacement of the lens. I teach all sufferers
from aphakia to accommodate in this manner. Let $F_1 = l' \phi'$ (Fig.
123 A) be

Fig. 123.

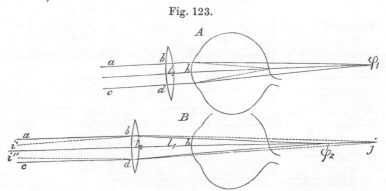

the focal distance of the lens required for distant vision, and the
distance $l_1 h$ be $= x$: then the rays $a b$ and $c d$, which, refracted at
h by the cornea (dotted lines), would meet on the retina, converge
towards ϕ_1, at $F_1 - x$ behind the cornea. If the same lens be now
$l_1 l_2 = x'$ removed farther from the cornea (compare Fig. B), ϕ_1
becomes equally removed forwards to ϕ_2 ($\phi_2 j = l_2 l_1 = x'$). Now
we know that rays, in order to be brought by the refraction of the
cornea on the retina, must be directed to j (corresponding to ϕ_1 of
A). Consequently they must proceed from a certain point i situated at
a finite distance, whence the rays $i' b$ and $i'' d$ are supposed to
diverge, and of which j is the conjugate focus. The distance
$i l_2 = y$ we therefore find from

$$\frac{1}{F_1} - \frac{1}{F_1 + x'} = \frac{1}{y}.$$

In order to find the distance of distinct vision to the cornea,
we must add to y, the distance $l_2 h = x + x'$ from the lens to the eye.

In the ordinary position the glass is about half-an-inch from the eye, and the spectacles can easily descend an inch farther on the nose. Now if a person in order to see at a distance, requires glasses of $1 : 3\frac{1}{2}$, placed at half-an-inch from the eye, let the spectacles be removed only half-an-inch more, and the above mode of calculation shows that accommodation has taken place for the distance of $29''$; let them be removed a whole inch more, and the point of distinct vision lies at $17\frac{1}{4}''$. If glasses of $1 : 3$, placed at half-an-inch from the eye, are necessary for distant vision, then, on removing the glasses to $1''$, the point of distinct vision lies at $22''$, on removing them to $1\frac{1}{2}''$ it lies at $13\frac{1}{2}''$, and some people then read exceedingly well.

Notwithstanding this artificial power of accommodation, it is in general advisable in aphakia to give two spectacles, one for distant, the other for close vision. Each pair of spectacles can then take on itself a part of the desired region of accommodation, and the necessary displacement may now be very slight. But in order to read or write anything for a moment, the spectacles usually worn for distant vision are simply displaced as may be necessary.

If, with good power of vision, aphakia exists in both eyes, we must carefully attend to the mutual distance of the axes of the two glasses. The greatest care is then required, in order, under different circumstances, to guard against double vision. Sometimes I have been obliged to have the glasses more or less ground on the outside, especially when the eyes stood particularly close to one another. Once too, for near vision, insufficiency of the musculi recti interni occurred to me, which was completely corrected by modifying the distance of the axes. The knowledge of the general laws must here be our guide in each particular case.

Finally, in altered curvature of the cornea, which is seen especially after prolapsus iridis in extraction, an oblique position of the glass is required, of which I shall speak more fully in treating of astigmatism.

A word, in conclusion, on examination with the ophthalmoscope in aphakia. In general a high degree of H exists in this condition. If the rays, in order to come to a focus on the retina, must converge in a point situated $3''$ behind the cornea, the rays proceeding in a diverging direction from the retina will appear, after having been refracted on the anterior surface of the cornea, to proceed from a point situated $3''$ behind the cornea. With myopia of nearly $1 : 3$, therefore, the observer can still examine the retina in the unreversed image.

2

We understand, moreover, that in order to see the fundus accurately in aphakia in an ordinary eye, an emmetropic eye must either remove, or accommodate strongly for near objects, or make use of positive glasses. We may also combine one plan with another. For the oculist it is important, that he should be aware of each change in his accommodative power, and that he should, under all circumstances, be able voluntarily completely to relax his power of accommodation. With this total relaxation the emmetropic eye sees, with glasses of 1 : 5, held at about 2″ from the observed eye, the fundus oculi in aphakia, with perfect acuteness. The rays then appear to proceed from a point, situated 3″ behind the cornea, and the eye investigated therefore re- quires glasses of 1 : 3½, at ½″ from the cornea, in order to be accommodated for parallel rays, that is, for distance. We can thus, from the observation with the ophthalmoscope, deduce the strength of the glasses required. This is not, however, attended with any essen- tial advantage. The patient himself states, more accurately than can be determined with the ophthalmoscope, the glasses which he requires for distant vision, and in general decides with great precision, at what distance, and with what inclination of the glasses, a remote point of light is most acutely seen. But the observation is im- portant in another point of view. In fact, it is known, that in the emmetropic eye the whole curvature of the retina lies in the focal surface of the dioptric system : with the ophthalmoscope we see, with unaltered accommodation, even the eccentric parts of the retina acutely defined in the unreversed image ; and in the eye of the white rabbit, removed from the head, I saw sharp images of remote objects glimmering through the entire sclerotic, so far as the latter bears a retina on its inner surface. Thomas Young connected the union of the rays on the retinal surface with the laminated structure of the lens. It is certain that this is not without influence upon it. We can, in fact, satisfy ourselves, as might be à *priori* inferred, that the retina, where aphakia exists, is not visible with equal accuracy in all directions through the same lens, unless the observer alters his accommodation or his distance from the eye.

Another question is, whether the forms perceptible in the fundus oculi also undergo a change, when we look into the eye under a tolerably great angle with the visual axis. I have satisfied myself that this is really the case. If we dilate the pupil in cases in which clearly visible, sharply-defined forms occur in the fundus oculi ; for example, where circumscribed deposits of pigment exist in the retina, we see the same figures, under the slight difference of direction, with which they continue visible, becoming elongated and shortened in various directions. It appears to me that thus also the form of an eccentric image must deviate from that which is produced by the same object near the axis of the eye on the retina. The direction of the projection must be modified accordingly, while yet the objects are seen also indirectly in their true form. Now it deserves remark, that in a case of pigmentary deposition on the retina, in which the lens was extracted, this change of form, connected with looking in different directions into the eye, was no longer observed, or at least was perceptible in only a very slight degree. We must therefore assume, that indirect vision, in aphakia, has undergone a change, in this sense, that the forms of the bodies are now represented more correctly in the retinal images, but are even therefore less correctly projected. However, the importance of this ceases with the use of tolerably strong glasses, which is almost invariably required; for when such glasses are employed, no sharply-defined images whatever can occur on the eccentric parts of the retina.

NOTE TO CHAPTER VI.

In the writings of the eighteenth century I have sought in vain for proofs that H was observed and recognised as such, or that the existence of this anomaly of refraction was even suspected. It is not until 1811 that we find a case communicated by Wells (*Philosophical Transactions*, vol. ciii. p. 380). It relates to his own eyes. At the age of 55 he remarked, that his presbyopia was attributable to loss (diminution) of accommodation, and that he required even glasses of 36 inches positive focal distance, in order to see acutely *at a distance*. This observation did not escape the learned Mackenzie (*A Practical Treatise on the Diseases of the Eye*, London, 1830, p. 729). " Although the eye," we read, " after middle life, loses the power of distinguishing near objects with correctness, it generally retains the sight of those that are distant. Instances, however, are not wanting of persons of advanced age requiring the aid of convex glasses to enable them to see distant, as well as near objects." As he, in addition, quotes the case of Wells, it follows from the above, that he considers the occurrence of the condition in question at a more advanced period of life as not unusual, and Wells himself was of the same opinion.

The cases here spoken of have, however, reference only to hypermetropia acquisita. If no other form occurred, hypermetropia would not be of any great importance. It would then really be coextensive with presbyopia, and we should have been able to concur in the use of the term *hyperpresbyopia*, which Stellwag von Carion, starting from such cases, has given in general to those eyes in which the focus lies behind the retina.

On the 19th November, 1812, James Ware read before the Royal Society his *Observations relative to the near and distant sight of different persons.* After having spoken of the senile changes of the eye, and having, in conclusion, quoted Wells' case of relative hypermetropia acquisita, he adds the following remarkable words : "There are also instances of young persons, who have so disproportionate a convexity of the cornea or crystalline, or of both, to the distance of these parts from the retina, that a glass of considerable convexity is required to enable them to see distinctly, not only near objects, but also those that are distant ; and it is remarkable, that the same glass will enable many such persons to see both near and distant objects ; thus proving that the defect in their sight is occasioned solely by too small a convexity in one of the parts above-mentioned, and that it does not influence the power by which their eyes are adapted to see at distances variously remote.   In this respect such persons differ from those who had the crystalline humour removed by an operation ; since the latter always require a glass to enable them to discern distant objects, different from that which they use to see those that are near " (*Philosophical Transactions of the Royal Society of London, for the year* 1813. London, 1813, p. 43).   In these few words James Ware entitles himself to be called the discoverer of hypermetropia.*   In a youthful eye, with sufficient accommodation, position of the focus behind the retina and need of convex glasses for seeing distant objects : the portrait is complete.   But not perceiving the great bearing of his discovery, Ware confines himself to this brief communication, which was either overlooked or not comprehended.   Even Mackenzie (*loc. cit.* 4th edition, p. 923) speaking of it in connexion with presbyopia can say only : " The cases related by Mr. Ware, as occurring in young persons, seem to partake more of the character of asthenopia than of presbyopia."   Hence his asthenopia might, *vice versâ*, have suggested to him the idea of hypermetropia.

With Ware our knowledge of H was lost. We next meet with Sichel (*Des lunettes et des états pathologiques, consecutifs à leur usage irrationel. Annales d'oculistique*, Tome xiii. pp. 5, 49, 109, 169. Tome xiv. pp. 14, 193. Bruxelles, 1845), whose doctrines have long exercised a great influence. Cases of an anomaly of such general occurrence could not escape so excellent an observer. As " une espèce d'amblyopie congénitale compliquée de presbytie et prise d'ordinaire pour un tres-haut degré de myopie," to which he gives the name of *amblyopie presbytique congénitale*, he sketches a distinct picture of high degrees of hypermetropia.   The nature

---

* While the above pages are passing through the press, I find that Janin too was acquainted with H. Thus I read, in an article by Muncke, in Gehler's *Physik. Wörterbuch*, B. iv., 1828, p. 1309, the following words :— " To the singular phenomena belongs lastly such a condition of the eyes, that neither near nor distant objects can be distinctly seen without convex glasses, as after the operation for cataract.   Now Janin (*Mem. et observ. sur l'œil*, Paris, 1772, 8vo., p. 429) has observed this defect, which he attributes to too great flatness of the lens." I have not had an opportunity of perusing Janin's communication in the original.

of the affection he did not, however, comprehend. He states, indeed, that negative glasses only incommode, that on the contrary, improvement is obtained by convex glasses, "avec lesquels ils n'ont pas besoin de rapprocher beaucoup plus les objets, et qui même, pour leur servir efficacement, doivent être d'une certaine force." But he was far from believing that they really required these. "Il serait dangereux toutefois," he says, "de les leur accorder trop tôt, ou de permettre qu'ils usent des verres trop puissants: *mieux vaut les en priver le plus longtems possible.*"—If hypermetropics, who had already worn convex spectacles, resorted to him, he did not hesitate to declare that the use of the glasses was the cause why they could not distinguish without such assistance, and already saw a dangerous amblyopia looming in the distance. He therefore unconditionally forbad the use of positive glasses for remote objects. This he did even in the case of old persons. Nay, he blames Mackenzie in this respect, who nevertheless certainly did not go too far. In this singular prejudice against the use of positive glasses is contained the proof, that the nature of the deviation remained a mystery to Sichel.

The same prejudice continued for a long time to be tolerably generally entertained. Even so late as 1853, White Cooper (*On Near Sight, Aged Sight, and Impaired Vision*, p. 97) describes the case of a girl, aged eight years, who used a convex glass, and with it was enabled to work at the distance of a foot. He adds that her parents had both been obliged to wear convex glasses at the age of thirty (hereditary H); and still he could give the poor child no better advice than to refrain from the use of spectacles. "There is good reason to believe," he says, "that as she grows older, and her eyes are more employed upon near objects, the distance of the point of distinct vision will decrease."—So little was it suspected, that the structure of the eye caused the focus to fall behind the retina, and that at any distance correction by means of a convex glass was therefore necessary.

When, after the discovery of the operation for strabismus, this form of disease had attracted such general attention, and in a short time became the subject of a long series of essays, it followed, as a matter of course, that the power of vision of squinters should be specially attended to. Many of these essays, however, do not bear the stamp of unprejudiced investigation. Almost always a special desire was manifested to show that by the operation not only was the deformity removed, but that the disturbance of vision was also gotten rid of. In general we find anomalies of refraction and of accommodation mixed up and confounded with diminution of acuteness of vision, while theories respecting the influence of the external muscles of the eye upon accommodation were made the basis of the explanation of what was observed, or even determined the observation. It is evident that a squinting hypermetropic eye, which moreover usually suffers from diminished acuteness of vision, amblyopia, can distinguish an ordinary type only when near, although even then with difficulty,—better at least than the same type at a greater distance. Meanwhile, this condition was almost universally considered to be myopia, and Baudens even calls a child extremely nearsighted *because* it could distinguish objects only with strongly convex glasses. Ludwig Böhm (*Das Schielen und der Sehnenschnitt in seinen Wirkungen auf*

Stellung und Sehkraft der Augen, Berlin, 1845), as an unprejudiced observer proved, that in strabismus the vision of near was better than that of distant objects (therefore M ?), and that nevertheless the patient could, with convex glasses, read at a greater distance (therefore presbyopia ?). Thus he saw himself brought into a difficult dilemma, from which he knew not how to escape. Evidently he did not consider, that even without accommodation for near objects, letters of definite magnitude, especially when amblyopia exists, are more easily recognised near the eye, than at a greater distance, simply because the retinal images are larger, and that convex glasses, by improving the images, make it possible under those circumstances, to distinguish at a greater distance. But beyond this we seek in vain for any proof from him, whence it might follow, that in any case he had satisfactorily proved the existence of hypermetropia. Indeed he always investigated only, with what convex glasses a distinct type of medium magnitude was best recognised, and nowhere is it stated, that this distance was greater than the focal distance of the glasses employed.

Among the cases of strabismus communicated by Ritterich (*Das Schielen und seine Heilung*, p. 73, Leipzig, 1843), we find one recorded in which the existence of H was demonstrated. " With a convex glass of No. 24," we read, " he saw (the subject was a boy of eleven years) both near and distant objects *better*." However, this condition was not more accurately determined or appreciated, nor was the case further observed. A similar case, described by Fronmüller (*Beobachtungen auf dem Gebiete der Augenheilkunde*, p. 54, Fürth, 1850), in which it is expressly stated, that " in order to be able to see well at a distance," the patient, who was twenty-two years of age, and was affected with strabismus, was obliged to make use of a strong convex glass No. 8 ; this case, I say, was in some incomprehensible manner confounded with the myopia at a distance of Kerst, which is nothing else than a slight degree of myopia.

In order to ascertain whether earlier writers had any idea of H, we had to search under the heading of presbyopia. Now in the works of many we find it stated, that some people early require convex glasses for reading and writing, and occasionally even very strong ones. Thus we read in Mackenzie (*A Treatise on the Diseases of the Eye*, p. 728. London, 1830) " Young men of twenty years sometimes cannot see to read or write without convex glasses of six or eight inches focus, while persons of eighty years and upwards are occasionally met with who are able to read even a small print without assistance. . . . . These, and similar differences, depend *upon the original formation of the eyes*, how they have been used, and the general health and constitution of the individual." Thus Smee (*The Eye in Health and in Disease*, p. 33. London, 1854) also says : " Although far sight occurs most commonly as a disease, yet I have been occasionally consulted by patients who have suffered from this abnormal state as a result of congenital defect. The patient in this case prefers to sit before a window with the light falling directly upon the pupil, so that by its contraction to a pin's point, only the central rays infringe upon the retina, and thus fair vision may be obtained. Congenital farsight may exist with most perfect power of adjustment." These last words are of great importance. When the power of accommodation is perfect, and nevertheless near objects cannot be seen, the condition can be none other than H. He adds: "the disease may be determined with great accuracy, instantly, by the optometer." But from the tables, in which the results of optometric observations obtained by calculation are collected, it does not appear that Smee was actually aware of the existence of H.

Thus no progress was as yet made beyond the point attained by Ware.

He who knows by experience how commonly H occurs, how necessary a knowledge of it is to the correct diagnosis of the various defects of the eye, and how deeply it affects the whole treatment of the oculist, will come to the sad conviction that an incredible number of patients have been tormented with all sorts of remedies, and have been given over to painful anxiety, who would have found immediate relief and deliverance in suitable spectacles. We may therefore look upon it as truly fortunate, that many had recourse simply to ordinary empirics, so-called opticians, who endeaour to give men those spectacles which render their vision persistently easier. Sichel's lamentation over the number of patients who had got convex spectacles for distant vision, satisfactorily proves that the opticians knew very well, that in some eyes distant vision is improved by convex glasses. And still every day almost the same thing occurs. But what is more, some of these opticians had more or less correct notions of hypermetropia. Thus we find, so early as in 1842, concealed under a chaos of confused ideas, a condition separately described and characterised by Mr. J. A. Hess (*Theoretisch en praktisch handboek der mechanische oogheelkunde*, p. 216, Zierikzee, 1842) under the name of presmyopia (sic!), of which he says: "the only certainty consists in this, that the vision of these eyes at all distances is improved by the addition of a convex glass," and thus H is evidently defined. Mr. Hess stated that this condition occurs in different degrees, that the power of accommodation (by him called extensibility and impressibility) may at the same time exist, and thought that in these eyes the lens is either wholly absent or must be partially degenerated, and that there is much hope of curing slight degrees of the affection.

At length in 1853, we find hypermetropia, for the first time, described in a scientific manual (Ruete. *Lehrbuch der Ophthalmologie für Aerzte und Studirende*, Bd. i. p. 234, Braunschweig) in the following words, under the name of *oversightedness (Uebersichtigkeit)*: "Oversightedness is the condition in which, on account of a peculiar, and as yet not sufficiently investigated, construction of the refracting media of the eye, neither near nor distant objects are distinctly seen. The eye appears in it to suffer from a total want of accommodating power, and to possess but a very slight refractive power. This defect of sight is in general congenital, or is at least developed in very early youth. Vision is considerably improved by the use of convex spectacles, whose focal distance must, however, vary according to the distance of the objects, so that those suffering from this defect are able even to read." The description still leaves much to be desired; the state is not accurately characterised; moreover, it is incorrectly supposed, that the power of accommodation is in these eyes almost wholly wanting. But still in these few words lies the germ of further investigation, and we thus see here also, as in many other points in ophthalmology, the impulse given by Ruete to our knowledge.

Two years later, namely on the 12th of April, 1855, Dr. Carl Stellwag von Carion laid before the Imperial Academy of Sciences at Vienna, a detailed essay entitled: *die Accommodationsfehler des Auges.* (*Sitzungsberichte der Kaiserlichen Akademie der Wissenschaften, Mathematisch-naturwissenschaftliche Classe,* Bd. xvi. pp. 187-281.) In it we find a correct definition in the following words: "the optical essence of oversightedness lies in this, that the focal range of the dioptric apparatus in perfect rest of the accommodating muscle is greater, than the distance of the layer of rods and bulbs from the optical centre of the refracting media." Stellwag too has the merit of having satisfactorily indicated the method of determining *r* in cases of H. Slight degrees of H he appears, however, scarcely to have recognised, the latent not at all (compare de Haas, *loc. cit.*); and on the whole, as the very name of hyperpresbyopia used by him shows, he has not strictly enough distinguished hypermetropia from presbyopia.

Only a few months after Stellwag von Carion had brought forward his investigations on defects of accommodation of the eye, we find in the *Archiv für Ophthalmologie* (Bd. ii., Abth. i. pp. 158-186) a paper by von Graefe, under the title of "Ueber Myopia in distans, nebst Betrachtungen über das Sehen jenseits der Grenzen unserer Accommodation," in which occurs a masterly description of the highest degrees of hypermetropia. Stellwag von Carion had observed, that "the oversighted person," in order to recognise an object, brings it very close to the eye, and singularly enough, he seems to imagine (compare p. 269) that it then appears more illuminated. Von Graefe has remarked the same, but has also, in part at least, indicated the cause, by proving mathematically, that in the hypermetropic eye, on approaching the objects, the angle under which they appear increases more rapidly than the circles of diffusion, and by imitating the effect on the eye made hypermetropic by negative glasses. He shows further, that this hypermetropic eye is clearly distinguishable in structure from the myopic eye, by the flatness of its anterior chamber and by the narrowness of the pupil; but he has not, any more than Stellwag von Carion, properly recognised and appreciated the slight and moderate degrees of hypermetropia.

In my first communication (*Nederlandsch Tijdschrift voor Geneeskunde,* Jaarg, 1858, pp. 465-476. *Archiv für Ophthalmologie,* Bd. iv., Abth. i., pp. 301-340), and likewise in the dissertation by MacGillavry (*Onderzoekingen over de hoegrootheid der accommodatie,* Utrecht, 1858), soon after written under my superintendence, the condition under consideration was indeed accurately distinguished from presbyopia, but the division into anomalies of refraction and of accommodation, and the opposition of myopia and hypermetropia, were not yet apparent. It was at the meeting held at Heidelberg in 1859, that I first showed, among other things, that presbyopia and the so-called hyperpresbyopia are, both in essence and in symptoms wholly different conditions, that the latter alone is opposed to M, that an eye may be even very hyperpresbyopic without being in the least affected with presbyopia, etc. I argued that, consequently, the name of hyperpresbyopia must be set aside, and Helmholtz, who was at the meeting, immediately proposed the term hyperopia. This coincided with the word "oversightedness" (*Uebersichtigkeit*) first used by Ruete, and quickly found acceptance with some. On more fully working out my system, I thought, however, that the term hypermetropia would be more in accordance with the nomenclature I had already employed in the words ametropia and emmetropia, and this name has since that time been most generally adopted.

My investigations respecting H are to be found in *Ametropie en hare gevolgen*, Utrecht, 1860, and in the *Archiv für Ophthalmologie*, Bd. vi., Abth. i., pp. 62-106, Abth. ii., pp. 210-243.

Since I published my researches, different writers have treated of the anomalies of refraction; among others Hasner (*Klinische Vorträge über Augenheilkunde*, Prag. 1860); Giraud-Teulon (*Physiologie et pathologie fonctionnelle de la vision binoculaire*, Paris, 1861); Happe (*Die Bestimmungen des Sehbereichs und dessen Correction*, Braunschweig, 1860), and Soelberg Wells (*On long, short, and weak Sight, and their Treatment.* London, 1862). Our knowledge of H has not, however, been increased by these works. That of Professor von Jaeger, Junr. (*Ueber die Einstellungen des dioptrischen Apparates im menschlichen Auge*, Wien, 1861) has also been fruitless in this respect. But the last-named writer has the merit of having been the first to make an attempt to trace the changes of the refractive condition of the eyes in the normal development of childhood. I think that less importance is to be attached in this respect to his measurements of the eyeball and of the crystalline lens after death, than to his derminations of the refractive condition of the eyes at different periods of life with the aid of the ophthalmoscope, especially when previously to the investigation he paralysed the accommodative system with atropia. Von Jaeger, following the example of Helmholtz (*Beschreibung eines Augen-Spiegels zur Untersuchung der Netzhaut im lebenden Auge*, p. 38, Berlin, 1851), early recommended the ophthalmoscope for the determination of the refraction of the eye (*Oesterreichische Zeitschrift für praktische Heilkunde*, No. 10, März, 1856), and he has undoubtedly acquired great expertness in the use of this method. His observations extend over more than 1600 eyes. The numbers noted by him are the following :—Of 100 eyes of

	Hypermetropic	Emmetropic	Myopic
Infants, from 9 to 16 days old, are . . .	17	5	78
Children, from an infant-school, of between 2 and 6 years of age	8	30	62
Boys, in the country, between 6 and 11 years old .	11	46	43
Girls, in the country, between 5 and 11 years of age	10	34	56
Boys, in an orphan house, between 7 and 14 years	12	33	55
Pupils, from a boarding-school, of from 9 to 16 years	2	18	80
Soldiers (Italian), from 20 to 25 years . .	1	57	42

In von Jaeger's table the degrees of ametropia are also stated.

CHAPTER VII.

MYOPIA. M.

§ 26. Dioptric Determination, Diagnosis, Degrees, Occurrence, Hereditariness, Development with Advancing Age.

Myopia we have already considered as the condition opposed to H. In the latter, the focus of the dioptric system lies behind, in M, on the contrary, it lies in front of the retina; in other words

Fig. 124.

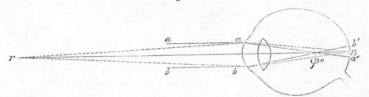

parallel rays (Fig. 124, $a\,a$, $b\,b$), derived from infinitely remote objects, unite in the myopic eye in front of the retina in ϕ'', and each infinitely remote point therefore forms upon the retina a circle of diffusion, $(a'\,b')$ of rays, which have already intersected. Hence it follows, that, in order to unite upon the retina in r_1 rays must proceed from a point r situated at a finite distance, and must therefore fall diverging upon the cornea (see the dotted lines).

The above is true of the eye in a state of rest. By tension of accommodation the emmetropic eye, and usually even the hypermetropic, can bring its focus for parallel rays in front of the retina; but it does not therefore become myopic. Even when by spasm of accommodation the focus comes to lie before the retina, and relaxation to E is not possible, the eye cannot be said to be myopic. M depends, just like H, on the structure of the eye, irrespectively of accommodation, or rather with actual relaxation.

In general M is easily recognised. The rule is, that near objects are accurately seen, while at a distance vision is, on the contrary, diffuse. So soon as letters of double magnitude are not recognised at double the distance, we are, in general, justified in assuming the existence of M. The criterion consists further in this, that with concave glasses distant vision becomes more acute. However, this is not true of all concave glasses. In slight degrees of M, vision is even worse with strong concave glasses than without glasses, and in the highest degrees of M, the effect of weak concave glasses is scarcely perceptible. The question is, therefore, with what glasses must we in a particular case commence the investigation, in order to satisfy ourselves of the existence of M; and this is answered by the first trials of the sight. From these trials we learn, namely, what is about the distance R of the farthest point of distinct vision. Almost always the myopic presents himself before us with the statement, that he can see near objects well, while he with difficulty distinguishes at a distance, and if we then place in his hand a book with small type, for example I or II of Snellen's Tests, the distance which he chooses itself indicates about the farthest point. We now, however, make him remove the book farther off, until he reads less easily and sees even somewhat larger letters less acutely, and we estimate the distance at which this diminution of acuteness commences. If this be 6″, we try at first glasses of $-\dfrac{1}{6}$; if it is 10″, glasses of $-\dfrac{1}{10}$, &c. Almost invariably vision at a distance is now better: of the table with CC to XX or less, letters will be recognised at a distance, which without spectacles are not distinguished, and the existence of M is thus proved. The matter is simple: at 6″, at 10″, vision is distinct ; and by glasses of $-\dfrac{1}{6}$, of $-\dfrac{1}{10}$, the parallel rays derived from remote objects acquire a direction, as if they had proceeded from a point situated at 6″, or at 10″ from the glass (compare p. 32), and distinguishing at a great distance has thus become possible.

We now investigate immediately and more accurately the *degree* of M; in other words, we determine R, the distance from *r* to *k′*. This is found by trying, what the *weakest negative glass* is, with which vision is as acute as possible. In order quickly to attain this object, we place the glasses supposed to be suitable in a frame, cause the patient to look through them at the table already mentioned, and now hold, while we raise the frame somewhat with the fingers, glasses before the eye, which are somewhat weaker, and ask whether with them vision is as good or even better: if he answers yes, we then place these in the frame, and compare them, in like manner, again with somewhat weaker glasses, repeating the trial until we receive for answer, that vision is not so acute with the glasses last tried. But we should even still try yet weaker glasses, and not be satisfied until we are told that vision is with them much less acute : experience has in fact taught me, that we cannot be too cautious; for with good accommodation the action of too strong glasses is easily enough overcome, and since with slight differences in strength the sight remains nearly the same, this equality may lead to its being said that the vision is less accurate. Thus I have with $M = \frac{1}{16}$ seen $-\frac{1}{8}$ preferred to $-\frac{1}{9}$ or $-\frac{1}{10}$, although $-\frac{1}{16}$ finally proved to be sufficient.—Not unfrequently, however, the glasses first tried are too weak, in which case, on comparison, the weaker are immediately rejected. This we find to occur especially with older myopes, who prefer reading at a comparatively great distance; while very young, and still in the possession of a great power of accommodation, they readily bring the object within the distance of their farthest point, and so, on the first trial, they cause a higher degree of M to be suspected. If we have now found that, in order to attain the greater acuteness of vision, a stronger glass is necessary, we go on until further strengthening no longer produces an improvement, and we then try once more, whether a somewhat weaker glass is not equally satisfactory. Thus the object is at length attained.—We have already observed, that the distance at which the glass is held from the eye, has an influence upon its action. While a convex glass, by removal from the eye, acts more and more strongly, the reverse obtains with regard to concave glasses. The thing is plain : parallel rays, refracted by a concave glass, appear to proceed from a point placed as far *before the glass*, as the focal distance amounts to, and that point lies still so much farther from the eye, as the distance between the eye and the glass. Thus a glass of $-\frac{1}{8}$, held an inch farther from the eye, is equal to a glass of $-\frac{1}{9}$, but with this difference, that the images are smaller : therefore $-\frac{1}{9}$, if held an inch closer to the eye, is chosen. Now, of the influence of distance on the action of glasses, we may often advantageously make use, in order to see quickly whether the glass tried is too strong or too weak. If it is too strong, removing it a little is no disadvantage; if it is too weak, the patient will hold it rather directly to the eye. However we must not be too sure on this point. Thus, the myope who has a good accommodating power, will hold even a too strong glass by preference close to the eye, because the retinal images are thus rendered larger. Therefore when vision is equally good or even better on the removal of the glass, we may infer that the latter is too strong, not *vice versâ*. In any case we should never be satisfied, until we have determined what is the weakest glass which, held close before the eye, is quite sufficient. By this the degree of M, and at the same time the acuteness of vision are known (compare p. 97).— The investigation may in general be undertaken with both eyes at the same time: almost invariably the M is sufficiently nearly equal in the two eyes, and what has been found for both eyes, may in a moment be tested for each eye separately. But if we have reason to suspect, *à priori*, inequality of the M in the two eyes, or if we obtain confused answers to the first tests of vision, we may first try the one eye and afterwards compare the other. We should always begin with the eye which the patient himself calls the best, the other should be gently closed with the hand.*

Many will possibly find the above directions tedious and too minute. And yet they are in many respects incomplete; so that, at the risk of incurring the displeasure of my readers, I will take leave to point out some additional sources of error. Let it be borne in mind that an incorrect determination of the degree of M may highly endanger the eyes.

In the first place some think, although they are not nearsighted, that they see distant objects more accurately with concave glasses: the smaller dimensions of letters and of other forms appear to them so flattering and agreeable, that they feel bound to boast of their distinctness. Therefore we should never be content with the

---

* Von Graefe has lately (see *Deutsche Klinik*, 1863, p. 10) had an optical instrument made, which, by a simple mechanism, can be so modified in its action as to represent lenses of very different focal distances. It may now, held before the eye, be so arranged that the ametropia is precisely corrected, and thus the tedious determination with different glasses may be dispensed with. Von Graefe praises it very much. I am sorry that I have not yet been able to try it. It appears to me that the influence on the magnitude of the images must give rise to some disturbance in the determination. In using this instrument, each eye is separately investigated.

declaration: " I see better;" but we should satisfy ourselves of its correctness, by making the patient name the letters.

In some cases objects are really better distinguished by using concave glasses, although the eye is free from M.   We meet with this especially in misty opacities of the cornea, when the narrower pupil, which is the result of the tension of accommodation made necessary by the concave glass, diminishes the diffused light.   Particularly when the turbidity is local, and is so situated that it disturbs direct vision only when the pupil is dilated, constricting the pupil by using a concave glass, produces a very considerable improvement of the power of vision.   It need not be said that the existence of a sufficient range of accommodation is here the *sine qua non* for obtaining improvement by means of negative glasses.—Further, one should beware of mistaking spasm of the ciliary muscle, with which the accommodation cannot be relaxed to E, although the vision of distant objects is improved by negative glasses, for M.   In speaking of the disturbances of accommodation, I shall revert to this subject.   Here it may suffice to state, that the sudden occurrence of the disturbance, in connexion with other phenomena (especially myosis), will lead us to suspect the existence of spasm, which is easily tested by paralysis by atropia. We shall further see, in the disturbances proceeding from high degrees of M, that a certain measure of spasm is not unfrequently combined therewith, and makes the degree of M be too highly estimated.

On the other hand, *actually existing* M *is not always indicated on ordinary investigation*.   This depends upon different causes.   In the first place, diminished S is to be noted.   If, as we have already seen (p. 254), without the presence of H, a convex glass is sometimes chosen for distance, because the advantage of magnifying the images may counterbalance the disadvantage of diminished acuteness, a concave glass, which diminishes the size and adds little to the distinctness, will, under similar circumstances, where M exists, be rejected.   Always too, in the highest degrees of M, a too weak glass is preferred above a completely compensating one, and often vision is better with it: the cause of this lies partly in the diminished S, partly in the fact, that the circles of diffusion prove particularly small in relation to the degree of the M still remaining with imperfect correction (compare the vision of myopes).—In the second place, a smaller pupil is to be noted.   The smaller the latter is, the less disturbance do the circles of diffusion cause in imperfect accommodation; and thus it is explained why, with incomplete atresia pupillæ, with very small pupilla artificialis, in either case with diminished S, nay, even with senile constriction of the pupil, neutralising a certain degree of M in general yields no advantage, and the neutralisation in such cases may therefore the more easily escape us. We should take particular care that in trying the glasses the eyelids be not squeezed together, as myopes are accustomed to do, and the circles of diffusion be so diminished.

Next to the examination with glasses is that with the ophthalmoscope. Of this we have already spoken in general (pp. 105 *et seq.*). If the pupil be wide, the investigator can determine high degrees of M in the unreversed image; with a narrower pupil this is more difficult, and the examination in the inverted image answers better, although the degree of M is not by it to be determined with accuracy. The ophthalmoscopic investigation yields essential service in the determination of the degree of myopia: 1°, when the eye is blind, and the nature of the morbid process may be connected with its structure. (Helmholtz* determined the M in such a case; it has often occurred to me to be able to give a favourable prognosis for the second eye, because the ophthalmoscope showed me, that the lost eye had been highly myopic). 2°, when, with diminished S, the ophthalmoscope is first used, which now directly gives us tolerably accurate information respecting the existing ametropia: † at the first

---

* *Beschreibung eines Augenspiegels.* Berlin, 1851, p. 38.

† It is desirable systematically to carry out the ophthalmoscopic investigation for each eye. The emmetropic individual should combine with his ophthalmoscope a glass of $\frac{1}{10}$, should look 10° or 15° to the outside of the visual axis directed on a given point, beginning at the distance of 10″, and should gradually approach, so as consecutively to see the cornea, pupil, lens, and vitreous humour; he should, in the investigation of the lens, especially make the patient look for a moment downwards (where the opacity usually begins); in the examination of the vitreous humour he should make him move the eye in different directions, and then suddenly stop at the originally fixed point (so as to see floating flakes); he should again remove, in order, with the interposition of a convex lens, to look into the inverted image; he should then begin again in the original direction, so as to see the entrance of the optic nerve; subsequently he should make him move slowly in different directions, and should look from different points, in order consecutively to pass through the whole fundus oculi; above all, he should not neglect for a moment to make him fix the light in the mirror (in order to judge of the macula lutea); and finally, he should examine, if there is indication for it or if

22

glance into the eye from a certain distance it is evident in strong M, that the inverted image stands before the eye; 3°, when we wish to determine the degree of M in indirect vision, or to establish the existence of locally exalted M, through locally increased staphylomatous distention : in either case the examination with glasses fails ;—4°, where simulated or concealed M is suspected; 5°, in children, from whom correct answers are not to be expected.

The degree of M is, as we have already seen (p. 91), expressed as

$$M = \frac{1}{R}.$$

R is the distance from the farthest point r to the nodal point k' in the eye, situated about $\frac{1''}{4}$ behind the cornea. The position of r is found by determining the glass, which neutralises the M : it lies so far in front of this glass as the focal distance amounts to. If, for example, the required glass is $= -\frac{1}{12}$, r lies 12″ in front of the glass, and if the glass stands $\frac{1''}{4}$ before the eye, and therefore $\frac{1''}{4} + \frac{1''}{4} = \frac{1}{2}$ in front of k', r lies 12½″ from k', and consequently R is $= 12\cdot5$ and M $= 1 : 12\cdot5$ (compare p. 32). We now understand distinctly, that the distance r (that from the glass to k') signifies little when the glass is weak : it is, in fact, nearly indifferent, whether a glass of $-\frac{1}{30}$ stands at $\frac{1''}{2}$ more or less before the eye, by which it changes at most from $-\frac{1}{30\cdot5}$ to $-\frac{1}{31}$. But $\frac{1''}{2}$ difference in distance acquires much importance, when strong glasses are in question; for example, glasses of $-\frac{1}{2}$, which may then act as glasses of $-\frac{1}{2\cdot5}$ or $-\frac{1}{3}$. Therefore, in the manner above pointed out, use can be made for strong glasses of the difference in distinctness by difference in distance, in order quickly to find the glass required, and therefore, where high degrees are concerned, in the determination of

strong magnifying be desired, with a weak object-lens in the inverted image and with the requisite glasses in the unreversed, or employ the method of Liebreich (Compare p. 367).

the M, the distance required for the neutralising glass must also be accurately taken into account. In order that it may appear from the note made, that attention has been paid to this distance, we are accustomed to add it separately after a $+$, and to write, for example, $M = \dfrac{1}{3 + \frac{1}{2}}$, which signifies that a glass of $-\dfrac{1}{3}$ at $\dfrac{1''}{2}$ from k' was necessary to neutralise the M.

The strongest concave glasses to be met with in spectacle boxes, are of $-\dfrac{1}{2}$. With these we can at most neutralise $M = 1 : 2\frac{1}{3}$. Now, not unfrequently, still higher degrees of M occur, and in order to determine these, we must place $-\dfrac{1}{2}$ as spectacles before the eye, and examine what glass must in addition be held in front of them, in order to produce complete neutralisation. Let this second glass $= -\dfrac{1}{3}$, then both combined give $-\left(\dfrac{1}{2} + \dfrac{1}{3}\right) = -1 : 1\cdot2$; and to this we have still to add the distance x from the strongest glass to k,* so that, with $x = \dfrac{1}{2}$, M is, in the case supposed $= 1 : 1\cdot7$.

M occurs in the most different degrees from E to $M = \dfrac{1}{1\cdot3}$, probably still higher. The highest degrees are, however, the rarest. For many thousand eyes of myopic patients who have consulted me, the degree of M has been noted. The following table thence calculated for one thousand eyes, gives a synoptical view of the relative occurrences of the different degrees.

* If great accuracy is desired, we must, in the calculation, also take into account the distance between the two glasses, and reckon, for example, $-\frac{1}{3}$, placed at $\frac{1}{4}''$ before $-\frac{1}{2}$, only as $1 : 3\frac{1}{4}$. We may then further, with sufficient precision, measure the distance to k', that is x, from the middle of the mass of the biconcave glass $-\frac{1}{2}$.

Degree of the Myopia.	Number of Cases in 1000.
$16:24 = 1:1\frac{1}{2}$	
	3
$15:24 = 1:1\frac{2}{3}$	
	4
$14:24 = 1:1\frac{5}{7}$	
	3
$13:24 = 1:1\frac{11}{13}$	
	5
$12:24 = 1:2$	
	13
$11:24 = 1:2\frac{2}{11}$	
	16
$10:24 = 1:2\frac{2}{5}$	
	24
$9:24 = 1:2\frac{2}{3}$	
	47
$8:24 = 1:3$	
	49
$7:24 = 1:3\frac{3}{7}$	
	68
$6:24 = 1:4$	
	83
$5:24 = 1:4\frac{4}{5}$	
	110
$4:24 = 1:6$	
	149
$3:24 = 1:8$	
	171
$2:24 = 1:12$	
	169
$1:24 = 1:24$	
	85
$0:24 = 1:\infty$	

At first, to begin with the highest degrees, for each $\frac{1}{24}$ M less, the number of cases increases. That the increase subsequently becomes slower, and finally even gives place to diminution, depends solely upon the fact that comparatively few of those affected with the slight degrees apply to the oculist. Nevertheless, I have endeavoured, in connexion with other observations, *approximatively* to express the relative occurrence of E and of the different degrees of M and H, among the Dutch population in general (Fig. 125). Along the figure are given, from $1:\infty$, above, the degrees of M to $M = 1:1\cdot3$, and beneath those of H to $H = 1:2\frac{2}{3}$, being the highest degrees observed by me. The lengths of the transverse lines correspond to the frequency of occurrence in the adjoining degrees, with this exception, however, that the lines a and a' next to $\dfrac{1}{\infty}$ must be supposed to be ten times longer. Since, therefore, the mutual distance of the lines represents $\dfrac{1}{96}$, the length (multiplied by ten) of the first line above $1:\infty$, being the line a, represents the number of cases from E to $M = \dfrac{1}{96}$, the (simple) length of the second line the number of cases between $M = \dfrac{1}{96}$ and $M = \dfrac{1}{48}$, the length of the third line the cases from $M = \dfrac{1}{48}$ to $M = \dfrac{1}{32}$, etc.—Of equal degrees of H, the occurrence is expressed by the lines following under $1:\infty$ (a' being again taken as tenfold). From the figure it now appears, that in the slightest

Fig. 125.

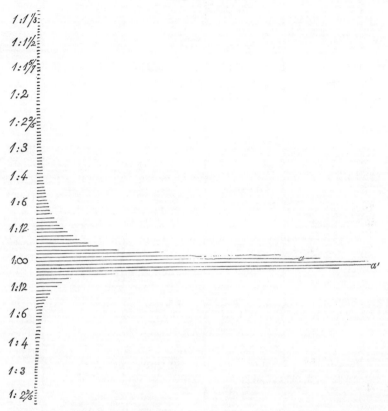

degrees H occurs more frequently than M, while the contrary obtains in the higher degrees : $M = \frac{1}{24}$ is already more frequent than $H = \frac{1}{24}$. The highest degrees of both are so rare, that they can be expressed only by a point. From this figure it is very clear, that the emmetropic is the normal eye. If we bring M and H in their almost imperceptible degrees from $\frac{1}{96}$ to E, E gives 1650 mm. length in lines, while all the other lines, representing H and M, amount to only 350; and these are reduced to 200 against 1800, when we take M and H at $\frac{1}{48}$ under the E.

On the distribution of M, position in society has a great influence. It is remarkable how much in the registers of my private patients (the more wealthy) the M,—in those of my hospital patients, on the contrary, the H predominates. To be correct, I must say, that among those in easy circumstances not much less H, but much more M occurs. That, moreover, the inhabitants of towns suffer more from M than those of the country is a matter of general observation. Ware*, upwards of 50 years ago, directed his attention to this fact.

"I have inquired," he says, "for instance, of the surgeons of the three regiments of Foot-Guards, which consist of nearly 10,000 men; and the result has been that myopia among the privates is almost utterly unknown. Not half-a-dozen men have been discharged, nor have a dozen recruits been rejected, on account of this imperfection, in the space of nearly 20 years." In the Military School at Chelsea, among 1300 children, no complaint was made; three only experienced some inconvenience. On the contrary, in the colleges of Oxford and Cambridge a considerable proportion of myopes was met with, in one college at Oxford, 32 out of 127. In all writers on the subject we find the same thing stated.† I must, however, remark, that in the country and amongst the least civilized ranks, even the highest degrees of M are exceptionally observed in particular families, and I will here add, that even among sailors, who never strain their eyes in looking at near objects, I found a few cases of progressive M.

Further, I believe that M is not equally prevalent in all countries. It is certainly more specially proper to cultivated nations. Furnari‡ tells us that among the Kabyles no myopes occur, and among the States of Europe visited by me, I, both in general life and in the cliniques, nowhere met with relatively so many myopes as in Germany. It would be of great importance, to possess accurate statistics of the ametropia occurring, at a given time, in a particular

---

* *Observations relative to near and distant sights of different persons* Read before the Royal Society, 1812.

† Conf. Szokalski, *Prager Vierteljahrschrift*, B. xvii.; von Hasner, *Klin. Vorträge ueber Augenheilkunde.* Prag. 1860, 1, p. 36.

‡ *Annales d'Oculistique*, T. X., p. 145.

category of men, especially, for example, among the students of a university, in order to be able to compare them with the results of repeated investigations at subsequent periods.   If it were thus found—and I can scarcely doubt that it would be so,—that the M is progressive in cultivated society, this would be a very serious phenomenon, and we should earnestly think of means of arresting this progression.   Not only is the myope not in a condition to discharge all civil duties, not only is he limited in the choice of his position in society, but in the higher degrees M leads to disturbance of the power of vision, and threatens its subject with incurable blindness.

The distribution of M, chiefly in the cultivated ranks, points directly to its principal cause : tension of the eyes for near objects. Respecting this fact there can be no doubt.   But the explanation of it is not so evident.   In tension of accommodation for near objects the crystalline lens, as we are aware, becomes more convex : now if myopia also depended on greater convexity of the crystalline lens, it might be considered as the permanent result of a frequently repeated state, and the M would thus be explained.   But the M depends upon a prolongation of the visual axis, and this is not altered in accommodation for near objects.   How then is this prolongation to be explained ?   Three factors may here come under observation : 1°, pressure of the muscles on the eyeball in strong convergence of the visual axes ; 2°, increased pressure of the fluids, resulting from accumulation of blood in the eyes in the stooping position; 3°, congestive processes in the fundus oculi, which, leading to softening, even in the normal, but still more under the increased pressure of the fluids of the eye, give rise to extension of the membranes.   That in increased pressure the extension occurs principally at the posterior pole, is explained by the want of support from the muscles of the eye at that part.   With the imperfect elasticity of fibrous membranes we understand, moreover, that of each in itself imperceptible extension above the normal limits a minimum each time remains.   Now in connexion with the causes mentioned, the injurious effect of fine work is, by imperfect illumination, still more increased : for thus it is rendered necessary that the work be brought closer to the eyes, and that consequently the convergence be stronger, and the tendency to the stooping position of the head, particularly in reading and writing, is also increased.   To this it is to be ascribed, that in schools, especially in boarding-schools, where, by bad light the pupils

read bad print in the evening, or write with pale ink, the foundation
of M is mainly laid, which, in fact, is usually developed during
these years.   On the contrary, in watchmakers, although they sit the
whole day with a magnifying-glass in one eye, we observe no development of M, undoubtedly because they fix their work only with one
eye, and therefore converge but little, and because they usually avoid
a very stooping position.

The same causes, which give rise to M, are still more favourable to
its further development.   I have always, with great care, watched the
course of myopia.   I attach to it a special importance.   The well-
known fact that myopes, with little light, can recognise small objects, and especially the circumstance that at an advanced period of
life, they need no glasses to enable them to see near objects,
procured almost general acceptance for the prejudice, that near-
sighted eyes are to be considered as particularly strong.   Many
medical men even participate in this error.   But the oculist has only
too often been convinced by sad experience, of the contrary.   I have
no hesitation in saying, that a near-sighted eye is not a sound eye.
In it there exists more than a simple anomaly of refraction.   The
optical characteristic of myopia may consist in this, the anatomical
is a prolongation of the visual axis, and the latter depends upon
morbid extension of the membranes.   If this extension has attained
to a certain degree, the membranes are so attenuated, and the resistance is so diminished, that the extension cannot remain stationary,
the less so, because in the myopic eye the pressure of the fluids is
usually increased.   In this progressive extension progressive myopia
is included, which is a true disease of the eye.

From what has here been said, it will easily be understood, that
high degrees of myopia are less likely to remain stationary than
slight degrees are; at a more advanced time of life they even continue to be developed, with increasing atrophy of the membranes.
In youth almost every myopia is progressive; the increase is then
often combined with symptoms of irritation.   This is the critical
period for the myopic eye : if the myopia does not increase too much,
it may become stationary, and may even decrease in advanced age ;
if it is developed in a high degree, it is subsequently difficult to set
bounds to it.   At this period, therefore, the above-mentioned promoting causes should be especially avoided.   On this point I cannot
lay sufficient stress.   Every progressive myopia is threatening with

respect to the future. If it continues progressive, the eye will soon, with troublesome symptoms, become less available, and not unfrequently at the age of 50 or 60, if not much earlier, the power of vision is irrevocably lost, whether through separation of the retina from the choroid, from effusion of blood, or from atrophy and degeneration of the yellow spot. In a subsequent section I shall have to treat of these sad results of M.

The number of myopes most accurately examined by me, amounts to more than 2500. Each time the degree of the myopia was accurately determined and noted. If after months or years the myope consulted me again, the determination was repeated. I thus came to the conviction, that almost always the myopia is somewhat progressive, that such is the rule between the 15th and 25th years, and that the highest degrees often exhibit the greatest increase. I have never in the periods of youth or manhood proved diminution of the myopia, except in the rare cases in which spasm of the accommodating system had temporarily increased it, and where, therefore, anomaly, not simply of refraction, but also of accommodation was present. Even at a more advanced time of life diminution of the degree of the myopia seldom occurs. Undoubtedly in the near-sighted eye the dioptric system undergoes the same change as in the normal (compare 204); but when at the same time the visual axis increases in length, as is very usual in near-sighted eyes, this change is wholly or partially compensated, and the myopia may even continue progressive at an advanced time of life.—All this is the result of direct experience, which, however, with respect to the same persons, extends only over some few years. In order, therefore, to get a satisfactory idea of the course of the myopia through the whole of life, the recorded experience of many patients must be made use of. I have attached especial importance to this when, by the production of such spectacles as were formerly found sufficient for distant vision, their report was confirmed. The test has in such cases not failed.

When in this manner the ordinary course of the farthest point, that is the degree of the myopia through all periods of life, had been ascertained, it was not difficult to infer the course of the nearest point, as has been done in Figs. 125, 126, and 127. For this it was only necessary to know the range of accommodation proper to each time of life. With respect to this, I have arrived at the conclusion, that in myopes it is about equal to that of normal eyes. In very high degrees only it is less; and here the whole eye, particularly the anterior part, the m. ciliaris included, is extended, which may be noted as a sufficient cause thereof.

These observations are illustrated in the sketches of Figs. 126, 127, and 128, the meaning of which, after what has been said respecting Fig. 104, needs no further explanation. They represent three categories of myopia, in its course of development, as it mostly occurs. Fig. 126 is a *stationary*, Fig. 127 a *temporarily progressive*, Fig. 128 a *permanently progressive* myopia. The course of the myopia is shown by the line *r r'*, which represents the farthest point, with parallel visual lines. The range of accommodation, proper to each time of life, is expressed by the distance between *r r'* and *p p'*. I must allow myself to make some observations respecting each of these categories.

Fig. 126 is called *stationary myopia*. Yet we see the myopia

Fig. 126.

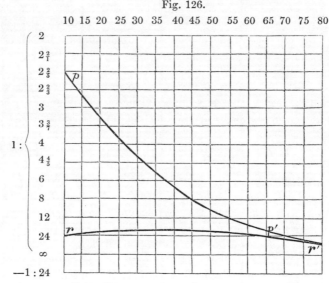

ascend from $\frac{1}{24}$ to $\frac{1}{16}$. As I have above remarked, such ascent is, in the years of development, to be considered as the rule. Consequently if the ascent be not more remarkable, the myopia may, in contrast to the progressive, be called stationary. In general the slight degrees belong to this form.   For this reason, a myopia of only $\frac{1}{24}$ was chosen for Fig. 126.   However, on the one hand, an originally high degree of myopia may continue stationary, and, on the other, the slightest degree may become permanently progressive, and thus, finally, attain a very considerable height.   This last we observe especially, when in the parents or other members of the family, a high degree of myopia occurs, while, moreover, the mode of life, especially stooping and strong convergence of the visual lines, promote its further development.   In the most favourable course of the myopia (Fig. 126), it remains quite stationary during the period of manhood, and may, on the approach of old age, even diminish a little, as the figure shows.   This, however, seems to occur but very rarely.   The generally received opinion, that with the increase of years the degree of myopia usually diminishes, is an error, based partly upon the incorrect idea, that the degree of the myopia is determined by the nearest point, partly on the incontestable fact, that vision at a great distance gradually becomes more distinct, which is, however, to be attributed rather to the increasing constriction of the pupil.

The *temporarily progressive* myopia is represented in Fig. 127.

Fig. 127.

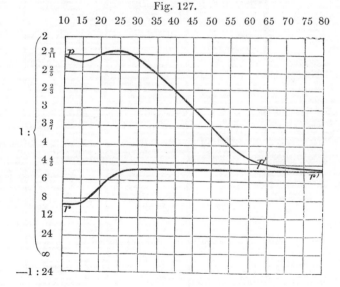

In this case the progression lies mostly between the 12th and 25th years. It is fortunate when the myopia becomes stationary at least before the 30th year. In Fig 127 it ascends from the 13th to the 35th year from $\frac{1}{8}$ to $\frac{1}{5}$; from the 18th to the 22nd year the ascent is the most rapid. After that it here becomes stationary. But, in fact, it is only exceptionally that, after having once attained this degree, it becomes perfectly stationary. High degrees of near-sightedness appear never to be congenital, unless we would refer congenital buphthalmos to that head. I cannot even decide whether, when the nearsightedness is hereditary, it is also in a certain degree congenital. I scarcely believe it is. I have too often seen here-ditary myopia which, in the 12th or 15th year was present in a very slight degree, for example $\frac{1}{16}$, subsequently become rapidly developed to a high degree of $\frac{1}{5}$ or $\frac{1}{4}$, to think it impossible, that in the first years of life it was not almost wholly absent. On the other hand, I have extremely rarely seen near-sightedness arise after the 15th and never after the 20th year in eyes, which were previously normal. It is true it is often supposed by the patients that such is the case, but this is only because the primitive slight degree of myopia was overlooked. In this primitive degree, trifling as it was, lay the germ of the affection; the complaints of various kinds are not made until the myopia becomes progressive. The myopia is most progressive when even in the 15th year it was rather considerable, for example $= \frac{1}{8}$, as is assumed in Fig. 127. The course represented in Fig. 127, is therefore still to be considered comparatively favour-able. It now seldom becomes in manhood completely stationary; still more rarely does it diminish in advanced old age. Often it continues to increase, at least in some degree, and thus approaches to the

Permanently progressive myopia, represented in Fig. 128. In the majority of cases belonging to this category, the myopia is con-siderable even at the age of 15 years. Therefore it is here assumed $= \frac{1}{6}$. It ascends most rapidly to the 25th, indeed even to the 35th year, more slowly at a more advanced period, incessantly, as it appears, but still often in jumps. The line $r\ r'$ gives a view of this.

It may ascend to ½ and more. The worst is then to be feared. It

Fig. 128.

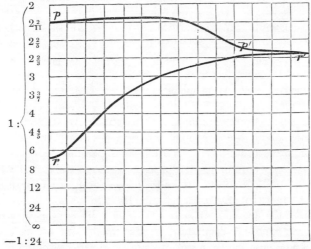

is rare at 60 years of age to find a tolerably useful eye, with myopia of 1 : 2½ or even of 1 : 3. Diminution of such degrees of myopia at an advanced time of life, is not to be thought of: the influence of the increasing distention of the eye in the direction of the visual axis, is never overcome, and is even not compensated by the diminishing refraction of the lens.

From the progression of the M it follows, that the higher degrees occur proportionately most frequently at a more advanced time of life. How far very young children are affected by it, has not been accurately investigated. A commencement in this direction was made by Ed. v. Jaeger, who has also stated his intention of following the course of the refraction in the same persons through their whole life. We wish him for that purpose a long life and faithful patients. He should, however, not have neglected the value of the method, followed by me, of throwing some light on this subject.

If the above-mentioned causes are capable of giving rise to M and of further developing it, the predisposition thereto is very different. I have already stated that I have never seen an hypermetropically constructed eye become near-sighted. Even on many emmetropic eyes, simple tension of accommodation for near objects has but little

effect.   In fact the predisposition is almost invariably congenital,
and in that case it is, moreover, nearly always hereditary.   Beer,
Jüngken, Böhm, von Hasner, and many others, have referred to its
hereditary nature; I believe, even, that from time immemorial the
conviction thereof has been general among the people.   At least, at
present the patients are accustomed at once to state, that their father or
mother was near-sighted, and that the same condition was found
among brothers and sisters.   I cannot, with any accuracy, give the proportion in which hereditary cases occur; but this I may say, that where
I found near-sightedness in one or more of the children, and had an
opportunity of examining both parents, I only exceptionally saw M
wholly wanting in both, while, on the other hand, when one and equally
when both parents were myopic, the predisposition almost always
passed on, at least to some of the children, perhaps more specially
to the younger (v. Artha).   Experience shows further, that where
only a trace of M is present in youth, it inevitably becomes further
developed, and that the greatest care leads to nothing more than
limitation of the degree.   In statements of its diminution in youth,
I have never met with accurate determinations of the degree of M,
and we know how lightly assertions are in general made as to the
increase and diminution of M.   A consideration of all these facts
leads us to the conclusion, that fundamentally emmetropic eyes seldom,
fundamentally hypermetropic eyes perhaps never, become myopic;
but that, having once occurred, the M is often transmitted as predisposition to posterity, and under fresh exciting causes is developed
to its higher degrees.   Thus the hereditary principle accumulates in
the posterity the effect of the causes repeated in every generation.
In some families the M therefore has attained a high degree, and the
danger is the greater, because, according to experience, the hereditary
tendency manifests itself the more certainly, the more the myopia has
already been transmitted through a number of generations, and has
assumed a typical character.

A double distinction has been made in M, in which I cannot agree.   Two
classes have been formed with respect to the degree and to the congenital or
non-congenital nature of the affection.   As to the degree, since observers
had based their idea of M upon the fact, that in it acute vision could exist
only close to the eye, they were puzzled by those cases in which there was
distinct vision at a distance of 2, 3, and 4 feet, and nevertheless at the distance of from 15 to 20 feet letters of the magnitude of an inch could no
longer be easily distinguished.   They did not perceive that in such cases

they had to do with slight degrees of myopia, with degrees of $\frac{1}{24}$, $\frac{1}{36}$, $\frac{1}{48}$, in which the farthest point lay at about 24, 36, or 48 inches from the eye. At the distance of 15 feet the circles of diffusion are then already pretty considerable, at least when the pupil is tolerably wide.

The confusion produced by an incorrect comprehension of these cases is incredibly great. Dr. Kerst met among the young men who presented themselves as pupils at the school of military surgery at Utrecht, some who easily read ordinary print at the distance of from 15 to 20 inches, and nevertheless at the distance of from 12 to 20 feet could not distinguish letters of the size of 3 or 4 inches. He wrote on the subject to Cunier, and concluded by asking, whether this condition was not a sort of myopia, although no mention was made of it in the various works on diseases of the eye, under the head of myopia. Cunier communicated this letter to Sichel (*Leçons cliniques sur les lunettes*, etc. Bruxelles, 1848, p. 99), and the latter most properly answered Dr. Kerst's question in the *affirmative*. However, as it appears from the lengthy reasoning of the writer, it was not clear to Sichel that in such instances we have to do simply with a degree of myopia, in which the farthest point of distinct vision lies at from 15 to 20 inches.

Some years later Fronmüller treats, in reference to this point, of "a variety of short-sightedness," and gives to it the name of "*myopia at a distance.*" Sichel and Kerst, he says, first drew attention to it. However, Fronmüller describes (*Beobachtungen auf dem Gebiete der Augenheilkunde*, Fürth, 1850, p. 54), as an example of his myopia at a distance, a case of hypermetropia—as appears from the circumstance, that with a convex glass distant vision was distinct and easy, while concave glasses made vision at any distance more indistinct. Fronmüller has, therefore, confounded a moderate degree of hypermetropia, with which ordinary print could still be read at a distance of 10″ (as is not unusual), with the cases of slight myopia, to which Kerst had directed attention, and has given it the name of *myopia at a distance*. Nevertheless, even Kerst himself subsequently applied the name of "myopia at a distance" to slight degrees of myopia.

Finally, von Graefe (*Archiv f. Ophthalmologie*, B. ii. Abth. 1, p. 158), not knowing at the time, as he acknowledges, where and by whom the name of M at a distance was introduced into science, makes a rational use of it to characterise those cases in which, *with reference to the degree of myopia, the distinguishing of remote objects is very defective*. He investigated and analysed a case of the kind with great accuracy, whence it appears that this condition may depend on an involuntary action of the muscles of accommodation, which is spasmodically combined with every effort to see farther than the naturally farthest point.

Such cases, however, are certainly of extremely rare occurrence. Among more than a thousand myopes I have not met with a single instance of the kind. The too great indistinctness of remote objects, with reference to the degree of myopia, was always to be explained by a more than ordinary size of the pupil. This does not prevent vision being perfectly acute at the distance for which the eye is accommodated; but on account of the magnitude of the circles of diffusion increasing with the diameter of the pupil, it makes the observation beyond the boundaries of accommodation very imperfect. In this, too, as we have seen, lies one of the causes, why many think, that with the advance of years their myopia has diminished, even when this is not the case: their pupil has become smaller, and they consequently see better at a distance. If we cause the so-called myopes at a distance to look through an opening with a diameter of 5 mm., the disproportion has disappeared. Let us beware, therefore, of explaining every disproportion between the degree of myopia and the observation at a distance, by spasm of the muscles of accommodation. The size of the pupil will almost always account for it. Therefore, too, in my opinion, the term myopia at a distance, which has already given rise to so much confusion, may very well be dispensed with in science. Neither the slight degrees of myopia, which are as well defined by $\frac{1}{R}$ as the high, nor hypermetropia, which is the opposite of myopia, deserve this name, and the rare form of disease, distinguished by von Graefe, might be denoted as spasm of the muscles of accommodation, produced by an effort at relaxation.

With respect, in the second place, to the origin of M, I have above stated the result of my experience. It amounts to this, that M is almost always hereditary, and is then further, at least as predisposition, congenital; but that it is also, exceptionally, without special predisposition developed in the emmetropic eye as the result of excessive tension of accommodation. This influence of extraordinary accommodation necessarily suggested the idea of change of form of the lens. Eighteen years ago (*Nederl. Lancet,* 1845) my argument was as follows: " M is the result of accommodation for near objects; examine what M *permanently* is, and you will know the change which the accommodation each time excites." By the discovery of the cause of M in a longer visual axis, and of the principle of accommodation in the greater convexity of the lens, my expectation was disappointed. But I never lost sight of the possibility, that in myopia, especially in the acquired variety, the lens should be really more convex. It would certainly not be strange that, especially during the periods of development, the influence of much accommodation for near objects should permanently affect the form of the lens, and that, *vice versâ*, want of this accommodation might lead to unusual flatness of the lens (compare p. 246). I have, however, in no way been able to satisfy myself of this.—Moreover, in the fact that M, almost without exception, is either connected with a peculiar posterior atrophy, or at least before the fortieth year becomes connected therewith, lies the proof, that at all events nearly without exception, another cause is in operation: this posterior atrophy is, namely, connected with a distention of the posterior part of the eyeball, which distention it either accompanies or rapidly follows. And in the rare cases in which this posterior atrophy is wanting, I have mostly found, by direct measurement with the ophthalmometer, a *morbidly* distended cornea, or I established the existence of morbid distention of the anterior part of the sclerotic, with prolonged visual axis, so that finally, no cases remained in which I was obliged to take refuge in extraordinary convexity of the crystalline lens. (See further the Section upon the anatomical changes in M.)

Moreover, in adults, and even in young people, provided they are absolutely free from M, simple tension of accommodation is not sufficient to excite M. Even wearing concave glasses does not give rise to it. Only in the artificial H produced by concave glasses, as well as in the natural, a part of this H finally becomes latent, that is, the eye accustoms itself in distant vision also to tension of the muscle of accommodation; but that no organic change of form of the lens is in operation appears from the fact that atropia, by paralysing the ciliary muscle, immediately suppresses the apparent M. The displacement of the relative range of accommodation in the use of glasses, which modify the connexion between convergence and accommodation, temporarily gives rise to some difficulty. This is true also even of positive glasses. Thus, after working with a magnifying glass, in which, perhaps, without wholly parallel lines, I am accustomed to relax my power of accommodation as much as possible, it is at first difficult for me again satisfactorily to accommodate at a convergence, for which I otherwise find no difficulty, without, however, the absolute points p and r being at all altered. The same is soon perceived, when, holding a weak prism with the angle inwards before the eye, we wish to see singly at a distance, and thus, with convergence, to accommodate for a distant object. The opposite is produced by concave glasses or by a prism with the angle turned outwards. Now, it is easily understood that at least prisms, which do not at all modify the accommodation, will exercise no permanent influence on the crystalline lens, and the effect of convex and concave glasses, within certain limits, completely agrees with that of prisms.

All the foregoing is most strongly opposed to the importance of the crystalline lens in the production of M. But although there was no argument against the latter, so long as it did not appear, from direct investigation, that by tension for near objects the lens permanently acquires greater convexity, it seems an ignoring of the requirements of science to admit a form of M based upon mere supposition, and to oppose this (writers have even given it the special name of *plesiopia*) as acquired M, to the almost invariably congenital myopic structure of the eye. Ed. von Jaeger (*l. c.* p. 28) says: "that in such individuals as are constantly occupied with tension of accommodation, fewer eyes do not in general occur with normal length of axis, than under opposite conditions, and that in those classes of the population who are not usually accustomed to fatigue their eyes by efforts of accommodation, at least as many, *nay, even more individuals* occur, who, in consequence of prolongation of the axis of the bulb (Staphyloma posticum), are short-sighted, than in the upper ranks of society." So far as the Netherlands are concerned, I can expressly contradict this assertion, and with all respect for the zeal of observation of von Jaeger, I cannot admit its truth even for Austria.

---

§ 27. Results of the Ophthalmoscopic Investigation of the Myopic Eye.

Since the ophthalmoscope has made the fundus oculi accessible to

23

examination during life, our idea of the anatomical basis of M has undergone a complete modification. Ophthalmoscopic investigation has shown that, almost without exception, even in moderate degrees of M, changes, especially in the chorioidea, are to be observed; and it has now further been found, that these changes are the expression of atrophy of the chorioidea, which, combined with atrophy of the sclerotic, is, as well as the latter, dependent on a distention of the posterior part of the eyeball. *Myopia* and *Staphyloma posticum* have thus become nearly synonymous.

Thousands of myopic eyes have been examined by me; of not less than 700 do I possess more or less detailed drawings or sketches, of some eyes more than one, with an interval of some years; and in every case sex, age, degree of M, and in many instances accommodation, movements of the eye, acuteness of vision, hereditariness and accessory disturbances have been noted. From these observations, which, communicated *in extenso*, would form a volume, the following description, and also the conclusions drawn, are in great part borrowed: much of the same is, however, already to be found in the writings of my predecessors. The principal changes are: *atrophy of the chorioidea, on the outside of the entrance of the optic nerve*, when highly developed, combined with *change of form of the nerve-surface, a straightened course of the vessels of the retina, incomplete diffuse atrophy of the chorioidea in other places*, and *morbid changes in the region of the yellow spot*. I commence with a description of the changes in general, and shall afterwards sketch their development, in connexion with the degree of M and of the time of life.

1°. *Atrophy of the chorioidea, principally to the outside of the entrance of the optic nerve*. The surface of the optic nerve of the normal emmetropic eye exhibits itself as a nearly round, rather strongly reflecting, slightly reddish plane, from which the retinal vessels set out; often an impression is to be seen on it. This plane is distinctly bounded by the commencement of the pigment of the chorioidea, to the inside of which we sometimes observe a thin, white, strongly reflecting line (the so-called sclerotic-boundary of Liebreich), to which the faintly-defined nerve-substance then succeeds. To this part of the fundus oculi we usually first direct the eye. At the first glance we recognise in it with tolerably great certainty the M (compare Fig. 129), distinguished by a crescentic, strongly reflecting surface (*c*) between the outside of the nerve (*n*) and the boundary of the pigment of the chorioidea. That surface is always poor in pigment.   Still it may, if it be slender, when there is

FIG. 129.

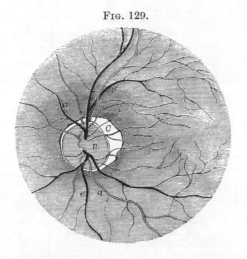

normal or even diminished fulness of the vessels, be proportionately red, but the colour is then also brighter than that of the rest of the fundus and approaches sometimes to orange; almost always, however, it soon acquires a whiter shade, on which at first the larger chorioideal vessels, extended in a horizontal or radiating direction, are visible, often even more distinctly than on the adjoining parts of the chorioidea abounding in pigment.   Between the straightened vessels the remaining pigment of the stroma is recognisable as oblong brownish-grey little spots.   The chorio-capillaris in this place now seems no longer to carry blood.   At length all blood-carrying vessels may disappear in the atrophied place, which now appears still grey or marbled and, finally, perfectly white, reflecting still more strongly than the nerve-surface itself, although the latter has also increased in whiteness.   However, even now some darker pigment-spots (pigment-epithelium) occasionally still remain in the atrophied place, especially near the margin, similar to those in the neighbouring red tissue.

The atrophied surface passes sometimes without defined boundaries into diffuse atrophy, and through this into normal tissue; in general it is, however, limited by a sharp, tolerably regularly curved boundary line (circumscribed atrophy).   This line is distinguished, at least here and there, by an abundance of dark pigment, as usually occurs on the boundaries of morbid changes of the chorioidea, as well as on

2

its normal limits.   Not unfrequently there is, at a certain distance, a second dark line, parallel to the boundary line, together with increased vascularity of the adjoining chorioideal tissue, or on the atrophied part traces of an innermost concentric line of pigment are to be seen.

The *form** of the circumscribed atrophy is almost always that of a crescent whose concave side encompasses the outside of the nerve-surface (crescentic atrophy).   In slight degrees scarcely to be recognised, sometimes only locally through a projecting dark point (Fig. 130), it extends usually the farther around the nerve-substance, the broader it is, that is, the longer the axis (*a a'* Fig. 132) of the crescent is (compare Figs. 130 to 132).   On further development the

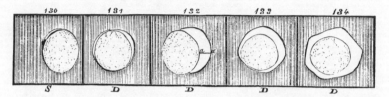

* I append some sketches merely for the determination of the forms of the atrophic place.   The above figures are taken from particular eyes.

No.	Sex.	Age.	Eye.	Degree of M.
130	F.	12	Left	1 : 7
131	F.	32	Right	1 : 12
132	M.	42	R.	1 : 6
133	M.	51	R.	1 : 9·6
134	M.	24	R.	1 : 4·75
135 *a*	F.	37	R.	1 : 2·5
b	F.	16	L.	1 : 3·8
c	M.	25	R.	1 : 2·7
136 *a*	M.	32	R.	1 : 2·14
b	M.	57	R.	1 : 4
137	M.	20	R.	1 : 3·5
138	M.	66	R.	1 : 3·1
139	F.	46	R.	1 : 2·3
140	F.	66	L.	1 : 3
141	M.	13	R.	1 : 5·6
142	M.	54	R.	1 : 7
143	F.	22	L.	1 : 3

Excellent representations of the fundus oculi of the myopic eye are given by many, among others by Dr. Ed. Jaeger (*Beiträge zur Pathologie des Auges*, Wien, 1855, Pl. 17 and 18; and *Ueber die Einstellungen des dioptr. Appar.*, Wien, 1861, Tab. 11); and by Liebreich (*Atlas d'ophthalmoscopie*, Paris, 1863, Tab. 111).

atrophy assumes very different forms. If the axis is longer, without proportionate extension around the papilla, the crescentic form passes into the semi-elliptical, of which various modifications occur (Fig. 135 *a*, *b*, *c*) ; if, on the contrary, the atrophy extends more around the nerve-surface, without proportionate prolongation of the axis, the semi-annular form arises (Fig. 133), and further, the annular (Fig. 134), which, when more extended, deserves the name of elliptical (Fig. 136 *a*) or circular (Fig. 136 *b*). In all these forms the ring is almost constantly broader on the outside than on the inside, where it is often

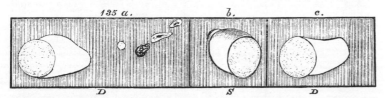

still slenderer than above and beneath. Finally, the atrophy may

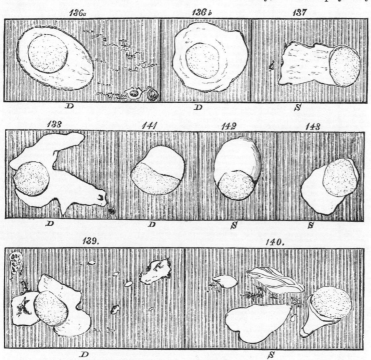

be very irregularly bounded, for example, it may have an angularly curved form (Fig. 137), may present ramifications (Fig. 138), sometimes in the form of a leaf of clover (Fig. 139), and may even have completely separated atrophic spots around it (Fig. 140). Thus the atrophy attains a considerable extent of three or even six mm. and more in different directions, in which cases still other parts of the chorioidea are in various modes morbidly affected.

In the emmetropic eye the yellow spot lies to the outside of the nerve (from the middle of its surface to a distance of about 4 mm.), almost always, however, somewhat lower. The axis of the atrophic crescent has a similar, but usually somewhat yet more descending direction, and is therefore turned towards the yellow spot. (The figures 129–140 are all drawn with the image inverted). Extremely rarely, however, even with the greatest development of the atrophy, does it reach directly to the yellow spot, which removes more and more from the nerve-surface; but it is very usual, as we shall see, in high degrees of atrophy, to find the yellow spot independently affected. Deviations from the direction described are, however, on the whole, not uncommon; the axis may descend much more directly (Fig. 141) and even be directed completely downwards (Fig. 142), or it may be horizontal, and may even ascend considerably (Fig. 143), but it is never directed straight upwards.

In rare cases the *atrophic part* is particularly strongly *excavated*, as may appear on its outer margin from a certain curvature of the retinal vessels; in general, however, the curvature is continued tolerably uniformly in the non-atrophied part.

2°. *The nerve-surface has, in high degrees of M, undergone a partly apparent, partly true change in form.*—As to the apparent, the horizontal dimension often appears comparatively smaller. The reason of this is evident: in the emmetropic eye the nerve-surface lies only a little to the inside of the axis of the cornea, and we therefore look through the pupil nearly directly on it; on the contrary, in the highly-distended myopic eye (compare Fig. 55), in which the nerve-surface is displaced more to the inside, the perpendicular to this surface is directed more strongly outwards, and this causing us to look obliquely on the nerve through the pupil, it appears shortened in the horizontal direction (Artl). But besides this apparent, there occurs a true change in form, which everyone had indeed seen, but to which, if I am not mistaken, Liebreich* was the first to direct

---

* *Archiv f. Ophthalmologie*, vii. 2, 124. *Atlas d'ophthalmoscopie*, Paris, 1863, p. 6.

attention : *the nerve-surface usually has, in extensive atrophy, the greatest diameter in a direction perpendicular to the axis of the atrophy*. Von Jaeger endeavours to attribute this also in great part to appearance ; but the fact is true (compare the above figures). To these, other changes supervene. In young myopes the nerve-surface is particularly red (capillary hyperæmia), otherwise it is not altered ; subsequently, in high degrees, on the contrary, it is almost always, wholly or partially, strongly reflecting, not unfrequently it is locally excavated, with a more distinct appearance of the (more superficially situated) lamina cribrosa ; also, perhaps, somewhat excavated over the whole surface, apparently atrophic and sometimes passing, without distinct boundaries, into the strongly reflecting atrophy. I have seen cases in which a retinal vessel appeared to come from an atrophied place, which we were therefore again inclined to refer rather to the nerve-surface.—Of the true dimensions of the nerve-surface it is difficult to judge, because the myopic structure has a very complicated influence on the magnitude of the inverted image. In the note to this section some further remarks will be found upon this subject.

3°. The *retinal vessels*, which are depicted with incomparable clearness on the atrophic surface, are distinguished in high degrees of M by their straight and little tortuous course; this is particularly true of the most atrophied places. This straightened course is evidently the result of the extension, which the retina also has undergone. In the calibre of the vessels there is seldom any great change.

4°. Much farther than the strongly reflecting and completely atrophied part we find, in high degrees of M, proofs of *extension and attenuation of the chorioidea*, both in the stronger reflexion and in the straighter course, with greater mutual distance of its vessels. Not unfrequently, too, the stroma-pigment, which occupies the intervascular spaces, is in these parts evidently diminished, and the epithelium of pigment-cells is unequally distributed. In the intervals the surface is now sometimes dotted with yellow or white, and reflects strongly. We often find this diffuse atrophy at the inside of the nerve-surface, but especially at the outside, and continuous with the complete atrophy, which is now less sharply defined. The region of the yellow spot has now also often passed into atrophy.

5°. *Circumscribed changes of the yellow spot and of the fovea centralis*.—These interfere with direct vision, and deserve all our attention. In high degrees of M we should therefore never neglect, after the investigation of the nerve and the parts around it, also to

examine the yellow spot, which we have in sight, when the observed
eye fixes the flame reflected by the mirror. The changes are connected with a continuation of the atrophy from the outside of the
optic nerve, or they exist independently and separately. They appear
as scattered irregular granular pigment, lying or not on one or more
oval or angular bright-red spots, surrounded by diffuse pigment,
or as some larger dark groups of pigment on a white ground or
alternating with white spots, or finally as one single, sharply-defined,
sometimes bluish and elevated spot, which may attain even the magnitude of the nerve-surface: this last form is probably connected
with extravasation of blood, which I have sometimes seen limited to
a part of the yellow spot.

6°. The further changes in the fundus oculi, which, without belonging to the essence of myopia, are apt to supervene in the highest
degrees of M, are *chorioiditis disseminata*, distinguished by white
and yellow spots of various sizes, with irregular deposition of pigment, scattered here and there; moreover, spots of extravasated
blood in the retina, whether one or more larger, or numerous smaller
ones, which, finally, pass over into pigment-spots,—and detachment of
the retina by blood, and much more frequently by exudation. A
movable, grey, slender, but tolerably long flake also sometimes extends
from the nerve-surface to which it is adherent, into the vitreous humour.
Lastly, we sometimes see, in the highly myopic eye, a particular
form of glaucoma arise with the changes peculiar to the same.

7°. In the more fluid *vitreous humour, movable flakes* are,
in the high degrees of M, among the most ordinary phenomena.
They are in part connected with the changes described under 6°.

8°. In high degrees of M we see more than ordinarily a commencement of obscuration of the lens. Where there is detachment
of the retina, whether with or without secondary iritis, obscuration
is often rapidly developed even in youth.

Of the changes just described the atrophic crescent on the outside of the nerve-surface is the most common and the most characteristic. This is, the time of life being equal, in general more fully
developed the higher the degree of M is, and for equal degrees of
M it is more developed the more advanced the age of the individual
is. The subjoined table exhibits the length of the axis (Fig. 132
a, b) of the atrophied part, in relation to the age and the degree of
M, deduced from observations on 1400 eyes.

LENGTH OF THE AXIS* OF THE ATROPHIC CRESCENT IN MILLIMETRES WITH

Age in years.	$M = \frac{1}{\infty}$ to $\frac{1}{12}$	$M = \frac{1}{12}$ to $\frac{1}{6}$	$M = \frac{1}{6}$ to $\frac{1}{4}$	$M = \frac{1}{4}$ to $\frac{1}{3}$	$M = \frac{1}{3}$ to $\frac{1}{2}$
10 to 30	0·1987 mm.	0·4255	0·5563	0·7431	1·25
30 to 50	0·2975	0·7035	0·9679	1·356	1·68
50 to 80	0·7059	1·046	1·183	1·795	2·127

The table exhibits most clearly the influence on the extent of the atrophy, both of age and of the degree of the myopia. Even when for less difference in degree and less difference in age the average of a certain number of cases is taken, the same regularity is still apparent. Nevertheless the individual observations differ very much, so that as minimum, in tolerably high degrees, only traces of atrophy occurred, and the maximum may amount to 6 mm. and more. The increase of the atrophy with age appears to be placed beyond all doubt. Taking into account that the degree of the myopia also, at least in most cases, increases, we may even infer that the atrophy increases with age still more rapidly than the numbers belonging to the same column indicate. Probably we approach the truth by reading off in the diagonal direction, and thus assuming that, when the axis of the atrophy at twenty years amounts to 0·1987 mm., this at 40 years increases to 0·7035, and at 65 to 1·183.

After the simple announcement of the facts, I shall now endeavour to give a sketch of the development of the atrophy and of its concomitant phenomena, as the ophthalmoscope reveals them in the myopic eye.

In a very young individual atrophy is, in moderate degrees of M, very rarely to be observed. Hasner† declares, however, that he has seen it remarkably developed at four or five years of age, and Ed. v. Jaeger has, from the examination of children in schools, even come

* The axis of the atrophic part was determined by measuring the sketches made of 700 cases of myopia. For actual magnitude the nerve-surface was used as a scale, whose diameter was assumed = 1·9 mm. In the annular and in the circular atrophy, the extent on both sides of the nerve-surface was assumed as axis. Imperfect and undefined atrophy are not included.

† *Klinische Vorträge über Augenheilkunde.* Prag, 1860.

to the conclusion, that a particular form of atrophy, which sometimes led him to recognise one child as brother or sister of the other,
differing in each of the two eyes, may be hereditary.   Even in
nurslings and new-born infants of myopic mothers, he saw the
tendency to atrophy of the same form.   I too have seen, without
particularly looking for them, some cases of distinctly developed
atrophy at the ages of five and seven years, though in simple M the
intervention of the oculist is seldom invoked at so early an
age.   The rule is, however, that even in those, in whom we
may subsequently expect a high degree of M, during childhood only
slight traces of atrophy are at most to be seen.   There first appears
either an irregular, small projection, rich in pigment (compare Fig.
129), to the outside of the optic nerve, or a little crescent, distinguished from the adjoining fundus by a brighter red colour, its
boundary being somewhat darker at the outside than the contiguous
fundus.   In the first case the atrophy extends directly from the
margin of the nerve-surface, while the pigment, in a certain sense,
removes outwards, and a white strongly reflecting line, which soon
assumes the crescentic form, appears along the nerve-surface.   In
the second case the atrophy is, in a certain sense, directly terminated,
evidently from diminution of pigment, and its further development
consists at first rather in the becoming more perfect, than in the
extension of the atrophy. Often, however, we now see a second convex line of pigment arise at the outside of the original crescent.
While in adolescence myopia is gradually more and more developed,
there not unfrequently set in troublesome symptoms of irritation,
and on ophthalmoscopic examination we now often find the most
external boundary of the atrophy, as well as the nerve-surface itself,
in a congestive condition.   If the myopia seems likely to attain only
a slight degree, there occur in adolescence but the first traces of
atrophy, and where this is the case, a great development of the same
is to be apprehended only from an improper use of the eyes.   But
where myopia of $\frac{1}{6}$ or $\frac{1}{5}$ exists from the sixteenth to the twentieth
year, we find, almost without exception, a very decided, almost perfect
atrophy accurately defined under the form of a crescent, whence it
sometimes appears that precisely this part is more highly concave than
the rest of the fundus.   The pigment-epithelium has disappeared upon
this surface, the chorio-capillaris seems to be no longer present, the
greater chorioideal vessels are slender, extended, sometimes they have

almost wholly disappeared, while only brownish-grey spots still indicate the intervascular space.—From a combination of numerous
observations we may very well deduce the development of the
atrophy; but I have in addition, had the opportunity of examining
repeatedly in consecutive years many eyes, and this has shown me
that the atrophy sometimes advances more rapidly at intervals, but
that it very rarely continues long, for example, for one or two years,
unaltered. Especially in youth, when the adjoining tissue of the
chorioidea is particularly rich in blood, and long-continued tension
of the eyes is attended with inconvenience, the development proceeds
regularly. Apparently, the boundary of the pigment is thus displaced
outwards. In so far as the membranes at the outside of the nerve-
surface are extended, this is also really the case. But in addition we
must, in explanation of the process, assume that in the place where,
at the inner boundary of the hyperæmia, in consequence of extension
the atrophy begins, the pigment is absorbed, and at the same time
is more strongly formed on the hyperæmic line extending outwards.
In general the stronger formation of pigment is due to hyperæmia
of the chorioidea.* Now, if on the one hand, probably through a
more rapid course of the atrophy, the absorption of the pigment is
imperfect, and if black spots therefore remain in the atrophic part,
the hyperæmia on the other, extends in some points more outwards,
and here gives rise to increase of pigment. Thus it would appear
too, that the spots of pigment existing at both sides of the boundary
of the atrophy may be explained. A real displacement of the pigment over the surface of the chorioidea, as it occurs in exudative
chorioiditis, seems here not to be admissible.—The direction, in
which the atrophy at first extends, is at once conclusive as to the
form to be expected. This is indeed included in what has already
been said. Here we may remark only, that in slight degrees the
form is never annular, and that the annular and circular forms are
to be expected when the crescent rapidly extends far around the
nerve-surface, most of all, when also at the opposite inside of the
nerve-surface a second smaller crescent is early formed.

The atrophied part is for a long time regular in form, and beyond it
scarcely any change is to be seen in the fundus oculi: at most it may
be observed, when a strong pigment-epithelium does not prevent it,
that the chorioideal vessels are more separated, and arc in part more

* Compare Coccius. *Ueber Glaucom, Entzündung und Autoskopie mit
dem Augenspiegel*, 1859, p. 36.

slender than usual. But after the five-and-thirtieth, and particularly after the fortieth year, in high degrees of M, the changes above described begin here and there to occur (compare Figs. 132, 135, and 139). Now also the boundary line of the atrophy sometimes describes a more irregular form, or atrophic spots have formed next the original ones, which by the extension of both may subsequently coalesce. The most important change beyond the seat of the original atrophy is the degeneration in the region of the yellow spot, especially when it occupies the fovea centralis. It is true this may occur at any age even in non-myopic eyes, and on localised disturbance of the function in the same place, with or without perceptible organic change, a number of cases of ordinary amblyopia depend. But a particular morbid change, based upon extension and atrophy of the sclerotic and chorioidea, whereby the retina here also becomes secondarily disturbed in its function, is decidedly peculiar to high degrees of myopia. As we know that the yellow spot often corresponds to the apex of the staphyloma posticum, and that in high degrees the atrophy of the sclerotic and chorioidea is here the strongest, this can by no means surprise us. In the first place, there often arises, in $M = \frac{1}{4}$ or more, in advanced life, imperfect diffuse atrophy of the chorioidea, in a belt passing from the outside of the atrophy through the yellow spot, and recognisable by a disproportionately white or yellow-dotted grey, sometimes strongly reflecting almost glittering appearance, with interspersed pigment; and where this occurs, the region of the yellow spot never altogether escapes; but in addition, at a comparatively less advanced age, the above-described local degeneration of the yellow spot not unfrequently supervenes on the original atrophic crescent, while the part situated between this and the yellow spot still deviates but little from the normal. On one occasion I observed this in a patient aged fifteen; under thirty years of age it is, however, even in the highest degrees of M, still rare; after the thirtieth year it recurs with comparative frequency in myopia of $\frac{1}{3}$ or more, and at sixty the yellow spot, and even the fovea centralis, have in M of $\frac{1}{3}$, often, and in myopia of $2\frac{1}{2}$ and $\frac{1}{2}$, they have, I might almost say, always suffered. This occurs both when the original atrophy is annular or circular, and when it extends only to one side, sometimes even when the axis of the atrophy is still short, and is not directed to the yellow spot.

The above-described changes of the nerve-surface are distinctly seen only in comparatively high degrees of myopia, for example, higher than $\frac{1}{5}$, and in these degrees the straightened direction of the retinal vessels, especially at the side of the atrophy, is not to be mistaken. Particularly remarkable in this respect are those cases where, in the same person only the one eye is strongly myopic, or at least is much more strongly myopic than the other. On the whole the connexion between the degree of the myopia and of the different changes in the fundus oculi, independently of the time of life, is in these cases most strikingly brought to light.

Other deviations, to which highly myopic eyes are liable, as effusion of blood, detachment of the retina, glaucomatous degeneration of the nerve-surface and opacity of the lens, are not constant and not sufficiently peculiar to M, to justify their description here as the simple results of a further development of M. More correctly might chorioiditis disseminata, to be treated of in the following section, be referred to M.

Movable flocculi in the vitreous humour are, on the contrary, as I have remarked, but seldom absent in high degrees of M.

We have still, in conclusion, two important questions to treat of: first, how far the atrophy, above described, is constant in myopia; secondly, whether it occurs only in M, and is, therefore, characteristic of the latter?

Von Graefe established that in ten cases of high degrees of M, the atrophy alluded to (by him attributed to sclerotico-chorioiditis) occurs at least nine times. Ed. von Jaeger had perhaps earlier arrived at a similar result, and all other observers agree therein. According to my experience we may go still further.

As I have already remarked, slight degrees of myopia may exist in young persons without atrophy, but whether the myopia have remained stationary, or have been further developed, in the fortieth year traces of atrophy are usually no longer absent. Even after the thirtieth year I found with $M > \frac{1}{12}$ the atrophy only three times wholly absent, and still with $M > \frac{1}{20}$ it was present in every case but five. We are therefore justified in saying that *myopia depends on a condition in which the development of atrophy is included.* In the following section it will more fully appear that M may also exceptionally be produced by some other changes of form of the eyeball; but, singularly enough, in those cases in which morbidly developed greater convexity of the cornea contributed to the M, the atrophy peculiar to staphyloma posticum is found only extremely rarely entirely absent.

As to the second question, we cannot consider the atrophy described to be completely characteristic of M. We often see, at least in mature age, slight traces of atrophy at the outer margin of the nerve-surface, sometimes even an annular or circular atrophy, without M being present; twice I have observed it even with certain degrees of H. We cannot assume that in all of these cases M has existed at an earlier period, and has disappeared in consequence of senile changes in the eye (compare p. 205). In the second place, a peculiar form of atrophy not unfrequently occurs around the nerve-surface in glaucoma. This is annular, and attains only a moderate magnitude; evidently the chorioidea is here also atrophic, which atrophy appears to me to be connected with the excavation of the nerve-surface: probably in this case inflammation is also in operation.

NOTE TO SECTION 27.

The ophthalmoscopic investigation of strongly myopic individuals in the non-inverted image, for which the use of a highly negative eye-piece is necessary, requires a great deal of practice. Ed. von Jaeger thinks, however, that there is some advantage in this method, and in any case practice is desirable, because, as we have already seen, we may in the glass required find an indication of the degree of the myopia. But for ordinary cases, examination in the inverted image is quite sufficient. Without the use of an object-glass, the inverted image of the fundus oculi stands before the myopic eye, at the distance for which the latter is accommodated. With $M = \frac{1}{2}, \frac{1}{3}, \frac{1}{n}$, it will, therefore, stand about 2, 3, n inches before the eye, so that, in high degrees of M, removing somewhat more than usual, we can, without the intervention of any glasses whatever, looking directly through the opening of the mirror, see the image. But it is better to add a convex object-glass to the observed eye, whereby the field of vision becomes larger and, by movement of the glass in the vertical plane, extends alternately in different directions. In the choice of this object-glass we find ourselves, however, in a difficult dilemma: if we select one too strong, the image becomes quite too small; if we choose one too weak, we obtain too small a field of vision. The too small image we can partially counteract, by combining a pretty strong eye-piece with the ophthalmoscope, whereby the observer can, without any effort, see the little inverted image very .near, and magnified: in general, when the investigator is not myopic, such a convex glass is to be recommended. Therefore a pretty strong object-glass, with which the magnifying is less, but the field of vision is greater, is advantageous, and this is to be combined with a tolerably strong eye-piece.—Liebreich (*Archiv für Ophth.*, Bd. vii., 2, p. 130) has proposed a particular method of examining very highly myopic eyes. He uses no object-lens, but only a strong eye-piece, and with this approaches the eye so much that the iris lies nearly in the focus of this lens, so that the iris, in a certain sense, disappears and a very large field of vision is obtained. At the same time, the inverted image must come to lie between the eye observed and the lens, in order that it may be seen through the latter. This is to be attained in M $= \frac{1}{n}$ with a lens of nearly $\frac{1}{n+1}$. Then we have really the advantage of seeing a large field of vision under a strong magnifying power.

In ophthalmosopic investigation in the inverted image, we look as through a compound microscope, whereof the dioptric system of the observed eye, with the lens held before it, is the object-glass, while the lens held before the opening of the mirror is the eye-piece, through which the eye of the observer views the inverted image of the fundus oculi formed by the object-glass. The weaker the object-glass is, the shorter is the distance g'' from the fundus oculi B to the resulting nodal point k', and the greater the distance g'' from the image β to the resulting nodal point k''.—Now, as $\beta : B = g' : g''$, it appears that the magnifying $\frac{\beta}{B}$ of the inverted image is greater, the weaker the object-glass is. But in this it is further included, that the increased length of the visual axis in M, as determining especially the magnitude of g', is co-operating cause of the slight magnifying of the inverted image. If, indeed, a shorter radius of curvature of the surface of the cornea or of the lens, without any change in the length of the visual axis, were the cause of the M, g' would be less; and if now, while the inverted image was at the same distance from the eye, g'' continued unchanged, the magnifying $\frac{g''}{g'}$ would prove greater.

If there was any object of known and constantly equal magnitude in the fundus oculi, it would be a problem from the size and position of its inverted image to deduce the length of the visual axis in life.

---

§ 28. Anatomy of the Myopic Eye.

In the preceding paragraphs we have seen, that M depends almost exclusively upon the prolongation of the visual axis, connected with staphyloma posticum. We have therefore here little more to do than, in the first place, to describe the changes, which, under these circumstances, occur in the eye, and in the second place to trace their development. This will therefore form the subject-matter of this paragraph. But if we comprise all together, which may lead to

M in the dioptric sense of the word, that is, to a condition of the
eye in which the focus lies in front of the retina, we may distinguish
the following deviations :—

1. *More than ordinary convexity of the cornea.*

It is evident that, when, all parts of the eye being equal, the cornea
is more convex, M must be the result. Now, until the most recent
period M was therefore by many attributed to a greater convexity of
the cornea. Our measurements have, however, led to the unexpected
result, that myopes have, on an average, a less convex cornea than
emmetropes (compare p. 89), and we may add, that in the most
highly myopic persons, the cornea is the flattest. If, for example,
we divide the 34 eyes measured by us into three classes: the first of

$M = 1:1{\cdot}6$ to $1:4$; the second from $1:4$ to $1:10$; the third from $\dfrac{1}{10}$

to $\dfrac{1}{80}$, we find:

in the first class, the radius in the visual line $\rho^\circ = 7{\cdot}93$
   „   second „   „   „   „   „ $\rho^\circ = 7{\cdot}829$
   „   third „   „   „   „   „ $\rho^\circ = 7{\cdot}867$

In emmetropes I found on an average $\rho^\circ = 7{\cdot}785.$

In the most highly myopic individuals a long radius of the cornea
is, in fact, the rule. We had formerly measured the following
cases :—

    With $M = 1:1{\cdot}648$ ………… $\rho^\circ = 8{\cdot}21$
      „ $= 1:2{\cdot}625$ ………… $\rho^\circ = 7{\cdot}885$
      „ $= 1:2{\cdot}66$ ……… $\rho^\circ = 8{\cdot}06$
      „ $= 1:2{\cdot}83$ ………… $\rho^\circ = 7{\cdot}68$
      „ $= 1:2{\cdot}875$ ……… … $\rho^\circ = 7{\cdot}67$
      „ $= 1:3{\cdot}5$ ………… $\rho^\circ = 7{\cdot}84$
      „ $= 1.3{\cdot}75$ ………… $\rho^\circ = 8{\cdot}07$
      „ $= 1:3{\cdot}75$ ………… $\rho^\circ = 7{\cdot}97$
      „ $= 1:3{\cdot}75$ ………… $\rho^\circ = 8{\cdot}02$
      „ $= 1:4$ ……… …. $\rho^\circ = 7{\cdot}96,$

and subsequent observations have confirmed our result. This particularly great radius with very high M is connected with the
distended form of the eye; in ordinary cases we may say, that in
myopes similar differences occur in the radius of the cornea as in
emmetropes.—Nevertheless a *morbid* condition of the cornea may
make the focus of an otherwise normal eye fall in front of the retina.
In the first place, the increased convexity of the cornea occurs as a

result of inflammation, whereby the transparency is rendered imperfect, and the curvature is usually so irregular that under the astigmatism thence derived the acuteness of vision suffers. In the second place, there is the peculiar morbid process known under the name of conical cornea, of which I shall have to speak in treating of irregular astigmatism. In the commencement this simulates an ordinary M with amblyopia.

2. *Short focal distance of the crystalline lens.*—Determinations during life, with the aid of the ophthalmometer, and direct measurements after death, prove that, with respect to the crystalline lens, as well as to the cornea, individual differences occur; but if it has appeared that the cornea, except in its morbid changes, plays no part in M,—of the crystalline lens, it is at least not proved, that it should have a shorter focal distance in myopic, than in emmetropic eyes. So far as measurements exist, rather the contrary has appeared to be the case. Percy and Reveillé-Parise (*Hygiène oculaire*, p. 32) state expressly, that in myopes the crystalline lens is not more convex. The distinguishing a *particular form* of M, as has been assumed by Stellwag von Carion and Ed. von Jaeger, as the result of partial accommodation for near objects, we have formerly, as I think upon good grounds, opposed (compare p. 353).

3. *Dislocation of the crystalline lens.*—Two cases have occurred to me in which partial laceration of the zonula Zinnii, the one the result of concussion, the other of actual injury, gave rise to a slight degree of M. The one case, in which the crystalline lens acquired a somewhat oblique position, is described in the following Chapter, treating of Astigmatism. These cases are in favour of Helmholtz' view that, under the influence of tension of the zonula Zinnii, the crystalline lens is flatter.

4. *Displacement or more anterior position of the crystalline lens.*—This might really give rise to a certain degree of M. But we know that in the hypermetropic eye the lens lies closer to the cornea, while in the myopic it is, on the contrary, more remote from it. Hence it is sufficiently evident, how little right we have to bring M into connexion with it. Two cases may here be briefly related. One is, that of luxation of the crystalline lens, in consequence of a violent concussion of the eye, whereby it was forced through the pupil into the anterior chamber, and placed itself very regularly immediately behind the cornea. In this case M had actually arisen, in part probably in consequence of increased convexity. The man

24

did not comply with my request to place himself at once under treatment, and when he, not knowing what to do, appeared a couple of months later, the eye was painful, hard as a stone, and had become blind in consequence of the supervention of glaucoma. The lens was removed, but the eye continued, of course, blind.—The second case was that of a considerable degree of myopia, with rather soft eyeball and extraordinarily deep chamber, with the iris highly concave forwards. After this state had been long observed, without any known cause, in the course of twenty-four hours an altered position came on: the concave surface of the iris became convex anteriorly, whereby it came to lie, together with the lens, very close to the cornea. The myopia must therefore have somewhat increased; but in consequence of the slight accuracy of vision it was not possible to determine this with certainty. In the last position the eyeball had become firmer, and evidently the vitreous humour must now have been again secreted under higher pressure than the aqueous humour: the reverse had previously abnormally existed and the iris with the lens had been pushed backwards.

5. *Modifications in the coefficient of refraction of the different media* are indeed, rather hypothetically, assumed as causes of M.

6. *Inflammation of the anterior part of the sclerotic,* often combined with so-called kyklitis, may have given rise to extension of the anterior part of the sclerotic, and thus to prolongation of the visual axis, of which M is the result.

7. *Spasm of accommodation,* and therefore the several organic causes of this spasm, render the emmetropic eye myopic. To this head belong the cases of so-called intermitting M. Here an anomaly of accommodation, not of refraction, is in question.

After this enumeration of unusual deviations, which may form the basis of M, I now pass over to the consideration of the typical form of M, the eye with staphyloma posticum. It occurs under two varieties. There are, namely, cases, in which the eye is uniformly enlarged in almost all its axes, and in which its condition thus approaches to the congenital buphthalmos. In true buphthalmos we found a flat cornea and extensive atrophy in the fundus oculi, in a case with still tolerable power of vision, but with an extraordinary degree of M, so that the person who had buphthalmos on one side, had considered the eye so affected to be blind, until I showed him that at the distance of $1\frac{1}{2}''$ he was able to read with it.— In by far the great majority of cases, however, the visual axis has increased much more in length than the other axes, and the eye exhibits a tolerably regular ellipsoidal form, as has already been represented by Scarpa.*

I here append the ascertained lengths of the different axes in some myopic eyes.

Visual axis.	Horizontal axis.	Vertical axis.
33·0	26·8	25·6
31·7	26·0	24·7
31·0	26·5	26·0
30·0	27·5	25·4
28·5	24·3	24·0

Von Jaeger† has also measured a great number, in which, too, the prolongation in the visual axis was always the most remarkable.   In most cases the apex of the sclerotic ellipsoid corresponds about to the axis of the cornea,‡ and from the relaxation of the membranes in this place it appears, that the atrophy has here attained the highest degree; sometimes along with the original distention a second is here present, where apparently the membranes have offered still less resistance to the pressure. While, therefore, the apex corresponds more or less perfectly to the region of the yellow spot, which has approached the axis of the cornea, the optic nerve has removed more than ordinarily towards the inside (Compare Fig. 144).   In other cases the apex lies farther from the axis of the cornea, and indeed in different directions, but especially inwards, whereby it may coincide about with the optic nerve.   Sometimes the latter is said to be here implanted as on a second distention.   I have never seen this ; but there rather occurs at the base of the optic nerve, from yielding of its external fibrous sheath, a thickening to 8 mm. and more, which suggests the idea of a second distention of the sclerotic (compare Fig. 146). Von Jaeger says he has found the apex of the enlargement even to the inside of the optic nerve.

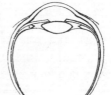

Fig. 144.

In high degrees of staphyloma posticum the eye when taken out rapidly becomes soft and flaccid; and near the posterior pole the membranes are so thin and transparent, that there the well-known

---

* *Traité pratique des maladies des yeux.* Traduit par Leveillé. Paris, chez Bertrand, 1807, Tome II., p. 190.   † *l. c.,* p. 262.

‡ Compare also Dr. Josef Ritter von Hasner, *Klinische Vorträge über Augenheilkunde,* Prag, 1860, p 19.   2

bluish appearance occurs which is peculiar to staphyloma scleroticæ anticum.   Turning the distended part to the light, we see through the pupil the fundus oculi quite clearly illuminated.   Even in life, when the cornea is strongly turned inwards, the bluish colour of the staphyloma posticum is sometimes visible; and a case occurred to me, in which the whole visible sclerotic had, through general attenuation, acquired a very disagreeable uniformly blue appearance.

In order now to examine the eye further, we make, either in the fresh state or after hardening in a solution of chromic acid, a section in a plane passing through the middle of the cornea and of the optic nerve, taking care that it does not pass the apex of the staphyloma.   It now appears that the *sclerotic* has everywhere become thinner, and indeed increasingly so towards the posterior pole; that it is in general more attenuated at the outside of the globe of the eye than at the inside, and that near the apex of the ellipsoid it is, in the highest degrees, not much thicker than a sheet of paper, nay that in some points its fibres are even separated from one another.   In the second place, we observe that the *iris* and the *lens* are moved more backwards.   The same is true of the *processus ciliaris,* and more than once I have seen that the *musculus ciliaris* also, with prolongation and attenuation of the vitreous fibres, which, derived from the membrana Descemetii, serve as origin to the muscle in question, commenced farther from the cornea than in the normal eye, and was at the same time longer, flatter, and more or less atrophic.   This we find decidedly when the anterior part of the sclerotic also is considerably attenuated, which is, however, by no means the rule.   In like manner, in ordinary cases, the anterior part of the *chorioidea* is almost quite normal, and is only towards the back part progressively attenuated and discoloured.   In general the chorioidea can with tolerable ease be separated from the sclerotic, but in proportion as we approach the atrophic parts, it must be removed with the greater care, because the membrane, while it increases in thinness and fineness, becomes at the same time more homogeneous and more easily torn. On all sides we can, however, recognise and isolate the chorioidea, atrophic as it may be.   Von Jaeger has found this to be the case in numerous eyes, and even in 1856 I saw it, in the collection of Stellwag von Carion, illustrated by excellent preparations.   The chorioidea usually exhibits the greatest attenuation immediately at the optic nerve, from which it is now easily separated ; the sclerotic, on the contrary, is thinnest at the posterior pole. According to von Hasner, the retina is more intimately connected with the chorioidea at the margin of the atrophy.—We view the chorioidea on its inner surface, after having carefully removed the vitreous humour and the crystalline lens together with the retina. It is seldom that in the eye hardened anteriorly any pigment continues adherent to it; but, on the other hand, in two eyes examined by me, a part of the outer layer of the retina remained connected with the pigment, especially in the region of the equator of the eye: they were taken from a woman aged 66; in other eyes examined by me, I have not seen this. In this woman occurred also the well-known elevations (compare p. 192) on the vitreous membrane of the chorioidea, which, where the chorioidea is not yet very atrophic, can always be easily isolated. If we now bring under the microscope, a long slender portion of the chorioidea, extending from the ora serrata to the optic nerve, isolated from the sclerotic and carefully treated, so that no pigment is lost, with the inner surface upwards, we can study the transitions from the normal condition to the most perfect atrophy. In the first place it appears, that the pigment-epithelium is less uniformly coloured, and that the cells are larger, and perhaps also flatter than in the normal eye; outside the highly reflecting atrophic crescent, where they are actually wanting, they form, however, a perfect layer. If the atrophy be diffuse, transition forms occur, and we observe that the cells gradually disappear, leaving only pigment-granules more or less collected in groups. The dark black spots, which we observe with the naked eye or with a magnifying glass, particularly in this diffuse form, scattered here and there, exhibit no regular cells, but perfectly black, irregular, angular, mutually coherent masses, between which, and also around which, we sometimes find colourless atrophic chorioideal tissue. Grey spots, on the contrary, surrounded by similar black pigment, I saw resting on normal chorioideal tissue, which glimmered more feebly through them.—If the cell membranes disappear from the pigment-epithelium, while the pigment-granules remain, the reverse holds good with respect to the *pigment*, belonging to the *stroma of the chorioidea*. This is observed most distinctly when the pigment-epithelium has been washed away with a pencil. In the first place it then appears that, even in cases of circumscribed crescent, the stroma has already got remarkably pale, where it was still sufficiently covered with pigment-epithelium; and in these decolorized parts the ramified pigment-cells of the intervascular spaces are equally distinctly visible, but are poor in pigment-granules, which towards the atrophied side progressively diminish and finally disappear, while the ramified cells themselves, nevertheless, continue present. In the darker places, on the contrary, where the chorioidea also has maintained about its regular thickness, the pig-ment-cells appear perfectly normal.—The *large vessels* of the outer layer of the *chorioidea* I found in the normal and little atrophied parts very highly congested with blood, more so than is usually the case under ordinary circumstances in normal eyes. In consequence of this the membrane had a red, striped appearance. The same sanguineous congestion was exhibited in the same place in the most remarkable manner by the chorio-capillaris; but in proportion as we approached the atrophied part, the blood diminished in the vessels, and at length wholly disappeared. Here the thin membrane which remained from the chorioidea gradually acquires such homogeneousness, that it is difficult to suppose that the vessels should have retained any calibre, although, with a strong magnifying power, we can still very well per-ceive the large vessels, and sometimes even the chorio-capillaris, surrounded with granular matter. Besides, the larger chorioideal vessels long continue to carry blood, when the chorio-capillaris is already closed. I am sure that on the white reflecting crescent, on which we often still see some larger chorioideal vessels running, the chorio-capillaris is wanting, not only because it was not filled on a very successful injection, but also because we do not see it in life. If there be a red or dark background, it is invisible when magnified by the ophthalmoscope on account of the transparency and the slight reflecting power of the thin layer of blood; but if the background be white, it ought to manifest itself by a reddish tint, and even to be visible as a network.

The foregoing description has, in general, reference to the highest degrees of staphyloma posticum, in which the defined atrophy, per-ceptible with the ophthalmoscope, has already visibly connected itself with a diffuse atrophy. It has, however, seemed to me, that diffuse atrophy occurs also where, on account of the tolerably perfect pigment-epithelium, it appears during life only from the great mu-tual distance of the still blood-carrying larger vessels of the chorioidea.

In staphyloma posticum *the place where the optic nerve enters the eye* is important. Some years ago I investigated this place in the normal eye.* It then appeared to me, that the *trunk* of the optic

* *Archiv für Ophthal.*, Bd. i. h. 2, pp. 82 *et seq.* 1855.

nerve is already divided by fibrous tissue into the numerous small bundles into which it at once separates on issuing as retina, and thus differs essentially in its structure from other gradually ramifying nerve-trunks; that it possesses a *double fibrous sheath,* an external and thicker one, *a* (Fig. 145), which is continued at *a′* into the

Fig. 145.

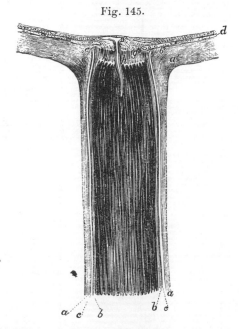

most external part of the sclerotic, and an internal one *b*, which envelopes the trunk as far as the chorioidea *d*, is connected with the latter, and bends close to it into the there pigment-containing sclerotic *b′*, while at the same time the lamina cribrosa *g* for the most part proceeds therefrom, and is only to a small extent formed by the chorioidea. Between the two fibrous sheaths, *a* and *b*, is a thin layer of loose connective tissue, the *connective-tissue-sheath c*, consisting of a network of sharply-defined fasciculi, which ascends to *c′* close to the lamina cribrosa. Even beneath the lamina cribrosa at *h* the nerve-fibres, as Bowman[*] first stated, lose their *medullary sheath,* whereby the nerve becomes thinner and at the same time transparent.

[*] *Lectures on the parts concerned in the operations on the Eye.* London, 1849, p. 82.

These thinner fasciculi now pass through the so-called lamina cribrosa, which may be regarded as a strengthening of the neurilemma of the separate bundles, and of which a fine continuation can be traced between the bundles of the fibrous layer of the retina. The *chorioidea* appears to terminate abruptly at the margin of the nerve, because the pigment, which is here largely accumulated, actually ceases, nor are the chorioideal vessels continued further; but its tissue nevertheless surrounds the fasciculi of the optic nerve, and thus really contributes to the formation of the *lamina cribrosa*. So the *chorioidea*, both through its connexion with the internal sheath *b'* of the optic nerve, and by its prolongation among the nerve-tissue, is here firmly attached. Almost directly at the place, where its pigment commences, the elements of the deeper retinal layers begin to show themselves, over which the nerve-layer now expands.—If with this we compare the section of the entrance of the optic nerve in highly-developed staphyloma posticum (Fig. 146) it will appear

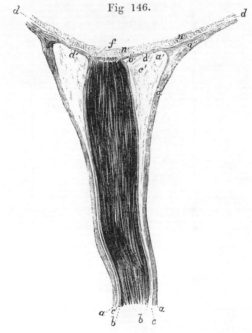

Fig 146.

that the *external sheath*, *a*, escapes near the sclerotic from the nerve, that a small part, *a'*, here turns inwards, but that the greatest part, *a"*, inclines outwards towards the sclerotic; that, on the contrary, the inner sheath, *b*, continues closely to surround the nerve; near the nerve-surface *f* forms the lamina cribrosa, and now passes at *b'* outwards into the sclerotic, running to meet the fasciculus, *a'*, of the outer sheath turning inwards. This thin fasciculus, *a' b'*, bounds the loose connective tissue, *c*, which here, *c'*, has acquired a great breadth, and is therefore evidently very much extended. The sclerotic consequently here consists almost exclusively of a thin fasciculus, *a' b'*, derived from the two nerve-sheaths, and this is covered anteriorly by the completely atrophic pigmentless chorioidea, *d'*. It appears, that the nerve, which here exhibits superiorly a perhaps accidental thickening, after its fibres have lost the medullary sheath, is still thinner than in ordinary cases, and thus goes inwards, through a smaller opening in the chorioidea, sometimes in an oblique direction, in order immediately as retina, *n n*, to spread itself over the anterior surface of the atrophic chorioidea. In the instructive drawings given by von Jaeger,[*] one of which I have here copied (Fig. 147), the sheath of connective tissue has for the most part not only extended upwards, but an extremity of it also stretches between the layers of the sclerotic. Von Jaeger further remarks, that the internal extremity of the nerve, with early bending and spreading of its fibres, appears as it were drawn within the eye: in Fig. 147 (after Jaeger) the lamina cribrosa and

Fig. 147.

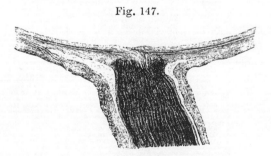

the place where the nerve-fibres lose their medullary fibres, really appear to have approached nearer to the retina.

The *retina* has in general a normal appearance. It is hard to say whether it is more or less attenuated in one place or another; but thus much is certain, that the atrophy in this membrane cannot be

[*] *Ueber die Einstellungen*, etc. Wien, 1861, Tab. i. and ii.

compared with that in the sclerotic and chorioidea. The extended course of the vessels, already ophthalmoscopically seen, can be easily proved : how far the proper tissue is altered, it is difficult to say. Coccius,* who often examined the retina in staphyloma scleroticæ, in consequence of chorioiditis postica, found, with the exception of some empty places on the posterior layer (the layer of rods and bulbs), no changes in it. H. Mueller† thinks that in one case he found the tissue looser; but he himself adds, that it is necessary to be particularly careful in one's judgment on this point. In my notes I find, that in isolating the retina, the nerve-substance on the nerve-surface very easily separated from the lamina cribrosa and remained connected with the retina; that in the tolerably fresh eye the yellow spot was sometimes scarcely visible; that the plica was formed as usual; that the fibrous layer appeared normal; that on sections of hardened retinas the different layers, with the exception of that of the rods, were admirably to be seen; that at the edges radiating fibres with adherent granules from the two granular layers occurred already isolated; that in the region of the yellow spot the different cell-layers were distinctly visible, and that viewing the recently removed retina on the outer surface, a tolerably good image of the layer of rods and bulbs, which could be isolated in the ordinary way, was usually obtained. But, what here has particular bearing : how far morbid changes occurred in these percipient elements, how far they were more separated than in the normal eye, how the bulbs in the yellow spot, and particularly in the fovea centralis, are circumstanced in high degrees of atrophy—on these points I cannot speak with certainty.

Respecting the vitreous humour I have only to state, that in high degrees of staphyloma posticum it is fluid and not perfectly clear. The flocculi present in it have a fibrous, granular appearance without any distinct structure.

If we now endeavour, from the facts which have been observed, to form an idea of the development of staphyloma posticum, the optic nerve with the membranes of the eye and the nerve-surface itself, will, in the first place, attract our attention. According to ophthalmoscopic examination, we have in these parts to seek the

---

* *Ueber Glaucom*, etc. Leipzig, 1859, p. 40.

† *Verhandlungen der phys.-med. Gesellschaft.* Würzburg, B. ix. S. liii. 1859.

commencement of the affection, and in many instances anatomy at
least does not oppose this view.   We have then to suppose that in
these cases the disposition consists in this, that the sclerotic near the
optic nerve is more extensible, particularly to its outside, and that by
this extension the outer sheath of the optic nerve is soon a little removed
from the latter, and the sheath of connective tissue is so extended (compare Figs. 145 c' and 146 c').   So soon as this happens, the thin layer
of sclerotic tissue, b', situated in front of the sheath mentioned, must
be very much attenuated, and the same is true of the chorioidea, d',
connected therewith, and forming, with the fibrous layer mentioned,
the so-called lamina cribrosa, between the nerve-fasciculi.   At the
side of the nerve-surface, therefore, the retina now rests on an extended
and attenuated chorioidea and sclerotic, which posteriorly further lose
all support.   It is not until we come somewhat more outward that
we find the external sheath of the optic nerve, a, strengthening the
sclerotic.   With this extension, in the immediate neighbourhood of
the optic nerve, the origin of the atrophic crescent seems to be
really connected : the chorioidea, d', is here united with the nerve,
both immediately through the fibres, which are continued between
the fasciculi of the nerve, and mediately through their connexion with the inner sheath of the nerve.   At the borders of
this attachment its vessels cease ; on any extension, therefore,
obstruction to the circulation in the extreme terminations of the
chorio-capillaris must easily arise, and thus the condition for incipient
atrophy is supplied.   We find something similar in the origin of
emphysema of the lungs from atrophy of the most distended pul-
monary vesicles, which thereby also finally lose both their capillary
network and their pigment.   Now, if the excessive extension has here
once begun, and the resistance is thus diminished, it is more unlikely
that the condition should become stationary, than that it should be
progressively developed ; and it actually is the rule that the atrophy
of the chorioidea advances more and more, without the visual axis,
in slight degrees of staphyloma, necessarily becoming persistently
longer and longer.—The extension at the margin of the optic nerve
takes place often only at one side, and indeed principally at the
outside, with which the atrophic crescent keeps pace at the same
side.   The number of my observations is not sufficiently great to
enable me to form a positive opinion,—but it appears to me very
likely that, if the apex of the staphyloma falls nearly in the optic
nerve, the outer sheath has given way at all sides of the nerve,

and that to this the annular and circular atrophy of the chorioidea then also correspond: in the eye, from which Fig. 146 was taken, the atrophy was really circular. If, as is usually the case, the apex of the staphyloma is situated at the outside of the optic nerve, atrophy of the chorioidea is also found especially at this side, and even the fact, that the yellow spot, to which the apex of the staphyloma often corresponds, is situated at the outside of and a little beneath the nerve-surface, and that the axis of the atrophic crescent usually extends in this same direction, indicates most distinctly, that there is a connexion between the apex in question and the direction in which the atrophy of the chorioidea advances. Whether the sharply-defined atrophy of the chorioidea does not reach further than over the extended connective tissue, b', I cannot decide. Von Jaeger does not admit even any such intimate connexion, and he asserts that the direction of the atrophy does not at all correspond to the side where the sheath of cellular tissue has given way. As to the narrowing of the nerve-surface in a direction perpendicular to the axis of the crescent, observed with the ophthalmoscope, I can give no satisfactory explanation.—Now, in the ordinary cases, where the optic nerve does not lie in the apex of the staphyloma, it may be a question, whether the extension does not commence rather in the region of the yellow spot, and only secondarily become communicated to the outside of the optic nerve. This view is the more admissible, not only because by it the position of the optic nerve at the inside of the ellipsoid would be explained, but also because in very young persons, with comparatively high degrees of M, the crescentic atrophy of the chorioidea is still often absent, or at least is very slight. We can also very easily imagine, how extension in the region of the yellow spot gives rise to the atrophy. In the yellow spot the chorioidea, which here abounds in pigment, is more intimately connected with the sclerotic. If the membranes here give way backwards, the extension will be equal on all sides, and the chorioidea will, moreover, the more easily maintain its connexion with the sclerotic, because precisely here it is more intimately connected with it. If now the sclerotic too gradually extends in the direction of the optic nerve, the chorioidea becomes very tense over this part, for we may assume the yellow spot and the outer margin of the optic nerve to be two fixed points: at the attachment, therefore, to the outside of the nerve-surface the chorioidea is particularly strongly drawn, and considering that the chorioideal vessels terminate pre-

cisely at this boundary, the production of atrophy by extension cannot surprise us; according to the direction of the tension which
takes place it is even easy to understand why the atrophy should
assume the crescentic form.   The atrophy at this place will now
certainly be still promoted, so soon as also in the immediate neighbourhood of the nerve the sclerotic is extended, and thus the
outer sheath of the optic nerve gives way outwardly.   This giving
way can almost without exception be demonstrated, and it is attended
with the necessary consequence, that the arterial circle, known even
to Zinn, occurring in the sclerotic around the optic nerve, as Jaeger*
has shown, is removed from the nerve.   On the whole, the outer
half of the sclerotic is extended in a higher degree than the part
situated at the inside of the nerve : there it is consequently also in
general thinner.   With this is connected the fact that, as we have
already seen (compare p. 182), the yellow spot removes towards the
inside, so that it may even go beyond the axis of the cornea, whereby
the visual line cuts the cornea to the outside of its axis.   That in
this extension atrophy does not occur at the outside of the yellow
spot in the anterior part of the chorioidea so readily as at the inside,
is easily explained from the great extensibility of the chorioidea in
this direction.   It appears, moreover, gradually to move a little
over the surface of the sclerotic : thus, at least, I think the retrogression of the iris, of the ciliary process and of the chorioidea
itself, with the ciliary muscle must be explained, in those cases in
which the anterior part of the sclerotic has retained almost its normal
thickness.   However, there exists everywhere more or less extension
of the chorioidea, and that this gives rise to diffuse atrophy and to
diminution of the elastic resistance, needs no proof.   To the elastic
resistance of the chorioidea, I think essential importance must be
attached.   If the membranes of the normal eye be all cut through
together, the chorioidea is seen to retract, leaving the sclerotic bare
at the edge.   This proves that the chorioidea may be displaced, and
moreover, proves its tension.   During life, in consequence of the
vessels being full, of the tone of the blood-vessels, and of muscular
fibres† scattered here and there, the tension of the chorioidea is un-

---

* l. c. p. 52.

† H. Müller (*Verhandl. der phys.-med. Gesellschaft*, Würzburg, B. x.
p. 179) has pointed out these muscular fibres, and also ganglionic cells in
the chorioidea, of the presence of which Kölliker satisfied himself, in Müller's

doubtedly still greater. By virtue of this tension it bears a part of the pressure of the fluids of the eye, which now does not act entirely upon the sclerotic, and it is evident that where an atrophic condition has set in, and the chorioidea has given place to a thin, brittle membrane, the full pressure comes to bear upon the already extended sclerotic. Consequently a tolerably advanced staphyloma does not easily become stationary, the less so because the pressure of the fluids in the myopic eye is in general somewhat increased. Therefore, also, in staphyloma the blood-vessels and the inequalities of the chorioidea, as well as the elongated, but not easily atrophied, ciliary nerves,* make deep impressions on the inner surface of the atrophic sclerotic. More than once this has attracted my attention. Various circumstances may, moreover, contribute to cause that, in one instance in one part, in another in a different part, the extension, and with it the atrophy, is particularly great. Especially *in the region of the yellow spot* it frequently attains a maximum, because, from whatever cause it may be, the apex of the ellipsoid is usually often found here. On this excessive extension the above-described local changes mainly depend, whereby the function of the retina comes to suffer. It is easy to see, although it has not been proved by accurate microscopic investigation, that under such extension the outermost layer, which consists of radiatingly placed very small bulbs, must suffer ; that these bulbs at least must be separated, irregularly distributed and made oblique, and that they must easily be actually destroyed. In other parts, too, of the retina, the rods and bulbs, as we have seen, appeared to be more separated. That, on the contrary, in the fibrous layer little or no disturbance occurs, will not appear strange, when we consider how well the structure and function of nerves in general resist extension by morbid tumours or from other causes. Where there is vital metamorphosis of matter, change of form much more readily takes place under the molecular change, without disturbance, than in solid fibrous parts, and in this respect the retina has a great advantage over the sclerotic.

The changes in the *vitreous humour* may have a different origin. They may depend upon extravasations of blood, which, perfect as the absorption may be, never leave behind them an absolutely clear vitreous humour. Solution of the as yet so badly explained connexion of the vitreous humour, gives rise to turbidity, as is seen in preparations. Schweigger's preparations also appeared to me to be conclusive.

* Compare also Heymann, in *Archiv f. Ophthal.*, ii. 1, 131.

traumatic injuries, and where foreign bodies are present: a slight thread of india-rubber carried with a needle in the region of the equator transversely through the eye of a rabbit, strongly extended by pulling the ends, and while in the extended state cut off at both sides close to the eye, contracted (in an experiment by my assistant, Dr. Brondgeest) to a small body, visible with the ophthalmoscope in the centre of the vitreous humour, and around it a considerable turbidity was developed, while the little wound of the membranes regularly cicatrised. Now the considerable distention of the vitreous humour in staphyloma posticum probably also causes laceration, at least synchysis, and some turbidity is consequently to be expected.* Finally, in some cases, an irritative or inflammatory condition of the retina and chorioidea is also certainly in operation.

We have now approached an important point. The question is, how far staphyloma posticum is connected with inflammation. It is known that von Graefe at first thought the practical idea of sclerotico-chorioiditis posterior applicable to it; but that he in vain sought, in two eyes which he had the opportunity of examining anatomically, the proofs of preceding inflammation. Von Graefe's opinion was disputed in various quarters. Stellwag von Carion adhered from the beginning to another opinion, and Ed. von Jaeger soon followed him in the same. According to them staphyloma posticum is only the result of a congenital condition, and the atrophy connected with it increases, according to von Jaeger, even with the eyeball itself, until at a certain point it often becomes stationary. There is, indeed, some truth in this statement. Thus much is certain, that the staphyloma posticum cannot be considered as a simple result of sclerotico-chorioiditis, and that without the disposition, and that usually of an hereditary nature, it is not easily developed. Moreover, it must be admitted that without symptoms of irritation or inflammation staphyloma posticum may attain a tolerably high degree. But, on the other hand, there is no doubt that the morbid distention very often leads to irritation and inflammation, and finds therein, with softening of the membranes, a condition of rapid development. It appears to me to be an error not to consider the eye with staphyloma posticum, combined with simple atrophy, as morbid, and a still greater error to overlook the fact, that when highly developed, this condition almost without exception induces symptoms of irritation, which still further threaten the integrity of the power of vision. Von Jaeger's doubt, whether chorioiditis dissemi-

* Compare, on this subject, also von Hasner, *l. c.* p. 21.

nata occurs more frequently in highly myopic eyes than in others, indeed surprises me. In high degrees of M this inflammation is at a certain time of life the rule. In the course of the morbid distention inflammation is readily developed, which cannot be considered as a new condition, but usually makes itself known, at an early period, as more or less distinct irritation. Even in youth, as Hasner also observes, symptoms of irritation are usually present even in slight degrees of M, and ophthalmoscopic investigation now reveals to us capillary redness of the nerve-surface, and, what is remarkable, sometimes only over the half of its extent. Probably there is in this case, in consequence of tension of the chorioideal ring and of the lamina cribrosa, some mechanical irritation, perhaps even pressure on the small fasciculi of the optic nerve. Subsequently, as the extent becomes greater, and the disproportionate tension is augmented, the phenomena of irritation increase, and at the boundaries of the circumscribed atrophy hyperæmia exists, showing that the chorioidea before atrophying, here also passes through a period of irritation. Therefore I cannot admit the existence of well-defined limits between the further development of the crescent, and the occurrence of remote atrophied spots, which last exclusively von Jaeger considers as products of inflammation. Even the abundant deposition of pigment on the boundaries of the crescent, again absorbed in the progress of the atrophy, in order to be anew deposited more externally, is in favour of a state of irritation. At a later period the subjective phenomena, also, become more characteristic, and in different parts of the fundus oculi atrophic spots are formed, preceded by inflammatory action : chorioiditis disseminata, I repeat it, is in the highest degrees of M at a more advanced age, connected with its normal development. Our conclusion is, therefore, briefly as follows :—that almost without exception the predisposition to the development of staphyloma posticum exists at birth ; that it is developed with symptoms of irritation, which in moderate degrees of staphyloma do not attain any great clinical importance; but that in the higher degrees an inflammatory state almost always occurs, at least at a somewhat more advanced time of life, as a result and as a co-operative cause of the further development of the distention and of the atrophy.

This conclusion is certainly not inconsistent with the fact, that after death so few products of inflammation are to be met with. For these products pass, as well as the normal tissue, into a state of atrophy. In this way false membranes, as we see in the synechia of the iris, in adhesions between the pleuræ, and in other places, become atrophied and absorbed when extended. Even on the capsule of the lens sometimes nothing else remains of the inflammatory products of iritis than some spots of pigment. In staphyloma posticum the inflammation exists almost as the transition period to atrophy. That in general no adhesion of the membranes is met with is also easily reconcileable to this view. Adhesions are, however, sometimes found, and it is questionable, whether, in general, the separation would be so easily obtained if the chorioidea before passing into the atrophic form, had not been imbibed with parenchymatous exudation. Moreover, as H. Mueller[*] states, the tissue of the chorioidea in the intervascular spaces exhibits in staphyloma posticum, groups of cellular bodies, which he considers to be also in favour of the pre-existence of inflammation. Finally, the analogy with staphyloma anticum, which is evidently the result of inflammation, is not to be denied.

Another important question is, in what the predisposition to staphyloma posticum may consist. It appears to be as yet not satisfactorily solved; at least I have no decided opinion on the subject. The relative number of adults in whom we can ophthalmoscopically perceive more or less atrophy, is much greater than that in children. Von Jaeger is certainly quite right in asserting that something of atrophy is occasionally to be seen in young children; I even readily admit, that he has himself found defined crescentic atrophy in newly-born infants, both during life and in the dead body; but the rule is, that we see nothing of the kind, although atrophy at a later period makes its appearance, and though in all probability there was an hereditary tendency to it. This leads us, I think, to the conclusion, that in these cases, the resistance at the outside of the optic nerve was originally less than in the unpredisposed eye. Now, this predisposition has been brought into connexion with the history of the development of the eye. If we look at the drawing given in the *Archiv für Ophthalmologie* (Bd. IV. I. 39) by von Ammon, of the *protu-berantia scleralis*, described by him thirty-five years previously, as existing at a certain period of the fœtal eye, which is here reproduced as Fig. 148, the form of staphyloma posticum is at once suggested to the mind. Von Ammon states, that in an early period of fœtal existence the sclera is still open at the cerebral side;

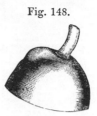

Fig. 148.

* *Verhandl. der phys. med. Gesellschaft*, Bd. ix. s. liii. 1859.

25

that it then has the form of a cup, and is connected by an oval opening with the anterior cerebral cell. This opening is closed by a tissue proceeding from the margins, and as the eye becomes larger, the supplementary tissue forms the protuberance in question, which is, according to von Ammon, directed at first downwards, but subsequently backwards and outwards, as it is here represented. Von Ammon adds, that the different membranes close the said opening nearly at the same time. In the first place, there is brought into connexion with this mode of development the coloboma chorioideæ, which as a defect of the chorioidea, proceeding from the nerve-surface, extends inferiorly, whether over only a small extent, or over the whole chorioidea, and may now unite even with coloboma iridis.* We have here, therefore, an ordinary *arrest of development*. And as such Stellwag von Carion and Ed. von Jaeger also consider the disposition to staphyloma posticum, and in a certain sense staphyloma posticum itself. The arrest of development is here only much less, and might be limited even to a slight remnant of the protuberantia scleralis. The direction of the atrophy, indeed, corresponds to that of the already fully-closed protuberantia scleralis.

As I was already about to observe, I am unable, for want of personal investigation, to give any opinion upon the subject. I, however, feel myself called on to remark, that it appears to be chiefly this idea which has led Stellwag von Carion and von Jaeger to consider acquired myopia as another condition, and to start from the supposition that congenital myopia is in no way connected with the use of the eyes, and that it should be equally distributed among all classes of society. Against this view I have already raised difficulties (p. 352), and I shall again revert to them. In this place I cannot avoid observing, that if the connexion with the protuberantia scleralis really exists, and if congenital staphyloma posticum, as well as the predisposition to the same, may be considered as an arrest of development, this view does not invalidate my statement, that the undue use of the eyes promotes the occurrence of staphyloma posticum. Indeed, it is certain that if, with slight predisposition, the eyes are much used for close work, the staphyloma becomes more fully developed, and direct experience as well as analogy shows, that

* Compare Liebreich, *Archiv für Ophthalmologie*, Bd. v. ii. 241, and *Atlas d'Ophthalmoscopie*, Tab. xii. Fig. 5; and Nagel, *Archiv für Ophthalmologie*, Bd. vi. i. 170.

in such a case the probability of transmission to posterity, even in a higher degree, is greater than when the staphyloma was not brought under promoting circumstances to a state of further development.

§ 29.—The Vision of Myopes.

The vision of myopes, without the aid of spectacles (of which alone I am here speaking), is characterised by comparatively less acuteness for remote than for near objects. We are already aware that this depends upon the circles of diffusion formed upon the retina by the rays proceeding from remote points. Myopes have a farthest point of distinct vision, and the rays proceeding from a point situated there, can unite upon the retina into one point; with respect to more remote points, the circles of diffusion become greater, and vision consequently becomes more indistinct, the greater the distance is. In slight degrees of M this indistinctness is so trifling that the persons affected with it have not observed it, and it is not until they employ a weak concave glass that it appears that they are thus enabled to see more distinctly at a distance, and are consequently myopic. In these slight degrees myopia is attended with no inconvenience. Against the disadvantage, that at a great distance vision is not perfectly accurate, is the advantage that, the range of accommodation being equal, very small objects brought closer to the eye, and therefore, under a greater visual angle, can be better distinguished, and that when at a more advanced period of life the range of accommodation is diminished, ordinary work can be still longer performed without spectacles. Even with a myopia of $\frac{1}{18}$, in which, at the distance of eighteen inches, accurate images are still obtained, the anomaly is, in most kinds of work, attended with no inconvenience. In somewhat higher degrees myopes have, at least in youth, with perfect accommodation, a tendency to approach closer than is necessary to the objects, and thus, particularly at sedentary work, to assume a stooping position. If the myopia amounts to $\frac{1}{10}$ to $\frac{1}{8}$, or more, this occurs without exception; of course, to a greater extent, the higher the degree of the myopia is. With increasing myopia, too, the fancy increases of occupying one's-self with small objects: persons so affected read by preference small

2

print; they accustom themselves to small handwriting, and as much as possible avoid long lines. It is evident that in doing so they are able to see more at once, and, for example, in reading, they need not move the eyes and head so much as when they have broad pages and large letters before them. It is not until the objects diminish in magnitude in proportion as the distance becomes less, that myopic are on a par with non-myopic individuals, and with equal acuteness of vision distinguish those objects equally well. However, as we shall hereafter see more fully, in the highest degrees of myopia the acuteness of vision is imperfect, and although those labouring under them can distinguish very small objects still better than non-myopes, these must in reference to the distance be really somewhat larger; it is, moreover, a very great inconvenience, that a bent position, and, if binocular vision is not sacrificed, particularly great convergence, are not to be avoided, an inconvenience which is attended with actual injury, inasmuch as the further development of the myopia is thereby promoted.

Much greater still, in these high degrees of M, is the inconvenience of indistinct vision at a distance. The emmetrope can form an idea of it by holding before his eye a strongly convex glass, and he will be surprised how quietly myopes usually submit to their fate. But at the same time, many peculiarities developed in myopes, unless they early accustom themselves to the use of spectacles, will no longer be an enigma to him.

The circles of diffusion in vision at a distance are the greater, because in myopes the diameter of the pupil, as even Porterfield and Jurin were aware, is in general larger than in non-myopic persons, and to this magnitude the circles of diffusion are proportionate. Therefore myopes under mydriasis see very badly at a distance. With a bright light they see remote objects much more distinctly, and therefore also at a more advanced time of life, the degree of M being unchanged, they distinguish better at a distance, which often makes them incorrectly infer that the degree of the myopia is diminished. Myopes now also distinguish much more accurately beyond their farthest point, when they look through a small opening, and in the highest degrees of myopia, as will hereafter be seen, even practical use may be made of this fact. The Calabar bean, too, which, dropped in solution into the eye, has the remarkable property of constricting the pupil, is thus serviceable to them: on very slight action of this agent the pupil becomes narrow, without increasing the myopia, and when the remedy acts more powerfully, the farthest point, which had at first approached the eye, after an hour returns to its normal condition. Among the early scholars many myopes were to be found. In this number was Dechales,* a Jesuit of the seventeenth century, who has with wonderful accuracy described many peculiarities of myopic vision. In church he saw very remote little flames as round circles of diffusion, and thereupon studied his entoptic spectrum, which he perfectly understood. He was also aware, and explained the fact very correctly by the diminution of the circles of diffusion, that myopes distinguish more accurately through a small opening, and with respect to the influence of the approximation of the eyelids he communicates some particulars, which are not to be met with even in later writers. Thus, regarding this point, he observes, that, properly speaking, only the vertical dimension of the circles of diffusion thereby disappears, so that horizontal lines are better seen, but that also the horizontal extension of vertical lines is somewhat divided by the cilia, so that a number of images are seen close to one another, of which one is usually distinguished by particular clearness. Many myopes have so very much accustomed themselves to approximate the eyelids that it actually belongs to their physiognomy, and that they persevere in doing so, even when the use of concave spectacles makes it superfluous : this reminds us of the involuntary tension of accommodation, sometimes even combined with strabismus, of young persons whose H has been corrected by a convex glass. In strong myopia the imperfect vision has, even at a short distance, peculiar results. Those affected with it seldom fix the persons to whom they speak, because they imperfectly distinguish their features; they have in general no correct idea of the impression which their person and their words make upon another, and, according to their original disposition, a peculiar freeness and too great self-confidence, or else, what is rarer, a more than ordinary bashfulness, are thence not unfrequently developed. In their bearing, and often also in their gait, a certain awkwardness is frequently manifested, by which some are recognised at a distance. Finally, much more of what passes in the world escapes them than they themselves are aware of, and with respect to a number of things their knowledge is less correct, because they fill up what is deficient through the operation of a brisk imagination. Cardanus asserts that myopes are particularly amorous, because that not observing defects, they look upon human

* *Cursus s. mundus mathematicus*, T. III. p. 393.

beings' as angels. The starry heavens they also see in extraordinary splendour.

In point of acuteness of vision myopes are in general inferior to emmetropes. In low degrees of M the difference is extremely slight, but in the higher degrees it is, at least in advancing years, considerable, even without the myopia being combined with unusual morbid changes. Where M is $> \frac{1}{6}$, S is often imperfect, unless the myopia is congenital, and the individual is still very young. In myopia $> \frac{1}{5}$ imperfection is the rule; in myopia $> \frac{1}{4}$ it is the rule probably without out exception. Especially in high degrees of myopia S decreases with the increase of years much more rapidly than in E. Where $M = \frac{1}{4}$ or $\frac{1}{3}$, S at sixty years of age usually amounts to not more than $\frac{1}{3}$. The cause of diminished S in myopes is evident. In M the retinal images, indeed, are larger for equal angles, under which the objects are seen, because the distance from the nodal point to the retina is greater; but, on the other hand, the surface of the retina is also larger, and therefore in a given plane comprises fewer percipient elements. Where there is perfect compensation of these two factors an equal number of percipient elements could now, the visual angles being equal, be impinged upon, and S may thus remain equal. But the extension affects especially the posterior pole, also occupies principally the region of the yellow spot, and for direct vision, therefore, perfect compensation is not to be expected, even when the extension produces no further disturbance in the function of the different elements. We had here in view the determination of the acuteness of vision applied to objects situated within the farthest point of distinct vision. The determination with the aid of objects situated at a greater distance, and seen with correcting glasses, proves still more disadvantageous, because k'' thereby approaches the retina.

With the increase of the myopia, the same objects at an equal distance are undoubtedly seen by degrees with a smaller portion of the percipient elements. As this has occurred gradually, the eye has, during its occurrence, accustomed itself to it, and the magnitude of an object is now also, even on the fixing of a single point, invariably correctly estimated, and the finger, when it is wished to touch it, goes right to its boundaries. The extension has, moreover, had this result, that the original connexion between the amount of the muscular action required and the number of percipient elements, which thereby consecutively receive the image of a certain point, is modified, and nevertheless the harmony has been preserved, so that on movement of the eye no apparent movement of the object is seen. We cannot therefore, properly say, that the myope, who sees the same object at an equal distance with fewer percipient elements, actually *projects it smaller in appearance outwards;* he undoubtedly sees it *less acutely,* but the idea which he forms of the magnitude is not determined simply by the number of affected percipient elements, but is the result of a very complicated psychical process, to which a number of factors contribute. In any case we are justified in coming to the remarkable conclusion, that in consequence of slowly progressive displacement by extension, a point of the retina is projected outwards in a direction different from that originally belonging to it, and we hence infer that the direction of projection is not absolutely congenital, but that it has been developed in connexion with other means of observation.

That myopes are possessed of a normal power of accommodation could be overlooked only by confounding the region and the range of accommodation. Some early writers have fully comprehended this, and even in Smith * we find it expressly stated. It is also satisfactorily seen when we neutralise the myopia, whereupon young myopes see near objects perfectly well, distinguish acutely at a few inches from the eye, and are at the same time in a condition to see remote objects accurately. We have, too, already remarked that the range of accommodation of myopes appears to be equal to that of emmetropes; but in the highest degrees, in which the musculus ciliaris and sometimes also the nervi ciliares are atrophied, the power of accommodation diminishes and is at last wholly annihilated: this, however, happens at an age when, moreover, this power has been almost quite lost. We have, too, already calculated what range of accommodation, with difference in length of the visual axis, corresponds to a certain change of the crystalline lens, and we found that myopes, on account of their longer visual axis, are in this respect somewhat in the background (Compare pp. 95, 96). On the other hand, the use of concave glasses has an advantageous influence, and therefore has a compensating effect. Such small quantities are here, however, in question, that this cannot

Complete System of Optics, Cambridge, 1738.

appear in practice.   Of much greater importance is the difference in
the relative range of accommodation between emmetropic and ametropic eyes, which I have fully explained (pp. 119, *et seq*.).   Under a
somewhat different form it may here be briefly remarked in reference to
this point, that myopes (contrary to what we find in hypermetropes)
with slight convergence can manage a comparatively small part of
their power of accommodation; but are therefore also in a better
state, with convergence for their farthest point of distinct vision, to
omit all tension of accommodation : their effort was of course always to
keep the binocular farthest point removed as far as possible from the
eye.—In myopes, moreover, the range of accommodation diminishes
with age in the same manner as in emmetropes.   A glance at Figures
125, 126, and 127 shows this directly.   True presbyopia, which we
made to commence when p_2 lies farther than 8″ from the eye, can of
course occur only when M is $< \dfrac{1}{8}$.

§ 30.   Complaints and Disturbances in Myopia.

Slight degrees of M give rise to no complaints.   In youth the inferior acuteness of vision at a distance passes almost unobserved, and
at the fiftieth, sometimes at the sixtieth year, when the narrower
pupil makes remote objects more distinct, we hear only boasting and
praise of the excellent vision for near objects.   Myopic eyes have
consequently acquired the reputation of strength and excellence,
which, on unprejudiced examination, they cannot maintain.   A slight
degree of M may have its advantages for men engaged in study or
minute work, high degrees are combined with disturbances which
often make themselves only too plainly felt at an advanced period
of life.   The condition itself, in youth may be very tolerable; the
prospect is often gloomy.

But even in youth many myopes complain of inconvenience from
continued tension.   There is then a state of irritation which appears to
be combined with hyperæmia, both of the external eye and of the
internal parts.   At a later period, especially when the eyes are very
prominent, and probably, in consequence of tension of the extended
muscles, are somewhat harder than is normally the case, such a
state of irritation may become habitual, and may even be combined
with a troublesome irritation of the eyelids.   Especially when the
myopia in a certain period rapidly attains a higher degree, pain and

fatigue of the eyes, particularly by artificial light, are much complained of.

Where high degrees of M are in question, there is added to this state of irritation a certain spasm of accommodation, so that now a still higher degree of M is met with, which on the yielding of the irritation, especially after a Heurteloupian abstraction of blood, and a stay in the dark, again gives way. Professor Junge, of Petersburg, has called my attention to this fact, and I have, in different instances, found it confirmed. In other cases the myopia gradually attains a very high degree, without the occurrence of any other disturbance than imperfect vision at a distance. Indeed, when we consider the changes which the fundus oculi has undergone, we are often surprised at the slight disturbance connected therewith. The explanation of this is to be sought in the fact that when important structural changes of the chorioidea arise slowly, the retina undergoes but little disturbance, and that, moreover, diminished acuteness of sight on indirect vision is not apt to cause much inconvenience. Even with the marbled atrophic white and yellow-speckled appearance, extending in a girdle from the outside of the crescent through the region of the yellow spot, direct vision sometimes still retains its normal acuteness, and the imperfection of indirect vision is scarcely observed. However, in extensive diffuse atrophy beyond the crescent this is exceptional. But the disturbance of vision is much greater when, as is often the case, the existing tension and extension give rise to a state of general irritation of the retina. This is the proper amblyopia of myopes. It sometimes attains in a short time a tolerably high degree, and is again capable of improvement on the employment of suitable treatment. Von Graefe* considers the prognosis in this form of amblyopia to be even comparatively very favourable, and I quite agree with him if our object be limited to obtaining a temporary improvement. But in high degrees of myopia, relapse and eventual aggravation of the affection are always to be expected. Besides the diminished S, the rapid supervention of fatigue, a feeling of tension in the eye, sometimes pain on pressure, and moreover photopsia and muscæ volitantes are connected with this condition. These last two phenomena often in myopia constitute a permanent source of complaint, even when no particular state of irritation and no extraordinary diminution of the sharpness of vision exist. Ordinary muscæ volitantes, as I have already

* *Archiv f. Ophthalmol.*, B. ii.

explained (pp. 197 *et seq.*), are not attended with any essential inconvenience : they are dependent on microscopically small bodies, which in every one float in the vitreous humour. Myopes are, however, troubled with them more than others. In the circles of diffusion of smaller surfaces of light, they exhibit themselves with extraordinary distinctness, and in general the more diffuse uniform aspect of the objects is a condition under which they appear more distinct. In non-myopes they are seen indeed also mostly on uniformly illuminated surfaces, while no other forms are depicted on the retina. Therefore, too, myopes find a diminution of this symptom from the use of concave glasses, which remove the uniform diffuse appearance of the objects. But often the complaints continue, especially when the patients are uneasy about the symptom, and have once accustomed themselves to attend to it. I have seen instances in which anxiety about muscæ volitantes amounted to true monomania, against which all reasoning and the most direct demonstrations were in vain. This is especially the case when morbid changes in the vitreous humour have supervened. We must admit the existence of morbid changes so soon as we can with the ophthalmoscope perceive turbidities in the vitreous humour. To these a real pathological importance is to be attached. The ordinary corpuscles are too small to be ophthalmoscopically visible, and therefore whenever forms appear, we must admit the existence of abnormal products, the origin of which has been above explained (§ 28). In inflammatory irritation they are certainly almost always to be considered as the results of exudation. Such forms, also, arise and disappear, independently of myopia, in consequence of kyklitis and chorioiditis anterior; in myopia they are usually situated more deeply in the vitreous humour, sometimes even in connexion with the surface of the optic nerve,* and they scarcely ever disappear. In order to see them, the observed eye should be directed downwards, and suddenly raised to the point at which we again look through the plane of the pupil, in which case we usually observe them rapidly floating past. The depth of their position can be determined from the glass with which they are seen, and from the distance from the eye at which the observer must place himself. Usually, they are long and fibrous, or granular, sometimes also

* In reference to this situation, I have occasionally thought there might be a remnant of the artery running in the fœtal state to the capsule of the lens, which has been seen by some, but the brown flake did not extend far in the vitreous body.

perhaps membranous.—The second complaint we mentioned was photopsia. This in general accompanies the more acute amblyopic symptoms of myopes; but sometimes it continues constantly present in high degrees of myopia, and yields to no treatment whatever. Ophthalmoscopically we then usually observe diffuse atrophy, combined with white spots and so-called pigment-maceration, the origin of which is also not unconnected with inflammatory action.—Nervous persons are sometimes very much depressed by the constant phenomena of light, which are still more troublesome in the dark than in the daylight. I believe, too, that they must be looked upon as an unfavourable sign, because they in every case indicate persistent irritation from increasing tension and distention, or from inflammatory action; but still I have found that the power of vision may with them long remain tolerably uniform. The principal point will be, how far the atrophy extends in the region of the yellow spot.

Besides the amblyopia dependent on supervening irritation, the acuteness of vision is in general, as we remarked in the preceding paragraph, diminished in high degrees of myopia; but on this point little complaint is made. As myopes can hold objects so much closer to the eye, and thus look under a greater visual angle, they can still very long sufficiently distinguish them, and from distant vision they have never required much. In general, therefore, they do not apply to the oculist, until a disproportionate disturbance takes place in direct vision. They then complain of obscurity in reading and writing, of a dimness or glimmering which lies over the letters, of truncated letters, or of total absence of others; of total inability to see correctly what they fix. Often this is preceded by the curved appearance of lines, which indicates a disproportionate displacement or transposition forwards of a part of the percipient elements. Where these complaints arise in myopes, we always find also one or other of the above-described changes in the yellow spot. In this region there are almost invariably to be seen whitish spots, little accumulations of pigment, and other proofs of atrophic degeneration, even before any complaint is made. Usually the degeneration of the yellow spot sets in much earlier in one than in the other eye; but while we see it tolerably complete in the one, precisely the changes just mentioned appear in the second eye, and foretell but too certainly, that after a few years direct vision will here also be lost. Against the progress of this degeneration we can by hygienic measures do comparatively little, and by proper medical

treatment nothing whatever.   It is true that even now the acuteness
of vision sometimes improves ; but in this case we must suppose that
the disturbance was dependent rather on irritation of the retina,
supervening on the atrophy : the atrophy itself runs regularly
through its course, and combating the attendant symptoms of irritation can at most retard this course.   The dimness which was complained of, sometimes continues for a long time almost unchanged,
until in a few days or weeks reading becomes wholly impossible.   This
does not always indicate a really quicker development.   The latter,
indeed, occurs, and sometimes even a local effusion of blood in the
yellow spot puts an end at once to direct vision ; but in general it is
only the extension to the fovea centralis, which so rapidly injures the
acuteness of vision.   In fact, there have been almost always long
before numerous little blind spots scattered here and there in the
retina, and particularly around the fovea centralis.   They sometimes
even extend into a part of the fovea centralis, which in another part
still continues available.   Peculiar phenomena may be produced by
these groups of scotomata : thus I have seen cases in which very
small print was more easily and more quickly read than a larger one,
because of the latter a whole word was never seen at once, and even
larger letters were only partly visible.   The glimmering complained
of is entirely due to the fact, that in slight movements of the eye the
letters form their images alternately on sensitive and insensitive parts,
and thus each time come and disappear, sometimes with change of
form, according to irregular displacement of the percipient elements.
So long as the fovea centralis still fixes, the patients can themselves
very well project their scotomata on a surface, for example, on a
sheet of paper, and fixing a given point, can circumscribe the
boundaries of the blind spots with a strongly-contrasting object.   In
this manner we can satisfy ourselves as to the existence of these
groups of scotomata in the region of the yellow spot, without the
fovea centralis being as yet affected and reading having become an
impossibility.

The scotomata in question are little limitations of the field of
vision.   We should suppose that they must exhibit themselves as
black spots.   This, however, they do not : almost invariably they
are seen only more or less distinctly as grey spots.   They approach
in this respect the *undefined non-vision*, the hiatus in the field of
vision, which is projected through the nerve-surface, and this is, in
fact, to be compared with the portion of space lying beyond our

field of vision, for example, behind us ; we do not see it black, we see it *not*. That, however, local scotomata of the retina also should not appear black, is certainly strange, the more so because that with respect to them, we cannot think of subjective action, which must exhibit itself in the dark or in closed eyes as light.

In connexion with scotomata, it seems fit here to state some facts with reference to limitation of the field of vision in general. Even long ago some knowledge existed on this subject. Mariotte discovered the blind spot named after him, which discovery attracted much attention at the time, and gave rise to various theories. Latterly, too, it has often been treated of. Determinations of its magnitude and position might have led to the inference, that it corresponds to the nerve-surface, before I had shown that a little image of a flame, thrown with the ophthalmoscope upon this surface, actually does not become visible to the eye under examination, until it passes the bounds of the nerve-surface. It was known, too, that the field of vision is sometimes partly lost, and hemiopia and visus dimidiatus were spoken of. But I believe I am correct in stating that the systematic investigation of the limits of the field of vision in amblyopia was first introduced into practice by von Graefe.* Dr. Snellen subsequently applied himself to show, that in many cases of amblyopia, without actual limitation and without scotomata, particularly where ophthalmoscopic investigation exhibited no morbid changes, direct vision is almost always very much diminished in the whole region of the yellow spot : the boundary where the duller vision begins, is in these cases often tolerably accurately indicated on the projected field of vision.— The limitation of the field of vision is in general examined in the way in which Mariotte demonstrated the lacuna discovered by him. However, the projection takes place at a shorter distance (which in myopes is indeed necessary), in general at the distance of a foot, unless a high degree of myopia requires still greater proximity. In order to be able to preserve the result obtained, we, on each trial, make use of a separate sheet of paper, of a dark-blue colour, 70 centimetres (27½ English inches) in breadth, and 60 (23½ English inches) in height, which is fixed in a frame and is thus hung up vertically. On this a little white cross is now drawn, and a small piece of clean white chalk fastened in a long, dark handle (the colour of the paper), is then moved in all direc-

* *Archiv für Ophthalmologie*, B. ii.

tions from the periphery of the field of vision, with a slight shaking
motion, towards the fixed cross, and the point is marked where the
chalk seems to disappear.   If a blind place is thus found, we proceed
with the chalk in all directions from it, and mark the points where
the chalk begins to be seen.   These points we connect with a line,
which now indicates the boundaries of the limitation.   The ascertained
field of vision is then copied on a small scale in the record of the
patient's case, and the blind part is blackened.   If a part of
the field of vision is found to be in-
sensible to the white chalk, but not to
stronger impressions of light, for example,
to those of a little flame, this is indicated
by streaks (compare Fig. 149, being the
projection, consequently the inverted
image of a right eye with $M = \frac{1}{3}$, S
$= \frac{14}{70}$, and limitation of the field of vision

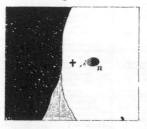

Fig. 149.

by detachment of the retina,—the projection reduced for a distance
of about 18 mm., and therefore the distance between the nodal point
and the retina being assumed to be equal to 18 mm., of the natural
size, at least for the central parts): the little cross signifies the
fixed point, that is, the projection of the fovea centralis; n, the
blind spot of Mariotte.   It is evident that in the method described
the most external part of the field of vision is not examined.   In
general, this is done with sufficient accuracy, according to the mode
stated at page 193.

   As limitations more properly peculiar to myopia, we have, in addition to the above-mentioned scotomata, still to mention chiefly those
which occur as amplifications of the spot of Mariotte; as well as
those which depend on atrophic spots developed with inflammatory
symptoms; on detachment of the retina, in consequence of exudation
and sometimes of extravasation of blood; on extravasation of blood
also in the tissue of the retina; finally, on glaucoma.—As to the
spot of Mariotte, von Graefe states that a magnifying of its surface
in the sclerotico-chorioiditis (the staphyloma posticum) of myopes can
always be demonstrated.   Von Hasner and others state the same.
Von Jaeger attributes this to the displacing inwards of the optic nerve
assumed by him, with which, of course, the percipient layer must be
defective at the margin of the chorioideal opening.   My investigations have shown that with a slight development of the crescent, as

we can observe ophthalmoscopically with a little image of light, the perception of light is not deficient there, but that in high degrees with complete atrophy it really wholly, or almost entirely, disappears (compare Fig. 148 n) : sometimes even we find again tolerably accurately in the projected form that of the crescent. It is also in a physiological point of view not unimportant, that even in those cases the conduction of the more peripherically received stimulus of the retina is not deficient over the atrophic crescent,—whence it appears, that the fibrous layer of the retina, through which this conduction must take place, has not essentially suffered.—Respecting the smaller and larger scotomata of the atrophic spots, we have no more to say; it is enough that those, too, do not interrupt the conduction from more peripheric parts.—Detachment of the retina is one of the worst morbid forms, to which the myopic eye is much more liable than any other; it is met with chiefly in the lowermost half, which according to von Graefe is to be ascribed to the fact, that when it occurs in high parts, it may, by sinking of the fluid be transmitted downwards. Sometimes it is only to a slight extent, and the retina is but little removed from the chorioidea. In other instances a great part, nay even the whole retina, may be detached, and it then, according to the very correct expression of Arlt, assumes the form of a convolvulus-flower, whose stem is the optic nerve. When the detached portion is of moderate size it projects far enough into the vitreous humour to be seen, even in considerable M, not inverted, without a negative, or even with a positive glass. We recognize it at once by its grey colour, and by the moveable folds of the membrane, on which the retinal vessels are very distinctly visible, at first even with difference of colour of the arteries and veins. It is remarkable that the perception of light has then not yet ceased, so that we must suppose that the layer of rods has separated with the retina, and may in this state continue sensitive to the impressions of light. A striking case of this kind occurred to me. A girl, aged fifteen, with $M = \dfrac{1}{2\frac{1}{2}}$ in both eyes, on a sudden cried out with joy that she could see the people at the other side of the street before the window, and could even recognise them. Her joy was, however, of short duration. Three days later the eye was quite blind, and I discovered a detachment of the retina, extending through the yellow spot, whereby the latter was pushed forward almost into the posterior focus of the eye. Whether, in general, in detachment of the retina, the disturbance is very important, depends chiefly on its seat : if the

yellow spot is implicated, the eye is to be considered as nearly lost;
if it has remained free it is nevertheless often deranged in its function, especially when the detachment extends into the vicinity of
the spot; but this disturbance may, under proper management, again
in great part give way.   Not unfrequently, however, the detachment
sooner or later extends still further.   Von Graefe thinks he has observed that this takes place chiefly when, with staphyloma posticum,
extensive atrophy exists in the fundus oculi, and I believe I must
agree with him in that opinion.   But still I have seen a few cases,
where, with advanced atrophy, a partial detachment of the retina
was for many years stationary, and the acuteness of vision in the
yellow spot was maintained.   Well-established cases of recovery by
the spontaneous replacement of the retina are very rare.   I have
seen only one, in which, too, a relapse occurred, and Liebreich also
has described one.*   This melancholy result certainly justified the
attempt to effect an improvement by means of operation, and such
has really in some cases been obtained.   If the detached retina has
once become atrophic,—and this is pretty often the case, as is apparent
from the disproportionate loading of the vessels, with perceptibly
metamorphosed blood, the presence of pigment spots, the loss of
colour and a certain transparency,—discharge of the fluid, or section,
can have no other object than to prevent, so far as possible, the further extension of the lesion.   Almost always the fluid situated behind
the retina is of a serous nature, more or less turbid, and subject to
further metamorphosis.   Such fluid will here occur, when it can be
exuded from the vessels under higher pressure than that to which
the vitreous humour is exposed.   The condition for its formation we
know not, but it is certain that when the retina is detached the bulb is
usually soft.   It is very plausible to assume that the extension which
the retina undergoes in staphyloma posticum may cause it to
be more easily separated from the chorioidea, and it seems certain
that increasing staphyloma must promote its further detachment.
In this state now the limitation of the field of vision is and continues
to be the principal phenomenon.   In the commencement especially
the limitation is still more extensive than the detachment, and often
it seems that direct vision is almost destroyed, while, nevertheless, it
subsequently appears that the yellow spot is not involved in the
process.   Exceptionally, too, effusion of blood is the cause of detachment of the retina.   This is true, not only of myopic, but also of

* *Archiv f. Ophthalmologie*, B. v. 2. p. 251.

other eyes. Occasionally one or more relapses of hæmorrhage of the chorioidea occur, with perforation of the retina, after which the blood effused in the vitreous humour, each time in proportion as the eye has meanwhile become softer, appears in greater quantity, to be each time again more or less perfectly absorbed. Finally, on a fresh relapse, the blood remains now also behind the retina, and separates it from the chorioidea. At the same time it may partly be again effused in the vitreous humour. In general, the detached retina cannot be distinguished so well when blood occurs behind it ; and when there is simultaneous effusion into the vitreous humour, the diagnosis is at first often very uncertain, and the investigation, in what directions perception of light has remained, is, on account of the opacity of the blood accumulated in the lower parts of the vitreous humour, very deceptive. — The hæmorrhages here spoken of, certainly occur more frequently in myopic than in other eyes, and it is easy to understand that while in atrophy the larger bloodvessels of the chorioidea continue long filled with blood, the disposition to laceration through further extension must exist. However, on account of the frequent occurrence of detachment by a serous fluid, precisely in myopic eyes, the separation of the retina is in them comparatively still more rarely the result of effusion of blood, than in other eyes. To effusions of blood in the retina itself, and from the retinal vessels, the myopic eye is also very much inclined. The circumscribed extravasation of blood, sometimes to be seen in the yellow spot, and in some measure elevating the latter, is certainly derived from effusion from a chorioideal vessel; on the other hand, we not unfrequently see in the retina itself a number of smaller extravasations near the retinal vessels, and apparently derived from the latter. Of some larger retinal sanguineous infiltrations it is also more than probable that they took their origin from retinal vessels. The chief symptom in these cases is the scotoma, or the interruption of the field of vision, which is always more remarked and more troublesome, the closer it is to the yellow spot.

With all these morbid changes in the fundus oculi occur, to a greater than ordinary extent, changes in the vitreous humour, which in general give rise only to flakes floating before the field of vision, but, nevertheless, in some instances, especially when they are of a membranous nature, very essentially interfere with the power of vision ; and with these changes of the vitreous humour is combined the disposition to opacity of the lens, which, undoubtedly, is greater

26

in myopes than in emmetropes. It is remarkable that in the commencement of cataract myopes imagine that it is only their myopia which is increasing. As they see objects at a short distance from the eye under great angles, they do not so immediately experience much inconvenience, for example, in reading. Therefore, they remark at most that with respect to distinguishing at a distance they are retrograding, and they are surprised only that their myopia, which ought to improve with years, as it is said, is on the increase.

In connexion, finally, with high degrees of staphyloma posticum, glaucoma is not unfrequently developed, especially at a more advanced period of life; this, however, in its typical form, belongs rather to the emmetropic and to the hypermetropic eye. When combined with high degrees of M, it appears as if it ought, even in its origin, to be considered as a distinct form of disease, having for the most part, in common with ordinary glaucoma, only increased tension of the eyeball and excavation of the optic nerve. It is glaucoma simplex in so far as the ordinary inflammatory symptoms proper to glaucoma are wanting, but beyond this it is distinguished from ordinary glaucoma by less hardness of the eyeball, oblique direction of the excavation, unusual limitation of the field of vision, and the absence of other symptoms; while, moreover, we cannot in these cases reckon so certainly upon the results to be obtained by iridectomy, as in the ordinary cases of glaucoma.—Lastly, we have still to observe, in connexion with this subject, that in apparent strabismus convergens (the result of displacement of the visual line) the mobility of strongly myopic eyes is often somewhat limited, that especially sufficient convergence for binocular vision is not attained, so that perseverance in the attempt to effect it leads to muscular asthenopia, and therefore those who are highly myopic usually read only with one eye, and that not unfrequently relative, and at length absolute diverging strabismus is the result. Of this I think it more convenient to speak in a separate paragraph.

§ 31. Insufficiency of the internal Muscles and Diverging Strabismus, both Results of M.

Diverging strabismus is in general combined with M. In the commencement of my statistical investigations, I had become aware of the connexion between hypermetropia and strabismus convergens;

but I was far from suspecting that myopia stands in almost as close a relation to strabismus divergens. Systematic investigation first brought this to light.

The nature of the connexion is not, however, in each case the same. If hypermetropia produces strabismus convergens, this takes place in fact in virtue of the tension of accommodation required in consequence of the anomaly of refraction. If strabismus divergens arises, in connexion with myopia, the anomaly of refraction, as such, is not indeed wholly without action, but the anatomical element has the chief causal influence, I mean *the distention and the altered form of the eyeball*: therefore where myopia exceptionally depends on other causes, consequent strabismus is not to be expected. In the ordinary forms of M, the greater dimensions in general in themselves interfere with the mobility of the eye, but still it is chiefly the ellipsoidal form, which, in turning round the short axes in a cavity of similar shape, in consequence of the required change of form, gives rise to great resistance. Besides, the centre of motion has removed not only from the anterior but also from the posterior surface of the eye. Besides its position is in general not unfavourable. Investigations made in concert with Dr. Doÿer showed, namely, that it is situated behind the middle of the visual axis, and indeed in such proportion, that the part in front of the centre of motion is to the part of the visual axis behind this centre as $57\cdot32 : 42\cdot46$, that is about $= 15 : 11$. But almost the same proportion was found also in the longer visual axis of myopes: it is in the latter on an average even somewhat less favourable, namely, $= 56\cdot83 : 43\cdot17$. The annexed table, in which the angle a is also introduced (compare p. 181), contains the results of observation in detail.

No.	Age.	Eye.	M	Length of the Visual Axis		Position of the Centre of Motion		a
				To the Retina.	To the Posterior Surface of the Sclerotic.	Behind the Anterior Surface of the Cornea.	Before the Posterior Surface of the Sclerotic.	
1	32	D	1 : 16	22·96	24·16	13·49	10·67	5°·00
2	26	D	1 : 10	23·43	24·53	13·49	11·04	4°·00
,,	,,	S	1 : 10	23·43	24·53	13·59	10·94	5°·25
3	27	S	1 : 9·25	23·53	24·63	15·22	9·41	4°·00
,,	,,	D	1 : 6·25	24·24	25·04	14·19	10·85	4°·00
4	35	D	1 : 6·25	24·24	25·04	13·18	11·86	—1°·50
5	18	D	1 : 6·25	24·24	25·04	14·97	10·07	4°·75
6	26	D	1 : 5·25	24·69	25·39	13·77	11·62	1°·50
,,	,,	S	1 : 5·25	24·69	25·39	14·78	10·61	1°·00
7	49	D	1 : 4·75	24·99	25·59	14·90	10·69	—1°·25
8	19	D	1 : 4·75	24·99	25·59	14·64	10·95	—1°·00
,,	,,	S	1 : 4·75	24·99	25·59	14·52	11·07	—1°·00
4	35	S	1 : 4·25	25·39	25·89	13·79	12·10	1°·75
9	18	S	1 : 4·25	25·39	25·89	15·52	10·37	4°·50
10	23	S	1 : 4·25	25·39	25·89	15·97	9·92	2°·00
11	9	D	1 : 3·75	25·91	26·31	14·91	11·40	2°·00
10	23	D	1 : 2·25	29·56	29·76	15·86	13·90	—1°·50

The table shows that, with a single exception, the centre of motion in the myopic eye is absolutely farther from the posterior surface of the sclerotic than in the emmetropic (= 9·99 mm.), and in general the more so, the higher the degree of M is; and almost invariably, too, the *relative* position in the visual axis is more unfavourable. Moreover the angle a (between the axis of the cornea and visual line) is particularly small, and in five cases is even negative, that is, it is situated to the outside of the axis of the cornea.

As a result of the greater distance from the centre of motion to the posterior surface of the sclerotic, the excursions are in these cases greater for equal degrees of rotation, and turning is therefore necessarily limited. This limitation would be still greater, if the entrance of the optic nerve was not, in consequence of disproportionate extension of the *external* posterior part of the segment, usually transferred more inwards, and thus removed comparatively less from the centre of motion. Besides, the greater distance between the centre of motion and the points of insertion of the muscles, to which distance the arc of rotation, obtained with a given shortening of the muscles, is inversely proportional, may contribute to produce limitation.

Meanwhile, apart from all this, the longer eyeball, as such, sufficiently accounts for the existing limitation. This is true of movement both inwards and outwards. In myopes it is so general, that of the seventeen eyes nine fell so short, that in the determination of the centre of motion our method (compare p. 185), requiring an excursion inwards and outwards of not more than 28°, was not applicable without modification.   The limited movement outward has, in the first place, no other result than that the lateral excursions for distant binocular vision are less, and that turning the head more rapidly must supplement it, which besides is necessary in wearing spectacles.   But the insufficiency of the turning inwards has other and more important results, which we have consecutively to consider, in order to arrive at the occurrence of absolute diverging strabismus, as its ultimate effect.

Insufficiency of the inward movement we assume, when the visual lines cannot be brought to intersect at a distance of $2''\cdot5$, at which they cut one another under an angle of about 51°.   In high degrees of myopia this insufficiency exists almost without exception. For this a double cause may be assigned. In the first place, the mobility is, as we have seen, actually diminished by distention and modification of form, and the insufficiency is so far to be considered *absolute*.   But, in the second place, in order to bring the visual lines to intersect at the distance of $2''\cdot5$, the angle a being small, the axes of the cornea must be brought under still *stronger* convergence than in emmetropic eyes.   We thus understand that even where the inward movement does not fall absolutely too short, it must at least relatively do so.

Now the insufficiency of which we are here speaking, leads in some instances to fatigue in vision, when the work requires a certain convergence to be maintained for a long consecutive period (*asthenopia muscularis*).

Cases have occurred to me, in which there was at first vision with both eyes, but where, on fatigue, the one eye gave way, and the work was then attended with less difficulty ; others where precisely that giving way caused trouble and was complained of.   This latter state I met with where the degree of M was comparatively slight, and where, therefore, besides the resistance of the eye, a certain weakness of the muscles (not only insufficiency of movement, but true *insufficiency of the musculi recti interni*) must be understood : a condition, which in moderate degrees of M, I have found to be hereditary, with the phenomena just described.   With this giving way on continued tension *relative diverging strabismus* is already admitted : at a greater distance the visual lines are properly directed; in close work only one eye is used.

Relative diverging strabismus is here represented as the result, in some sense as a further development, of the insufficiency of the inward movement. To a certain extent this is correct. But if we endeavour to define this relative strabismus, it appears that it is inseparable from high degrees of M, and that if the movement were not at the same time limited, the strabismus would nevertheless be present. Relative diverging strabismus, in fact, exists, so soon as the proximity required for acute sight excludes binocular vision. In unlimited convergence also it therefore occurs, so soon as the farthest point of distinct vision has approached to within the point of convergence of the eyes. Taken in this sense, relative diverging strabismus is, for example, with $M > \dfrac{1}{2 \cdot 5}$ necessarily present: always indeed (cases of strabismus convergens excepted), when there is acute vision without glasses, the one eye has deviated outwards.

In the foregoing it is included that relative diverging strabismus may arise: on the one hand, where there is considerable insufficiency of the musculi recti interni, without any myopia; on the other, in high degrees of myopia, without any insufficiency. In fact, it occurs in its most important forms, when M and insufficiency are combined in a moderate degree. Myopia must here be our starting-point. If the myopia be absent, the insufficiency usually produces only muscular asthenopia, and is seldom developed to strabismus divergens. If M be present, a number of causes coincide, to produce strabismus divergens, at least relative, and precisely thus to prevent asthenopia muscularis.*

The formula is simple, and has already been given above in reference to insufficiency: myopia requires more convergence of the visual lines, because vision takes place closer to the eye, and precisely in M the convergence is for two reasons more difficult, first, on account of the impeded movement, and secondly, on account of the altered direction of the visual lines (the smaller angle a).

* Thus we read also in von Graefe (*Archiv f. Oph.* B. viii. p. 343):— "It has been already mentioned that myopia supplies an important, but not absolutely preponderating contingent (in muscular asthenopia). The latter would indeed be the case, *if those who are highly myopic did not pass through the period of asthenopia into strabismus divergens, much more rapidly* than hypermetropes and emmetropes."

That relative diverging strabismus occurs preferentially in M, follows from these facts as a matter of course. And this is still more the case because the need of binocular vision and the aversion to double images, here afford no important counterbalancing power. It is almost always a small object that the myope wishes to see acutely : he approximates it to the eye that he wishes to use, and the other is meanwhile directed to remote objects which, on account of the myopia, supply very diffuse, and therefore but very slightly disturbing images. If now vision once takes place with deviation, there can be little tendency to make the tension required for convergence;—the less so, because at the same time the distance R (that of the farthest point of distinct vision) would become smaller, and the object should therefore be held still closer to the eye. Precisely when difficulty in convergence begins to be experienced, does the associated tension of accommodation become particularly great.

In progressive myopia we often observe how binocular vision attempts to maintain itself against the relative diverging strabismus. It is, however, usually obliged speedily to give way to the fatigue arising from the tension. Reading, for example, is at first binocular, but after some time one eye yields, involuntarily and unconsciously, so that the complaint is made that one page moves over the other. We can now establish numerous transitions. If an object be approximated more and more to the eyes, the convergence increases to nearly its maximum. If the object remains here, one eye yields the more speedily, the nearer the object had approached to the maximum of convergence. It immediately gives way when the object is brought to within the maximum of convergence. This happens likewise directly when in strong convergence the one eye is covered with the hand. If the covering hand is now removed, the yielding of the convergence nevertheless continues. Even when the object was approximated to the eye, while before the other open eye the hand is held, the convergence is seldom sufficient: the endeavour to maintain the binocular vision commenced at a greater distance, was the absolute condition under which the convergence was developed; in perfectly established relative diverging strabismus, even under that condition, it is absent. The greatest difficulty is always experienced when the eyes are directed upwards. As a transition we observe, that in fatigue there is no convergence, while the latter appears after rest has been enjoyed.

On the boundaries between alternating and confirmed relative diverging strabismus lies a practically important condition, to which I formerly directed attention.* The condition is this : there is still tendency to convergence, this is seen on approximating an object : but even before the distance of distinct vision is attained, or at least soon after, the one eye deviates. If we now give concave spectacles, which bring the binocular farthest point to 8″, 10″, or 12″, vision again takes place with both eyes. Often, however, complaints are now heard of the occurrence of fatigue, and examination shows, that not the tension of accommodation, but the convergence required, slight as it is, is the cause thereof. Consequently, asthenopia muscularis is in operation, so that, in order to make binocular vision possible, a combination of the concave with a prismatic glass is required. In these cases it is especially evident, that the cause of the relative diverging strabismus is to be sought solely in the impeded movement inwards, while the tendency to co-operation of the two retinas for the sake of binocular vision may continue undisturbed. It is only in absolute diverging strabismus that that tendency is, as shall hereafter appear, not unfrequently removed.

We have above seen, how in progressive M binocular vision for near objects usually in vain endeavours to maintain itself. To this there are, however, exceptions. " A powerful simultaneous action of the recti interni" even belongs, according to von Graefe,† to a "relative normal shortsightedness." He goes so far as to assert, that it is to be considered as a *pathological condition*, " when the increase in the power of tension of the internal muscles of the eye does not continue in harmonic development with the increase of the refractive condition (of the myopia)." Indeed, even in high degrees of M, whether on account of a favourable size of the eyeball, or of an original or acquired preponderance of the internal recti muscles, the visual lines may sometimes be properly directed in close vision, and may without effort be kept in that direction. But this in many cases is obtained only at the expense of the mobility outwards. Limitation of the latter is, in such instances, rarely absent, and it may now attain to that degree, that the visual lines cannot in distant vision be brought to parallelism, which constitutes relative converging strabismus. And if with increasing M in these cases the convergence for near objects also becomes insufficient, we have the singular combination of relative diverging strabismus, in vision for near objects, with relative converging strabismus in distant vision, while

* *Archiv für Ophthalm.* B. vii. Abth. 1, p. 83.
† *Archiv*, B. iii., 1, p. 309.

at a medium distance a certain margin has remained for binocular vision.   It reminds us of the combination of M with presbyopia.— However, as I have observed, this is all exceptional.   The rule is, that the facility of convergence does not keep pace with the development of the myopia, and that the tendency to relative diverging strabismus rapidly becomes remarkable.   I satisfied myself by investigation, that, proceeding from the visual lines, in M the mobility inwards is in a great number of cases very soon limited,* while that outwards is in no way impeded, nay, that under the influence of a prism, the visual lines can generally be brought even under greater divergence than in non-myopes. It appeared, indeed, to be in favour of the more ready convergence of myopes, that, as my determinations of the relative range of accommodation showed, certain degrees of convergence are possible, without proportionate tension of accommodation. This, however, furnishes no absolute proof. From this we learn only that, by practice, the association of accommodative tension may, up to a certain degree, become independent of the effort at convergence, without preventing its reappearance when the effort is stronger.

The *absolute diverging strabismus* is distinguished by divergence of the visual lines in distant vision.   In close vision the divergence sometimes remains unchanged; generally it diminishes, or even gives place to a certain degree of convergence, but not being sufficient, binocular vision is still excluded.   In a few cases, however, I observed, that in looking to a great distance divergence existed, but that, on looking to the distance of some feet or some inches, this gave way to *sufficient* convergence, which was then, however, not to be maintained. The fact is remarkable. The explanation may be, that binocular vision is much more important for the estimation of near, than for that of remote, objects.—At first, diverging strabismus exists usually in a slight degree, and only slowly increases. Sometimes it continues in but a slight degree during the whole of life. I have, indeed, found that precisely the highest degrees of diverging strabismus not unfrequently have another origin than simple myopia.

It is commonly the custom to apply the term squint exclusively to the absolute form.   In this sense it is less frequent than strabismus convergens.   And if, nevertheless, a certain number

---

* On this subject still further investigations have been made by one of our students, Mr. Schuerman : the mobility of the eyes, the maximum of convergence, the relation to prismatic glasses, &c., have been, in connexion with the axis of the cornea and the visual line, with determination, at the same time, of the position of the centre of motion, investigated in eyes of different refraction.

of cases, about equal to that in strabismus convergens, is to be
explained by primary disturbance of the muscles (paralysis, inflammation, spasm, complicated congenital anomalies, &c., a blind eye
also often deviates outwards), myopia cannot occupy the same prominent position as an etiological element, that hypermetropia does
in reference to strabismus convergens ; nevertheless, in about two-
thirds of the cases of *absolute* diverging strabismus, myopia was
met with. But if, on the other hand, we take *relative* diverging strabismus also into account, the diverging form is as frequent, if not
more frequent than the converging; and now, moreover, the extraordinary causes, originally proceeding from the muscles or from blindness in one eye, fall into the background : therefore in at least 90 per
cent. of the cases of *relative* diverging strabismus we find M.—It
is often remarked that while strabismus convergens usually occurs
in childhood, strabismus divergens is most frequently not developed
until a later period. The observation is correct. The fact is connected with the cause of its occurrence : *progressive myopia.*

Now if, in general, absolute diverging strabismus proceeds from
relative, it is far from being the case, as appears even from the
relations described, that the relative should always be followed by
the absolute form. This appears to be rather the exception. We
here meet with a like relation to the cause as in converging strabismus. Thus, as most hypermetropes are spared from the latter
affection, we certainly find many myopes with relative diverging
strabismus, without the absolute form being developed from it.
Here, therefore, the question also arises : What accessory circumstance causes the true absolute diverging strabismus to occur ?

Perhaps we may be able to invert this question, if we first consider why, in general, the relative deviation predisposes to the absolute. The result of this consideration may be thus formulised :—

Relative diverging strabismus gives dissimilar images on the two
yellow spots, particularly in close vision. The need of equality of
impressions, the effort at simple binocular vision must, in general,
be consequently weakened. A commencement of deviation, having
arisen where much advanced convergence was required, immediately
attains a tolerably high degree, by simply yielding to the natural tension of the muscles,—partly also, perhaps, although unconsciously,
in order to make the double images more remote from each other,
or to exclude the tension of accommodation associated with diffi-

cult convergence, and thus to remove the farthest point of distinct vision from the eye.   In general, when, for example, with blindness of one eye, the internal recti muscles are no longer for the sake of binocular vision of near objects stimulated to contraction, they soon, through diminished energy, become ineffectual, and strabismus divergens is the usual result thereof.   Relative diverging strabismus now leads to similar inaction, likewise followed by diminished energy. Thus two important factors coincide : slight resistance to double images, and diminished force of the internal muscles.   It can, therefore, not be a matter of surprise that, in distant vision also, the action of the latter soon fails.   And this must occur the sooner in myopes, because the angle a is particularly small, and therefore distant vision requires a slighter divergence of the corneal axes than in emmetropes.   Now, if the action of the internal muscles be once weakened, the effort to overcome the tendency to divergence will easily make the farthest point of distinct vision approach the eye, will thus render the retinal images of remote objects still more diffuse, and instinctively this effort will therefore not occur, or it will be removed.

Thus, undoubtedly, the origin of absolute diverging strabismus is satisfactorily explained.   If I am not mistaken, we must now really, as I foresaw, invert the foregoing question.   We ask no longer: What accessory circumstance, where relative diverging strabismus exists, leads to the development of the absolute variety ?   We rather inquire : What is the reason that not every relative diverging strabismus is followed by the absolute form ?

In the first place, I remark that absolute diverging strabismus is, as I find more and more every day, in high degrees of myopia very general, much more general than is supposed.   Slight degrees pass unobserved, because, although the visual lines diverge, the corneal axes exhibit no particular divergence, often certainly still less than in non-squinting hypermetropes : it is not until the properly directed eye is covered, that it appears that the visual line of the other was directed too much outwards.   But I repeat the question : What is the reason why not *every* relative diverging strabismus is followed by the absolute form ?

The cause of this lies partly in the maintenance of binocular vision.   Although, in consequence of relative diverging strabismus, the attempt to obtain equal impressions on the two yellow spots and on further corresponding points is weakened, it is not extinguished.

This attempt alone sometimes restrains the deviation. In many the one eye actually turns outwards behind the hand, to reassume a proper direction when uncovered. And where this giving way does not take place, it is sufficient to hold a weak prismatic glass, with the refracting angle towards the nose, before the eye, to satisfy ourselves of the attempt at binocular vision : we immediately see a convergence set in, correcting the action of the prism. Only in the highest degrees of myopia, where even no strongly-marked object forms comparable images, is the convergence absent in this experiment. It thus also appears that acute sight is not an absolute condition for, if possible, maintaining single vision.

Further, we seek the cause of the absence of absolute strabismus in limited mobility of the eyes. Turning the great ellipsoidal eyeball of myopes is impeded not only inwards, but sometimes also outwards. This obstruction may go so far that, as I have above remarked, relative converging strabismus in distant vision may be combined with relative diverging strabismus in near vision. But even if it does not attain this degree, it really hinders an excessive deviation outwards, especially when it is allied to the need of binocular vision.

Thus then, just as in converging strabismus, different impelling and resisting forces contend with one another, and it is in fact difficult to say under what conditions the first acquire the preponderance. Experience did not at least immediately reveal them.

Undoubtedly, however, there come under observation : a, circumstances which promote movement outwards ; b, such as deprive binocular vision of its value. Among the first we include an original preponderance of the external recti muscles, more than ordinary displacement of the visual lines, in consequence of myopia (extraordinarily slight or even negative value of the angle a), further a favourable form for outward movement, and superficial position of the eyeball. Among the latter may be reckoned, diminished acuteness of vision in the one eye, and especially a difference of refraction in the two eyes. This last occurs as an influential factor. If the difference of refraction is great, the one eye highly myopic, the other scarcely so or even emmetropic, the rule is perhaps that in distant vision the myopic eye has deviated outwards. These cases furnish a peculiar form of strabismus divergens, which certainly deserves to be thoroughly investigated and separately described. Sometimes, especially at first, the squint is intermittent, and manifests itself only either on fatigue or under certain states of mind; in other cases it may, even when highly developed, be overcome by the will, particularly for near objects, for a short interval, although not without rapidly supervening fatigue, and at all events without essential advantage to the sight. Not unfrequently, too, the one eye is used in distant, the other in close vision. Usually each eye projects and judges correctly, while it sees independently, and notwithstanding it is declared that the same object seen with the one eye appears larger, with the other smaller. More that is remarkable still remains to be mentioned, and especially to be investigated, on this subject. As to its pathogeny, with which alone we are, properly speaking, at present concerned,—it is easy to see that, in the first place, binocular vision in these cases has not much value; secondly, that, particularly in distant vision, the double images of ordinary objects are scarcely observed, and the patient thus easily abstracts from the impression of the strongly myopic eye; thirdly, that the limited mobility in this case affects only the one eye, and a relative deviation outwards must therefore meet with less difficulty; and finally, that so soon as any tension of the musculi recti interni is required, in order to prevent divergence of the visual lines, this tension will therefore be absent, because the weakly myopic or emmetropic eye seeing tolerably acutely at a distance, in consequence of the accompanying tension of accommodation, immediately perceives less perfectly.

It is well known that Buffon (*Sur la cause du strabisme ou des yeux louches*, in *Memoires de l'Académie*, 1743,—to be found also in Buffon, *Histoire*, &c., Supplém. iv., p. 416, Paris, 1777) sought the principal cause of squinting in a difference between the two eyes. That difference he calls rather indefinitely, "une inégalité de force dans les yeux." Evidently he had in view in his definition a difference in refraction; but in his examination of squinters this is sometimes confounded with a difference in acuteness of vision. Buffon especially endeavours to show, that unequal impressions of the same objects on corresponding parts of the retina are more disturbing than those of wholly different objects. The one eye would therefore instinctively deviate where there is a great difference between the eyes. In this he has had in view chiefly, I should almost say exclusively, strabismus convergens; but at the close of his essay he speaks also of some cases, "where one eye is used in looking at distant, the other at near objects, while the unused eye deviates either inwards or *outwards*." Besides, Buffon thinks that, so far as the regions of accommodation for the two eyes coincide, even when the boundaries of those regions differ, both eyes may receive sharp images of the same object, and that thus the tension of accommodation in each eye, independently of the other, can regulate itself according to the distance of the object. On this error a great deal of his demonstration rests.

Joh. Mueller (*Vergl. Physiologie*, etc., p. 228), admitting the fact, is not satisfied with Buffon's explanation. He gives us another, remarkable chiefly because in it a disturbed connexion between convergence and accommodation is assumed. We miss in Mueller the distinction between presbyopia and hypermetropia; nor does he ask whether strabismus convergens or divergens is to be explained, and a clear insight into the cause of the affection could not thus be acquired. But we find the experiment stated in which, by holding a concave glass before one of the eyes, strabismus convergens is excited, so soon as this eye is used for acute vision,—an experiment which explains the exceptional cases of strabismus convergens, where the properly-directed eye is hypermetropic, the deviating eye less hypermetropic, or even emmetropic, but originally amblyopic. Had Joh. Mueller held a negative glass before each eye, it would not have escaped him, that thus also a deviation inwards is readily produced, and probably his clear glance would at once have penetrated the character of hypermetropia and its connexion with strabismus.

Some (compare Böhm, *Das Schielen, l. c.*; Artl, *Die Krankheiten des Auges*, B. iii., pp. 306 *et seq.*, Prag, 1856) attach too much, others (compare Ruete, *Lehrbuch der Ophthalmologie*, B. ii., p. 524) attach too little value to difference between the two eyes, whether in acuteness of vision or refraction, in reference to the origin of strabismus. I think I have shown that the difference mentioned does not occur as the immediate cause of strabismus, but that it may be the reason why, with certain determining conditions, to be sought in the non-deviating eye, strabismus is produced.

The connexion, too, between myopia of the two eyes, and strabismus divergens was formerly not completely overlooked. Joh. Mueller (*Vergleichende Physiologie*, p. 237) even describes a *strabismus myopum*. "It is known," thus he commences the explanation of the mode of development, "that shortsighted people look at very near objects only with one eye, while the other eye, which is also nearsighted, completely turned away and directed to a distance, sees indistinctly or not at all." This is the state which we have called *relative diverging strabismus*. It has been described by Buffon, as occurring in his own eyes. In his own case he introduces the difference of the images in the two eyes into the explanation; but in general he finds in the extraordinary convergence required by myopes, the reason, "that the sight is fatigued and less distinct than in looking with a single eye." Mueller assigns the first place to the same cause, but in addition points to the increasing refraction produced by the convergence. However, in explaining why the visual axis subsequently deviates permanently also more or less from the normal direction, he thinks only of the neglect of one eye resulting from the deviation, nor do we then read that this deviation takes place positively *outwards*.—Ruete, too (*l. c.*, B. i. p. 226), speaks of the connexion between myopia and strabismus. We saw, that, while in general relative diverging strabismus and a tendency to absolute are connected with high degrees of progressive myopia, the convergence in close vision is exceptionally maintained, though at the expense of parallelism in distant vision. Now this exception, whereby converging strabismus—relative, if we will—is combined with progressive myopia, was recognised by Ruete, not the diverging strabismus, which is the rule. Even of the existence of *relative* diverging strabismus he could not satisfy himself, undoubtedly because he sought it in too slight degrees of myopia, where it is usually wanting.

On the whole, little satisfaction is obtained by consulting the more recent copious literature on strabismus, with reference to its causes. Strabismus divergens, in particular, is very imperfectly treated of. A distinction of the causes, according to the different forms, is not to be met with, and where the causes of strabismus in general are spoken of, the writers have evidently been filled with the idea of strabismus convergens. I have yet only to refer to the writings of von Graefe, with respect to the insufficiency of the internal recti muscles, in the numerous modifications of which the gradual transition to strabismus divergens is to be sought, and where it certainly has been sought for by von Graefe. " We may in general"—thus we read in his latest essay (*Archiv f. Ophth.*, B. viii., Abth. 2)—"define the insufficiency as a dynamic *outward squint*, varying according to the distances of the object, which is *at the time* overcome by the attempt at single vision." If we reflect that, even according to von Graefe, this effort must in myopia often give way, it is as if we, under certain conditions, already see before us the development of absolute diverging strabismus.

Our investigations have thus led us to a striking result, which may be expressed in the following antithesis :—

Hypermetropia causes accommodative asthenopia, to be actively overcome by strabismus convergens.

Myopia leads to muscular asthenopia, passively yielding to strabismus divergens.

----

§ 32. Hygiene.—Treatment.—Spectacles.—Illustrative Cases.—History of Myopia.

The cure of myopia belongs to the *pia vota*. The more our knowledge of the basis of this anomaly has been established, the more certainly does any expectation in that direction appear to be destroyed, even with respect to the future. So long as it was thought that the cause of myopia might be found in increased convexity of the cornea, the endeavour to restore the latter, by pressure, to its normal curvature (Purkinje* and Ruete) appeared perhaps not altogether to be rejected ; but the idea, that the extended, attenuated,

* *Neue l'eiträge z. Physiologie des Sehens in subjectiver Hinsicht*, p. 147.

atrophic membranes in myopia, might be brought back to their natural condition is simply absurd. We should not even be able to approve of the practice of those, who, in order to compensate for the excessive length of the visual axis, endeavoured to bring the arching of the cornea below the normal. Systematic pressure is an excellent auxiliary in preventing a staphylomatous prominence of the cornea in morbid softening during the process of recovery; but, leaving out of the question, whether a healthy cornea would be affected by it, we should remember, that no more is to be expected from a compensating flattening than from a negative glass: the peculiar morbid process, on which the myopia depends, and which in high degrees threatens the destruction of the eye, would remain unchanged. Treatment is, alas, partly a matter of fashion. Thus discharging the aqueous humour from the anterior chamber of the eye, is now the order of the day. Some have even spoken of applying this method in myopia. If it be intended thereby to make the cornea flatter, the object will not be attained in this way, which is the less to be regretted, because, as I have already remarked, the myope would not be benefited by it : besides the paracentesis referred to is not always itself equally harmless. We formerly lived under the rule of the myotomists. Rendered rash by ignorance, some have actually employed their operation for the relief of myopia, and have even persuaded themselves that they had thus accomplished a cure. The truth is, that they in general subjected not myopic, but rather hypermetropic, eyes, which they mistook for myopic, to the operation, and that even in these the latter was ineffective. However, in another point of view, where myopia really exists, tenotomy may sometimes be applicable. If the muscles are, as a result of extension, permanently too much upon the stretch, and if the bulb is consequently harder, the displacement backwards of the insertions by tenotomy might diminish the pressure, and thus one of the conditions for further development might be removed. Division of the tendon of the rectus externus, is, as we saw in the preceding section, not unfrequently indicated for promoting convergence in high degrees of myopia, and by that division the bulb also acquires less tension; now it has been proposed to divide the tendons of the rectus internus and rectus externus, in order to diminish the existing tension, and in some cases this has actually been done. Further experience must decide as to the value of the plan.—Lastly, the removal of the crystalline lens has also been suggested. When in a case of highly myopic structure of the eye, a lens affected with cataract has been successfully extracted, and a nearly emmetropic condition has been obtained, the operator has been exposed to the temptation of endeavouring, by the abstraction of a normal lens, to remove the myopia. A patient, who was an amateur in dioptrics, endeavoured to induce me to perform this operation !

But I need not say, that such a momentous undertaking, doubly dangerous where a myopic eye and a transparent lens are concerned, without that, even in the most favourable case, any real advantage is to be expected, would exhibit culpable rashness. Not only would the staphyloma posticum continue equally threatening, but we should also have sacrificed the accommodation—an advantage which that of somewhat larger images than would be obtainable by neutralising glasses, could by no means counterbalance.

From the above it follows, that the idea of curing high degrees of myopia with developed staphyloma posticum must be abandoned. The question is, whether slight degrees can really be cured. That, through senile metamorphosis at an advanced period of life, they may give way, we have already seen. In young persons, on the contrary, I have never established the fact of any diminution of the myopia. Where the latter appeared, on superficial observation, to have taken place, spasm of accommodation had been in operation. It has, however, often been asserted that slight degrees of myopia have yielded to the employment of suitable measures. Some years ago Berthold* proposed the use of a certain desk, called *myopodiorthoticon* (!) by which the myope was compelled to remain at a great distance from what he was reading, while this distance was systematically increased. Burow†, however, shows clearly, that no diminution of the myopia is to be expected from this plan, as the accommodation for the farthest point is only a passive, and not an active operation, and he supplies the proof from the experience of his own eyes. Berthold's desk was also tried in vain at Köningsberg; and according to von Hasner the attempt at Prague was attended with no better result. However, the last-named writer expressly states, that myopia depending upon slight degrees of staphyloma scleroticæ, may, particularly in the commencement, be again diminished by restraining the eye from looking at near objects. Respect for Hasner's accuracy cannot prevent me from doubting the correctness of this assertion. I have, *under all circumstances*, found steady increase of M in young indi-

* Das Myopodiorthoticon, 1840.
† *l. c.* p. 49.

27

viduals; its diminution I have never observed. Many cases quoted here and there lose all value as proofs, because it does not appear that the farthest point of distinct vision, on which our judgment in this instance depends, was determined with the requisite accuracy. Even in presence of the case quoted by von Hasner, where the myopia is said to have given way after typhus, I cannot abandon my scepticism. Had spasm, perhaps, previously existed, which was now removed? Had myosis followed, which now made reading at a greater distance possible?—However this may be, we may safely doubt the diminution of the staphyloma posticum, and require convincing observations from those who assert the contrary.

The task of the oculist in myopia resolves itself into the following:—

1. To prevent the further development of the myopia, and the occurrence of secondary disturbances.

2. By means of suitable glasses to render the use of the myopic eye easier and safer.

3. To remove the asthenopia muscularis by the use of glasses or by tenotomy.

4. To combat the secondary disturbances of the M.

I. In the exposition already given lies, I think, the proof, that where predisposition exists, continued accommodation for near objects promotes the development of staphyloma posticum. Where this predisposition occurs we must be aware of it even from youth. We have remarked that accommodation, as such, is not in this case in operation, for in it only the form of the crystalline lens is changed, and in M the latter has undergone no change. In a mediate way, therefore, through accessory circumstances, it must be, that accommodation for near objects promotes staphyloma posticum. Of such circumstances two especially come under observation: *strong convergence and a stooping position.* As to the first, in order to see acutely, myopes must bring the object within the region of accommodation, and where M is somewhat advanced, binocular vision under these circumstances requires a strong convergence. Children and young myopes, with great power of accommodation, are even accustomed, particularly in bad light, to bring the objects much nearer to the eyes than the degree of the myopia, properly speaking, requires. This strong convergence increases the tension of the eyeball by pressure of the muscles, perhaps also by pressure against the surrounding

tissues, and increased pressure promotes the staphylomatous distention. Especially when commencing insufficiency of the mm. recti
interni renders the convergence difficult, the latter is combined with
great tension of the eyeball. Now strong convergence may be
avoided in various ways. In the first place we cause the patient to
look much at a distance. But we cannot absolutely forbid looking
at near objects, and we therefore give spectacles which bring the
farthest point, r, to a sufficient distance; for example, to from 16 to
18 inches. At the same time the patient is to be strongly recommended not to look at a shorter distance than 16" or 14", to which
young people have the greatest tendency; a ruler of this length may
serve as a measure to parents and masters as well as to the myope
himself. Moreover, it is desirable that often (for example, every half-
hour) work should be discontinued for a couple of minutes.—In very
high degrees of M, only one eye is usually employed in vision, and
thus convergence is excluded. This appears to me to be often a desirable condition : in strong M binocular vision loses its value, and the
tension which would be required for it cannot be otherwise than injurious. Now, in such cases, for reading no spectacles are given; in
the first place, because the acuteness of vision has usually somewhat
decreased, and the diminution of concave glasses is now troublesome ;
in the second place, because with the retrocession of r injurious efforts
at convergence and at binocular vision might be excited. In any
case the spectacles should be so weak as to avoid these results.

A stooping position was also mentioned as a promoting cause of
M. This position of necessity leads to accumulation of blood in the
eye : under the influence of gravitation, the afflux of blood takes place,
in fact, under higher pressure, and until the efflux, too, more pressure
remains in the veins; and with the augmented pressure of blood the
tension of the fluids in the eye increases. The symptoms of irritation
connected with hyperæmia, which in young people usually accompany progressive myopia are, I think, for the most part also to be
ascribed to the cause just mentioned. Even in non-myopes an unpleasant feeling of pressure in the eyes speedily occurs when the face
is held horizontally. Now the increased tension of the fluids certainly
promotes, as such, the development of staphyloma. But in yet another way the accumulation of blood is still more injurious, namely,
by promoting, perhaps even by exciting, the inflammatory affections
under whose influence the staphyloma is so rapidly developed. In
the hygiene of myopia, therefore, the very first point is to guard

2

against working in a stooping position. While most work takes place in a horizontal plane, myopes are only too much inclined to it. Such a habit is usually opposed on the supposition that the thoracic organs suffer from it. Without denying this, I think, however, that it must be forbidden chiefly for the sake of the eyes. In general everything will be useful for this purpose which was recommended for the avoidance of strong convergence : to keep objects removed as far as the degree of myopia permits; to intermit work frequently; by suitable glasses to bring r to a sufficient distance. But we may also add : to read with the book in the hand, and in writing to use a high and sloping desk. To this last I attach much importance. Rectilinear drawing on a horizontal surface is decidedly very injurious to myopes. Again, with respect to the thoracic organs, many think that in writing a standing position is to be recommended. For that I see no particular reason. It is sufficient that the height of the desk suit the height of the head, and that the inclination be as great as circumstances permit : in writing the limits are when the ink no longer flows from the pen, but even then a pencil may be used.—Further, those who are highly myopic must be earnestly dissuaded from everything which gives rise to increased action of the heart, and to tendency of blood to the head, with a view both to limit the progress of the myopia, and to prevent the occurrence of secondary affections.

II. The prescribing of spectacles for myopes is a matter of great importance. While emmetropic and hypermetropic eyes do not readily experience any injury from the use of unsuitable glasses, this may in myopes, particularly on account of the morbidly distended condition of the eyeball, and of the tendency to get worse, be very dangerous.

There exists in general a dread of the use of too strong glasses. It is laid down as a rule : rather too weak, or no glasses, than too strong. In this rule the necessary distinction is lost sight of. Too strong glasses make hypermetropic eyes myopic, and myopic eyes hypermetropic. The rule, therefore, cannot be equally true for both. In fact, it is in general much less injurious to produce a certain degree of myopia than of hypermetropia, in which last particularly much is required of the accommodative power. The rule would therefore be more correctly stated thus : in hypermetropia we must beware of giving too weak, in myopia of giving too strong, glasses; a rule the second part of which we should especially insist upon. But even by this little is gained. Not using glasses, or using too weak glasses, may also be injurious to myopes. All the circumstances must therefore be studied, which can exercise an influence on the choice of glasses. It is difficult to reduce these to definite rules. But to attempt to do so is our task.

On a superficial view, we should suppose that we have only completely to neutralise each degree of myopia, in order to obtain all the advantages connected with the emmetropic eye. The case is, however, quite different. If in neutralised myopia the eye is equal in its farthest point to the emmetropic, with respect to the relative limits of accommodation for each convergence there is a great difference, and in acuteness of vision, too, it usually fails. These differences alone would in themselves be sufficient very much to limit the indication for perfect neutralisation, and we shall become acquainted with other circumstances still, which positively forbid it. The indication exists only :

1°. *When the glasses are used exclusively for distant vision,* for example, in a double eye-glass, which is only at intervals held before the eyes. Evidently, in looking to a great distance with such a glass the accommodation is in a state of rest, and its use can therefore never cause any injury. But so soon as the same glasses are used for shorter distances in looking at drawings, plates, &c., the exceptions, of which I shall hereafter speak, come under observation.

2°. *When the myopia is slight in reference to the range of accommodation, and the eye is otherwise healthy.* In this case, neutralising glasses may be worn as spectacles, and may be used even in reading and writing. I think it is even desirable that this should be done. When persons with moderate degrees of myopia have in youth accustomed themselves to the use of neutralising spectacles, the eyes are in all respects similar to emmetropic eyes, and the myopia is, under such circumstances, remarkably little progressive. I am acquainted with numerous examples of this even among those of my friends, who have passed their lives in study. Glasses of $-\frac{1}{10}$, adopted at seventeen years of age, are often still sufficient at forty-five years, both for seeing acutely at a distance and for ordinary close work. Not until the age at which emmetropes need convex spectacles, and often even some years later, do the neutralising spectacles become rather too strong for close work, and it is desirable to procure somewhat weaker ones, which, with the narrower pupil peculiar to that time of life, are now nearly sufficient for distance also. At a still more advanced age, according to the degree of the myopia, sufficiently correcting spectacles may be worn, and laid aside for work.— In order to obtain all the advantages of concave glasses, the myope must begin early with them. If the myopia amounts only to a fourth or a third of the range of accommodation, we may immediately wholly neutralise it. If it amounts to more, we must usually begin with weaker glasses, and replace the latter at the end of six months with stronger. If we have, without the necessary transitions, given too strong spectacles, this may be immediately evident from too great a distance of the binocular nearest point, but in any case it will be manifested by the occurrence of fatigue (asthenopia) in close work. In this respect great individual differences exist, chiefly dependent on the position of the relative range of accommodation. If this be unfavourable, we must more slowly increase the strength of the glasses. The effect of wearing glasses is, in fact, that the relative range of accommodation is displaced, becoming gradually the same as the position proper to emmetropic eyes, and therefore the binocular farthest point approaches the eye, while the absolute farthest point r by no means does so.—The myopia thus neutralised is less progressive, because both too strong convergence and a stooping position are avoided. But if the tendency to these is so great that they still occur in neutralised myopia, the use of glasses is dangerous, and must be discontinued, so soon as it appears that the myopia is particularly progressive. In this case it is necessary for a time to forbid all close work.—Besides, if in the cases mentioned the use of concave glasses is desirable, it is not so necessary that we should always be compelled to adopt them. Women particularly have a right to be allowed some liberty in the matter.

Many circumstances forbid the complete neutralisation of the myopia. They are connected with:

a. The degree of the myopia.—In very slight degrees, from $\frac{1}{60}$ to $\frac{1}{18}$, we may leave the myope to himself; in higher degrees the neutralisation, as I explained under 2°, is desirable. In the highest degrees, from $\frac{1}{5}$ upwards, perfect neutralisation is not pleasant for close work, because, with regard to the usual diminution of the acuteness of vision, the images become too small. We should then rather bring r to 12 or 16 inches,* and let the patient wear these spectacles, with which a lorgnette with glasses of $-\dfrac{1}{12}, -\dfrac{1}{16}$, respectively, is also given, which may for distant vision be held before the spectacles. The idea that there is anything injurious in this combination is an unfounded prejudice. We may also, with weaker spectacles for working, give stronger to be worn; but completely neutralising glasses are not pleasant for a constancy, because the myopia is usually less in indirect than in direct vision. If in general too strong glasses are to be carefully avoided in myopia, the danger to be apprehended from their use is greater the higher the degree of the myopia is.

b. The range of accommodation.—If the range of accommodation be, as is usually the case, proportionate to the time of life, the proper mode of proceeding is included in what has been said under 2°. In saying this, however, we take for granted that nearly neutralising glasses have been used from youth. If this has not been the case, the peculiar position of the relative range of accommodation is attended with difficulties. Moderate degrees of myopia, for example of $\dfrac{1}{10}$, we can no longer completely neutralise at thirty-five years of age. So long as only distant objects are viewed with neutralising spectacles, all is tolerably well; but even in speaking with people we hear complaints of the tension required in order to see the eyes and face acutely, and work is, on the whole, not to be maintained with them. We should then confine ourselves to glasses, which bring r to about 24″, giving, if necessary, still weaker ones for working, and at the end of six months or more, we should examine whether we can increase a little, without causing asthenopia.—Of the optical aids in actual disturbances of accommodation, I shall treat in speaking of the anomalies of accommodation.

c. Acuteness of vision.—This has a great influence in the choice of glasses. We know that in the highest degrees, the acuteness of vision is usually diminished, and therefore we must be very careful.

---

* To bring r, instead of to ∞, to n inches, we give glasses which are $\dfrac{1}{n}$ weaker than those required for complete neutralisation of the myopia. If strong glasses are in question, the distance from the eye is also to be taken into account in the calculation.

Von Graefe has forcibly insisted on the great danger of giving strong glasses for near objects, where the acuteness of vision is diminished. The objects, especially letters in reading, then appear smaller, and from the need of seeing them under a greater visual angle, such shortsighted amblyopes, in order to be able to bring them nearer, put their accommodative power with all their might upon the stretch, and both thus, and by the accompanying convergence, promote the existing staphyloma. But, on the other hand, without glasses, the convergence is still stronger, and the tendency to the bent position is still greater. We thus find ourselves in a sad dilemma, which is to be avoided only by, in great part, forbidding close work. The most favourable circumstance is when in near vision convergence does not take place, and thus only one eye is used. Less injury is then to be expected from reading without spectacles, with the book in the hand, but writing must be avoided. In the same cases we may permit older persons to wear partially neutralising spectacles, and with these spectacles, aided by a reading-glass, occasionally to peruse something, which may in this way be done at a greater distance (compare pp. 229 *et seq.*). Smee advises that his amplifier should, under these circumstances, be used. In any case we should insist upon moderation in reading, and on the selection of large print, although the latter is also attended with particular difficulties.—For the purpose of distinguishing pretty well at a distance in the highest degrees of myopia with diminished acuteness of vision, there is no other means than the use of a double eye-glass, or of the very portable glass-conus of Steinheil* for a single eye. In such cases, a wholly neutralising concave glass makes the distant images appear so small, and the objects so remote, that vision is by no means satisfactory. Imperfectly neutralising glasses in a stenopæic frame, which limits the remaining circles of diffusion, answer still better.

d. Age.—The influence of age is, for the most part, comprised in the diminution of the range of accommodation, and of the acuteness of vision. At a very advanced time of life, we need attend less to the future than to the present. We may therefore, in order with diminished acuteness of vision to make reading still possible,

---

* A simple solid conus of glass, about one inch long, the base convex, the opposite surface concave, with a smaller radius than the convex. It acts as a Galilean telescope: parallel rays, refracted on the convex surface, are converging in the glass, and, refracted again on the concave surface, obtain a diverging direction, and can also unite on the retina of a corresponding myopic eye. The magnifying power increases for the glass-coni, required in high degrees of myopia. Such coni are to be had of Steinheil, Munich.

in the slighter degrees of myopia, even with convex glasses, bring r to 6″, 5″, and even closer to the eye.   We should give only such a form of glasses as the patient can easily see over.   Old people seldom know how to derive much benefit from glasses à *double foyer*.

e. The nature of the work, and the distance at which it is to be performed.—He who in youth neutralises his myopia, can, if his sight be otherwise good, also, later in life, perform ordinary work at any distance required.   He who, on the contrary, either could not or would not wear spectacles, retains the relative range of accommodation peculiar to myopes, and now, when for any particular object vision is required at a somewhat greater distance, he cannot use completely neutralising spectacles.   The rule is with the glasses, therefore, to bring the farthest point precisely to the distance at which acute vision is needed.   The necessity for this is felt most in ladies, for the reading of music, when r must be brought to from 18″ to 24″.   Meanwhile, they can, for distant vision, use a neutralising eyeglass.   It is also in general desirable in writing (in reading it is less necessary), in order to prevent a stooping position and strong convergence, to bring r to from 14″ to 16″, sometimes even to 18″, to make ledger-work possible.   Lastly, in order to see the writing in lectures, especially in the pulpit, the farthest point must be brought precisely to the requisite distance.   Particular attention is necessary—even though spectacles were always worn—in the case of elderly people, who have lost their power of accommodation, and have not perfect accuracy of vision,—in general in those whose myopia cannot be neutralised.   More especially where there is diminished acuteness of vision we meet with difficulties, which by diminishing the distance as much as possible, and giving proportionately weaker glasses, we cannot always overcome.   Persons so circumstanced are not satisfied. They read the smallest writing at 3″ or 4″ distance, and are surprised that they cannot with spectacles see much larger writing at 18″. They do not consider that the distance is from four to six times greater, and that by the concave glasses the images are still further diminished.   Consequently there is nothing to be done, but to write particularly large.

We have, in a separate section, treated of the vision of myopes. We have also examined the direct influence of glasses on observation, and on the estimation of what is observed (pp. 143 *et seq.*), and we need the less to return to the subject, because many points bearing upon it came again under our notice in speaking of the indications and contra-indications of concave glasses. As to the indirect influence (the result of longer use), we became acquainted with the displacement of the relative range of accommodation, and the approximation of the binocular nearest point. We may still add that the at first incorrect estimation of magnitude, distance, and form, is tolerably quickly lost. It is remarkable how myopes, when using spectacles, immediately begin, unconsciously, to write larger than before, and how, after some time, they involuntarily resume their smaller handwriting, unless with considerable energy they resist the tendency to do so. Another result of wearing spectacles is, that by being accustomed to look nearly through the axes of the glasses, the eyes gradually limit their movements. After the removal of the spectacles, too, this limitation continues, and the movements of the head especially provide for the necessity just mentioned, giving a peculiar bearing to myopes who are accustomed to wear glasses.

III.—We have already seen that in high degrees of myopia the internal recti muscles are often insufficient, and that this insufficiency may be developed through different degrees to relative, and even to absolute diverging strabismus (§ 31). The insufficiency first makes itself known by asthenopia muscularis in binocular vision for near objects. Sometimes we find (at least temporarily) the proper remedy for this state of things in concave glasses, which bring r_2 to from $12''$ to $14''$, and we may try these, if there is no contraindication for other reasons against them. In using them we may, if it seems necessary, somewhat diminish the mutual distance of the glasses, by which less is required of the internal muscles (compare p. 167). In other cases the use of spectacles may itself give rise to asthenopia muscularis. Thus, in very high degrees of myopia relative diverging strabismus is a very common occurrence: for the short distance, at which vision is distinct, the convergence is, in fact, insufficient, and therefore only one eye is used, while the other deviates outwards. When, in such cases, r is by concave glasses brought to a greater distance, the effort at binocular vision sometimes returns; and the musculi recti interni are then obliged to exert themselves so powerfully, that asthenopia muscularis is unavoidable. Now this is not only troublesome and fatiguing, but it is also injurious, as it affects the further development of the myopia. If the one eye, so soon as it is covered, perceptibly deviates outwards, and on removing the hand again turns inwards, in order to resume its former direction, we may expect the occurrence of asthenopia muscularis.   It is often difficult enough to decide what is to be done in such cases.   For the rules applicable to insufficiency of the internal muscles in non-myopes, by no means hold good in the asthenopia muscularis of myopic individuals.   In the former the condition referred to is, in the first place, free from danger, and it is even allowable to try by systematic practice with prismatic glasses to excite the energy of the internal muscles.   In myopia, on the contrary, cure of the insufficiency of the internal recti muscles is not to be thought of.   Once begun, the insufficiency develops itself more and more, in double proportion, when, as is usual, the myopia is progressive.   Often no other result is possible, than the exclusion of the one eye, with diverging strabismus. In the worst cases the mobility is even so limited, that it is insuffi-cient both inwardly and outwardly.   Both these conditions have been distinctly enough put forward in the preceding paragraph. Seeing the danger connected with strong action of the musculi recti interni, and the prospect of not being able to prevent the progress of the insufficiency, I have often asked myself, whether we must not simply submit to the tendency to outward deviation, which removes the asthenopia muscularis by the intervention of relative strabismus divergens.   Von Graefe* is of opinion that we should decide upon this sacrifice only in excessive myopia, in order to avoid asthenopia. A middle course may, however, also be adopted: we may allow reading without glasses, that is with the exclusion of one eye; but for writing and other work, which, to prevent a stooping position, must be performed at a somewhat greater distance, we should give prismatic-concave glasses.   The concavity of these should be such as to bring the farthest point to from 12″ to 16″, and the angle of the prism should be so great that in looking to a distance of from 12″ to 16″, covering one eye should no longer be followed by any outward movement.   Von Graefe is a great advocate of this com-bination, which, if it is arranged with strict care for individual cases, really renders binocular vision, without asthenopia, possible.   If we are particularly successful we may allow these glasses to be used also in reading; if the difficulties are not altogether removed, their use must be limited to writing, but even in this moderation must be ob-served; and if, after repeated efforts, the patient continues to com-plain, we should not hesitate to sacrifice the one eye.

" The proper principal remedy," says von Graefe, " is above all

* *Archiv für Ophthalmologie*, B. viii. Abth. 2, p. 314.

tenotomy of the musculus rectus externus." Even where myopia is the cause of the affection it may sometimes yield excellent results. In such cases it is, however, comparatively rarely adopted, so long as there is merely simple insufficiency of the recti muscles, without strabismus divergens. The cause of this is the limited mobility of the eyes in the high degrees of myopia, the basis of which we have already indicated. It will, in fact, in general be admissible only when, after the operation, no permanent converging strabismus in distant vision, even in looking somewhat towards the side operated on, is to be expected. Von Graefe has from this point of view established the indications with great accuracy. The condition, *sine qua non*, for tenotomy is this : that under the attempt at single vision, a sufficient divergence of the visual lines should appear to be possible. This should be tried (after neutralisation of the myopia by concave glasses placed at a proper distance from each other) with prismatic glasses; we should investigate, with what prismatic glasses, held with the refracting angle outwards before the eyes, single distant vision is still attainable. The strongest glasses then, which can still be overcome, give the measure of the possible divergence. It is allowable now so to perform tenotomy that this possible divergence shall be completely removed. Even convergence of from 1 to $1\frac{1}{2}$ mm. may at first, in looking straight forward, be obtained, which, after cicatrisation, again gives way. When, without the employment of prismatic glasses, in distant vision divergence of the visual lines already exists, there is not the slightest difficulty in the way of tenotomy, although we should still even then endeavour to determine the effect to be obtained by the maximum of the prisms to be overcome. But we must not suppose that with the removal of the possible divergence, we have always made binocular vision for near objects easy : when deviation of the eye behind the hand, at the distance at which binocular vision is desired, is much greater than the utmost divergence which we are allowed to correct by tenotomy, we shall, after this correction, retain an insufficiency for this distance, which, with binocular vision, if it is not wholly absent, will still give rise to asthenopia. We must, therefore, in such cases bear in mind that after tenotomy, the correction must be supplied by prismatic-concave glasses. Hence, therefore, it also follows, that when in distant vision only comparatively very weak prisms can be overcome, the operation certainly effects almost nothing, and where it appears that no divergence is possible, tenotomy is absolutely contra-indicated. Certain rules for regulating the effect of tenotomy according to the degree of the deviation, are laid down by von Graefe. Personal experience is, however, also necessary.   In general, I found in strongly myopic individuals the effect of tenotomy to be less.

IV. *Therapeutic Treatment.*—For myopia, as such, there is no therapeutic treatment.   Myopia consists in an anomaly of form capable of no improvement, and of which only hygienic measures must, if possible, prevent the further development.   But it is not un-frequently complicated with symptoms of irritation and inflammation, and with other pathological deviations of different kinds, which partly proceed from it, partly promote its further development; and with respect to these it is the duty of the therapeutist, to the best of his ability, to interfere.   It is not part of the plan of this work to enter into detailed discussions respecting therapeutic questions. While it treats of anomalies of refraction, it must make known the dioptric remedies which counteract them; but it cannot treat *in extenso* of complications, which neither necessarily belong to the essence of these anomalies, nor are characteristic of them—much less still of their treatment.   Consequently, only brief indications are to be ex-pected here, respecting treatment, in connexion with some prognostic hints.

In the foreground appear symptoms of irritation at the period of puberty, characterised by capillary hyperæmia of the nerve-surface (and of the retina), and by fatigue and pain in the eyes, especially on exertion in the evening.   Under such circumstances we should be particularly strict with respect to the hygienic directions (com-pare p. 408), which are in themselves in many cases sufficient.   It is also of great importance to keep the feet warm.   Often, too, a douche on the closed eyelids is agreeable.   If the symptoms do not give way, we may, with avoidance of a stimulating diet, combine some derivation on the intestinal canal, and we may in addition recommend the application, to the frontal and temporal regions, of a stimulating embrocation, composed, if there be any coexisting external irritation of the eyes, rather of non-volatile ingredients.   At the same time, especially when it appears that the myopia is rapidly pro-gressive, all tension must be avoided.   So far as work is permitted, this must be accomplished in slight degrees of myopia without spec-tacles, and in higher degrees r must be brought accurately to twelve inches.   If fatigue or pain should occur, work must in either case be suspended; and if the use of spectacles appears more rapidly to cause fatigue, we should not lay stress upon their adoption, but take care only that the patient maintains a proper position in whatever work he still performs. If it be suspected that the symptoms of irritation have excited spasm of accommodation, as often occurs in high degrees of myopia in youth, we should employ sulphate of atropia, partly to test the truth of the supposition, partly to remove the spasm and to prevent it returning on each effort to see. We may then even continue this application for some days, whereby the myope becomes accustomed to look at the greatest distance of distinct vision; unnecessary convergence is thus prevented, and from this plan no injury is to be apprehended, provided we cause the patient to avoid strong light, or to moderate it by means of grey glasses. In case of a relapse of the symptoms of irritation, with spasm of accommodation, the application of Heurteloup's artificial leeches to the temples, followed by twenty-four hours' stay in the dark, with gradual transition to light, has been found very useful.— In spite of all efforts, however, these symptoms of irritation in some constantly recur. If, moreover, the myopia is rapidly progressive, the patient's state is serious enough to make it necessary to warn him against choosing an occupation in which close work would be constantly required; above all, such myopes should not be office-clerks. But such cases are rare: with few exceptions the inconveniences disappear before the twentieth year.

At a later period of life, the acuteness of vision sometimes diminishes in high degrees of myopia in a few months in a manner to cause considerable uneasiness. In these cases the hyperæmia at the borders of the atrophy often leads us to suspect the existence of progressive myopia, while to this state of things other signs of irritation are usually added. If, in such instances, no organic changes are ophthalmoscopically to be observed in the region of the yellow spot, we almost always obtain, within a few weeks, a considerable improvement of the acuteness of vision, by the weekly abstraction of blood after Heurteloup's method, by keeping the patient in a moderate light, and by making him avoid tension of the eyes, combining this plan, according to circumstances, with the use of the douche and of a stimulating embrocation, with derivation by the intestinal canal and stimulating pediluvia. Even when there are perceptible morbid changes in the yellow spot we need not despair, so long as subjectively a defined scotoma does not remove direct vision. In persons of 60 years and upwards, with myopia of $\frac{1}{5}$ and even of $\frac{1}{4}$, I have, by following the above directions, seen the acuteness of vision rise from $\frac{1}{30}$ or $\frac{1}{20}$, to $\frac{1}{4}$ or $\frac{1}{3}$, and thus become quite sufficient for writing and reading. It is quite a different thing when a circumscribed scotoma, ophthalmoscopically perceptible in the yellow spot, is also perceptible to the patient. This indicates a profound disturbance in the seat of direct vision. Blindness is in general not particularly threatened thereby; but improvement of direct vision is not to be expected, and if both eyes are equally affected, the patient must prepare himself for the impossibility of reading, writing, or performing minute work.—In cases of accessory chorioiditis disseminata the same directions are to be observed. In such we must expect repeated improvement and aggravation of the affection. After many years, however, the result usually becomes so unfavourable, that ordinary work can no longer be performed. Motes are at the same time often present in the vitreous humour; of the cause of these I have already treated. Especially under these circumstances it is usual to prescribe a long course of small doses of preparations of iodine or mercury. I too, have repeatedly done this, but I would not venture absolutely to assert, that I have seen favourable results from it. Many patients give themselves more trouble about these motes than they deserve. If no definite morbid changes threaten the yellow spot, we may give a comparatively favourable prognosis; we should advise that the attention should be as much as possible withdrawn from them, and the attempt to do this should be seconded by causing the patient to wear nearly neutralising glasses, made so as at the same time to moderate the light, and thus to make the shadows of the motes appear less defined.*— Complaints of persistent photopsia are yet louder, but are fortunately rarer. It occurs chiefly in diffuse atrophy, and indicates a state of irritation of the optic nerve. I have, in addition to the above-described treatment, tried numerous remedies against it, among others, narcotics, but, so far as I recollect, always in vain. The complaints were, in some cases, especially in nervous women, lamentable, and it has often surprised me, that, with such signs of continual irritation, the acuteness of vision was, in the course even of some years, but slightly diminished.—Against the most melancholy complications of myopia, effusion of blood, and detachment of the retina,

* Opaque membranes in the vitreous humour cause more disturbance. The most recent experience of von Graefe raises the question whether some results are not in these cases to be obtained by operation.

treatment is almost powerless.   In cases of effusion of blood in the
vitreous humour, we may expect absorption, leaving behind it some
opaque motes and membranes.   The metamorphosis, under which the
absorption takes place, is a spontaneous process, which treatment cannot promote, and the physician has therefore to confine himself to
hygienic rules, and to such derivative or constitutional treatment as
may appear to be adapted to each individual case.   Pressure, by means
of a bandage applied at intervals, might probably favour absorption,
but when the bandage is taken off the tension of the fluids is
diminished, and, as appears on ophthalmoscopic investigation, the
vessels are distended, whereby the danger of fresh effusion must necessarily be increased.   After repeated relapses, the vitreous humour
remains opaque, and the fundus oculi is sometimes wholly invisible.—
Occasionally, after repeated effusion of blood in the vitreous humour,
local detachment of the retina occurs, in some cases certainly in
consequence of blood accumulated between the retina and the
chorioidea.   Partial absorption is here also to be expected, but the
detached portion of the retina never again resumes its functions.
The prognosis in detachment of the retina by a serous fluid, such as
often occurs in high degrees of myopia, is somewhat less unfavourable.
Irritation of the chorioidea and diminished connexion by displacement of the retina over the disproportionately extending atrophy of
the chorioidea, must tend to promote this.   In very rare cases absorption may occur, which many endeavour to promote by means of
all kinds of remedies (mercurials, preparations of iodine, derivants,
sudorifics), very problematical in their action; but in general improvement of the sight depends upon the fluid sinking to beneath
the seat of direct vision, or upon a diminished morbid condition of
the parts of the retina bordering upon the detachment.   Rupture of
the retina * is so far advantageous, as the danger of further detachment appears thereby to be lessened.   This fact it was which chiefly
suggested the idea of dividing the detached part by incision.   Sichel
had already at an earlier period advised the discharge externally of the
effused fluid, by puncturing the sclerotic in the seat of the detachment.
This is attended with no difficulty whatever; but it does not appear that
any advantage is obtained by it.   The incision of the detached part was
performed chiefly by Adolf Weber and by von Graefe,† with a two-

---

* Liebreich gives a good representation of it, *Atlas d'Ophthalmoscopie,*
Tab. vii. Fig. 1.

† Compare *Archiv f. Ophthalmologie,* B. ix. p. 85.

edged needle, carried from the inside through the vitreous humour. In this manner a communication was established between the fluid accumulated behind the retina and the vitreous humour, with which it mingled; and the difference of pressure, which plays a part in the origin and further development of the affection, was thus removed. No injurious effect resulted from the operation; in some cases, at least at first, some improvement was observed; but experience has as yet by no means decided, whether, and in what cases, permanent benefit is to be obtained by this method: hitherto it has been employed almost exclusively in old and nearly hopeless cases. It has, indeed, appeared, that in staphyloma posticum the danger of extension of incipient detachment, and consequently of increasing destruction of sight, is greatest. This therefore justifies the practitioner in more boldly attacking precisely these cases in the commencement.—In all cases of recent detachment of the retina, in addition to the ordinary hygiene of the eye, jolting, vibration, &c. (in carriages and on railways), as well as violent exertion in fatiguing work, are to be strictly forbidden.

For the sake of illustration I will, in conclusion, endeavour to sketch, in a few lines, the most frequently-occurring types of myopia.

Slight degrees of myopia escape the observation of the patient himself.

1. Mr. S. brings me his son, a boy of 15 years, who has been rejected for nearsightedness at the Military Academy. "The lad is not nearsighted, he reads the smallest writing still farther than he can reach." At twenty feet he sees only No. 60, with $-\frac{1}{22}$ No. 20, with $-\frac{1}{20}$ no better, with $-\frac{1}{24}$ and particularly with $-\frac{1}{26}$ less acutely. He has therefore M $= \frac{1}{22}$, and the rejection is legitimate. Ophthalmoscopically scarcely a trace of atrophy is found, but the papillæ are red. He has latterly worked very hard, in the evening, too, with moderate light, in order to prepare himself for his examination. In doing so he found no inconvenience. He had indeed last year observed, that he could not recognise people so far off as before, but he did not attribute this to nearsightedness, because he could see the finest object sharply at the distance of two feet.

My opinion is: that the myopia will increase a little. To prevent it increasing much, let him work by good light (by preference by daylight), holding up his head, at the distance of from 14″ to 16″, on an inclined plane, with intervals of some minutes every half-hour. I add, "Be of good

28

cheer, my young friend, you can be whatever you wish, except a soldier ;*
towards your eighteenth year (with M about $= \frac{1}{16}$), you will get spectacles
to wear and to work with, and you will put these off for work about the
age at which others begin to wear glasses."

In higher degrees young people must forthwith accustom themselves to the use of spectacles.

II. H. comes in his eighteenth year to the University. He is nearsighted,
and would now, if allowed, gladly wear spectacles, in order to see better
at a distance. On examination, I find $M = \frac{1}{11}$, $S = \frac{22}{20}$, a slender crescent at the optic nerves, good range of accommodation, and also in other
respects, sound eyes. With $-\frac{1}{11}$ he sees acutely at 4″, and reads, under my
inspection, for a quarter of an hour without trouble. In order, however,
with certainty to avoid asthenopia, when reading for a longer time, he gets
for the present only $-\frac{1}{16}$, with which he is quite content, and a year
later, $-\frac{1}{11}$. After three years he thought he did not see at a distance so
acutely with these glasses. I now found $M = \frac{1}{10}$, and did not hesitate to
give him glasses of $-\frac{1}{10}$. Under no circumstances does he, in using these
glasses, experience any inconvenience to his eyes, and I venture to pro-
gnosticate that his myopia will not increase much more.

With diminished range of accommodation the myopia can no
longer be neutralised.

III. Dr. L., aged 37, with myopia $= \frac{1}{9}$ and otherwise sound eyes, has
for the last twelve years, now and then, worn spectacles, which corrected
about from ½ to ⅔ of his myopia, but he has always read and written without glasses. The degree of the myopia has at this time somewhat, but certainly not much increased. Not long ago he consulted an optician, who
gave him $-\frac{1}{9}$ to wear, with the advice to continue to work without
spectacles. Dr. L. immediately found that these glasses were disagreeable
to him ; walking and looking at a distance, he found all very well, but at
the distance of two feet he could not see acutely without an effort, which
inconvenienced him at table, in speaking to people whom he wished to look
at, and under many other circumstances. He asked me what he was to do.
My answer was : " If you had commenced in your twenty-fifth year with neutralising spectacles, or if you had, at least, used your weaker glasses also at
your work, you would now find no trouble with neutralising spectacles with

---

* In England, M does not disqualify an officer.

convergence at two feet, and even at one foot, in accommodating for that distance. You are now obliged to keep to weaker glasses, for example, $-\frac{1}{12}$ with which you still see perfectly sharply at three feet, and also sufficiently well at a great distance. You are tall, and are therefore inclined to stoop forward, and it is consequently desirable that at work you should accustom yourself to spectacles, which, however, must certainly for the present not be stronger than $-\frac{1}{20}$; by degrees their strength may be somewhat increased, and perhaps you may succeed, within a couple of years, in accustoming yourself to $-\frac{1}{12}$, without their use being attended with symptoms of asthenopia, in which case you may, without any injury, easily keep the same glasses of $-\frac{1}{12}$, under all circumstances, for half a score of years,"

When symptoms of irritation occur, myopic eyes have need of rest.

IV. Miss v. D., aged 18, is much addicted to reading, and not less so to working, and has in both respects fully indulged her inclination, even when her eyes were tender and rather intolerant of light. She now, particularly in the evening, on exertion, quickly gets pain in the eyes, and she has applied for advice. I establish the existence of $M = \frac{1}{7}$, of $S = \frac{18}{20}$, of capillary hyperæmia of the optic nerves, of a small, doubly-contoured, half-atrophic crescent, with very red edges, and, externally, of some injection of the subconjunctival vessels; the lateral movements of the eyes, as well as the convergence, are ample and free. Her mother has $M = \frac{1}{4}$. The young lady remembers to have formerly had much more acute vision for distant objects, and particularly during the last two years to have lost ground in this respect.—She must for the present neither read nor work; she must avoid strong light; she must get spectacles with round, blue glasses, and must, three times a-day, for five minutes on each occasion, apply a douche upon the closed eyelids; she must sit up straight, take care to keep her feet warm, go to bed early, and avoid all stimulants. A month later the symptoms of irritation seem to have yielded. Upon her own authority she lays aside the spectacles and again begins to work, with the result, that in a couple of days the pain reappears. After a fresh period of rest she gets leave, on condition of steadily observing the other directions, and of using glasses of $-\frac{1}{11}$, with which she sees acutely at 18″, to play the piano for two hours daily, the music being placed at precisely 18″,—but on the further condition that every quarter of an hour she rests for some minutes. After the lapse of a month, she may gradually begin to read a little. Fine work is permanently forbidden, and writing is very much restricted, the more so because she will not use spectacles, and therefore must always strongly converge, and be inclined to stoop forward. She was strictly enjoined to hold every object at the greatest distance of distinct vision.—A year subsequently she again presents herself. The myopia is increased to $\frac{1}{6}$; now and then some sensibility had stimulated her to a stricter observance of the directions, and more severe symptoms were thus prevented.—Moderate reading, with the book in the hand, and piano-playing, with the use of the spectacles, are the only indulgences at present permitted; for distant vision a glass of $-\frac{1}{7}$ is given her.—With great care, the inconvenience will gradually lessen, but it is to be expected that at fifty years of age the myopia will have increased to $\frac{1}{4}$, and that at a more advanced period the acuteness of vision will have more than ordinarily diminished, while her eyes will be liable also to other accidents.

Spasm of accommodation may supervene upon the symptoms of irritation.

v. T. W., aged 17, was nearsighted from childhood, and has for some time been unable to continue working, in consequence of rapidly-increasing pain in the eyes, which are also permanently sensitive. I found myopia of $\frac{1}{2.7}$, somewhat stronger still in the left eye; moreover, capillary hyperæmia of the optic disc; at its outside a perfectly atrophic, white, sharply-defined crescent, 0.8 mm. broad in the transverse direction (the axis), straightened retinal vessels, no trace of chorioiditis, rather small pupil, easy convergence of the visual lines up to $2\frac{1}{2}''$ (he then also read binocularly), scarcely any subconjunctival injection, no prominence of the eyes, eyelids healthy, but a tendency to approximate them, not merely in order to see better, but also on account of some intolerance of light. He showed me spectacles of $-\frac{1}{9}$, which he had worn, and had also used at work, but by the advice of others, he had afterwards laid them aside, and he had since not got on better. The acuteness of vision amounted to only $\frac{13}{20}$. This latter circumstance chiefly induced me to prescribe a Heurteloupian abstraction of blood * from both temples, and to make him remain for twenty-four hours afterwards in the dark. After gradual transition to the light, the degree of myopia was again, with the aid of glasses, determined in the most accurate manner, and was found $= \frac{1}{3.4}$; at the same time the acuteness of

---

* Heurteloupian abstraction of blood is accomplished by means of an artificial leech making a circular wound, and yielding much blood on exhaustion by means of a glass cylinder. (The instrument is to be had at Luer's, Paris. Its price is fifty francs.)

vision had increased to $\frac{17}{20}$. Instillation of sulphate of atropia now brought

the myopia to $\frac{1}{3\cdot7}$. The patient was still kept some days in a half-darkened apartment; subsequently the double abstraction of blood was again had recourse to, and the hygienic rules which have already been repeatedly mentioned, were strictly enjoined. Thus at the end of a month the acute-

ness of vision had risen to $\frac{18}{20}$, and the myopia was established as $\frac{1}{3\cdot6}$. He

now got spectacles of $-\frac{1}{5}$, both to wear and also in order occasionally to

read and write for a quarter of an hour, which *could* thus be done at the distance of about 10″, and therefore *must* be done. From time to time slight attacks of pain still occurred, which disappeared on strict rest. The

spectacles were subsequently strengthened to $-\frac{1}{4\cdot5}$. These glasses, held

close to the eye, brought the farthest point to 14″, which was quite sufficient. —The strong convergence and bad position, not completely corrected by the

glasses of $-\frac{1}{9}$ previously used, had, with original highly myopic structure,

been followed by congestion of the optic nerve, with diminished acuteness of vision, spasm of accommodation and other symptoms. They yielded to the rather energetic treatment, and by avoiding strong convergence, &c., with the use of suitable spectacles, they did not return with equal violence. It is, however, to be anticipated that the myopia will continue permanently progressive, and that at a more advanced age, the acuteness of vision will suffer. The eyes must therefore always be watched, and a position in life is to be preferred which will not require much close work.

Even in youth a very high degree of myopia may produce profound disturbance.

VI. Miss S., a little deformed personage, aged 27, has prominent eyes, with considerable enlargement of all axes (buphthalmic form), apparently small cornea, somewhat bluish sclerotic, with widely-open eye-

lids, with myopia $= \frac{1}{1\cdot8}$; and, on correction of the myopia, acuteness of

vision at a distance of only $\frac{9}{100}$. Even in her twelfth year the nearsighted-

ness was inconvenient, and it constantly increased until now she cannot attempt writing, and can read only comparatively large print, held close to the eye, of course only with one eye, without convergence; she complains also of motes floating before her eyes, and of flashes of light, particularly in the dark. Ophthalmoscopically we find an apparently small optic disc, of a white colour, with irregularly bound edhalf-elliptical atrophy, straightened retinal vessels, a light-red fundus, here and there some-what spotted with yellow and grey, with separate chorioideal vessels. The employment of Heurteloup's abstractions of blood and strict hygiene of the eyes produced scarcely any improvement. The patient does not wish to wear spectacles, which, in comparison to the diminution, add but little distinctness to the objects ; she also finds it equally fatiguing when she endeavours to read large print with spectacles, and she finally consents to confine herself to coarse work, which she can perform by feeling. Some words she reads without spectacles, with one eye. For distant objects she finds a stenopæic eyeglass of $-\frac{1}{25}$ the most satisfactory. In this unfortunate condition nothing but impairment is to be expected, the progress of which may, by the known rules of ocular hygiene, be indeed retarded, but not prevented. If the symptoms of irritation increase, Heurteloup's method of abstracting blood may still occasionally be useful.

The occurrence of fatigue during work indicates the existence of insufficiency of the musculi recti interni.

VII. Miss v. R., aged 18, has for some years been constantly obliged to suspend her work, in consequence of a feeling of fatigue and tension. She has in vain tried various spectacles. I establish $M = \frac{1}{7}$, $S = 1$, with the ordinary crescentic atrophy ; the eyes are otherwise sound and the eyelids healthy. I suspect insufficiency of the recti interni. While she reads at 6″ with both eyes, I bring a small screen before the left, and observe it deviate outwards behind the screen. On removing the screen the eye again converges sufficiently. Having made some inquiries, I find that, after having read for half-an-hour, the left eye is always drawn outwards, that this gives her an unpleasant sensation, and that the effort to overcome the deviation fatigues her still more. Thus, she had herself already remarked the insufficiency, without having been able clearly to account for it, and without having spoken of it. On approximating an object, she converges up to 4″, after which the left eye rapidly and strongly deviates. However, on lateral movements the excursions appear normal ; towards distant objects the eyes are also properly directed, and they maintain this direction when one eye is covered ; a prism, too, placed before one of the eyes, with the angle upwards, gives double images of a remote light, without lateral deviation, one of the images being almost directly above the other ; while a prism of 6°, with the angle outwards, gives intersected double images, which do not disappear. Thus it is evident that our patient can diverge little more than normally, and yet that she has comparatively much too great difficulty in converging. With glasses of from $-\frac{1}{12}$ to $-\frac{1}{8}$ she can, looking at from 13″ to 16″, maintain the convergence much longer, but yet not sufficiently : the covered eye now always deviates also, still directly outwards. By combining $-\frac{1}{12}$ with a prism of 8° the difficulties appear to be removed, and the now covered eye actually scarcely any longer alters its direction. Besides such glasses, she receives a double eye-glass with simple glasses of

$- \frac{1}{7}$. With this she is exceedingly pleased, but the prismatic combination wearies her. She would willingly undergo tenotomy, which was spoken of, but as, undoubtedly, even in looking straight, and particularly in looking to the left, double images at a distance would remain, I do not think the operation indicated. Finally, I give her glasses of $- \frac{1}{7}$, with the axes closer to one another than the axes of the two eyes; and if she has to work only one hour, she gives the preference to these, above the prismatic combination. She has to be particularly careful not to use these spectacles in looking at remote objects: on account of the position of the glasses she would in doing so be compelled to diverge somewhat, which could not act otherwise than injuriously upon the power of the recti interni.

The insufficiency may sometimes be completely corrected by tenotomy.

viii. Mr. C., a mechanic, with $M = \frac{1}{8}$, has, except the ordinary crescent, sound, sharpseeing eyes. Yet his work fatigues him after a short time, and he thinks it not well to continue using his sight. His looking at a distance did not exhibit the ordinary apparent convergence, but rather gave the impression of divergence. This immediately suggested to me the idea of insufficiency of the recti interni. On examination, it appeared that in unconscious distant vision he had the tendency to divergence, which was absent when he saw acutely through glasses of $- \frac{1}{8}$; that he, however, aided with $- \frac{1}{8}$, for the sake of single vision, could overcome a prism of 12° with the angle outwards, and consequently could considerably diverge. When, in reading at a distance of 8″, a screen was brought before the one eye, this evidently deviated outwards, to turn again inwards on the removal of the screen, and it appeared that this movement was scarcely greater than that which was observed after the removal of the prism of 12°, in looking at a distance. Consequently the insufficiency with a certain convergence, made itself not much more strongly felt than in distant vision. Tenotomy was therefore indicated. It was immediately performed, first, on the left eye, the effect of which was still unsatisfactory; then also on the right eye, when it was at first too great, so that remote objects appeared single only in the direction to the right of the middle line; but forthwith convergence to 8″ took place, with the greatest ease, and after some weeks the double images ceased also at a distance. The success was complete. Fatigue was no longer mentioned, particularly not after our patient, by my advice, had begun to wear glasses of $- \frac{1}{16}$, and to use them at his work.

Even in elderly people myopic amblyopia may, in a great measure, yield to suitable treatment.

IX. Mr. M., a banker, aged 63, has spent his life writing, " has," as he says, " carefully refrained from the use of spectacles, and has, nevertheless, by degrees nearly lost his sight." For a long time he had still been able to read with the left eye, but some time ago this became worse than the right. I establish in the left eye, $M = \frac{1}{5}$ with $S = \frac{1}{14}$; in the right, $M = \frac{1}{5.5}$, with $S = \frac{1}{8}$. The latter eye had also so much opacity of the lens, that without it the acuteness of vision would still have been pretty good; in the left eye, on the contrary, rather well-marked diffuse atrophy, with an atrophic belt through the region of the yellow spot, was to be seen. I stated my regret, that both defects did not exist in the same eye; but, at the same time, my hope that in the left eye, in which within some weeks the sight had so very much diminished (without effusion of blood, without detachment of the retina, and without local scotoma of the yellow spot), improvement was still to be obtained. I gave a stimulating liniment, to be applied above the eyes, pediluvia with mineral acids, rhamnus to keep the bowels open, ordered rest of the eyes, avoidance of strong light, prescribed grey glasses, and had a Heurteloup's leech applied to the left temple every week. At the end of three weeks the acuteness of vision had risen again to $\frac{1}{4}$, and it subsequently attained, under a continuance of the treatment, with abstraction of blood every fortnight, nearly to $\frac{1}{3}$, so that he could again very well read ordinary print. He was forbidden to write. He read without spectacles, with the book in the hand, at the distance of 5″, while the right eye deviated outwards. For distance he got a double eyeglass, with a glass of $-\frac{1}{5}$, to be used sparingly. He had lived so far without using spectacles, and I found no indication to give them to him in his sixty-third year; otherwise he could, without inconvenience, have worn glasses of $-\frac{1}{7}$; but with the diminished acuteness of vision he ought not to read except without spectacles, and fortunately convergence did not then take place.

Scotomata in the yellow spot make reading and writing impossible, but do not threaten blindness.

X. The Consul M., aged 47, presents in his whole bearing the characters of a highly myopic person: stooping neck, closely-knit eyelids, large eyes, of the long axes of which we can easily satisfy ourselves. His myopia has existed from youth, and is of hereditary origin. He has always read and written much, usually with comparatively weak spectacles. In the right eye the myopia now amounts to — $\frac{1}{3\cdot3}$ with $\frac{3}{8}$ acuteness of vision; in the left the myopia is not less; but it cannot be accurately determined on account of a scotoma in the yellow spot. In the space of two months this had developed itself, so that he could not see what he fixed. He was in a sad state of mind, and put the question to me, " Must I become blind ? " Ophthalmoscopically I found in the left eye a tolerably extensive circumscribed crescent, here and there traces of diffuse atrophy, and in the yellow spot a pale granular fold, furnished with, and partly bounded by, larger, irregular, sharply-defined, dark pigment-spots. In the right eye, too, the crescent was about equal to that in the left; and in the yellow spot the pigment was slightly granular, and was irregularly distributed upon a paler ground. I could now answer him : " Do not fear blindness, but abstain from all exertion of the eyes. Confine your reading and writing to what is absolutely necessary, and let them be continued only for a few minutes occasionally. I cannot conceal from you that the left eye is for ever useless for fine work, the right eye would become so by exertion." I am accustomed unreservedly to state the danger of the patient's state, only when he has to act accordingly. This was the case in this instance. But nevertheless, I did not attain my object, " his circumstances did not permit it." There was no reason to add that, in my opinion, even if he left off all work, the further development of the scotoma in the right eye could not be permanently arrested. Dissatisfied with my opinion, the patient repaired to a foreign oculist, who promised him, and also made him believe, that he would cure even the left eye. A full year the patient spent with him, always in hope and confidence. But when the second eye commenced to refuse its service for reading, his confidence began to waver. Two years later he paid me a second visit. On the right eye, also, a scotoma was now so far developed, that he could scarcely decipher a single word. He appeared dissatisfied with himself for not having followed my advice. I gave him the ordinary hygienic directions, and I was able to comfort him with the hope that his condition would not become much worse. It is, in fact my opinion, that he will permanently continue in a state to move about freely and to distinguish large objects. He receives spectacles of — $\frac{1}{3\cdot5}$.

In loosening of the retina the prospect is very gloomy.

XI. Mr. S., aged 43, was, as well as his father, extremely nearsighted from youth. In his thirty-second year he lost in a great measure the power of vision in his right eye, in which cataract became developed. Extraction was followed by atrophy of the eye. Sight now suddenly became obscure in the left eye also. The following day he called upon me. I ascertained the existence of detachment of the inner part of the retina, extending into the neighbourhood of the yellow spot. Large letters he could still read, but at one moment much better than at another. I perceived that loosening of the retina must, at an earlier period, have existed in the right eye also, followed by secondary cataract, upon which, misled by the remaining perception of light, his medical advisers had operated—with what result, has already been seen. Blood was immediately abstracted by Heurteloup's method, rest in the horizontal position was enjoined, and derivation by the intestinal canal and lower extremities was prescribed. The abstraction of blood was again twice repeated, and by these means the patient was able, after the lapse of a week, to read satisfactorily ; the limitation, however, still continued. By degrees he resumed his place in society ; blood is still from time to time abstracted ; he leads a very regular life, avoids fatigue, over exertion, riding in jolting carriages, and travels, if necessary, in the canal-boat ; but he continues to read his price-current and other more necessary matters, and prefers not to go out with grey glasses, " because with them he cannot see by the way." There really exists some torpor and more limitation in weak light. At the end of six months the detachment has, by gravitation, removed farther downwards ; and at the same time the limitation has altered its place ; it still, however, at the inside directly adjoins the fovea centralis.—After the lapse of a year reading is more difficult, and is but little improved by the employment of artificial abstraction of blood. Now, nearly two years after the occurrence of detachment of the retina, distinct traces of cataract exist ; motes in the vitreous humour had already been seen at an earlier period, without laceration of the retina having been perceptible. The progress of the cataract is certainly not to be prevented. When it is fully developed our duty will be to try extraction (by preference with Waldau's spoon), at least if it does not appear that the detachment has extended much farther. We must, however, at the same time, give an unfavourable prognosis. We can scarcely hope that absolute blindness can be permanently averted.

A defined detachment of the retina may for a long time remain stationary.

xii. Mr. v. d. W., aged 23, has $M = \frac{1}{5}$ in both eyes, with small, sharply-defined, completely atrophic crescent. For years work has been difficult to him, and he did not like his spectacles. Some months ago his right eye became much worse, and he can scarcely read with it. I here find a red optic disc and a small, roundish, circumscribed, plaited and movable projection of the retina of a bluish colour, with a corresponding limitation. By artificial leeching to the temple, and strict ocular hygiene, the acuteness of vision increases within a month from $\frac{1}{7}$ to $\frac{1}{2}$. In the other eye it amounts to rather more than $\frac{2}{3}$. I earnestly represent to him that it is only by a regular life and a sparing use of his eyes, that he can retain his sight. I permit him at most to read four times a-day for half-an-hour each time, which he does, binocularly, with glasses of $-\frac{1}{10}$. The same glasses he may wear permanently, superadding for a moment for distant vision a double eyeglass with glasses of $-\frac{1}{10}$. At the end of two years he returns: his condition is not altered. Shortly afterwards the question is put to me by parents whose daughter he had asked in marriage, whether there is danger of blindness. My answer, which I stated that I would give only with the patient's consent, amounted to this: "Mr. v. d. W. is rather highly myopic. In connection with this nearsightedness a defect has arisen in the right eye, which, if further developed, might destroy the power of vision. It has, however, been stationary for two years, and we may hope that it will very long, perhaps to old age, remain stationary. The left eye presents no defect except the nearsightedness; but experience shows that with detachment of the retina in one eye, the other, when it is equally nearsighted, is not unfrequently attacked by the same defect. Considering the existing degree of the nearsightedness, and its stationary character, it is, however, not probable that, if the directions given be faithfully followed, the left eye will in this case become affected."—Six months later Mr. v. d. W. presented to me his young wife. I once more impressed upon him how necessary it was that he should *in every respect* take care of himself. Rather more than seven years have elapsed since that time, and his state is in general stationary; the myopia, too, having but very slightly increased.

He who, with moderate myopia, treats his eyes fairly, has nothing to fear at a more advanced time of life.

XIII. Mr. M., aged 52, who reads and writes much, has for many years used in doing so spectacles of $-\frac{1}{9}$, with which his myopia is exactly neutralised. For distant objects his acuteness of vision is at the same time $= 1$. Hitherto he has also seen every near object he required with his spectacles; it was only when he wanted to distinguish anything when it was half-dark, or for which others would need a magnifying glass, that he put off his spectacles for a few minutes. Latterly, he observes that he involuntarily raises his glasses to look sharply at smaller objects when near. "Do you still work in the evening without trouble with your spectacles?" As I expected, his answer was, "Only in good light, and when the print is not too small." "Then the time is approaching," I replied, "for diminishing the concavity of your glasses in proportion to the degree of the convex glasses which, at your age, you would require, if you were not myopic. Take, therefore, in the evening $-\frac{1}{10}$, and soon glasses somewhat weaker, and you will be content perhaps also to wear the same glasses habitually, though you will not see distant objects quite so acutely as with $-\frac{1}{9}$. When you are an old man, you will use two spectacles, $-\frac{1}{24}$, to work with, and $-\frac{1}{12}$ to wear habitually, and, finally, you will read without spectacles, and you will probably, when the acuteness of vision diminishes, come even to convex glasses: your myopia will, in fact, diminish somewhat, perhaps to $\frac{1}{12}$. Then may you, as a very old, but strong and healthy man, feel yourself still quite satisfied in wearing spectacles with glasses of $-\frac{1}{16}$ or $-\frac{1}{18}$.

NOTE TO CHAPTER VII.

We are indebted to Kepler for the earliest knowledge of the nature o myopia. He laid the foundations of dioptrics in general, and in particular of physiological dioptrics. The influence which spectacle-glasses have exercised in this direction is extremely remarkable. We have already alluded to these glasses as among the most indispensable instruments for man (p. 170). Their great importance in the history of science was demonstrated in the observation that they had led to the invention both of the microscope and of the telescope. After perusing the works of Kepler, I go still further, and think I may maintain that the development of physiological dioptrics has proceeded from spectacle-glasses. Alhazen showed about 1100 (*Opticæ thesaurus:* Basileæ, 1572), that the eye is not the source of light, but that the light proceeds from visible objects and enters the eye. With respect to the formation of pictures in the eye, he conceived wholly incorrect ideas. It is still stranger that we must say the same of Johannes Baptista Porta, who, although he compared the eye with the camera obscura invented by him, was of opinion that the pictures were formed on the anterior surface of the lens (see his *Magia Naturalis,* 1558 (?), and his work, *de Refractione, optices parte,* libri novem. Neap. 1593). His contemporary, Maurolycus (*Photismi de lumine et umbrâ,* Ven. 1575) arrived at more correct conclusions. This writer comprehends that the crystalline lens is to be compared with an ordinary convex lens, looks upon it as more convex in myopes, flatter in presbyopes, explains the action of convex and concave glasses, but nevertheless gives, in order to avoid the inversion of the images upon the retina, a totally confused idea of the action of the lens, and makes the images fall on the plane of the optic nerve, without mentioning the retina.

It was in 1601, Kepler himself informs us, that D. Ludovicus L. B. a Dietrichstein, put the question to him, why farsighted people distinguished near objects better through convex glasses, while nearsighted people saw distant objects more distinctly with the aid of concave glasses. Kepler was not acquainted with the work of Maurolycus. The only answer which he was at first able to give was, that convex glasses magnified near objects. But von Dietrichstein, not content with that, rejoined, that the question did not relate to magnitude, but to distinctness: for that concave glasses, which make objects smaller for all eyes, could otherwise assist no one. When, after three years' study, Kepler is at length in a position to give an answer: "responsum," he says, "si non satis clarum et indubium, satis certe tardum," his thankful tone testifies of the stimulus which he had received from the question of the man whom he calls, "Mæcenatum meorum præcipuus." That answer we find in his *Paralipomena ad Vitellionem quibus Astronomiæ pars optica traditur*, etc., Francofurti, 1604, p. 201. But we find more here. It is evident, and Kepler himself says it, that he could not at first answer the question proposed to him, because he had no correct·idea respecting vision. Here, now for the first time, we find the formation of inverted images upon the retina (some years later demonstrated in the curious experiments of Scheiner), contended for upon good grounds, and explained by the meeting of the rays, proceeding from each point of the object, again, in one point, upon the retina, in consequence of refraction by the cornea, and especially by the crystalline lens. Kepler knew also, that in order to form a sharply-defined image upon the retina, the object must be at a given distance (Propositio XXVIII); and with this is connected the answer respecting the action of spectacles, namely : that,—while in nearsighted persons the cones of rays, derived from each point of near objects, unite upon the retina, in farsighted persons, on the contrary, those derived from remote objects,—the rays of each cone, refracted by concave glasses, acquire a direction as if they had proceeded from a near point, and inversely, as if from a more remote point, after refraction by convex glasses. The explanation, as we see, leaves nothing to be desired.—The *Astronomiæ pars optica* is called by Montucla "un ouvrage plein d'idées neuves et digne d'un homme de génie, mais dans lequel il ne faut pas chercher cette précision ui caracterise ceux de notre siècle." This last cannot be said of Kepler's *Dioptrice seu Demonstratio eorum quæ visui et visibilibus propter Conspicilla non ita pridem inventa accidunt.* Augustæ Vindelicorum, 1611,—a work, as it seems, less known,—I found it quoted neither by Montucla nor by Priestley (The History and Present State of Discoveries relating to Vision, Light, and Colours, London, 1772),—but in which dioptrics, and especially physiological dioptrics, are treated of with conciseness and clearness. For the first time we here find the necessity of change of form in accommodation demonstrated. "It is not possible," thus runs Propositio LXIII, "that the retina maintaining the same position in the eye should receive a defined image both from near and from remote objects," and after this statement we read as Propositio LXIV : "Some see remote objects distinctly, near objects confusedly (presbyopes); others see near objects distinctly, remote objects confusedly (myopes); others see near and remote objects confusedly (morbid conditions); some, finally, see both distinctly." Of these last he says : "Oculum et sanum habent et *figura mobilem*," that is, they accommodate for different distances by altering the form of the eye. "Qui vero alterutra," thus he continues, "solum distincte vident, oculum habent sanum quidem, sed jam indurescentem, adsuefactum et quasi senilem." This he applies both to myopes and presbyopes. He places both in one line. He has thus, although himself myopic, overlooked the accommodation of myopes. Kepler developes his idea respecting the mode of origin still more fully in the following manner : He who in youth practises himself for distance and for near objects, in old age, becomes presbyopic, because practice diminishes with advancing years, and the parallel condition of the visual axes is the most natural; "but he who is from childhood occupied with study or fine work, speedily becomes accustomed to the vision of near objects, and with the advance of years this increases, so that remote objects are more and more imperfectly seen." Thus in Kepler's view nearsightedness consists in the condition of accommodation for near objects having become unalterable through partial or one-sided practice (oculus indurescens, adsuefactus et quasi senilis). And what does he suppose this condition to be ? He explains the accommodation by the retina changing its place and approaching to or removing from the crystalline lens, and he must therefore have supposed that in myopes the retina was at a greater distance from the lens.

Thus we see that Kepler looked upon myopia and presbyopia as opposite conditions, and this was in his position perfectly logical, for he admitted no accommodation in either state.

This vision of myopes was still farther investigated and explained by Scheiner (1625, see his work entitled *Oculus*), and subsequently, especially by Dechales (compare p. 389 of this book). But still Kepler's error always remained, or, if we choose, the hiatus left by him continued : observers were not aware of the accommodation of myopes. It is almost incomprehensible that, with the distribution of neutralising spectacles, for which rather correct directions were given, oculists should have overlooked the accommodation in young people ; but yet I have not been able to satisfy myself that any writer of the seventeenth century directly mentions it. It is by Robert Smith (see the *Author's Remarks*, p. 2, at the end of his *Complete System of Optics*, Cambridge, 1738, vol. ii.) that we first find it clearly expressed. He not only remarks that a myope sees distant and near objects acutely through the same glasses, but he also shows that no more accommodation is required for that purpose than for the short range which the myopic eye possesses without spectacles.—With the demonstration of the accommodation of myopes, the opposition of myopia and presbyopia should at once have disappeared (compare p. 80).

The most important point which remained to be investigated was the organic basis, the *efficient cause* of myopia. With respect to this we find among the earlier writers no definite idea. Evidently they did not attach due importance to it. Therefore they neglected to investigate the point, and contented themselves with enumerating all the deviations, which if they existed, would give rise to myopia, but the existence of which was not proven. Among the abnormities more prominently mentioned, we find a thicker lens, a more convex cornea, and a longer visual axis; altered coefficient of refraction and unusual position of the lens are also spoken of, and when not merely the physicists, but also the oculists began to take part in the discussion, thickening of the posterior surface of the cornea, increased coefficient of refraction of the vitreous humour (which ought to produce precisely the contrary), a wide pupil, and even a turgor vitalis were added to the list. Of all these arbitrary opinions history has no further notice to take. Only so far as they were based partly upon observation, do they deserve to be remembered, and this was not altogether wanting. Thus Boerhaave (1708), in his lectures *de Morbis Oculorum, prælectiones publicæ*, editio altera, p. 211, Göttingæ, 1750, published by Haller from manuscripts of different hearers, said : " Infinita sunt in oculo, nec unquam explicanda quæ hos effectus (myopiam) facere possunt, duas vero saltem sæpissime *observatas* causas hic proponemus," and, as such, he names : 1°. *Nimia oculi longitudo ;* 2°. *Corneæ convexitas nimia.* These two were indeed more than a mere optical fiction. Deceived by the greater depth of the chamber of the eye, observers thought that, viewed in profile, they saw a more convex cornea in myopes. And certainly it was also a matter of observation that in highly myopic individuals the eye-balls are often large and prominent. We find this fact already mentioned by much earlier writers than Boerhaave. By others, following him, mention is made even of the ellipsoidal figure (*figure "ovale"*) of the myopic eye (*Gendron, Traité des Maladies des Yeux.* Paris, 1770, tome ii., p. 359). But still this cause was in general not sufficiently put forward, and until a few years ago no decided opinion whatever was adopted. Von Graefe even acknow-ledges that previously to his examination of eyes with staphyloma posticum (*Archiv f. Ophthal.*, 1854, B. 1., H. 1., p. 399), he thought that the cause of myopia was to be sought in the vitreous humour. We notice also that Mackenzie, in 1830 (*A Practical Treatise on the Diseases of the Eye*, 1st Edition, p. 718), informs us, that " preternatural elongation of the eyeball" belongs to the " efficient causes of myopia," " and has even been regarded by *some* as the *only admissible cause*," but I know not who are meant by these *some.*

Now we are aware that it was an advance when, putting aside other causes, writers adhered to the increased length of the visual axis. Such an elonga-tion was anatomically first found (compare p. 371) by Scarpa (1801), in two female eyes, and was described by him under the name of *sta-phyloma*, because it appeared to be a *morbid distention.* This was per-haps the reason why it did not occur to Scarpa to bring the deviation he had established into connexion with myopia, for observers were at that time far from suspecting that an atrophic condition was con-nected with myopia. Subsequently, von Ammon remarks (*Zeitschrift für Ophthalmologie*, 1832), that the staphyloma posticum of Scarpa is not of such rare occurrence as had been supposed, and that the dis-tention is usually greatest at the posterior pole,—always without seek-ing a connexion with myopia. The first who states that he had found in the dead body the eye of a nearsighted person *pear-shaped*, is Ritterich (1839) ; but it was in the dissections of Arlt (1856), who, in various eyes of myopes, found an evident elongation of the visual axis, formed at the expense of the posterior wall, that the great importance of this distention with respect to myopia was studied and generally recognised. To this it certainly contributed much, that after the invention of the ophthalmoscope, the peculiar changes in the fundus oculi of myopes were discovered in different quarters (von Graefe, *loc. cit. ;* Jaeger, *Sitzungsberichte der Akademie*, 27th April, 1854), which changes were unmistakably connected with the posterior distention of the bulb. Von Graefe, too, had even already examined two eyes (*Archiv für Ophthalmologie*, 1854, B. I., p. 394), in which the peculiar atrophy (" sclerotico-chorioiditis posterior") was recognis-able with the ophthalmoscope, and where the length of the visual axis was found to be 29 and 30·5 mm.—Then the question arose, whether myopia must in every case be attributed to elongation of the visual axis. In the highest degrees of the affection no doubt could exist upon this point. Von Graefe forthwith stated, that, of those who need glasses of from $-\frac{1}{6}$ to $-\frac{1}{2}$, to neutralise their myopia, at all events $90^0/_0$ exhibit the peculiar change in the fundus oculi. Others confirmed this frequent occurrence, or found it independently of von Graefe. I very soon even thought that the proportion is much nearer to $100^0/_0$. It appeared to me, in fact, that, rare cases of *morbid* distention of the cornea excepted, the atrophic crescent is not absent in higher degrees of myopia, and that when in moderate degrees the atrophy may in youth still be wanting, it is developed, even without increase of the myopia, at a more advanced time of life, which leads to the inference, that in these cases also the longer visual axis was originally present. In this way it became very improbable that cornea or lens had any part in myopia. That the cornea has not, was now proved by numerous measurements (compare p. 89). That the lens should have it, or that a particular form of acquired myopia (plesiopia) should be dependent thereon (Stellwag von Carion, von Jaeger), appears to be still very problematical (p. 352). Thus much is certain, that the typical myopia depends upon elongation of the visual axis.—As to the mode of origin, von Graefe considered it at first to be the result of distention by inflammation. Stellwag von Carion (*Die Accommodationsfehler des Auges*, Wien, 1855, in the *Sitzungsberichte der kais. Akademie*, B. xvi.), showed that it may depend upon a congenital defect in form. The secondary morbid changes were seen and recognised simultaneously by many.—The position of the centre of motion in myopic eyes I determined with Dr. Doijer (Conf. §§ 15 and 31).—I had previously seen, and brought into connexion with the position of the eyes (p. 182), the change in the direction of the visual line by displacement of the yellow spot (p. 381).—The movements of the myopic eye, and the connexion of myopia and asthenopia muscularis were investigated by von Graefe (*Archiv*, 1862); to the connexion of strabismus divergens I also gave some contributions (§ 31). Lastly, the investigation of the relative range of accommodation in myopes was commenced under my direction by Mac-Gillavry (*Over de hoegrootheid van het accommodatie-vermogen*, Utrecht, 1858), was continued by me and applied to the indication for spectacles.—Of the anatomical examination of myopic eyes, to which Arlt and Ed. von Jaeger have made important contributions, we still have great need.

CHAPTER VIII.

§ 33. Definition of Astigmatism. — Regular and Irregular Astigmatism.

Ametropia, comprising the lesions of refraction, is resolved, according to § 6, into two opposite conditions : myopia and hypermetropia. Every lesion of refraction belongs to one of these two. Sometimes, however, it happens that in the several meridians of the same eye the refraction is very different. In one meridian the same eye may be emmetropic, in the other ametropic; in the several meridians a difference in the degree and even in the form of ametropia may occur.

The asymmetry, on which this difference depends, is proper to all eyes. Usually it exists in so slight a degree, that the acuteness of vision is not essentially impaired by it. But exceptionally it becomes considerable, and occasions an aberration of the rays of light, which interferes with the sharpness of sight.

This aberration, dependent on an asymmetry of the eye, may be designated as *astigmatism*. To make it clear, we must glance at the aberrations of light in general.

Rays of light which, sufficiently prolonged, all meet at one side in the same point, form *homocentric** light : they have a common centre. The diverging light, emitted from a point of any object, is therefore homocentric; a bundle of parallel rays, derived from a point situated at an infinite distance, is also homocentric. Consequently the rays of light, proceeding from any object, and received by the cornea, form cones of homocentric light. Only when the rays between the object and the eye are by some cause or other more or less diverted from their course, do the cones of light cease to consist of homocentric light.

In general, we may say that homocentric light, refracted by a spherical surface, continues homocentric : that, namely, the rays behind the refracting surface either unite again into one point, or

* Listing, *Beitrag zur physiologischen Optik.* Göttingen, 1845.

29

proceed in a direction as if they all were derived directly from a point situated before the refracting surface.

The homocentricity has, however, not continued perfect. The rays, in fact, are no longer directed precisely to one point, but are only nearly so. To this deviation from homocentricity the name of "aberration" is given; and we distinguish two aberrations of different origins: the *chromatic* and the *spherical*. The first depends on the nature of the light, the second on the form of the refracting surface.

Chromatic aberration is the result of a difference in refrangibility of the rays of light. Rays which were originally parallel to the axis of the light-refracting surface, and at the same time at an equal distance from that axis, undergo no aberration in consequence of sphericity, and should therefore remain directed exactly to one point, if they were all of like nature. Rays of unlike nature, on the contrary, find their focus in the axis, at different distances from the refracting surface, the violet and blue rays at a shorter, the red at a longer, distance.—The dioptric system of the eye also necessarily presents this chromatic aberration. Under ordinary circumstances, however, the latter scarcely interferes with the sharpness of vision.[*] I shall not dwell further upon it, as it has no essential connexion with our subject.

Rays of light of equal length of undulation, and as such, of equal refrangibility, form homogeneous light; the light is also of similar colour, and is therefore called *monochromatic*. If such rays fall parallel on a spherical surface, and at the same time at an equal distance from its axis, they are refracted in an equal degree from or towards the axis, and thus continue directed to one point: the homocentricity is perfect. But if, although parallel to the axis, they strike the surface at different distances from the axis, they cease to be directed exactly to one point: the farther from the axis they strike the surface, the nearer to the surface do they cut the axis. This deviation is called *spherical aberration:* it is the *monochromatic aberration* (that is, the aberration of rays of like colour) belonging to refraction by a spherical surface.

The dioptric system of the eye also has a monochromatic aberra-

---

[*] Helmholtz, *Physiologische Optik*, in *Allgemeine Encyklopædie der Physik*, herausgegeben von Gustav Karsten. Leipzig, 1856, 1 Lief. pp. 137 *et seq.*

tion. The latter is in it even rather considerable, and is highly complicated. For our purpose it is to be distinguished as—

a. An aberration, which has reference to the rays refracted in one and the same meridian.

b. An aberration, dependent on the difference in focal length of the different meridians of the light-refracting system.

The first represents *irregular* astigmatism. It is dependent chiefly on the structure of the lens, and its leading phenomenon is the polyopia uniocularis. Morbid deviations may also produce irregular astigmatism. Of these I shall speak in the last section of this chapter. The second gives rise to *regular* astigmatism, which is capable of correction. It is the principal subject of this chapter.

The Rev. Dr. Whewell has, as Mackenzie (*A Practical Treatise on the Diseases of the Eye*, London, 1854, p. 927) informs us, designated the defect, described by Airy as existing in his left eye, by the name of astigmatism. This word is derived from *a* priv. and στιγμα, from στιζω, pungo, and signifies that rays, derived from one point, do not again unite into one point. The entire monochromatic deviation in the eye we may therefore call astigmatism, and this meaning I have given to the term in question. Whewell had applied the name only to the regular form. By the word astigmatism, used without more precise definition, regular astigmatism will, in the sequel of this work, be understood.

§ 34. REGULAR ASTIGMATISM IN THE NORMAL EYE.

If we determine successively the farthest point, at which fine horizontal and fine vertical threads or stripes are acutely seen, we obtain unequal distances. The great majority of eyes discover a shorter distance for horizontal than for vertical stripes.

A similar difference is met with in determining the nearest point of distinct vision. The difference then, however, comes out too great, because the two determinations are not made under similar convergence, and with greater convergence the eyes accommodate more strongly.

Two threads, which cross in a plane, the one being vertical and the other horizontal, are not seen with equal sharpness. If we see the horizontal one acutely, the vertical thread, to be distinctly seen, must be removed from the eye; if we accommodate for the vertical, the horizontal must, in order to obtain equal sharpness, be brought nearer to the eye. A similar difference is maintained with each degree of tension of accommodation.

2

These experiments prove, that the points of the refracting meridians are not symmetrically arranged around one axis. The asymmetry is of such a nature that the focal distance is shorter in the vertical meridian than in the horizontal. In order, namely, to see a vertical stripe acutely, the rays, which in a horizontal plane diverge from each point of the line, must be brought to a focus on the retina : it is not necessary that those diverging in a vertical plane should also previously converge into one point, as the diffusion-images still existing in a vertical direction cover one another on the vertical stripe. On the other hand, in order to see a horizontal stripe acutely, it is necessary only that the rays of light diverging in a vertical plane should unite in one point upon the retina. Now horizontal stripes are acutely seen, as I have remarked, at a shorter distance than vertical ones : consequently rays situated in a vertical plane, which are refracted in the vertical meridian of the eye, are more speedily brought to a focus than those of equal divergence situated in a horizontal plane; and the vertical meridian, therefore, has a shorter focal distance than the horizontal.

The correctness of this view appears further from the form of the diffusion-images of a point of light. In accurate accommodation the diffusion-spot is very small and nearly round, while a nearer point appears extended in breadth, and a more remote one seems to be extended in height.

The signification of this phenomenon must be clearly understood, and appears, therefore, to demand more particular explanation.

Let us suppose the total deviation of light in the eye to be produced by a single convex refracting surface, with the shortest radius of curvature in the vertical, and the longest in the horizontal meridian. These two are then the principal meridians. Through a central round opening, Fig. 150, $v\,v'\,h\,h'$, let a cone of rays, proceeding from a point situated in the prolongation of the axis of vision, fall upon this surface ; of this cone let us consider only the rays, situated in the vertical plane $v\,v'$, and the rays situated in the horizontal plane $h\,h'$, whereof respectively the points $v\,v'$ and $h\,h'$ are the most external. After the refraction both approach the visual axis (which perpendicular to the plane of the drawing passes through a), $v\,v'$ does so, however, more rapidly than $h\,h'$. Before union they therefore lie, in the

Fig. 150.

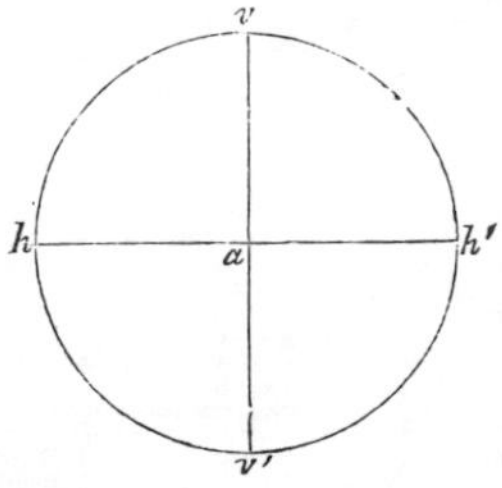

ellipse A, as in Fig. 151, and where $v\ v'$ meet in one point B, $h\ h'$ have not yet come to a focus. Thereupon we now find in

Fig. 151.

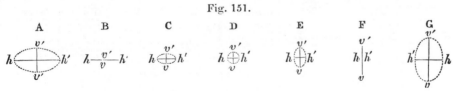

succession $v\ v'$ already intersected, $h\ h'$ approached to one another, C, D, and E; further, $h\ h'$ united in one point, and $v'\ v$ after intersection more widely separated, F; finally, both intersected, G. The focus of $v\ v'$ therefore lies most anteriorly, that of $h\ h'$ most posteriorly, in the axis. The space between these two points, where rays of different meridians intersect, may be called focal interval (*intervalle focal*, or *Brennstrecke* of Sturm).

From the above figures it is now evident, what successive forms the section of the cone of light will exhibit. In the middle of the focal interval, D, it will be nearly round, and anteriorly through oblate ellipses, C, with increasing eccentricity, it will pass into a horizontal line, B; posteriorly through prolate ellipses, E, it will come to form a vertical line, F, while before the focal interval a larger oblate ellipse, A, and behind it, a larger prolate ellipse, G, will be found.

To this, as we have seen, the diffusion-images of the eye in general correspond. They thus find their explanation, when the dioptric system of the eye is considered as a single refracting surface, with a difference of radius of curvature in its several meridians, and it will more fully appear that we are justified in so considering it.

Moreover, through the form of the diffusion-images, in refraction by such a surface, what I have stated respecting the difference in the distance of distinct vision of stripes of different direction is fully explained. Horizontal and vertical stripes, namely, are acutely seen, when the diffusion-images of all the points of the stripe form respectively horizontal and vertical lines, which cover one another in the stripe; and this will be the case when the beginning and the end of the focal interval correspond respectively to the percipient surface of the retina.

To make the description easier, we have thus far assumed that the maximum of curvature coincides with the vertical, the minimum with the horizontal meridian. And the rule in fact is, that they nearly do so. But to this rule there are numerous exceptions. Not unfrequently the deviation from the ordinary direction is very considerable ; and it even occurs that the maximum of curvature coincides nearly with the horizontal, the minimum with the vertical meridian. So Thomas Young, the discoverer of astigmatism, found it in his own eye, and I too have met with some cases of this nature.

In general there is no difficulty in determining the direction of the principal meridians (those of the maximum and minimum of curva-

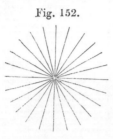

Fig. 152.

ture). The mode of doing so is included in the experiments above described, in proof of the existence of astigmatism. Were we so perfectly conscious of our accommodation that we could accurately state, what lines in the annexed figure are seen quite sharply at the maximum, and what at the minimum of augmented tension, the directions of the maximum and minimum of curvature would at the same time be known. That consciousness is, however, seldom very accurate.

A more certain mode of determination is supplied by the direction in which the diffusion-images of a point of light appear extended on this, and on that side of the distance of distinct vision. With the head perpendicular, the eye brought by glasses to a state of myopia of about $\frac{1}{9}$, let a point of light (for example, a very small opening in a black plate, turned towards the sky or towards the globe of a lamp) be brought in a horizontal plane successively *short of* and *beyond* the distance of distinct vision : it will exhibit itself in these two positions elongated in opposite directions, the longest dimension corresponding in the first position to the direction of the minimum of curvature, that in the second, to the direction of the maximum of curvature.

The result is often surprising when the eye, made slightly myopic $\left(\text{for example } \frac{1}{60}\right)$ by a glass (whose axis must coincide with the visual axis), is made to look towards a remote point of light (a small round opening in a black screen turned towards the light), and a negative glass $\left(\text{for example} - \frac{1}{30}\right)$ is alternately held before the eye and taken away. The diffusion-image then is extended in each time two opposite directions—with the addition of $-\frac{1}{30}$ in the meridian of the minimum of curvature, without this addition in that of the maximum of curvature. By quickly pushing the glass to and fro, the two images are (in consequence of the persistence of the impressions) persistently and simultaneously seen, and in some then exhibit the form of a cross.

The estimation of the direction may sometimes be doubtful in the experiment just described, when the *irregular* astigmatism is extraordinarily developed, and the diffusion-images are consequently highly complicated. We then, however, attain certainty by giving to a weak cylindrical glass, for ordinary cases of $\frac{1}{80}$, such a direction that letters or other small figures are most acutely seen : in the most advantageous position we obtain only the *difference* of the astigmatic effects of the cylindrical lens and of the eye ; in the most disadvantageous, on the contrary, we obtain the *sum*. The glass is placed with its axis directed vertically, in a ring, which turns in a second ring fixed on a plate : on this plate the position of the axis chosen can be read off in degrees. By this experiment we can satisfy any one that his eye is not free from astigmatism : if it were so, the vision of compound figures would be interfered with equally in every position of the axis. But this is by no means the case : most people even find an improvement of vision when a certain direction is given to the glass.

The cause of regular astigmatism is to be sought partly in the cornea. Numerous measurements have shown, that the cornea in its several meridians has a different radius of curvature ; and what holds good for the dioptric system of the whole eye, namely, that the maximum of curvature usually lies closer to the vertical meridian than to the horizontal, is equally applicable to the cornea, taken by itself. It is thus established, in the first place, that the cornea on account of its form produces astigmatism ; in the second place, that even if the crystalline lens has an influence, the direction given to it by the cornea in general preponderates.

On the lens depends irregular astigmatism ; to it polyopia uniocularis, to it the rays of the diffusion-images of a point of light owe their origin. The direct proof of this is furnished by the fact, that in the condition of aphakia, when the lens is wholly absent from the eye, all these phenomena of irregular astigmatism are removed. In numerous cases I have satisfied myself of this. The boundaries of the focal space, and the transition-forms of the diffusion-image (Fig.

151) are, when aphakia exists, exhibited with an accuracy and definition, which satisfy the most rigid requirements of the theory.

However, the crystalline lens modifies also regular astigmatism, whether in virtue of the form of its surfaces, or through oblique position. Therefore the regular astigmatism of the whole system corresponds exactly neither in direction nor in degree to the form of the cornea.

Astigmatism, the result of a positive cylindrical lens, may be removed by a second of equal focal distance, either by a negative, whose axis is parallel to the first, or by a positive, whose axis stands perpendicular to that of the first. Thus, also, the astigmatism of the eye may be corrected by a cylindrical lens; and, according to the principle laid down in § 6, for the determination of the degree of anomalies of refraction, the focal distance of the cylindrical lens required for this purpose defines the degree of the astigmatism: it is inversely proportionate to the focal distance of the correcting lens, expressed in Parisian inches.

So long as astigmatism does not essentially diminish the acuteness of vision, we call it normal. It is abnormal so soon as disturbance occurs. If it amounts to $\frac{1}{40}$ or more, it must be considered as abnormal. · The reason that Dr. Knapp found no disturbance with higher degrees would appear to be, that he deduced the degree from the determination of the nearest points, whereby too high values are obtained (see p. 451).

The asymmetry of the dioptric system of the eye was first observed by Thomas Young (*Philosophical Transactions* for 1793, vol. lxxxiii., p. 169, and *Miscellaneous Works* of the late Thomas Young, edited by Peacock, London, 1855, vol. i., p. 26), in his own person. The distinguished natural philosopher, whose brilliant merits in the domain of physiological optics were first duly estimated by Helmholtz, was himself nearsighted. In relaxation of the eye, consequently in determination of the farthest point, he saw in his optometer, held in a horizontal position, the double images of the thread intersect one another at seven inches from the eye, on the contrary at ten inches, when in a vertical position. This indicates, on reducing the English to Parisian inches, an astigmatism of about $\frac{1}{25}$; and it is therefore strange that Young, as he himself remarks, had experienced no disturbance from it. The optician Cary, to whom Young communicated his discovery, stated to him that he had before often found that nearsighted people distinguished objects much more acutely, when the glasses suited to them were held in a particular oblique direction before the eye: now by this manœuvre, at least when strong glasses are necessary, a certain degree of astigmatism may be corrected.—Young, too, had already studied and delineated the form of the diffusion-spots. The source of astigmatism he sought in the crystalline lens, because it continued when he plunged his cornea into water, and replaced its action by that of a convex lens. He now assumed an oblique position of the crystalline lens as the cause, and even thought that from the diffusion-images of a point of light it might be deduced, that the two surfaces of his lens were not centred.—In a double point of view, therefore, Young's eye presented an exception: the refraction was stronger in the horizontal than in the vertical meridian, and the cause lay principally in the lens.

Fick (*Zeitschrift f. ration. Medizin.* N. F. VI., p. 83.) found in himself an astigmatism of $\frac{1}{319}$; Helmholtz (*Physiol. Optik. l. c.,* p. 145.) of $\frac{1}{119}$. Bruecke, as I believe, could not observe anything of the kind. In my right eye it amounts to $\frac{1}{100}$, in my left to $\frac{1}{95}$. Sharp eyes have generally not more than from $\frac{1}{140}$ to $\frac{1}{60}$. If it amounts to more, the power of vision will be under some circumstances (compare the following §) already disturbed.

The theory of refraction by asymmetrical surfaces was developed many years ago by Sturm (*Comptes rendus de l'Académie des Sciences de Paris,* t. xx., pp. 554, 761, 1238, and Poggendorff's *Annalen* B. 65. 116. Compare Fick, *Mediz. Physik,* p. 327, whence the accompanying figure is borrowed). He showed that when a homocentric bundle of light falls on a very small circularly-defined portion (Fig. 153, *o*) of a convex asymmetrical surface, after the refraction it no longer continues homocentric, but that the refracted fasciculus of rays forms a certain skew surface (surface gauche), which, except through the small opening *o*, is bounded by two right lines *h h'* and *v v'*, intersecting in the space, and which do not lie in the same plane: if *h h'* be supposed to be in the plane of the figure, *v v'* is to be considered as the projection of a perpendicular line standing on the same. The space between *h h'* and *v v'* is the focal interval of Sturm.

FIG. 153.

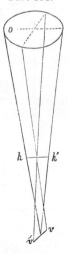

I have above remarked, that the forms of the diffusion-images of the dioptric system of the eye in general correspond to what the foregoing theory would require, excepting peculiar complications. It needs to be further investigated in what the asymmetry of the system consists.

In the first place, then, the cornea is asymmetrical. It may, as numerous measurements prove, be considered as the top segment of an ellipsoid with three unequal axes. The long axis corresponds to the visual axis; the two short axes lie in general nearly horizontally and vertically. All meridional sections, carried through the long axis, are nearly ellipses,

but of unequal eccentricity and of unequal radius of curvature (conf.
Knapp, *l. c.*).   The maximum and minimum of radius of curvature correspond to the principal sections which are carried through the long axis and
one of the short axes, the maximum usually corresponding to the horizontal, the minimum to the vertical principal section.   Now, to such an
ellipsoid the theory of Sturm is applicable.   That a focal space thus arises,
and what form its perpendicular sections have, is above conspicuously represented (Fig. 151).   I think it necessary here to introduce a fuller explanation, after Helmholtz.   In Fig. 154, let the line *g b* be an axis of the

Fig. 154.

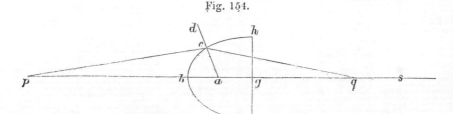

ellipsoid, in the prolongation of which at *p* is the point of light.   Let the
plane of the diagram be a *principal* section of the ellipsoid, so that a *second*
axis *g h* lies in this plane.   The normals of all points of an ellipsoidal plane,
which are met by a *principal section*, lie likewise in the principal section
of the ellipsoid.   And as a refracted ray remains in the plane, in which it
lay with the normal, so rays, incident in a principal section, also remain
after refraction, in the principal section.   When therefore a ray from *p*
falls upon the point *c*, the refracted ray remains in the plane of the diagram
(in which the ray and the plumbline *d a* lie), and cuts the axis *b g* in one of
its points *q*.   The refracted ray is thereby more accurately defined through
the condition that

$$sin\ a\ c\ q \text{ must be} = \frac{1}{n}\ sin\ p\ c\ d,$$

wherein *n* signifies the coefficient of refraction.   This condition is the same
as for symmetrical or rotation surfaces.   The almost perpendicular rays
incident at *b* have therefore a common focus in the axis, whose distance
depends on the radius of curvature, *r*, of the curved line *b c h* in *b*.   If *p* lies
at an infinite distance, the posterior focal length for the given principal
section is

$$F'' = \frac{n\ r'}{n-1}.$$

The rays which, proceeding from *p*, run in the other principal section,
which is determined by *b q* and the third axis, are in all respects similarly
related ; only the radius of curvature in the top of the plane has another
value *r''*, and the focal distance in this second principal section is

$$\frac{n\ r''}{n-1}.$$

The ray *p q* is therefore cut by the rays, which in the plane of the diagram border immediately upon it, in a point, for example in q; on the contrary, by the rays bordering thereon in a plane situate perpendicularly to the plane of the diagram, not in the same point q, but in another point, for example, in s.

It is now evident, that, in the point q of the axis, the rays, lying in a plane, perpendicular to the diagram, have still a linear extension in that plane; that, on the other hand, the rays, lying in the plane of the diagram and uniting in q, having arrived at the point s of the axis, have again acquired a linear extension: in q and s therefore lie the limits of the focal interval.— From the representation above given, all this may have been already ascertained. But now, for the first time becomes evident, what was above designedly left out of view, that in this consideration only the rays, coincident with the two principal sections of the tri-axial ellipsoids, are included. For only in these principal sections do the normals pass through the principal axis; in all other meridional sections the normals do not intersect the axis, consequently the incident rays are not refracted in a plane, in which the principal axis lies, and the rays therefore do not intersect in a point of the axis.—Hence it appears, that we cannot assume that in the focal interval a series of foci should lie on the axis. This obtains only for the beginning and end of this interval. The fasciculus is, as Sturm taught, contained in a skew surface, and hence it is to be deduced that all the rays refracted in the different meridians cut one another in the two intersecting lines, bounding the beginning and end of the focal interval, and that the above-described transition-forms of the sections of the bundle of light are found in the focal interval.

In a recently published essay, Dr. J. H. Knapp (*Archiv f. Ophthalmologie*, B. viii. Abth. 2, p. 108), led by a remark of Professor Kirchhoff, that by simple analytical geometry of space we can prove, that a bundle of rays refracted by asymmetrically curved surfaces, must pass through two right lines, has mathematically determined the form of the whole refracted bundle of rays.

The form of the cornea leads us to expect, that it in itself must produce an astigmatism, completely agreeing with that here

Fig. 155,

described. This I have, on investigation, found confirmed. For this purpose I have chosen cases in which, in congenital cataract, the lens had been absorbed after numerous punctures (so that the question of an alteration of form of the cornea in consequence of operation could not be entertained), and where the pupil had remained quite round. Without exception, the limits of the focal interval were by these eyes quite accurately defined as fine lines, and the changes of form of the diffusion-images were also given, agreeably to the theory. From the direction of the lines bounding the focal interval, the maximum and minimum of curvature of the cornea were immediately deducible. Fig. 155 indicates the direction found in cases of aphakia in young subjects; D represents a right, S a left eye; $h\ h'$ is the diffusion-image at the anterior, $v\ v'$ at the posterior boundary of the focal interval. It hence appears that only once (IX.) was the radius of curvature greater in the vertical meridian than that in the horizontal, once, while $h\ h'$ and $v\ v'$ both form an angle of about 45°, nearly equal to it (VIII.), and that in the seven other cases the vertical meridian evidently had a shorter radius of curvature, and four times even nearly coincided with the shortest.

To a similar result did the radii of curvature of the cornea in a horizontal and in a vertical plane, carried through the line of vision, ascertained with the aid of the ophthalmometer, lead. The following Table may be consulted :—

Observers.	hor. rad.	vert. rad.	F″ hor.	F″ vertic.	As = 1 :
	mm.	mm.	In Parisian inches.		
1	7·74	7·74	1·1356	1·1356	∞
2	8·20	8·12	1·2031	1·1914	88
3	8·34	8·19	1·2237	1·2107	85
4	7·23	7·23	1·0608	1·0608	∞
5	8·27	8·30	1·2134	1·2178	— 250
6	7·73	7·69	1·1342	1·1283	160
7	8·15	7·94	1·1958	1·1650	34
8	8·08	7·81	1·1855	1·1457	29
9	8·02	7·92	1·1767	1·1626	76
10	7·42	7·30	1·0887	1·0711	50
11	7·49	7·51	1·0987	1·1019	— 280
12	7·49	7·45	1·0987	1·0931	160
13	7·84	7·46	1·1503	1·0946	16·9
14	7·75	7·33	1·1371	1·0755	14·9
15	7·60	7·53	1·1151	1·1048	89
16	7·55	7·60	1·1078	1·1151	— 127
16	7·80	7·91	1·1445	1·1605	— 62
17	8·07	8·26	1·1840	1·2120	— 40
18	7·23	7·385	1·0608	1·0835	— 38
19	7·22	7·08	1·0593	1·0388	40
20	7·74	7·71	1.1356	1·1313	220

(Observers 1–16 are grouped under "Donders and Doyer."; observers 16–20 under "Knapp.")

In the second column the radii of curvature found for the horizontal, in the third those found for the vertical plane, are indicated, expressed in mm.; in the fourth and fifth columns the posterior focal distances, F″, of the cornea in the two planes are contained, calculated according to the formula

$$F'' = \frac{n \quad r}{n-1}$$

n being assumed = 1·3365. They are expressed in Parisian inches, and thence, according to the formula

$$f' = \frac{F'\,f''}{f''-F''}$$

the focal distance is calculated of a cylindrical lens which, applied to the horizontal meridian, should in this make the posterior focus coincide with the focus for the vertical meridian. In this formula, F′ (= F″ : n) is the *anterior* focal distance of the cornea in the horizontal plane, f″ the posterior focal distance in the vertical plane, f′ the distance from the plane of the cornea to a point in the axis, to which the rays in a horizontal plane must be directed, to find their point of union in the focus of the vertical surface. If the radius of curvature in the horizontal plane be greater than in the vertical, then is f″ < F″, and consequently f′ is negative, which signifies that the rays must converge towards a point, situated behind the cornea, and that the cylindrical lens must therefore be a positive one. If the radius of curvature be greater in the vertical plane, the reverse is the case, and the cylindrical lens must in this instance be negative. Therefore if f′ be negative, a positive lens is necessary, and *vice versâ*. The negative sign is placed in the Table, where a negative lens was necessary. Moreover, we find on calculation that (the lens being supposed to be immediately at the cornea) a negative lens, which shall alter the focal distance of the strongest curvature into that of the weakest, must have the same focal distance as a positive lens, which can do the opposite.

From the Table it appears in the first place, that among the fifteen cases examined by us, only three times was a shorter radius found in the horizontal plane than in the vertical, and that each time the difference was extremely slight. Among the five cases of Knapp (the last five), on the contrary, it happens that not less than three occur, in which the horizontal plane has a shorter radius of curvature than the vertical.

In general the calculated astigmatism is slight. At the same time it is also to be observed, that No. 14, with an astigmatism of the cornea of $\frac{1}{14\cdot9}$, had considerably diminished sharpness of vision, capable of improvement by a cylindrical glass, and that this probably was the case also with some others. No. 13, the left eye of the same person to whom No. 14 belongs, is an eye in which, with much astigmatism of the cornea, the whole system (on account of compensation by the lens) exhibited only a slight degree, which did not interfere with the acuteness of vision.

I have not endeavoured in these cases to compare the astigmatism for each eye in particular, proceeding from the cornea, with the total astigmatism of the dioptric system. No useful result was to be expected from doing so. In order, in fact, to be able to calculate what astigmatism the crystalline lens possesses, the direction and degree of astigmatism for the whole system, and for the cornea the radii of curvature in its *axis, and indeed in the meridians of maximum and minimum*, must have been known. Now we may admit that the radii of curvature in the visual line deviate little from those in the axis of the cornea, and the principal meridians usually approach to the horizontal and vertical directions, so that, in general, from the measurements made it can be estimated, how much astigmatism proceeds from the asymmetry of the cornea; but still I considered the deviation too great to allow of our determining the *slight* astigmatism of the crystalline lens (as difference between the total and that found for the cornea) *by simple subtraction.*

A more accurate investigation, formerly promised (*Astigmatisme en cylindrische glazen*, p. 68, Utrecht 1862), and now accomplished with the zealous co-operation of Dr. Middelburg (*de Zitplaats van het astigmatisme*, Utrecht, 1863), has shown, indeed, that such substraction is not admissible.

Hitherto the radius of curvature was determined only in the visual line, and principally in the horizontal plane (see, for the method followed, p. 18, comparing Fig. 75, and for the results obtained, p. 89); and in order to find the radius in another plane, for example in the vertical (as for the above Table), the head was simply held to the side. It is evident that in this way no reliable results were to be obtained. In the first place, it is certainly extremely difficult, if not impossible, with any accuracy, to give the head precisely the desired degree of inclination, and, in the second place, the visual line was always directed simply towards the ophthalmometer, and was therefore, properly speaking, not measured in the plane of a meridian, for the meridians do not cut the visual line, but the axis of the cornea.

A proper system of measurements seemed therefore to be obtainable only, if it were possible to make the lights themselves turn, in a vertical plane, round a point on which the common axis of the cornea and ophthalmometer is directed, in order by so doing to make the lights shine consecutively in the different meridians of the cornea, while a corresponding inclination is given to the glass-plates of the ophthalmometer. To attain this object, a vertically-placed ring,

Fig. 156.

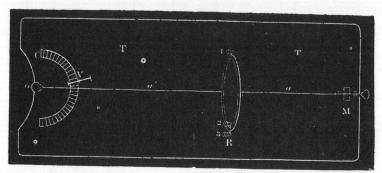

R, to whose centre the axis $a'\,a$ of the ophthalmometer stands perpendicular, and around which ring the lamps 1, 2, 3, here represented as lying in a horizontal line, can be turned, was steadily fixed on the oblong table (Fig. 156, T T), between the ophthalmometer M and the investigated eye, O. This ring, more accurately represented as Fig. 157, rests upon a pillar, S, which,

Fig. 157.

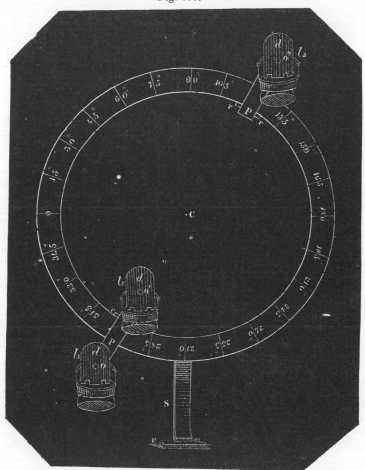

by means of its bending, does not impede the turning of the lamps, and is, by a broad foot-piece, v, firmly placed upon the table. The centre of the ring, c, is situated at one metre (= 3·28 English feet) from the eye; the diameter of the ring, measured to the outer margin, amounts to 388 mm. (15·27 English inches). On this ring turn two copper-plates P P', which, at the contact of two bent rims, $r\,r$, with the outsides of the ring, lie in the direction of the radii of the ring. To one of these copper-plates, P′, a lamp, l_3, is attached at the outside ; to the other bar, P, are fastened two similar lamps, l_1 at the outside, l_2 at the inside (indicated in Fig. 156 as 1, 2, and 3) ; each lamp is covered by a diaphragm, d, in which is an opening, o, 5·5 mm. large, and is movable in a hoop, so that in each position of the plates it assumes a vertical direction, turning round an axis, which passes exactly through the middle of the openings mentioned. The lamps are filled with oil, and have a flat wick, the flame of which completely illuminates the whole surface of the openings, seen from O. Now, in every position of the lamps the illuminated openings maintain unchangeably the same distance, namely, from o to o' = 144 5 mm., and from o' to o'' = 343·5 mm. Of course the two plates must always be diametrically opposite to each other, for example, P at 120°, and P′ at 300°, as in Fig, 157. In order to keep the flame steady, cases open in front are brought around the lamps, and when the latter are in a vertical position, a flat screen is held horizontally above the two lower ones, in order to prevent too great heating and the ascent of the current of air.

As has already been remarked, the axis of the ophthalmometer is directed to the centre, c, of the ring, and at the same time to the centre of the opening, in front of which the observed eye is. In taking the observation the axis of the cornea must also coincide therewith : therefore the first thing we have to do is to inquire what point the visual line must fix. From former observations it appeared that the axis of the cornea corresponds nearly to the centre of the cornea ; we now seek the centre first in the horizontal meridian, by the method followed by Dr. Doijer and myself (compare p. 186). For this purpose a light is placed directly before the centre, c (Fig. 157), of the ring, and the point is sought, which must be fixed in order to make the reflected image of this light correspond precisely to the middle of the cornea. In order to find that point, a flat copper arc, whose centre of curvature is situated in the nodal point of the eye O (Fig. 156), and to which a sight, v, is movably attached, is fastened on the oblong table in c. Now if for the horizontal meridian, the required position of the sight is found, the ophthalmometer is turned 90° round its axis, and it is thus determined with what direction of the visual line, above or below the horizontal plane, the edges of the cornea doubled in a vertical direction, respectively above and beneath, reach simultaneously the reflected image of a flame placed in the horizontal plane next the axis of the ophthalmometer : the direction is determined by moving the sight, which has the form of a slender cross, as much as necessary upwards or downwards.

In the position of the sight thus found, in whose fixation the axis of the ophthalmometer coincides with the axis of the cornea, the radius of curvature is in the first place determined ; and to ascertain whether the radius, thus measured, actually corresponds to the apex of the ellipsoid of the cornea, the sight is moved, consecutively in the horizontal and in the vertical plane, an equal number of degrees (usually ten), alternately to each side. And if it now appeared that in the two planes with equal deviation in two opposite directions a similar radius of curvature was found, it was assumed that the axis of the cornea was really properly directed. But if the difference amounted to more than was to be explained by error of observation, another direction was given to the sight, until repeated measurement proved the correctness of the position. It now appeared, that in the horizontal direction, the axis of the cornea usually passes through the centre of the section of the cornea, but that, when placed vertically, a deviation in this respect not unfrequently occurs.

With this determination of the axis of the cornea, the radius of the curvature at 0° and at 90° is already found.

While the point of sight continued the same, and the head was held in a vertical position, at least five measurements were now further made in each of the meridians, at intervals of 15 degrees. This was done simply by giving the required inclinations simultaneously to the three lamps and to the ophthalmometer.

The magnitudes, which corresponded to the degrees found on the ophthalmometer, had already been previously empirically determined, and thence the radii of curvature were now calculated.

No.	Name	Sex. Age.	Eye	Refrac-tion.	Radius of Curvature (in Millimetres) of the Apex of the Cornea in Meridian												Estimated Direction of M_e.	Ascertained Direction of M_o.	Remarks.	Observers.
					0°	15°	30°	45°	60°	75°	90°	105°	120°	135°	150°	165°				
1	M.	m. 24	L.	M $\frac{1}{30}$	7.94	7.96	7.84	7.66	7.70	7.73	7.71	7.90	7.86	7.82	7.85	7.88	90°	72°	$\mathrm{As} = \frac{1}{92}$	Hamer.
2	II.	m. 25	R.	E	8.22	8.02	7.99	7.96	7.98	8.11	8.05	8.09	8.09	8.22	8.24	8.31	55°	92½°	$\mathrm{As} = \frac{1}{92}$	Middelburg.
3	H.	m. 25	L.	M $\frac{1}{80}$	8.14 / 8.16	8.17	8.16	8.13	8.22	8.09	8.06 / 8.14 / 8.10	8.07	8.01	7.98	8.08	8.13	135°	87½°	$\mathrm{As} = \frac{1}{33}$	Donders.
4	v. D.	m. 26	R.	E	8.13	7.85	7.85	7.77	7.89	7.84	7.97	7.90	7.97	8.03	7.98	8.14	66°	102°		Middelburg.
5	v. D.	m. 28	L.	E	8.08	8.03 / 7.92	8.02 / 7.91	8.12 / 7.91	8.01 / 7.91	7.91	7.89 / 7.89	8.01 / 7.88	8.01 / 7.92	7.95 / 7.84	8.06 / 7.83	8.16 / 7.99	105°	17°		Donders.
6	P. G.	m. 36	R.	E	8.13	8.33	8.39	8.35	8.25	8.14	8.02	8.07	8.01	8.09	8.03	8.14	120°	62°	$\mathrm{As} = V\frac{1}{100}$	Middelburg.
7	P. G.	m. 36	L.	E	8.47	8.41	8.36	8.35	8.33	8.24	8.18	8.14	8.13	8.09	8.15	8.23	120°	97°	$\mathrm{As} = V\frac{1}{100}$	Middelburg.
8	O.	m. 16	R.	E	7.93	7.88	7.62	7.56	7.63	7.63	7.85	7.76	7.84	7.96	7.88	7.98	55°	95°	$\mathrm{As} = V\frac{1}{100}$; $\mathrm{S} =$	Middelburg.
9	O.	m. 16	L.	H $\frac{1}{50}$	7.92	7.91	7.87	7.85	7.78	7.62	7.68	7.62	7.53	7.48	7.63	7.68	120°	90°	$\mathrm{As} = V\frac{1}{100}$; $\mathrm{S} = \frac{30}{25}$	Hamer.
10	Gr.	m. 32	R.	H $\frac{1}{55}$	8.36	8.26	8.11	8.12	8.09	8.09	8.06	8.14	8.13	8.12	8.30	8.41	80°	90°		Middelburg.
11	v. R.	f. 28	R.	E	8.19	8.02	7.98	7.88	7.88	7.84	7.84	7.91	8.01	8.00	8.14	8.16	75°	90°		Middelburg.
12	v. H.	f. 21	R.	E	8.08	7.89	7.88	7.77	8.01	7.92	7.73	7.93	7.99	8.07	8.09	8.09	75°	72°		Middelburg.
13	W.	f. 18	R.	E	8.06	7.83	7.82	7.80	7.82	7.85	7.89	7.99	7.91	8.11	8.00	8.11	55°	2°		Middelburg.
14	S.	m. 50	R.	H $\frac{1}{40}$	8.07 / 8.09	7.96 / 7.90	7.93 / 7.84	7.84	7.97	7.86	7.94 / 8.02	7.96 / 7.86	8.00 / 7.93	7.96 / 8.03	7.97 / 8.03	8.04 / 8.13	?	172°		Hamer.
15	S.	m. 50	L.	H $\frac{1}{36}$	7.97 / 8.02	7.98	7.84	8.05	8.10	8.10	7.98 / 8.05	7.90	7.82	8.00	7.96	7.97	?	93°		Middelburg.

The results thus obtained with 15 eyes, are to be found in the foregoing Table. The latter requires some explanation. The direction of the meridian of maximum of curvature for the cornea M_c, communicated in column G, was estimated from the observations contained in column F. Before the number in degrees we have for each eye indicated its direction by a short stroke : while the broad intervening line represents the nose, the direction of M_c in the right eye is indicated before, in the left behind, the said line, by the slighter short stroke.   In column H we find indicated the direction of the meridian of maximum curvature determined for the dioptric system of the whole eye, M_o.   For the determination of the direction we use, according to the method above pointed out, a very weak cylindrical glass, whose required position was accurately noted.   It is more difficult to establish the degree of the astigmatism, where this is very slight.   In column I, we have indicated this for some eyes, in which we were convinced that sufficient accuracy was attained.

From the Table it now appears :—

1°. That of fifteen eyes the radius of curvature is in thirteen less in the vertical meridian than in the horizontal, while in two eyes, Nos. 14 and 15, both belonging to the same person, this is uncertain.   The measurements in No. 14 were made by Dr. Middelburg, and in the absence of decisive results with respect to the position of the principal meridians, I desired that Mr. Hamer should make a system of measurements upon the same eye : now these do not entirely agree with those of Dr. Middelburg ; but the direction of M_c is still as far from being determined.   Moreover, on the left eye of the same person, No. 15, numerous measurements were made at 0° and 90°, in which the average varies so little, that for this eye also we cannot with certainty decide in which of these two positions the curvature is greater.

2°. In harmony with 1°, we find on calculation M_c always approaching more nearly to 90° than to 0°.   Only in No. 3 did we find 135°, which is the medium between 90° and 0° (or 180°).   The directions here found for M_c, show plainly enough how little right we have to seek the maximum of curvature exactly at 90°.   We here find a deviation in each direction, about such as I found for aphakia, where the direction of the sole remaining astigmatism, that of the cornea, could be determined so accurately by a point of light (compare Fig. 155).

3°. The direction of the astigmatism for the whole eye, M_o, was found also, in most cases, nearer to 90° than to 0° ; only Nos. 5, 13, and 14 present exceptions in this respect.   In No. 5 and No. 13, consequently, M_o has quite a different direction from M_c; for No. 14 M_c could not be determined.   Meanwhile, where M_o and M_c were both nearer to 90° than to 0°, their directions still often differ considerably, namely from 3° (No. 12), to 58° (No. 6.).

Hence it now appears, that we have no right whatever to consider M_c and M_o as coincident.   Moreover, apart from the degree of M_c, in reference to M_o, it follows that, in normal astigmatism, the crystalline lens, too, plays a very decided part.   When the directions of M_o and M_c are opposed to one another, as in No. 5 and No. 13, the crystalline

2

lens must have the strongest influence. Had we wished to calculate this, it would have been necessary, from the measurements in twelve meridians for each eye, to calculate, according to the method communicated in treating of abnormal astigmatism, both the values M_c and As_c; furthermore, with the greatest accuracy not only M_o, but also As_o, in order finally, by rather complex formulæ, to be communicated in speaking of abnormal astigmatism, to calculate what direction of M_l (meridian of maximum curvature of the crystalline lens), and what degree of As_l (astigmatism of the crystalline lens), should be capable of modifying M_c and As_c to M_o and As_o. But we have thought well to omit this calculation, because our data in the slighter degrees of normal astigmatism do not possess sufficient accuracy to give much confidence in the result of the calculation. We need now scarcely remark, how far we are from being able, by subtracting the astigmatism found for the cornea, from that of the whole eye, both only in the horizontal and vertical directions, to find that of the crystalline lens.

If the crystalline lens takes part in regular astigmatism, it may do so in either of two ways. In the first place, by the form of the surfaces of curvature : these might very well be ellipsoids with unequal axes, of which the maximum and minimum need not coincide with those of the cornea ; respecting this, however, nothing is with certainty known. In the second place, by an oblique position of the lens, which would have a corresponding influence. That this influence sometimes exists, at least in higher degrees of astigmatism, is, as shall hereafter appear, directly proved. And that it obtains in the crystalline lenses of my own eyes, the study of the diffusion-images of a point of light have convinced me : before and behind the central part of the focal space the intersection of the fasciculus of rays, derived from a point of light, has precisely such divergent forms as take place, in an oblique position of a convex lens, upon a screen ; and with this is partly connected the fact, that the eye, in reduction for a point too near (not by accommodation, but by lenses, so that the pupil in both cases maintains an equal diameter), sees much more accurately, than in reduction for a too remote point: in the first case, although the diffusion-image is extended, many rays continue for a long time to form a much clearer nucleus. Partly, too, spherical aberration may be the cause of it (Conf. *irregular astigmatism*).

It would be instructive to be able to receive rays, refracted at the top of an ellipsoid with three unequal axes, on a screen. As this is, however, not a rotation-body, it will scarcely be possible to grind it of such a form. But we may obtain nearly the same by combining with an ordinary spherical lens a cylindrical one of much greater focal distance.

Such combinations are to be found in the boxes made at my suggestion by Nachet and Son, of Paris, for the investigation of astigmatism.

The light should first be allowed to fall on the symmetrical spherical lens, separated from the cylindrical one by a diaphragm with a round opening. As a cylindrical lens we should use a combination of two plano-cylindrical lenses, a positive and a negative of equal focal distance (lens of Stokes), one of which can turn round the axis of the case. We thus obtain the effect of a single cylindrical lens, whose astigmatic power is $= 0$, when the axes of the cylindrical surfaces of curvature are parallel, and on turning to $90°$

gradually ascends to that of the sum of the two lenses. By thus connecting the combined cylindrical with the spherical lens, we can communicate to it all the degrees of astigmatism. It then appears, on moving the screen, that the focal interval is greater, that the lines bounding it are longer, and the sections of the fasciculus of light in the course of the focal interval are greater, according as the cylindrical lens is stronger, that is, as the astigmatism is greater. If the latter be slight, we still obtain in the focal interval tolerably good images, which, in proportion as it becomes greater, gives way to such as are more and more diffuse. The whole form of the refracted bundle of light is very strikingly seen in tobacco-smoke, when the solar image is used as object.

Sturm assumed that the focal interval, which is the result of asymmetry, should make any accommodation of the eye for different distances superfluous. This opinion no longer needs refutation. Its inaccuracy becomes at once apparent when we reflect, that the focal interval for the dioptric system of the eye would be much too small, to contain in itself the whole range of accommodation, and that, were it long enough, the acuteness of vision would suffer considerably by the great diffusion-images, as in a high degree of astigmatism is actually the case. But thus far is there truth in Sturm's idea, that objects, whose distance from the eye differs so little, that their focal intervals still fall within one another, are seen with nearly equal distinctness. The accommodation-line of Czermak, which has been incorrectly connected with the length of the rods, is to be explained in this way: it depends upon the asymmetry of the refracting system of the eye, and is a function of the length of the focal interval.

I have indicated as an effect of asymmetry, that the posterior focus in the meridian of greatest curvature is least remote from the cornea, in that of slightest curvature is most so. To this evidently corresponds a difference in position of all the cardinal points. In treating of high degrees of astigmatism, we shall revert to this fact and to its consequences with respect to vision.

§ 35. Disturbances and Phenomena in High Degrees of Astigmatism.

We have seen that a certain degree of regular astigmatism occurs in all eyes, and therefore cannot be considered as abnormal. We do not call it abnormal until it attains to such a degree that the accuracy of vision perceptibly suffers from it. For equal lengths of the focal interval, this is the case sooner, in proportion as the pupil is larger. Our observations should therefore be made with an average size of the pupil, under sufficient illumination.

1. The disturbance manifests itself first, when stripes of different directions lying in the same plane have to be distinguished. If these stand far from one another, the accommodation usually regulates itself almost involuntarily, in order to see them acutely alternately, and the disturbance may still be unobserved. If they are close together, the diffusion-images of the one direction fall over the defined images of the other, for which the subject is accommodated, and confusion ensues. In most capital Roman letters this soon occurs.

Now in the most accurate accommodation, with or without spherical glasses, the eye never has, with abnormal astigmatism, in determination with letters, $S = 1$. It not unfrequently descends to $S = \frac{1}{5}$. If $S = \frac{1}{2}$ the disturbance is already the source of considerable inconvenience.

2. There exists a certain indifference for spectacle-glasses of nearly equal power. It is impossible to make a definite choice. Glasses of $\frac{1}{8}$ and of $\frac{1}{8}$ are found to be equally good. In diminished acuteness of vision, proceeding from other causes, this indifference does not exist, or at least it is present in a much less degree. This phenomenon led me long ago to suspect that the diminished acuteness of vision, often peculiar to hypermetropia, might be dependent on abnormal astigmatism. The phenomenon finds its explanation in the long focal interval, whose sections as diffusion-images are nearly equally disturbing, and in whose range, with moderate difference of glasses, the retina easily maintains its position (compare p. 453).

3. The diffusion-image of a point of light alters, in modification of accommodation, not only in size, but also in form. Only when the middle of the focal space corresponds to the plane of perception is the image nearly round; in every other state of accommodation it is extended in one or other direction. This is already the case in the ordinary degree of regular astigmatism, as we have seen, but at high degrees thereof it is particularly striking. In such we soon find a spherical glass, with which a point of light at a distance exhibits itself as a stripe of light, and at the same time a modifying spherical glass (whether positive or negative), which, placed before the first, makes the stripe of light assume a precisely opposite direction. In the required strength of this modifying glass we possess a means of determining the degree of astigmatism. By the alteration of direction of the stripe of light, on alternately placing the second glass in front, astigmatics

are especially impressed.*—He who has sufficient control over his accommodation, without using a modifying lens, can voluntarily produce similar changes of form of the diffusion-images.

4. The influence of the direction of stripes on their distinctness is exceedingly great. The strongest contrast is afforded by stripes corresponding to the direction of the lines of light described under 3, which rarely deviate much from the vertical and horizontal. It depends upon the state of refraction in the different meridians, which of these shall exhibit themselves most distinctly at a distance; but it is easy to find the positive or negative spherical glass, whereby either the first or the last are accurately seen: the greatest indistinctness of the stripes will correspond to the opposite direction. It is now also easy to find a modifying lens, with which these last become defined, and the first attain the highest degree of indistinctness. The higher the degree of astigmatism is, the greater will be this indistinctness, and the stronger must be the lens. The alternating distinctness of the stripes of opposite directions, on applying and removing the modifying glass, is very striking even in slighter degrees, while on a line, which cuts the two opposite stripes at an angle of 45°, it has scarcely any influence.

5. If the stripes of different directions consist of short lines as in the annexed Fig. (158), these at a certain distance coalesce for *all eyes*, and we therefore see only the principal stripe. On drawing near, the strongly astigmatic eye observes the transverse lines much sooner in the stripe which is most feebly seen, than in the clearest.

Fig. 158.

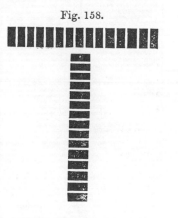

6. Lines of equal length in the two opposite directions do not appear equally long, and this gives rise to the incorrect estimation of the form of the objects: a square exhibits itself as an oblong.

* The stripes follow the lateral inclination of the head—a fresh proof that the vertical meridian of the eye assumes the same inclination as the head, and by no means remains vertical, in consequence of turning round the visual axis, as formerly assumed by Hueck. This we can likewise observe in the lines of the diffusion-image of a point of light (*Verslagen en Mededeelingen van de Kon. Acad. van Wetenschappen*, 1861, Dl. x. p. 192).

Here two different causes come into play. In the first place, in accurate accommodation, successively for erect and recumbent lines, those situated in the meridian of greatest curvature (in general the erect lines), for equal lengths, form longer images upon the retina. The cause is to be sought in the position of the nodal points, or rather of the second nodal point. The farther this point (relatively to the optical centre) lies from the retina, the larger will the retinal image be, and as the cause of astigmatism consists chiefly in a difference of curvature of the meridians of the cornea, the nodal point lies more anteriorly in the meridian of greatest curvature. In strong astigmatism this difference may amount to more than one mm., that is, about $\frac{1}{3}$ of the distance between the second nodal point and the retina.

In the second place, diffusion is to be taken into consideration. If a vertical line be acutely seen, a horizontal line presents a diffused appearance : it seems broader. Now the superior and inferior boundaries of a square may be considered as horizontal lines : consequently, when the eye is accommodated for the vertical limits of the square, the latter appears larger in the vertical dimension. As, moreover, on account of the difference of position of the nodal points, the distinct image is in this direction already greater than in the horizontal, so, in accommodation for the vertical boundary of a square, must the latter for a double reason appear higher, and the difference between height and breadth becomes considerable. On the other hand, when the eye is accommodated for the horizontal boundary, diffusion makes the square appear broader, and may thus compensate for the effect of the difference in position of the nodal points.—The effect of diffusion here described obtains in looking at a clearly illuminated square upon a dark ground; it is inverted in the case of a dark square, observed upon a brightly illumined ground.

7. The acuteness of vision is very considerably improved by looking through a slit of from one to two millimètres in breadth. In these experiments the stenopæic apparatus may be employed, the slit of which can be narrowed and widened at pleasure (p. 129). The improvement in the power of vision is greatest, when the slit is held in the direction of the maximum or minimum of curvature, which may have been ascertained from the direction in which the diffusion-image of a point of light is drawn (compare No. 3). The slit then coincides with a principal section, passing through two axes of the ellipsoid.—The improvement of the acuteness of vision, in

looking through a slit, is a very significant phenomenon. It affords a direct proof that the rays, refracted in the meridian of one of the principal sections, unite nearly in a point, and that consequently the existing disturbance of vision depends on asymmetry. What is more, we can determine the difference of the state of refraction in the meridian of the maximum and minimum of curvature in the way described, with the aid of spherical glasses, as shall be more particularly described in the following chapter.

It is also instructive that, in looking through a slit, not coincident with one of the principal sections, the objects are drawn out; partly because circles of diffusion still easily remain, which are elongated in the direction of the slit, partly because all the normals of a meridian, laid through only one axis, do not lie in one plane, and consequently all the refracted rays do not continue in the same plane.

8. In high degrees of astigmatism the phenomena of dispersion are very peculiar. Helmholtz* observed that, in general they are much more distinct when, instead of white light, such light is employed in the investigation as consists of only two prismatic colours of the greatest possible difference in refrangibility. Such light is most simply obtained by causing sunlight to pass through dark violet-coloured glasses. These glasses absorb the middle rays of the spectrum tolerably perfectly, and transmit only the outermost colours, red and violet.—In experimenting with the light of a lamp or of a wax-candle, a dark blue cobalt-glass, which transmits only the extreme red, with indigo and violet in large quantity, is quite sufficient. A more or less violet tint is, however, also preferable. Professor Dove showed me an excellent thick piece of glass of this nature; the glasses I had hitherto been able to procure must all give way to it. On looking with slight myopia (or accommodation for a near point) through such a cobalt-glass towards the flame of a candle, its edges are blue, and the centre reddish; in slight hypermetropia a beautiful red border is seen around the candle and the centre is blue.† On looking through a violet-glass at a small opening in a dark screen turned towards the daylight, we see, in accommodation for the violet rays, the opening surrounded by a red, in accommodation for the

---

* *Physiologische Optik, l. c.* p. 127.

† Slight degrees of ametropia are immediately distinguishable by this means. In high degrees the diffusion-images are too large, to enable us to observe the difference of colour with equal distinctness.

red we see it surrounded by a violet margin : in the latter case
the violet rays have not yet come to a focus in the retinal image, in
the former the red have already intersected, and are therefore on the
outside; a square opening is skirted in like manner. If, on the
contrary, an astigmatic person sees such an opening as acutely as
possible, and if, on the violet-glass being then pushed before his eye,
blue margins appear at the superior and inferior, and red at the two
vertical edges, the subject is shown to be myopic in the vertical, and
hypermetropic in the horizontal, meridian. If he sees the point of
light drawn out to a line (see under No. 3 of this Section), the
extremities and middle of the line are of different colours, and on
altering the direction of the lines of light by the modifying lens, the
colours also change.

All the above phenomena we may observe in ourselves. The only
thing necessary for this purpose is to make the eye astigmatic, and
this is effected by holding a cylindrical lens before it. The axis of the
cylindrical curvature should by preference be placed horizontally if
the lens be positive, vertically if it be negative : the observer then obtains in his eye the shortest focal distance in the vertical meridian,
just as astigmatics generally do. A cylinder-glass of $\frac{1}{20}$ or $-\frac{1}{20}$
(20″ focal distance, positive or negative) is sufficient. We may
therewith, by adding or not adding spherical glasses, combine every
degree of ametropia; the astigmatism always remains (apart from the
originally existing asymmetry) $= \frac{1}{20}$. To obtain in one's own person a simple and often-occurring case, we should make the horizontal
meridian hypermetropic, with emmetropia of the vertical. An emmetropic individual needs to this end only to hold before the eye a
cylindrical lens of $-\frac{1}{20}$ with the axis of the cylinder perpendicular.
But it is useful, subsequently to experiment also with ametropia
artificially produced in both meridians.

It appears superfluous to give further indications for the trials to
be made. All the above-described phenomena the observer will be
able without trouble to repeat. Two remarks only may be added :
the dispersion has appeared to me to be greater in such artificial
astigmatism than in the natural, and the difference in the size
of the retinal images in the two principal meridians is more con-

siderable. The explanation of the first of these facts would lead me too far. The reason of the second is evident: the cylindrical lens is, in fact, at some distance from the cornea, and its action here exercises more influence on the position of the nodal points, than if by modification of the corneal radius, the posterior focus had been equally displaced. Objects are therefore seen more drawn out, than in natural astigmatism of like degree.

Where regular astigmatism exists, it is requisite, in order to answer a number of questions, to determine the cardinal points in the two principal meridians. as if they formed two different systems. In the following I shall try this for a given case. Let us suppose an instance where the cause of the astigmatism lies exclusively in the cornea, the radius of curvature of which in the vertical meridian is, as not unfrequently occurs, 1 mm. shorter than in the horizontal. Let us take, to keep to a given case, No. 6 of the Table in my first treatise on astigmatism, where the radius in the vertical plane amounts to 7·38, that in the horizontal to 8·38 mm. : let the section in the vertical plane be v, that in the horizontal, H.

For the refracting surface of the cornea alone the cardinal points are easily determined : the principal point, h, lies in the apex of the plane of curvature, the nodal point, k, in the centre of curvature of the apex (respectively 7·38 and 8·38 mm. behind the apex); while the positions of the anterior focus φ', and of the posterior focus φ'' are calculated, according to the formula—

$$h \; \varphi' \text{ or } F' = \frac{r}{n-1},$$

$$h \; \varphi'' \text{ or } F'' = \frac{r \; n}{n-1},$$

by which, n being assumed $= 1\cdot3365$, we find

$$\text{for H} \begin{cases} F' = 24\cdot90 \\ F'' = 33\cdot28 \end{cases}$$

$$\text{for v} \begin{cases} F' = 21\cdot93 \\ F'' = 29\cdot31. \end{cases}$$

Thus the distances $h \; \varphi'$ and $h \; \varphi''$ are found. In Fig. 159 (in which c is

Fig. 159.

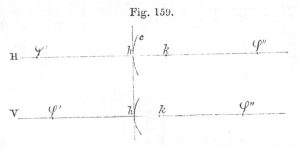

the cornea) the ascertained positions of the cardinal points are represented.

A simple calculation, given at p. 461, shows that in this case an infinitely thin cylindrical lens of $\frac{1}{6\cdot8}$, with a vertical position of the axis placed immediately at the cornea, can make the cardinal points in the two meridians coincide.

With this cornea let us now combine a symmetrical crystalline lens (that of the ideal eye of Helmholtz at rest) with focal distance = 43·707 mm., reciprocal distance of its two principal points = 0·2283, and distance of these principal points from the apex of the cornea = 5·7073 and 5·9356. The calculation of the combined system gives for the position of the cardinal points, reckoning from the apex of the cornea, in the two principal meridians H and V, the following results :—

		H.	V.
Anterior focus	ϕ'	— 13·2743	— 12·2967
First principal point	h'	1·9937	1·9443
Second principal point	h''	2·4359	2·2297
First nodal point	k'	7·1321	6·7359
Second nodal point	k''	7·5743	7·0213
Posterior focus	ϕ''	22·8423	21·2623

Consequently,

the posterior focal distance $F'' = h'' \phi''$	20·4064	19·0326
,, anterior ,, ,, $F' = h' \phi'$	15·268	14·241

In order to represent the systems diagramatically, I here add Fig. 160, showing, for H and V :—

    I. The cardinal points of the cornea ;

    II. Those of the crystalline lens ;

    III. The united dioptric system ;

and Fig 161, in which No. III of H and V stand one under the other, of double size, and are more easily compared.

The knowledge of the cardinal points places us in a position to be able to investigate the vision of astigmatic individuals in more than one respect.

In the first place, as concerns the acuteness of vision, in H ϕ'' lies 1·58 mm. behind ϕ'' of V. Therefore, if rays proceeding from a given point have come to a focus in V, in H they are still 1·58 mm. from their focus. It is evident, that the acuteness of vision must thence suffer very much. A more definite representation of this is obtained from the magnitude of the diffusion-images. We have them calculating (compare Helmholtz' method, *l. c.* p. 98), at an average size of the pupil of 4 mm. (corresponding to a magnitude of its lenticular image = 4·23 mm.), and a position of the plane of the pupil at 3·6 mm. (that of its lenticular image 3·713) behind the apex of the cornea. If the retina lies, in ϕ'' of V, at 21·26 mm. behind the cornea, parallel incident rays, converging in V, come to a focus on the retina, while those converging in H reach the retina at 1·58 mm. before their point of union. For their diffusion-image on the retina we found a length of 0·3494 mm., corresponding in this meridian to a visual angle of 1°24′·2.

If the retina lies in ϕ'' of H, at 22·1423 behind the retina, then the rays converging in V have already intersected at 1·58 mm. in front of the retina, and in the diameter and position of the pupil assumed above, the diffusion-

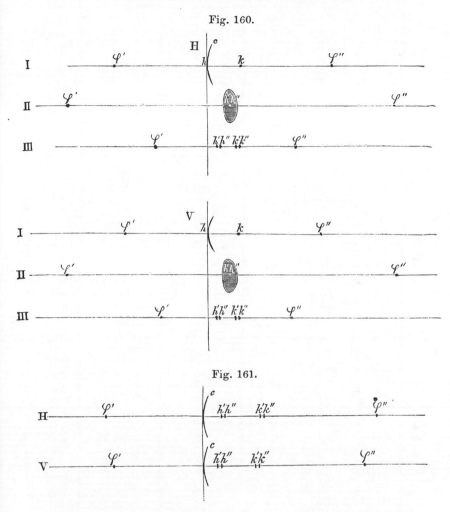

Fig. 160.

Fig. 161.

image is then $= 0\cdot3808$, corresponding in this meridian to a visual angle of $1°25'\cdot7$.

Finally, when the retina lies at $22\cdot018$ mm. behind the apex of the cornea, the linear diffusion-images in v and H are equal, amounting to $0\cdot18222$ mm. In this position, therefore, the retina receives that part of the focal interval where the diffusion-image is nearly a circle. The diameter thereof exhibits itself in the horizontal meridian under an angle of $41'\cdot8$, in the vertical under an angle of $43'\cdot4$. If we bear in mind that in perfect acuteness of vision letters are recognised under an angle of 5′, we can form an idea to what an extent the circles of diffusion mentioned must interfere with correct sight.

We shall obtain a still better point of comparison by calculating the accommodation required to make ϕ'' of H fall where, in the eye at rest, ϕ'' is found in V; in other words, to see with acuteness alternately vertical and horizontal lines.

Let us suppose the eye emmetropic in V (the retina lying at 21·2623 mm. behind the apex of the cornea) and consequently hypermetropic in H, and let us find that, to neutralise this degree of hypermetropia, a lens (standing in the air, its nodal point coinciding with k' of H) of 176·8 mm. = 6·53″ focal distance is required, consequently that there is hypermetropia of $\frac{1}{6·53}$, capable of being counteracted by an accommodation of $\frac{1}{6·53}$. But now the same accommodation necessarily takes place in V, whereby for this plane F′ becomes = 12·857 mm. and F″ = 17·183 mm., and horizontal lines appear distinct at the distance of 176·8 mm. = 6·53″. While, therefore, by accommodation of $\frac{1}{6·53}$, H became emmetropic, V assumed a myopia of $\frac{1}{6·53}$.

Hence it may be deduced, that in an accommodation of about $\frac{1}{13}$ the retina corresponds to the middle of the focal interval, the diffusion-image being a circle of diffusion of about the same magnitude as a symmetrical eye, accommodated for ∞, perceives of an object placed 13″ from the eye, or, when accommodated for the distance of 13″, sees of infinitely remote objects. By looking at distant objects, while the eye is by glasses rendered $\frac{1}{13}$ myopic or hypermetropic (and in the latter case refraining from tension of accommodation), we can observe in ourselves the disturbance proceeding from the circles of diffusion already mentioned. Obtained in this manner, it appears, however, to be somewhat greater than in astigmatics, which is partly to be ascribed to this, that the latter by some play of accommodation can make the diffusion-images alter their form and combine the vertical and horizontal lines thus alternately more distinctly perceived. Moreover, the light is less uniformly distributed in the diffusion-images of astigmatic individuals, and, in fact, more advantageously in the posterior part of the focal interval. In general, too, the diffusion-images, on account of their discontinuity (the result of the irregular astigmatism of the crystalline lens), may cause less disturbance than should be the case if they were homogeneous.

As has been above remarked, the retinal images are, for like dimensions of the objects, not of equal magnitude in a horizontal and vertical direction. If the projection corresponds in all meridians to the magnitudes of the retinal-images (which is doubtful), like dimensions of the objects do not appear equally large in the opposite meridians. The magnitude of the retinal images is, now that we have become acquainted with the position of the cardinal points, easily compared. As the distance of the objects is very considerable, relatively to the reciprocal distances of the nodal points and to the distance $k^c\ \phi''$, we may assume that the magnitudes of the retinal images, in alternate accommodation in the two principal meridians, are proportionate to the distances $k''\ \phi''$ in H and in V. Supposing that the retina lies 22·8432 mm. behind the cornea, the distances $k''\ \phi''$ in the two systems will be 14·241 and 15·268, therefore $= 1:1\cdot0721$. In this it is assumed that k'' in the accommodation continues bound to its place, which is not indeed exactly correct, but yet involves no inaccuracy of importance. The difference, therefore, in the two principal meridians, of the magnitude of the retinal images for equal dimensions of the objects seems, in accurate accommodation, to be considerable. That with this the change of the magnitudes, another depending on the diffusion-images may be combined (either increasing or compensating the difference), has been already above sufficiently explained.

---

§ 36. DIAGNOSIS OF ABNORMAL ASTIGMATISM, AND DETERMINATION OF ITS DEGREE.

In the phenomena, of which the preceding section gave a review, the diagnosis of astigmatism, and even the determination of its degree, is already included. It appeared to me, however, not superfluous to examine the methods of investigation thence deducible, with reference to their value and utility, and to indicate the course which leads easily and certainly to satisfactory knowledge.

In the anomaly under consideration, the subjective examination first presents itself. In the acuteness of vision under different conditions, we find the desired indication. Of this I shall, therefore, in the first place treat. Finally, I shall briefly point out the objective signs, which may cause the existence of astigmatism to be suspected, or even diagnosed with certainty.

A. *Subjective investigation.*—*Absence of the normal acuteness of vision* supplies the first indication. If the disturbance has existed from youth, almost unaltered and in equal degree, without striking variations, there is reason to suspect that astigmatism is the cause. It is even exceptional to find this suspicion refuted by investigation. If the practitioner choose, a few questions may be put, as to the distinctness of horizontal and of vertical lines, at a greater or less inclination of the head. Much time should not, however, be lost in doing so, but recourse should be had to the systematic investigation.

1. In every diminution of acuteness of vision, we begin by determining its degree (see p. 188). We must remember, that in high degrees of myopia, for more than one reason, perfect acuteness of

vision is usually not met with. A certain amount of imperfection in myopia, therefore, affords less reason to suspect abnormal astigmatism. Nevertheless the trial should be made.

2. Let then imperfect acuteness of vision be found. *We must now first determine, in what direction the principal meridians*, that is, *the maximum and minimum of curvature, are situated.* For this purpose we make use of a remote point of light. In my consultation-room one of the window-panes is of dull glass. In front of the centre of this glass is a black board, 35 centimètres (13·77 English inches) square: in the middle of the board is a perforated metallic plate, before which a diaphragm can be pushed, with openings of from ½ to 10 mm. in diameter. The patient should now be directed to look towards an opening of from 2 to 4 millimètres in diameter, at a distance of from 10 to 15 feet, while by means of glasses we cause slight myopia to alternate with hypermetropia (compare p. 470). Even in the normal eye, an extension of the diffusion-image is, on this examination, usually observed in two opposite directions, indicating the maximum and minimum of curvature. But in abnormal astigmatism this is particularly striking.—Subsequently I found, that we obtain a still better result by determining in what direction of the axis of the most neutralising cylindrical glass the patient sees best.

3. We have thus ascertained the direction of the principal meridians. We should now examine, *whether the rays, belonging to these, form more accurate images than those from the whole refracting surface.* For this purpose, we should hold, successively in each of the principal meridians, the slit of a stenopæic apparatus, set to the breadth of 1 or 2 mm., and ascertain whether the acuteness of vision be thereby increased. If not, we should then try the addition of ordinary positive and negative glasses, for the employment of which we shall already have found opportunity, in the examination mentioned under 1. If, even with the aid of these, no greater acuteness of vision be obtained, than existed without the use of the slit, it is almost certain that astigmatism is not to be considered as the cause of the disturbance. Only when the degree is slight, the acuteness of vision still amounting, for example, to ¾, can the result be uncertain; on the one hand, because looking through a slit in itself produces some disturbance, on the other, because in this experiment the astigmatism is not completely removed.

4. Let there be improvement of acuteness of vision; the existence

of abnormal astigmatism is thereby proved.   Now the question is :
what is the state of refraction in each of the principal meridians ?
This appears from the strength of the positive or negative glass,
with which in each of these meridians the greatest acuteness of vision
is obtained. We usually find for both a certain degree of ametropia.
It is now of importance, accurately to determine this degree.   By
this determination our object is attained.   The degree of astigmatism is included in it.   The determination is unattended with difficulty,
when a certain degree of myopia exists in both principal meridians :
the weakest negative glass, with which the greatest acuteness of
vision is obtained, is in that case a sufficient measure of it.   But if
hypermetropia be found in one or both meridians, it is, at least in
the case of young persons, probable, that, by the simple proof, the
degree is not accurately shown.   For involuntary, almost spasmodic
tension of accommodation conceals in part the existing hypermetropia,
and causes the indication of a too weakly positive glass for total correction.   Were the tension unaltered in the subsequent determination
for the two principal meridians, at least the difference of refraction,
and therewith the degree of astigmatism, would be known.   But this
equality of tension is not to be expected.   Moreover, it is not sufficient to know the degree of astigmatism, it is also necessary to know
that of the hypermetropia in the two principal meridians.   Now this
knowledge is certainly and accurately obtained only by repeating the
experiments during artificial paralysis of accommodation produced
by means of a mydriatic : the hypermetropia can then neither wholly
nor partially remain latent ; it necessarily exhibits itself entirely as
manifest hypermetropia.

5. In reference to astigmatism we desire to know :—

a, its existence ;

b, the direction of the principal meridians, those of the maximum
and minimum of refraction ;

c, the refractive condition of the eye in each of these meridians ;

d, the degree of the astigmatism.

Respecting *a* and *b*, we obtained information under 3, respecting *c*
under 4. It remains further to show how *d* is thence to be deduced.
The matter is simple : *the degree of astigmatism is found from the
difference of refraction in the two principal meridians.*   This shall
be illustrated by some examples, in connexion with the three forms
of astigmatism which, from the point of view of refraction, must, I
think, be established.

31

I.—*Myopic astigmatism*, to be distinguished into :—

a. Simple Am, with M in the one, E in the other meridian.

Thus let there be :—

> In the principal meridian н, emmetropia.
>
>   ,,   ,,   ,,   v, $M = \frac{1}{6}$,

then there exists simple myopic astigmatism

$$Am = \frac{1}{6} - \frac{1}{\infty} = \frac{1}{6}.$$

b. Compound myopic astigmatism, or myopia with astigmatism, M + Am, M existing in both principal meridians.

Thus let there be :

> In the principal meridian н, $M = \frac{1}{20}$,
>
>   ,,   ,,   ,,   v, $M = \frac{1}{10}$,

we then have $M = \dfrac{1}{20}$.

And moreover, $Am = \frac{1}{10} - \frac{1}{20} = \frac{1}{20}$, to be written as :

$$M = \frac{1}{20} + Am \; \frac{1}{20}.$$

II.—*Hypermetropic astigmatism*, likewise to be distinguished as :

a. Simple Ah, with H in the one, E in the other principal meridian.

In v let there be E.

In н let there be $H = \frac{1}{8}$,

then there exists simple hypermetropic astigmatism

$$Ah = \frac{1}{8} - \frac{1}{\infty} = \frac{1}{8}.$$

b. Compound, being H with astigmatism, H + Ah, H existing in the two principal meridians.

In н let $H = \frac{1}{8}$.

In v let $H = \frac{1}{18}$.

We thus find $H = \frac{1}{18}$.

and moreover, $Ah = \frac{1}{8} - \frac{1}{18} = \frac{1}{9}$,

and therefore write,

$$H \; \frac{1}{18} + Ah \; \frac{1}{9}.$$

III.—*Mixed astigmatism*, with M in the one, H in the other meridian.

Of this we may distinguish :

a. Mixed astigmatism, *with predominant myopia*, Amh.

In v let $M = \frac{1}{12}$.

In н let $H = \frac{1}{24}$.

Thus we find,

$$Amh = M\, \frac{1}{12} + H\, \frac{1}{24} = \frac{1}{8}.$$

b. Mixed astigmatism, *with predominant hypermetropia*, Ahm.

In v let $M = \frac{1}{24}$;

In н let $H = \frac{1}{12}$.

Therefore,

$$Ahm = \frac{1}{24}\, M + \frac{1}{12}\, H = \frac{1}{8}.$$

The above is in general sufficient for the diagnosis and deter-mination of the degree of astigmatism. The method recommends itself by its simplicity and facility of application. In general it deserves to be preferred to any of the following modes. Only the control described under 8 must not be omitted. This is, properly speaking, nothing more than trying whether the glasses employed in the investigation, described under 4, are really suitable. If the control proves accurate, the investigation in the condition of artifi-cial paralysis may, even where hypermetropia exists, for the most part be omitted.

The methods still to be described, come under consideration in particular cases. They cannot be passed over in silence, least of all that of Stokes, which, for its ingenuity, deserves to be known, and also sometimes yields good service. Employed as a control, it cer-tainly affords the most accurate indication.

6. *Modified method of* Young.—Young determined the distance at which the double images of the wire of his optometer, in accom-modation for the farthest point, held alternately vertically and hori-zontally, appeared to intersect. The method may be applied in myopic individuals, but gives too high a result (conf. p. 451). Moreover, the directions of the principal meridians must first be found, according to the method described under 2, in order to admit of the determination of the inclinations of the optometer, at which the observation is to be made.

7. *Method of* Airy.—This is applicable only where a tolerably high degree of myopia exists in the two principal meridians, which was the case with Airy. As point of light a small opening in an opaque disc is employed, turned towards the light of the sky, to-wards a dull glass or the globe of a lamp, and this is moved along a

2

graduated scale, for example, that of the optometer. We then find
a greatest distance, at which the point of light appears as the most
slender line, and a shortest distance at which it again becomes a thin
line, perpendicular to the first. The distances then give about the
degrees of myopia in the principal meridians.

If it be desired to apply this and the preceding methods to non-
myopic subjects, the eye must be rendered myopic by a suitable convex glass. In this, however, the difficulty presents itself, that, if
the axis of the lens does not accurately coincide with the visual axis,
the astigmatism undergoes a modification.

Moreover, in both cases the accommodation must remain at rest.
This can, however, scarcely ever be accomplished, and therefore
in the majority of instances, this method leads to incorrect results.

8. *Modified method* of Airy.—In order to meet the last difficulty,
the accommodation may be paralysed by means of a mydriatic. In
strong myopia Airy's method then affords tolerably fair results.
But if no, or if only slight myopia, exists, a remote point of light
deserves the preference. Thereby we avoid the trouble connected
with the use of strong lenses. To obtain a more accurate result,
I made use of a very small point of light, produced by the reflexion
of an illuminated little round opening upon a convex mirror. In
some cases it was then satisfactorily ascertained, with what spherical
glasses the point of light appeared as the slenderest streak, successively
in two opposite directions. In the majority of instances, on the
contrary, this remained undecided. The cause of this lies in the
irregular astigmatism, which excludes defined lines as diffusion-
images. Usually, secondary lines rapidly shot out, even before the
principal line had become slender, in different directions, preventing
an accurate determination of the glass required. Only in absence of
the crystalline lens, whereby the irregular astigmatism was removed,
did the results attain perfect accuracy.

Instead of a very small reflected point of light, we may employ an
opening of from 1 to 2 mm. in diameter, such as is to be obtained
by means of the board, described at page 45. Cases of aphakia excepted, the results thus obtained are not inferior to those where the
reflected point of light is used.

9. *Investigation with cylindrical lenses*.—While at a distance
letters without or with the best chosen spherical glass, are being seen
as distinctly as possible, we take a positive cylindrical glass of about
$\frac{1}{30}$, and turn it round before the eye. If astigmatism exists, it is

observed that, in a definite position of the glass (while the curvature of the cylindrical glass coincides with the meridian of strongest curvature), the acuteness of vision greatly diminishes, but that in a position perpendicular thereto, it, on the contrary, increases. The acuteness of vision now often becomes still greater on approximating the object: the cylindrical glass may, in correcting the astigmatism, have rendered the eye myopic. We may now further try, with what strength of cylindrical glass, always held in the most advantageous position, the greatest acuteness of vision is obtained, which must always be tested by difference of distance of the letters, or by combination with spherical glasses. We then, however, obtain at last, with the sacrifice of much time, only a moderate result.

The method, although thus in itself objectionable, is very well adapted to control the results obtained by that described under 4. The latter shows from what combination of spherical and cylindrical glasses the greatest acuteness of vision is to be expected, and we should never neglect to try this, nor omit a comparison with slight modification of the lenses. We shall thus always be able to congratulate ourselves on a more complete improvement of the acuteness of vision, than was obtained by the use of the slit, which, if it be too narrow, takes away much light and is obstructive by diffraction, and if it be too wide, very imperfectly corrects the astigmatism.

10. *Method of Stokes.*—The distinguished Secretary of the Royal Society had very well seen that Airy's method could lead to satisfactory results only when, together with the successive determination of the farthest points of distinct vision in the two principal meridians, the condition of accommodation of the eye underwent no change. By his method this difficulty is removed. He proposes to define the degree of astigmatism, by means of an astigmatic lens, the action of which can be regulated in a manner as simple as it is ingenious, so as to make it assume precisely the degree by which the astigmatism of the eye is corrected. I have had such lenses prepared, and give the description of the instrument, with the arrangement which appeared to me most advantageous: the principle is precisely that of the *astigmatic lens* of Stokes, which name may also be given to the instrument. It consists (Fig. 162B, exhibiting a section) of two cylindrical lenses, the one plano-convex l of $\frac{1}{10}$, the other plano-concave l' of $-\frac{1}{10}$. The first is fastened into a broad copper ring, K, the last into K', which rings at x are fitted to one

Fig. 162.

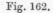

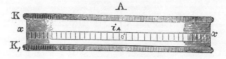

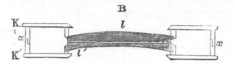

another, and can turn past one another around their axis. At the
same time, therefore, the lenses $l\,l'$ also rotate past one another;
they are turned with their flat surfaces towards each other, leaving
a very small interspace. Fig. 162 A, represents the instrument,
seen on the outer surface. It will be observed that on K an index i
occurs, on K' a graduated scale. If the index points to 0° or to 180°,
the axes of the two cylindrical lenses are parallel: the section of
the lenses appears then as in B, so that when united, they may be
regarded as a concavo-convex cylindrical lens, with equal radius of
curvature of the two planes, whose action is about = 0. If the
index points to 90° or to 270°, the axes of the cylindrical glasses
stand perpendicular to one another. At the same time the system
has its maximum m of astigmatic action: a plane of parallel rays
of light, coinciding with the axis of l, will undergo no deviation
through l, but through l' will be made convergent to its focus, situated at 10″; on the contrary, a plane of parallel rays, coinciding with
the axis of l', are made divergent through l, as if they came from a
point, situated 10″ in front of the lens, and through l' do not deviate further from this course. In the one meridian we thus obtain
an astigmatism of $\frac{1}{10}$, in the opposite of $-\frac{1}{10}$, and the astigmatism
m of rays, refracted in this position of the lenses, therefore amounts
to $\frac{1}{5}$. It thus appears, that by turning round from 0° to 90° the
astigmatism ascends from 0 to $\frac{1}{5}$, and by a simple formula,

$$As = m \sin a,$$

we can calculate the astigmatism for each angle a, which the axes of
the lenses make with one another. For the sake of convenience definite
degrees of astigmatism are directly given upon the instrument, rendering the calculation unnecessary.

It is easy to see the use which may be made of this instrument. If any one fails to obtain, with the most satisfactory accommodation or reduction for distance, the normal acuteness of vision, and if we suspect the existence of astigmatism, we set the instrument about at the degree of astigmatism, which the disturbance of vision leads us to suspect (rather somewhat too weak than too strong), and cause it, while the eye is steadily fixed upon the distant letters, to turn round before the eye. If improvement be now observed in a particular position, the action of the astigmatic lens can be increased or diminished in the manner above described, until the maximum of distinctness is obtained; but this change requires again another position.

We should not, however, imagine that our object has been thus altogether attained. The eye is now seldom properly adjusted for the distance at which the letters are. The astigmatic lens makes the eye in the meridian of maximum of curvature incline as much to hypermetropia, as it does in the meridian of minimum of curvature to myopia, and emmetropia (distinct vision at a distance) will therefore be obtained only when the eye, without the astigmatic lens, had selected a glass whereby it was reduced in its two principal meridians to an equal degree of ametropia (either myopia or hypermetropia). Sometimes this is completely accomplished, and the object is then immediately attained. But experience shows that this is the exception. In general, in correcting the astigmatism a slight degree of ametropia remains, and this again suggests the question, whether the astigmatism has been corrected as perfectly as possible, or not. If any myopia remains, this can immediately be demonstrated by approximating the object; and if the latter be now more acutely seen, the action of the astigmatic lens can be more accurately set and arranged: however, when in this manner, after a long search, an accurate result is obtained, a tolerably detailed calculation is still necessary to deduce, from the spherical glass used, from the astigmatic action of the lens and from the greatest distance at which, with this system, acute vision is obtained, the ametropia in the two principal meridians—a knowledge which we need. But if hypermetropia remains, there is, unless the accommodation provide for it, no distance discoverable, at which sufficiently acute vision is obtained, perfectly to regulate the astigmatic action of the lens, so that in that case the addition of a second spherical (positive) lens is required, to bring acuteness of vision at a distance to its maximum.

From all the foregoing it appears, that the method is not very

applicable in practice.   It answers best when the eye is by spherical
glasses reduced to a certain degree of myopia, and it is then tried for
near objects, with what action of the astigmatic lens the person can
best read.   In this, however, it is more difficult to take care that
the lenses be held perfectly centred before the eye; moreover, the
opinion as to the acuteness of vision is not quite certain, and at all
events we have learned only the degree of astigmatism, but by no
means the refraction in each of the principal meridians.

For all these reasons the method described under 4. deserves the
preference, and the astigmatic lens of Stokes is principally available
only as a means of control.   If, for example, we have deduced from
the results obtained, by what spherical glass the refraction in the
two principal meridians is reduced to equal degrees of ametropia
(either myopia or hypermetropia), we can, with the aid of the astigmatic lens, with great accuracy determine the degree of the astigmatism, and at the same time the instrument presents the advantage
of enabling us in a simple manner to regulate it in its action.   Its
precision will even enable us to discover and counteract little in-
accuracies in the result obtained by the above-mentioned methods.

This is the place to remind the reader, that above (p. 468) use
has already been made of the astigmatic lens of Stokes, in the construction of an instrument designed to make the phenomena of
astigmatism in very different degrees visible upon a screen.   What
was there said will have found its explanation in the statement here
given.

B.—We have now to treat briefly of the *objective signs* of
astigmatism.

They are so far inferior to the subjective, that they usually do not
exist with equal certainty, and never show accurately the degree of
the asymmetry.   But they derive a special value from the connexion
in which they stand to the cause of the affection.   They have partly
reference to the form of the eyeball.   Examination with the ophthalmoscope supplies a second series of objective signs.

1. Astigmatism occurs mostly in hypermetropic individuals.   If
diminished acuteness of vision exists in such persons, asymmetry is
generally in operation.   Hence the objective signs of hypermetropia
are already not without value (compare p. 252).   But the cornea
often affords more decisive signs.   Sometimes its asymmetry is
immediately recognised : it is either shorter than usual in the
vertical measurement, or it extends farther backwards (as the result

of greater curvature), so that the section between the cornea and the sclerotic does not lie in one plane. In other cases, the difference in magnitude of reflected images in the vertical and in the horizontal direction attracts attention. A square, for example the board, above mentioned (p. 480), is represented with a greater transverse dimension. The asymmetry of the cornea is then thus proved, and that of the entire system usually corresponds to it. Even in the form of the sclerotic we again find this difference: we shall often be able to convince ourselves even in the living subject, at least in hypermetropic individuals, that the vertical axis of the eyeball is considerably shorter than the horizontal.

2. Examination with the ophthalmoscope affords likewise in hypermetropic individuals the most certain indication of the existence of astigmatism. In a normal eye we see (unless the observer be himself astigmatic) the vessels, proceeding in different directions from the optic disc equally distinct with equal effort of our accommodation. In an astigmatic eye this is no longer the case. We then observe that, in order to see accurately in succession the vessels running in different directions near the optic disc, we must alter the state of accommodation of our eye. The rule is, that the emmetropic individual, in relaxation of his accommodation, observes accurately vessels running horizontally; on the contrary, to see vertical vessels distinctly, he must induce tension of accommodation. The explanation of this difference is evident. The vessels running vertically are not acutely seen until the rays thence diverging in a horizontal plane are brought to a focus in the eye of the observer, and if the observed eye be hypermetropic in the horizontal meridian, the rays belonging to this plane maintain outside the eye a diverging direction, so that tension of accommodation is required on the part of the observer to bring them to a focus. On the contrary, the rays proceeding from horizontal vessels in the vertical meridian will, in emmetropia in this plane, outside the observed eye be parallel, and these vessels will, therefore, without tension of accommodation, appear distinct.—In the inverted image of the fundus oculi the difference is also inverted, but, for more reasons than one, is less perceptible: omitting the slighter difference of required accommodation, it is too much influenced by the direction of the axis of the lens held before the eye, which even may correct the difference.

At the meeting held at Heidelberg in 1861, Dr. Knapp called attention to a second phenomenon in the fundus oculi in astigmatic

persons. I refer to the variable form of the optic disc. In the
direction of the meridian of greatest curvature the dimension, in
examining the non-inverted image appears more, in that of the
meridian of slightest curvature it appears less, magnified; the reverse
obtains in examining the inverted image. If, therefore, in examination by these two methods, the optic disc is elongated in opposite
directions, the existence of As is, as Schweigger* remarked, proved.†

§ 37. Cause and Seat of Abnormal Astigmatism.

Abnormal astigmatism is to be considered as a higher degree of
the same asymmetry, which belongs to normal eyes: similarity of
seat and conformity of direction of the principal meridians, in the
two cases, afford the proof thereof.

As to the normal, the *cause* is in general for the most part to be
sought in the cornea; and the direction of the principal meridians,
for the whole dioptric system, as well as for the cornea in particular,
is of that nature, that the meridian of maximum of curvature usually
approaches to the vertical, that of minimum, to the horizontal.

For abnormal degrees of asymmetry the same rules obtain. What
is more, they here present still less of exception. If in normal
astigmatism it is nothing unusual for the meridian of the maximum
of curvature to make a smaller angle with the horizontal than with
the vertical plane, in abnormal degrees I have found only a few
examples thereof. And, as to the seat—if we leave out of consideration a few cases of evident ectopia of the lens, to which I shall
revert—each disturbing degree of astigmatism was combined with an
extraordinary asymmetry of the cornea. Precisely the high degree
of this asymmetry explains, why it preponderates over the influence
of the lens.

The subjoined Table contains our first results of observation.

* *Archiv f. Ophthalmologie*, B. ix. p. 178.

† My friend Bowman recently informs me, that " he has been sometimes
led to the discovery of regular astigmatism of the cornea, and the direction
of the chief meridians, by using the mirror of the ophthalmoscope much in
the same way as for slight degrees of conical cornea. The observation is
more easy if the optic disc is in the line of sight and the pupil large. The
mirror is to be held at 2 feet distance, and its inclination rapidly varied, so
as to throw the light on the eye at small angles to the perpendicular, and
from opposite sides in succession, in successive meridians. The area of the
pupil then exhibits a somewhat linear shadow in some meridians rather
than in others."

No.	Name.	Sex.	Eye.	I. rad. hor.	II. rad. vert.	III. F″ horiz.	IV. F″ vertic.	V. As = 1 :
				mm.	mm.	In Parisian inches.		
1	Vl.	F.	R.	8·00	7·29	1·1737	1·0695	10·78
2	,,	,,	L.	7·80	7·48	1,14 i·4	1·0975	20·04
3	Vo.	M.	R.	8·29	7·56	1·2163	1·109	9·43
4	,,	,,	L.	8·14	7·67	1·1943	1·125	14·51
5	Rr.	M.	R.	8·32	7·30	1·221	1 071	6·374
6	,,	,,	L.	8·38	7·38	1·2295	1·083	6·800
7	Rr. Jr.	M.	L.	8·44	7·69	1·2383	1·1283	9·504
8	Fr.	M.	R.	8·72	7·13	1·2794	1·0461	4·293
9	,,	,,	L.	8·40	7·25	1·2325	1·0637	5·811
10	Pg.	M.	R.	7·93	7·50	1·1635	1·1004	15 18
11	Rm.	M.	L.	8·74	8·04	1·2814	1·1797	11·02
12	Im.	M.	R.	7·96	7·34	1·1679	1·0770	10·35
13	,,	,,	L.	8·28	7·33	1·2149	1·0755	7·013
14	Vg.	M.	L.	8·29	7·69	1·2163	1·1283	11·67
15	Dr.	M.	R.	7·69	7·25	1·1283	1·0637	13·90
16	,,	,,	L.	7·84	7·26	1·1503	1 0652	10·77
17	And.	M.	R.	8·19	7·50	1·2017	1·1004	9·767
18	,,	,,	L.	8·16	7·43	1·1973	1·0902	9·118
19	Ren.	M.	R.	8·11	7·23	1·1899	1·0607	7·310
20	Sch.	M.	R.	8·91	7·82	1·3073	1·1474	7·019
21	,,	,,	L.	8·81	7·96	1·2927	1·1679	9·051

It is made of like data, and calculated in the same manner as the Table occurring at p. 460, and referring to normal astigmatism. We find here 21 cases collected, in which diminished acuteness of vision existed, as the result of abnormal astigmatism.*

The Table requires little explanation. Of the five columns of figures,

I. Contains in millimètres the radius in a horizontal plane, carried through the visual line.

II. In millimètres the radius in a vertical plane, carried through the visual line.

* In the majority of these cases the measurements which are required for the calculation of the elements of the ellipse, were made both in the vertical and in the horizontal section. I pass them over here as being less pertinent to the matter in hand. I shall observe only that the eccentricity of the elliptical section in the vertical meridian usually proved particularly small. It also deserves to be mentioned that, especially when hypermetropia was in play, the visual line almost always made a great angle (7° to 9°) with the axis of the cornea, which must appear the less strange because, as numerous measurements, made in connexion with Dr. Doÿer, have shown (*Verslagen en Mededeelingen van de Koninkl. Akademie van Wetenschappen*, 1862), the angle between the visual line and the axis of the cornea is in general, in hypermetropic subjects, considerable (compare p. 299).

III. In Parisian inches, the posterior focal distance of the cornea in I.

IV. In Parisian inches, the posterior focal distance of the cornea in II.

V. In Parisian inches, the focal distance of the cylindrical lens, which, in the requisite direction, placed immediately before the cornea would make the focal distances III. and IV. equal. The degree of astigmatism, proceeding from the ascertained asymmetry of the cornea is therefore 1 : 10·78, 1 : 20·04, &c.—R. signifies the right, L. the left eye. In some persons both eyes, in others only one, are measured. M. stands for the male, F. for the female sex. On the whole, I have found the asymmetry more in men than in women; of the latter, however, comparatively fewer were submitted to measurement.

The eye discovers at a glance that in all the cases the radius of the cornea in the vertical plane is considerably less than that in the horizontal, that therefore the form of the cornea, without exception, accounts not only for a high degree of astigmatism, but also specially for an astigmatism with shorter focal distance in the vertical meridian, —quite in accordance with what, likewise without exception, was observed with respect to the whole dioptric system.

The great importance of the asymmetry of the cornea is particularly striking on comparing the Table to be found at p. 460, containing the results of observation of normal eyes, with sufficient acuteness of vision : the maximum of asymmetry occurring here is still below the minimum mentioned in the Table, in cases of abnormal astigmatism, if we leave out of view No. 2 of the abnormal, which had a relatively slight disturbance ($S = \frac{2}{3}$), and No. 14 of the normal, which, on closer examination, yielded no perfect acuteness of vision ($S = \frac{1}{3}$).

Another question is, how far the crystalline lens also has influence. In my original Essay upon Astigmatism, I was not in a position to give a satisfactory answer to this query. The investigations recently carried out with Dr. Middelburg, according to the method above described (see p. 462), have supplied me with the proof, *that with a high degree of asymmetry of the cornea asymmetry of the crystalline lens exists, acting in such a direction, that the astigmatism for the whole eye is nearly always less than that proceeding from the cornea.*

The subjoined Table (compare that at p. 493) contains the results of observation and of calculation, obtained for fifteen eyes, some of which were determined by more than one observer. The observations show :

Radius of Curvature through the apex of the Cornea in Meridian — measured table.

No.	Sex and Age	Eye	Refraction of the whole Eye in Mo.	Refraction mo.	0°	15°	30°	45°	60°	75°	90°	105°	120°	135°	150°	165°	Cornea: Mc.	Radius in Mc.	Radius in me.	Asc.	Whole Eye Mo.	Aso.	Lens Ml.	Asl.	Observers
1	m. 40	L.	—1:40	—1:12	7.97	8.06	7.95	7.79	7.79	7.47	7.61	7.72	7.93	8.18	8.25	8.14	63.4	7.63	8.26	1:11.	40°	1:17.14	173°.31	15.06	D.
2	,, 20	R.	—1:20	—1:8	8.47	8.18	8.02	7.68	7.67	7.54	7.56	7.67	7.90	8.09	8.34	8.37	78°	7.52	8.42	1:7.73	74°	1:13.33	174°.91	17.64	M.
3	m. 22	L.	—1:28	—1:56	8.81	8.74	8.59	8.27	8.10	7.99	7.95	7.66	8.02	8.16	8.37	8.46	92°	7.95	8.75	1:9.57	91°	1:7	87°.51	25.80	M.
4	m. 40	R.	E.	—1:19.6	8.76	8.72	8.60	8.42	8.12	8.10	8.01	8.16	8.16	8.37	8.47	8.56	91°	7.99	8.73	1:10.36	128°	1:19.6	89°.31	21.53	H.
5	,, 38	R.	1:24	—1:22	8.38	8.28	8.15	8.12	7.73	7.62	7.43	7.36	7.37	7.61	7.75	8.10	101°	7.38	8.36	1:6.92	104°	1:11.4	1°.11	8.22	M.
6	m. 38	R.	E.	—1:24	8.22	8.32	8.29	7.98	7.90	7.57	7.42	7.30	7.35	8.06	8.09	8.16	105°	7.33	8.33	1:6.71	90°	1:24.	17°.91	16.33	M.
7	m. 20	R.	—1:20	—1:7.5	8.44	8.45	8.54	8.28	7.97	7.76	7.60	7.67	7.84	7.89	7.94	8.10	85°	7.59	8.15	1:12.15	107°	1:12	171°.61	24.07	M. H.
8	m. 47	L.	E.	—1:17.5	8.43	8.43	8.35	8.22	7.97	7.93	7.85	7.82	7.67	7.89	8.15	8.37	102°	7.52	8.58	1:6.68	105°	1:17.5	6°.41	14.51	D.
9	f. 25	R.	—1:20	—1:8.66	8.56	8.56	8.40	8.18	7.94	7.87	7.63	7.84	7.89	7.94	7.98	8.22	101°	7.67	8.45	1:9.11	70°	1:15.3	6°.71	18.59	M.
10	,,	L.	—1:20	—1:13.5	8.06	7.94	8.12	7.97	7.80	7.67	7.50	7.56	7.84	7.93	8.03	8.16	73°	7.43	8.12	1:9.60	75°	1:41.	168°.71	25.02	M.
11	m. 18	R.	—1:15	—1:88	8.01	7.98	7.92	7.86	7.80	7.42	7.37	7.58	7.65	7.72	7.11	7.87	102°	7.56	7.99	1:19.46	91°	1:21.3	26°.11	23.78	M.
12	m. ,,	L.	—1:60	—1:60	7.92	7.80	7.80	7.61	7.51	7.25	7.23	7.30	7.36	7.57	7.82	7.77	86°	7.28	7.91	1:10.	73°	1:30.	171°.71	18.37	D.
13	m. 46	R.	—1:10	—1:10	7.71	7.77	7.86	7.57	7.27	7.17	7.23	7.30	7.36	7.68	7.68	7.77	94°.4	7.26	7.89	1:9.99	88°	1:26.3	129°.71	12.68	M.
14	m. 60	L.	—1:103	—1:16	7.81	7.82	7.91	7.91	7.91	7.84	7.84	7.68	7.63	7.68	7.73	7.80	148°	7.69	7.92	1:28.87	152°	1:28.8	174°.61	27.44	M. D.
15	m. 16	R.	—1:28	—1:14	8.42	7.70	7.75	7.93	7.78	7.48	7.69	7.73	7.92	7.55	7.68	7.63	123°.3	7.59	7.84	1:26.21	70°	1:28.	5°.11	28.47	M.

(Columns M., Mo., Ml., Mc., Mc. and the schematic meridian-direction marks shown in the original beneath each set of "Mc.", "Mo.", and "Ml." headings are indicated graphically in the source.)

1°. That the degree of astigmatism for the whole eye (column As$_o$) was in general not so high as had previously been found by Dr. Knapp and myself. It was on the present occasion ascertained by determination with the stenopæic slit, with cylindrical glasses, and with Stokes' lens, the average of the results obtained by these three methods being taken. These results, when the acuteness of vision was not particularly slight, usually differed but little from one another.

2°. That almost invariably (column D) hypermetropia existed in both meridians (the sign *minus*, placed before the numerical values of the refraction, signifies H).

3°. That the direction of the meridian of maximum of curvature (column G) is far from uniform, but yet in twelve cases deviates less than 20° from the perpendicular, and only in two cases is nearer to 0° than to 90°. (The determination was effected from the direction of the correcting glass required, according to the method described at p. 455, which is more accurate than that formerly used).

4°. That, in connexion with the most commonly occurring direction of M$_o$, with the exception only of No. 13, the radius of curvature of the cornea in 90° is less than in 0° (column E), and even in five cases the maximum of curvature is found very near 90°.

5°. That the average of the measurements, in each of the meridians obtained through intervals of 15 degrees (column E), No. 14 excepted, exhibits a very regular sequence in the ascertained values of the radius of curvature. (The lesser regularity found for the cornea with normal astigmatism (compare Table, p. 466), is undoubtedly to be ascribed to errors of observation, which, with the slight difference of the radius of curvature in the measured meridians, must of course be much more evident in the relation of the numbers.)

From the observations of the radius of curvature in the different meridians, it was now in the first place calculated, to what meridians maximum and minimum correspond and what are the values of maximum and minimum; whence, further, in a simple manner (compare p. 461) the degree of astigmatism caused by the cornea (see column F, under As$_c$) was then found.—In the second place, it was now calculated what the degree and the direction of the asymmetry of the crystalline lens must be, in order, in connexion with the values ascertained for the cornea, to elicit the direction and the degree of the astigmatism for the whole eye. In column H the results of this calculation for the lens are inserted. They will be found to be in accordance with the general result formulised at p. 492.

In particular, we still remark, that only in two cases does the meridian of maximum of curvature of the crystalline lens, M_1, approach more to the vertical than to the horizontal direction. In eleven cases it deviates even less than 10° from the horizontal direction. It thus appears that the maximum of curvature of the lens is still more constantly governed by the horizontal, than that of the cornea is by the vertical direction. Now with this is further connected the fact, that the astigmatism of the cornea is almost invariably greater than that of the whole eye. But at the same time it appears, that we should be far from the truth, if we made the compensating action of the crystalline lens equal to its actual astigmatism, and therefore assumed $As_1 = \dfrac{1}{As_c} - \dfrac{1}{As_o}$. The directions of the axes have too great an influence, as a single glance at the lines, by which they are indicated, at once makes evident.—We can therefore attach no particular value to the Table given by Knapp,* the less so, because the determinations of the astigmatism for the whole dioptric system must by his method come out too high (see p. 451).

I have called the astigmatism of the cornea greater than that of the crystalline lens : but, in fact, the astigmatism of the crystalline lens is greater than we have here found it. The calculation was made as if the crystalline lens were a single refracting surface, placed at an infinitely short distance from the anterior surface of the cornea ; and we can easily understand, that the deeper position of the crystalline lens must diminish its influence in astigmatism. I have thought a more accurate calculation on this point superfluous.

Lastly, the question still arises, whether, when asymmetry of the cornea exists, the radius in the horizontal meridian is greater, or that in the vertical is smaller, than that of the normal symmetrical eye. In the first place, I can to this answer, that that in the horizontal meridian is usually considerably greater. In measuring 120 eyes of men with perfect accuracy of vision, I found $\rho°$ in the horizontal meridian on an average 7.858 mm., the maximum being 8.396 and the minimum 7.291. Among these were many myopic and hypermetropic eyes, up to the highest degrees ; but they exhibited no difference of importance. The 21 asymmetrical eyes of men, collected in the Table (p. 491) give, on the contrary, $\rho°$ on an average 8·291, that is, nearly equal to the maximum found in symmetrical

* *Archiv f. Ophthalmologie*, B. viii. Abth. ii. p. 225.

eyes, and among them occur not fewer than five, which even exceed that maximum, namely, $\varrho^\circ = 8\cdot44$, $\varrho^\circ = 8\cdot72$, $\varrho^\circ = 8\cdot74$, $\varrho^\circ = 8\cdot81$, and $\varrho^\circ = 8.91$. As to ϱ° in the vertical meridian, this is in the asymmetrical eyes shorter than in the symmetrical, but the difference is here less considerable. On an average we found for the first (Table p. 491) ϱ° vertic. $= 7\cdot439$. Of ϱ° vertic. in symmetrical eyes I possess no determinations except those given at p. 460, which exhibit an average of $7\cdot695$. It therefore appears that, in asymmetry of the eye, ϱ° in the horizontal meridian usually ascends more above the normal, than ϱ° in the vertical descends below it. The same is to be deduced from the Table given at p. 493.

Besides congenital malformation of the cornea, various acquired conditions may give rise to abnormal astigmatism. These deserve separate consideration, and shall be spoken of in § 39, with the clinical forms, under which astigmatism occurs.

I here append the mode of calculating the part played by the crystalline lens in astigmatism, as it has been established, after consultation with my friends Professors Hoek and Buys Ballot.

In the first place it is necessary to establish for all the determinations made in twelve meridians a relative influence on the direction of M and m_c, as well as on the radius in M_c and m_c. From the observations must be calculated:—

1°. α the angle, which the horizontal plane makes with the plane m of the greatest radius of curvature.

2°. R, the least radius of curvature and r the greatest radius of curvature.

For this purpose, let the twelve observations be divided into three groups, and of the α, r and R, calculated from each group, let the mean be taken.

Let ρ_0 be the radius of curvature in the horizontal meridian, therefore making an angle $\alpha + 0$ with m, thus ρ_ϕ makes with m the angle $\alpha + \phi$. We thus obtain :

$$\frac{1}{\rho_0} = \frac{1}{R} \cos^2 \alpha + \frac{1}{r} \sin^2 \alpha,$$

to which another form is easily given,

$$\frac{2}{\rho_0} = \left(\frac{1}{R} + \frac{1}{r}\right) + \left(\frac{1}{R} - \frac{1}{r}\right) \cos 2\,\alpha \quad (1)$$

$$\frac{2}{\rho_\phi} = \left(\frac{1}{R} + \frac{1}{r}\right) + \left(\frac{1}{R} - \frac{1}{r}\right) \cos 2\,(\alpha + \phi).$$

The difference is

$$2\left(\frac{1}{\rho_\phi} - \frac{1}{\rho_0}\right) = \left(\frac{1}{R} - \frac{1}{r}\right) \left[\cos 2\,(\alpha + \phi) - \cos 2\,\alpha \right].$$

The difference of the two cosines, expressed by the product of two sines, we obtain

$$\frac{1}{\rho_o} - \frac{1}{\rho_\phi} = \left(\frac{1}{R} - \frac{1}{r}\right) \sin(2\alpha + \phi) \sin\phi \qquad (2)$$

and likewise

$$\frac{1}{\rho_{45}} - \frac{1}{\rho_{\phi+45}} = \left(\frac{1}{R} - \frac{1}{r}\right) \cos(2\alpha + \phi) \sin\phi \qquad (3)$$

Now the quotient of these proportions is:

$$\frac{\dfrac{1}{\rho_o} - \dfrac{1}{\rho_\phi}}{\dfrac{1}{\rho_{45}} - \dfrac{1}{\rho_{\phi+45}}} = \tan(2\alpha + \phi) \qquad (4)$$

and if we assume $\phi = 90°$, the simple formulas come

$$\frac{1}{\rho_o} - \frac{1}{\rho_\phi} = \left(\frac{1}{R} - \frac{1}{r}\right) \cos 2\alpha \qquad (2^*)$$

$$\frac{1}{\rho_{45}} - \frac{1}{\rho_{\phi+45}} = -\left(\frac{1}{R} - \frac{1}{r}\right) \sin 2\alpha \qquad (3^*)$$

$$\text{and} \quad \frac{\dfrac{1}{\rho_o} - \dfrac{1}{\rho_\phi}}{\dfrac{1}{\rho_{45}} - \dfrac{1}{\rho_{\phi+45}}} = -\cot 2\alpha \qquad (4^*)$$

If we apply this formula to the fourth line of the table, we find:
For the first combination of $\rho_o \, \rho_{90}$ and $\rho_{45} \, \rho_{135}$

$$\frac{\dfrac{1}{8\cdot01} - \dfrac{1}{8\cdot76}}{\dfrac{1}{8\cdot37} - \dfrac{1}{8\cdot42}} = \frac{-0\cdot0107}{-0\cdot0007} = -\cot 2\alpha$$

$$2a = -3°\,44'$$
$$a = -1°\,52'.$$

For the second combination of $\rho_{15} \, \rho_{105}$ and $\rho_{60} \, \rho_{150}$,

$$\frac{\dfrac{1}{8\cdot07} - \dfrac{1}{8\cdot72}}{\dfrac{1}{8\cdot14} - \dfrac{1}{8\cdot47}} = \frac{-0\cdot0092}{+0\cdot0056} = -\cot 2(a + 15°)$$

$$2(a + 15°) = 31°\,20'$$
$$a \qquad = \quad 40'.$$

For the third combination $\rho_{30} \, \rho_{120}$ and $\rho_{75} \, \rho_{165}$,

$$\frac{\dfrac{1}{8\cdot60} - \dfrac{1}{8\cdot16}}{\dfrac{1}{8\cdot02} - \dfrac{1}{8\cdot56}} = \frac{-0\cdot0063}{+0\cdot0079} = -\cot 2(a + 30)$$

$$2(a + 30) = 51°\,26'$$
$$a \quad = - \quad 4°\,17'.$$

As the mean of the three combinations, we now obtain:

$$a = \frac{-1°\,52' + 40' - 4°\,17'}{3} = -1°\,53',$$

which signifies that m lies at $1°\,53'$,
$$\text{M at } 91°\,53'.$$

In the second place we find R and r from the determinations of

32

$$\frac{1}{R} - \frac{1}{r} \text{ and } \frac{1}{R} + \frac{1}{r}.$$

For the first combination we find :

$$\frac{1}{R} + \frac{1}{r} = \frac{\left(\dfrac{1}{\rho_o} + \dfrac{1}{\rho_{90}}\right) + \left(\dfrac{1}{\rho_{45}} + \dfrac{1}{\rho_{135}}\right)}{2} = 0.2387.$$

For the second combination :

$$\frac{1}{R} + \frac{1}{r} = \frac{\left(\dfrac{1}{\rho_{15}} + \dfrac{1}{\rho_{105}}\right) + \left(\dfrac{1}{\rho_{60}} + \dfrac{1}{\rho_{150}}\right)}{2} = 0.2402.$$

For the third combination :

$$\frac{1}{R} + \frac{1}{r} = \frac{\left(\dfrac{1}{\rho_{30}} + \dfrac{1}{\rho_{120}}\right) + \left(\dfrac{1}{\rho_{75}} + \dfrac{1}{\rho_{165}}\right)}{2} = 0.2402.$$

And

$$\frac{1}{R} - \frac{1}{r} \text{ is found as } (2\,*),$$

$$\frac{1}{R} - \frac{1}{r} = \frac{\dfrac{1}{\rho_0} - \dfrac{1}{\rho_\phi}}{\cos 2\,\alpha}.$$

This gives for the first combination,

$$\frac{1}{R} - \frac{1}{r} = \frac{0.0107}{\cos 3° 44'} = 0.0107.$$

For the second combination,

$$\frac{1}{R} - \frac{1}{r} = \frac{0.0092}{\cos 31° 40'} = 0.0108.$$

For the third combination,

$$\frac{1}{R} - \frac{1}{r} = \frac{0.0063}{\cos 51° 26'} = 0.0101.$$

By adding the values obtained for $\dfrac{1}{R} - \dfrac{1}{r}$ to the corresponding values of

$\dfrac{1}{R} + \dfrac{1}{r}$, we obtain the value $\dfrac{2}{R}$, and by subtracting them from the same

value $\dfrac{1}{R} + \dfrac{1}{r}$ the value of $\dfrac{2}{r}$.   In the first combination

$$\frac{2}{R} = 0.2387 + 0.0107 = 0.2494.$$

second combination $= 0.2510$

third   „ $= 0.2503$

$$\frac{6}{R} \quad = 0.7507$$

$$\frac{1}{R} \quad = 0.1251$$

$$R \quad = 7.99$$

And
$$\frac{2}{r} = 0\cdot2387 - 0\cdot0107 = 0\cdot2280$$

$$\text{second combination} = 0\cdot2294$$
$$\text{third combination} = 0\cdot2301$$

$$\frac{6}{r} = 0\cdot6875$$

$$\frac{1}{r} = 0\cdot1146$$

$$r = 8\cdot73.$$

In this manner now both M_c and the radius in M_c and in m_c are found, and entered in the Table. The ascertained values of the radii in M_c and m_c are reduced to Parisian inches, and thence the posterior focal distances F'' in the maximum of curvature and f'' in the minimum of curvature are calculated, whence, further, f' was found (see p. 461).

We thus obtain :
$$As_c = \frac{1}{f'}.$$

Now, if the direction of M_o be known by direct determination, that of M_c by calculation, and if the values of As_o and As_c have also been found, these may be considered as the focal distances of two positive cylindrical lenses, the direction of whose axes is perpendicular to M_o and to M_c. Hence, therefore, M_1 can be found as the direction of the axis, and As_1 as the strength of the cylindrical lens, which, added to M_c and As_c, gives for the resulting lens M_o and As_o.

The following is the question :—

If of two infinitely thin cylindrical lenses, I and III, are given the focal distances, or the radii r_1 and r_3 and the directions of the axes,—what is then the focal distance or the radius r_2 and the direction of the axis of a lens II, which, added to I, has III as resulting lens ?

Let $\rho_0 = R$ of the cylindrical lens be ∞ (therefore in the direction of the axis),

$\rho_{90} = r$ the least radius of curvature, α, β the azimuths of the plane of the axes for each of the cylindrical glasses.

γ the azimuth of the axis of the lens to be added, then, as in an angle ϕ with the axis $\dfrac{1}{\rho_0}$ is always $= \dfrac{1}{R} \cos^2 \phi + \dfrac{1}{r} \sin^2 \phi$,

for the cylinder $\dfrac{1}{\rho_0} = \dfrac{1}{r} \sin^2 \phi$ and $\dfrac{1}{\rho_0} = \dfrac{1}{r} \cos^2 \phi$

and therefore in an *arbitrary* azimuth δ, that makes the angles $\alpha - \delta$ with the axis of the first, $\beta - \delta$ with the axis of the second, $\gamma - \delta$ with the plane of the axis of the third lens,

$$\frac{\sin^2 (\alpha - \delta)}{r'} + \frac{\sin^2 (\beta - \delta)}{r''} = \frac{\sin^2 (\gamma - \delta)}{r'''} + \frac{1}{R} \quad (1)$$

$$\frac{\cos^2 (\alpha - \delta)}{r'} + \frac{\cos^2 (\beta - \delta)}{r''} = \frac{\cos^2 (\gamma - \delta)}{r'''} + \frac{1}{R} \quad (2)$$

R always the radius of the sphere, which must be added to the lens γ, in order wholly to comprise the system α and β.

(2) minus (1) gives, on account of
$$\cos^2 \phi - \sin^2 \phi = \cos 2\phi,$$

2

$$\frac{\cos 2\,(a-\delta)}{r'} + \frac{\cos 2\,(\beta-\delta)}{r''} = \frac{\cos 2\,(\gamma-\delta)}{r'''} \qquad (3)$$

The azimuth δ is arbitrary, for in *each* azimuth it must be quite the same, whether we take a or β, or γ into the sphere.

This we express in the following manner :—

$$\cos 2\,(a-\delta) = \cos 2\,a \cos 2\,\delta + \sin 2\,a \sin 2\,\delta.$$

If we do thus with the other terms, and write the one under the other what is multiplied with $\cos 2\,\delta$, and also the one under the other what is multiplied with $\sin 2\,\delta$, there results (3)

$$\left.\begin{array}{l} \dfrac{\cos 2\,a}{r'}\cos 2\,\delta + \dfrac{\sin 2\,a}{r'}\sin 2\,\delta \\[2mm] +\ \dfrac{\cos 2\,\beta}{r''}\cos 2\,\delta + \dfrac{\sin 2\,\beta}{r''}\sin 2\,\delta \\[2mm] -\ \dfrac{\cos 2\,\gamma}{r'''}\cos 2\,\delta - \dfrac{\sin 2\,\gamma}{r'''}\sin 2\,\delta = 0 \end{array}\right\} \quad (4)$$

In order to express the arbitrariness of δ, the coefficient of $\cos 2\,\delta$ and that of $\sin 2\,\delta$ must each separately be equal to zero. Thus (4) falls into (5) and (6).

$$\frac{\cos 2\,a}{r'} + \frac{\cos 2\,\beta}{r''} = \frac{\cos 2\,\gamma}{r'''} \qquad (5)$$

$$\frac{\sin 2\,a}{r'} + \frac{\sin 2\,\beta}{r''} = \frac{\sin 2\,\gamma}{r'''} \qquad (6)$$

(6) divided by (5) is :—

$$\tan 2\,\gamma = \frac{\dfrac{\sin 2\,a}{r'} + \dfrac{\sin 2\,\beta}{r''}}{\dfrac{\cos 2\,a}{r'} + \dfrac{\cos 2\,\beta}{r''}} \qquad (7)$$

and $(5)^2 + (6)^2$ gives

$$\frac{1}{r^2_{'''}} = \frac{1}{r^2_{,}} + \frac{1}{r^2_{,}} + \frac{2 \cos 2\,(a-\beta)}{r'\,r''}$$

Thus r''' and γ are found.

If r' or r'' and a or β to be found, while r''' and γ, and moreover r'' or r' and β or a are given, we write (5) and (6) thus :

$$\frac{\cos 2\,a}{r'} = \frac{\cos 2\,\gamma}{r'''} - \frac{\cos 2\,\beta}{r''} \qquad (9)$$

$$\frac{\sin 2\,a}{r'} = \frac{\sin 2\,\gamma}{r'''} - \frac{\sin 2\,\beta}{r''} \qquad (10)$$

$\dfrac{10}{9}$ gives :

$$\tan 2\,a = \frac{\dfrac{\sin 2\,\gamma}{r'''} - \dfrac{\sin 2\,\beta}{r''}}{\dfrac{\cos 2\,\gamma}{r'''} - \dfrac{\cos 2\,\beta}{r''}} = \frac{r'' \sin 2\,\gamma - r''' \sin 2\,\beta}{r'' \cos 2\,\gamma - r''' \cos 2\,\beta} \qquad (11)$$

$$\text{of } \frac{1}{r^2_{,}} = \frac{1}{r^2_{,,}}\, r^2 \left[r^2_{,} + r^2_{,,} - 2\,r_{,}\,r_{,,}\cos 2\,(\beta-\gamma) \right]$$

$$\text{of } r_{,} = \frac{r_{,}\,r_{,,}}{\sqrt{r^2_{,} + r^2_{,,} - 2\,r_{,}\,r_{,,}\cos 2\,(\beta-\gamma)}}.$$

According to these formulæ M_1 ($= a$) and r' (and with them As_1, as proportionate to them), are now found and filled into the Table.

---

§ 38. Cylindrical Lenses,[*] and General Rules for their Employment.

Regular astigmatism may, as has above been remarked, be produced by adding a cylindrical to a spherical lens.

The action of a cylindrical lens can, in its turn, be counteracted by a second such lens of equal focal distance. If these cylindrical lenses are both either positive or negative, the axes of the cylindrical surfaces must, in order to neutralise each other, stand perpendicular to one another; if, on the contrary, one be positive, and the other negative, the effect is attained with a parallel state of the axes. Of the latter case the astigmatic lens of Stokes furnishes an example (conf. p. 486) : its action is, in a parallel state of the axes, $= 0$. The first we find represented in the so-called watchmakers' lenses, which have two convex cylindrical surfaces of equal focal distance, whose action, by the intersection of the axes of these surfaces, nearly coincides with that of spherical biconvex lenses. If the two cylindrical surfaces be similar and concave, they give the action of a negative spherical lens, with removal of the astigmatism, when their axes intersect.

Now as the action of one cylindrical lens may be destroyed by that of another, regular astigmatism may be corrected by means of a cylindrical lens. In order to form a good idea of the correction, experiments should be tried with one's own eye. A cylindrical lens, for example of $\frac{1}{10}$, produces astigmatism, and gives rise to peculiar disturbances in vision already described. A second cylindrical lens of $- \frac{1}{10}$, with a similarly directed axis, completely neutralises the action of the first, so that the presence of glasses before the eye is now scarcely observed. If, on the contrary, the second cylindrical lens, as well as the first, is a positive lens of $\frac{1}{10}$, the astigmatism is corrected, if the axes of the cylindrical surfaces be directed perpendicularly to each other; but the eye has then at the same time become myopic, and that to such a degree, that the farthest

* To be had, among others, from Nachet and Son, Paris, and Paetz and Flohr, Berlin, on giving the formulæ to be hereafter communicated.

point of a previously ametropic eye (the distance from the glass to the eye not being taken into account) comes to lie at $10''$ ($M = \frac{1}{10}$).

The glasses required for the correction of the different forms of astigmatism, may be reduced to three kinds.

I. *Simple cylindrical glasses* (Fig. 163). Just as the spherical these have either a positive (A, B, C), or a negative focal distance (D, E, F) ; the first we call simply *positive*, the second *negative*. If both the surfaces are cylindrical, their axes are parallel. To give a correct idea of their form, they are represented both in a section perpendicular to the axis (Fig. 163, I), and in a section, carried through the axis (Fig. 163, II), the surfaces being distinguished as *a*, the anterior, and *p*, the posterior.

　a. To the *positive* belong :—
　　　1. The bi-convex (Fig. 163 A).
　　　2. The plano-convex (B).
　　　3. The concavo-convex or positive meniscus (C).
　b. To the *negative* belong :—
　　　1. The bi-concave (D).
　　　2. The plano-concave (E).
　　　3. The convex-concave or negative meniscus (F).

Fig. 163.

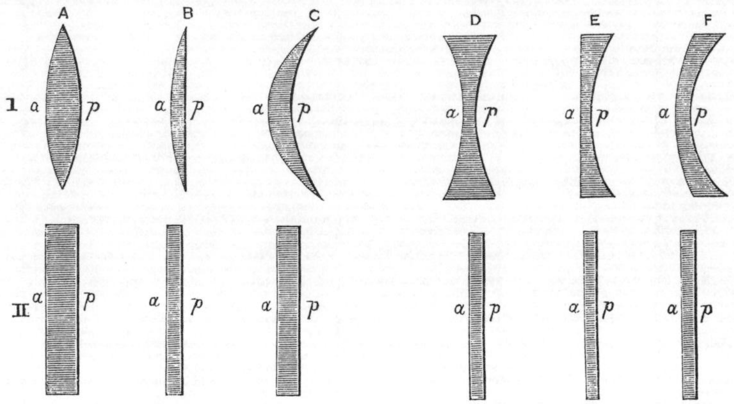

Practically the same is true of the cylindrical as of the spherical glasses : the plano-convex and plano-concave produce the greatest aberration, the bi-convex (provided it be not too powerful) and the bi-concave are in general very satisfactory, and the menisci have the advantage of being periscopic.

Of the simple cylindrical, glasses from $\frac{1}{50}c$ to $\frac{1}{5}c$, and from $-\frac{1}{50}c$ to $-\frac{1}{5}c$ are necessary, that is glasses of from 50 to 5 Parisian inches both negative and positive focal distance. That this focal distance obtains only for the surface perpendicular to the axis of the cylindrical curvature, and that, in a surface carried through the axes the focal distance is infinite, need scarcely be remarked here : they therefore leave in this last direction also, the focal distance of a dioptric system, wherewith they are combined, unaltered.

To express their nature and power we make use, as will have been seen, of the same formula as for the spherical glasses, with the addition of c.

II. *Bi-cylindrical glasses* (Fig. 164).—These have two cylindrical surfaces of curvature, whose axes are directed perpendicularly to one another (I a and II p). If the two surfaces are cylindrically ground, but their axes are parallel, they belong to the simple cylindrical, whether to the bi-convex, or bi-concave, or to the menisci, which have been already described above (Fig. 163, A, C, D and F). Of the bi-cylindrical one surface is in general convex, the other concave, as the two sections, taken in each of the two axes (Fig. 164, I a, II p),

Fig. 164.　　　　　Fig. 165.

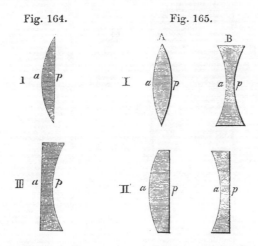

show. Such bi-cylindrical glasses, therefore, make parallel incident rays of light, after refraction, converge in the plane of the one axis,

and diverge in that of the other. Their action may be expressed by
the formula for each of the two planes, connected by the sign of a
right angle $\ulcorner$. A bi-cylindrical glass of 12″ positive focal distance
in a plane, perpendicular to the axis of the convex cylindrical
surface, and of 24″ negative focal distance in a plane, perpendicular to the axis of the concave cylindrical surface, is therefore expressed as :

$$\frac{1}{12}\,c\,\ulcorner\;-\;\frac{1}{24}\,c.$$

III. *Spherico-cylindrical glasses.*—Of these glasses the one surface has a spherical (Fig. 165, I and II $a\,a$), the other a cylindrical
curvature (I and II $p\,p$). Only those are used whose two surfaces are
either convex (A) or concave (B). These lenses may be considered
as the combination of a plano-cylindrical with a plano-spherical
lens, and we actually obtain both by cutting a spherico-cylindrical lens
in a plane, perpendicular to the axis of the spherical surface. Now
the action of a spherico-cylindrical lens is similar to that of the
combination mentioned, and it may be expressed by the formula for
each of the refracting surfaces, united by the sign of combination
$\smile$. If the spherical curvature, as a plano-convex lens, gives a focal
distance of 12″, the cylindrical curvature, as a plano-convex lens, a
focal distance of 24″, we write :

$$\frac{1}{12}\,s\,\smile\,\frac{1}{24}\,c,$$

signifying that the positive focal distance, in a section through the
axis of the cylindrical surface, amounts to 12″, in a section perpendicular to this surface, to $(\frac{1}{12}+\frac{1}{24}=\frac{1}{8})$ 8″. If the spherical
surface, as a plano-convex lens, represents $-\dfrac{1}{18}$, the cylindrical, as
a plano-cylindrical lens, $-\dfrac{1}{9}$, the combined spherico-cylindrical
lens gives :

$$-\frac{1}{18}\,s\,\smile\,-\frac{1}{9}\,c,$$

in which lens the negative focal distance, in the axis of the cylindrical surface, amounts to 18″, perpendicular to this axis to $(\frac{1}{18}+\frac{1}{9}$
$=\frac{1}{6})$ 6″.

It is now easy to see what cylindrical glasses remove the different
forms of astigmatism (compare p. 482). Suppose our object to be
to correct the ametropia at the same time with the astigmatism, that

is, to bring the farthest point of distinct vision to an infinite distance ($R = \infty$). We then find:

1. Simple myopic astigmatism is corrected by a simple negative cylindrical lens (Fig. 163, D, E, F) of a focal distance, corresponding to the degree of astigmatism:

$$Am = \frac{1}{6}$$

by glasses of $-\dfrac{1}{5\frac{1}{2}}$ c, placed at $\frac{1}{2}''$ from the nodal point.

2. Compound myopic astigmatism requires a negative sphericocylindrical lens. Thus, not taking the distance from glass to nodal point into account,

$$M \frac{1}{20} + Am \frac{1}{20}$$

is corrected by

$$-\frac{1}{20} s \bigcirc - \frac{1}{20} c \text{ (compare Fig. 165, B).}$$

3. Simple hypermetropic astigmatism, Ah, is corrected by simple positive cylindrical glasses (Fig. 163, A, B, C), corresponding to the degree of the astigmatism. For

$$Ah = \frac{1}{8},$$

a glass of

$$\frac{1}{8\frac{1}{2}} c$$

is therefore required, placed at $\frac{1}{2}''$ from the nodal point.

4. Compound hypermetropic astigmatism requires positive sphericocylindrical glasses:

$$H \frac{1}{18} + Ah \frac{1}{9}$$

is corrected (the distance from the glass to the nodal point not being taken into account) by:

$$\frac{1}{18} s \bigcirc \frac{1}{9} c.$$

5. Mixed astigmatism, lastly, yields to bi-cylindrical glasses:

$$Amh = \frac{1}{8},$$

composed of

$$M \frac{1}{12} + H \frac{1}{24},$$

by:

$$\frac{1}{24} c \ulcorner \; - \frac{1}{12} c,$$

and

$$\mathrm{Ahm} = \frac{1}{8},$$

composed of

$$\frac{1}{12} \mathrm{H} + \frac{1}{24} \mathrm{M},$$

by:

$$\frac{1}{12} c \ulcorner \quad \frac{1}{24} c.$$

These short examples will form a guide in the choice of glasses, when, with the astigmatism, ametropia is at the same time to be corrected. But it is not always desirable to attain this double object. Whilst by correction of astigmatism the power of vision is under all circumstances benefited, and we almost unconditionally can attain to it,— to reduce the eye at the same time to the state of emmetropia, is often not indicated. As to this reduction, the same rules apply in complication with astigmatism, as are applicable to ametropia in general, and which we have stated in detail when treating of hypermetropia (§ 23) and of myopia (§ 32).

It therefore only remains for us to show, how to find by calculation the necessary glass, in complication with astigmatism, when it is established to what distance R must be brought.

In the determination of the astigmatism, we proceeded from investigating the refraction in the two principal meridians. Hence the ametropia common to both meridians was deduced, and the degree of astigmatism was added as a separate value. Thus we found the formula for the compound astigmatism both hypermetropic and myopic. If we now revert to the two principal meridians, the method of finding the glasses which, neutralising the astigmatism, give the desired value to R in all meridians, is extremely simple. Giving to R a value of 40″, 20″, 12″ signifies nothing else than communicating to the eye a myopia of, or reducing the existing myopia to, $\frac{1}{40}, \frac{1}{20}, \frac{1}{12}$. We have therefore from the ascertained refraction in the two principal meridians only to deduct the desired degree of myopia, and if we give the glasses which completely correct the then remaining ametropia in each of the meridians, precisely this degree of myopia remains.

The following examples may serve to illustrate the foregoing :—

1. Let there be found :

In the principal meridian H, emmetropia,

$$,, \qquad ,, \qquad v, M = \frac{1}{6},$$

and let us desire to bring R to 18″, then we obtain by deduction :

$$\text{in H, emmetropia} - M \frac{1}{18} = H \frac{1}{18},$$

$$\text{in v, } M \frac{1}{6} - M \frac{1}{18} = M \frac{1}{9};$$

and to correct this a bi-cylindrical glass is required of :

$$\frac{1}{18} \, c \, \ulcorner \; - \frac{1}{9} \, c.$$

2. Let there be in the principal meridian H, $M = \frac{1}{20}$,

$$,, \qquad ,, \qquad v, M = \frac{1}{10};$$

and if we desire to bring R to 20″, we find, by deducting $M \frac{1}{20}$,

$$\text{in H, } M \frac{1}{20} - M \frac{1}{20} = \text{emmetropia,}$$

$$\text{in v, } M \frac{1}{10} - M \frac{1}{20} = M \frac{1}{20};$$

so that the object is attained by a simple cylindrical glass of $- \frac{1}{20} c$.

3. In H let $H = \frac{1}{6}$,

$$\text{in v let } H = \frac{1}{18};$$

if we desire, for reading, writing, &c., to bring R to 18″, we find by deduction :

$$\text{in H, H } \frac{1}{6} \quad M \frac{1}{18} = H - \frac{1}{4\frac{1}{2}},$$

$$\text{in v, H } \frac{1}{18} - M \frac{1}{18} = H - \frac{1}{9},$$

which (compare p. 505, under 4°) is corrected by :

$$\frac{1}{9} \, s \, \subset \frac{1}{9} \, c.$$

4. In a case of astigmatism let there be:

$$\text{in v, } M = \frac{1}{12},$$

$$\text{in H, } H = \frac{1}{24}.$$

And if we desire R at 24″, we obtain by deduction,

$$\text{in v, } M\,\frac{1}{12} - M\,\frac{1}{24} = M\,\frac{1}{24},$$

$$\text{in H, } H\,\frac{1}{24} - M\,\frac{1}{24} = H\,\frac{1}{12};$$

so that to obtain the proposed object, a bi-cylindrical glass is required of

$$\frac{1}{12}\,c\,\ulcorner\,-\,\frac{1}{24}\,c.$$

The rather complicated method here described may in all cases be adopted, but this is not always necessary. For when, together with compound myopic astigmatism, a high degree of myopia exists, which we wish partly to maintain, the myopia need only be reduced to the desired degree: for example, if in $M\,\frac{1}{6}$ + $Am\,\frac{1}{12}$, we wish to retain $M\,\frac{1}{18}$, this will be attained by sub-tracting $M\,\frac{1}{18}$, and thus correcting $M\,\frac{1}{9}$ + $Am\,\frac{1}{12}$ by $-\frac{1}{9}\,s$ $\bigcirc -\frac{1}{12}\,c$. In like manner we have in compound hypermetropic astigmatism only to increase the hypermetropia which is to be corrected by so much as corresponds to the desired value of R. Thus, in

$$H\,\frac{1}{18} + Ah\,\frac{1}{9}$$

R is to be brought to 18″ by

$$\frac{1}{9}\,s\,\bigcirc\,\frac{1}{9}\,c.$$

In all these calculations we have, for the sake of simplicity, omitted the correction proceeding from the distance between the glass and the nodal point: indeed, if particularly strong glasses are not required, its influence is so slight as to be in practice scarcely perceptible.

In the employment of cylindrical glasses, it is of the greatest importance that the axes of the surfaces of curvature should be situated in the principal meridians of the dioptric system of the eye. Even a slight deviation causes, especially when strong glasses are used, a very perceptible disturbance. The proposed end is now best attained by setting circular shaped glasses in a framework with rings, so that by turning round the glasses, the proper direction can easily be given to the axis of the cylindrical surface.   By slightly moving the whole arrangement, we soon observe in what direction the glass is to be turned; and the proof that it has acquired precisely the right direction consists in the correction becoming less perfect, the power of vision less acute, on gently inclining it to one side or the other. When once the correct direction has been found for the round glasses, we can, if it be preferred, still maintaining the directions of the axes, have them ground into oval glasses and placed in another framework.   That in the use of cylindrical glasses, it is above all things necessary to take care to have a well-adjusted and but slightly movable framework, is included in what has above been said.

The correction of regular astigmatism by means of cylindrical glasses is incapable of absolute perfection.   Apart from the amblyopia, which, independently of the light-refracting system, complicates many cases of astigmatism, the acuteness of vision must, even with the most accurate correction, leave something to be desired, because the asymmetry of the astigmatic eye cannot be completely counteracted by the presence of a cylindrical lens. Moreover, the correction is only of that nature that the posterior focal points for the different meridians are brought together without the same being true of the other cardinal points.   The absolute coincidence of the nodal points in the different meridians is scarcely attainable.   If they lie in the principal meridian of slightest curvature more posteriorly, correction with a bi-convex cylindrical lens brings them more forward, than those in the meridian of greatest curvature, and *vice versâ* if they be situated more anteriorly, on correction by a bi-concave cylindrical lens, they are moved more backward.   In this is implied that the form of bodies, on correction of astigmatism, is elongated in a direction opposite to that in which, before correction, elongation existed. This too great displacement of the nodal points becomes less, the closer the cylindrical glasses are to the cornea, and for this reason also it is desirable, in the use of spherico-cylindrical glasses, to turn that surface towards the eye, whereby the nodal point of the cylindrical surface lies closest to the organ.   If both be convex or concave, the one of least curvature should be turned towards the eye; if one be convex, the other concave, the concave one should be turned towards it.—The change of form, which is the result of cylindrical glasses, is also the cause, why, in looking for glasses of the required strength, we can less advantageously make use of the change in acuteness of vision on altering the distance between the glass and the eye, than when spherical glasses are in question: almost always the glass, both the convex, though it be too weak, and the concave, though it be too strong, is desired close to the eye. Moreover it is easily seen that, especially in using bi-cylindrical glasses, the distance from the eye ought to be short: indeed, in proportion as the distance increases, the images become in one direction smaller and smaller, in the opposite larger and larger, and under this double influence the change of form must make itself strongly felt. Furthermore, it is to be observed, that in some movements of the eye, which are connected with an obliquity of the vertical meridian, the direction of the axes of the cylindrical surfaces no longer coincides perfectly with the principal meridians, and the correction is therefore imperfect; whence it follows that in using cylindrical glasses the eye, in order to maintain the acuteness of vision, is somewhat limited in its movements. However, every spectacle-glass, as such, necessarily causes limitation, and, in fact, experience shows that in the use of cylindrical glasses this is productive of no particular inconvenience.

Finally, to omit nothing, I shall briefly state, that the accommodative changes in the astigmatic eye, especially after correction of the asymmetry, do not represent absolutely coincident ranges of accommodation in both principal meridians, so that the correction by definite glasses cannot be equally perfect in all states of accommodation. This difference is however so slight, that neither can it give rise to any practical difficulty.

As I have already stated, Airy was the first to discover abnormal astigmatism, in fact in his own left eye. At the same time he conceived that a cylindrical glass might correct the asymmetry, which he actually found to be the case, the disturbance of vision being corrected by such a glass. The form of his astigmatism was the compound myopic. Airy conceived that if he had two concave cylindrical surfaces ground, with axes directed perpendicularly to each other, each corresponding respectively to the degree of myopia to be corrected in the principal meridians, the object should be attained. But he correctly gave the preference to a negative spherico-cylindrical glass, whereof the concave spherical surface was to correct the common myopia of the two principal meridians, the concave cylindrical the still remaining simple astigmatism. And, in truth, bi-cylindrical glasses (with intersection of the axes), of which both surfaces should be either convex or concave, are never necessary : they may always be advantageously replaced by spherico-cylindrical glasses. The bi-cylindrical lenses used in Switzerland, and generally to be found with the watchmakers, whose convex surfaces, together with intersection of the axes, have a similar curvature, in their action closely resemble bi-convex spherical glasses. The watchmakers assert that they have a more extensive field : the truth is, that the field is wider in the direction of the axis of the surface turned towards the eye, but narrower in the opposite direction, so that the form of the distinct field of vision is an oval, which follows the movements of the lens in rotation. These lenses can the less vie with periscopic spherical glasses, as with them the forms of objects seen laterally appear in a peculiar manner distorted.

That astigmatism is, to a certain extent, capable of correction by convex and concave spherical glasses, when their axis is held before the eye at a certain angle with the visual line, was already known to Young and Cary. (See the quotation at p. 456.) It appears that others, especially in high degrees of myopia, have also made use of them. Thus we read in White Cooper (*on Near Sight*, etc., London, 1853, p. 199), that cases sometimes occur, in which, in consequence of a peculiarity in the form of the refracting media, or in the sensibility of the retina (?) the improvement caused by glasses is considerably increased " by sloping them or holding them obliquely," and that he had seen a striking example of this in a myopic patient. He adds, that in order to give the desired position to the glass, Carpenter and Westley made it turn in a second ring, contained in the ring of the spectacle frame. This means of correcting astigmatism is, however, capable of application only when relatively strong spherical glasses are required to neutralise the ametropia, and then, too, a more perfect correction will be attainable by cylindrical curvature of one of the surfaces. Only in aphakia can we advantageously, in my opinion, in order to correct a certain degree of astigmatism, make use of an oblique position of the glasses. Almost always it appears that when we give a certain inclination to the strongly convex glass, the acuteness of vision is improved, and the necessity of attending strictly to this point in every case of aphakia, is generally recognised.

Lastly, we must not omit to observe, that regular astigmatism might also be corrected by operation. Iriddesis, an operation brought into vogue chiefly by Critchett, would be serviceable in such cases, especially double iriddesis in opposite directions, as practised by Bowman and others in keratoconus (compare Critchett and Bowman, in *Reports of the London Ophthalmic Hospital*, 1859 and 1860). The pupil is thereby, in fact, changed into a narrow slit; and if the direction of this slit corresponds to one of the principal meridians, the aberration dependent on asymmetry would certainly be almost entirely excluded. The indication of this *double* iriddesis in keratoconus I cannot admit : in this case the cause of the loss of acuteness of vision is not the difference of curvature in the various meridians, but rather the conical curvature in each meridian; and, in connexion with that, Bowman has proposed some modifications of iriddesis (comp. the treatment of irregular astigmatism). But where there is only difference of curvature of the several meridians, that is in regular astigmatism, the narrow slit obtained by double iriddesis would undoubtedly very much promote acuteness of vision. However, considering that we have it in our power to obtain the desired correction by means of cylindrical glasses, I am, looking to the greater or less danger of the operation, and not less to the deformity which is the result of it, far from recommending its application.

---

§ 39. NOSOLOGY AND CLINICAL STUDY OF ASTIGMATISM.—HISTORY
OF OUR KNOWLEDGE OF THE SUBJECT.

Astigmatism is either congenital or acquired. In the great majority of cases it is congenital. If it be acquired, it is to be looked upon clinically as another form of disease, whose practical importance has become more and more evident to me, and of which I shall separately treat, after having first considered :—

1. *Congenital astigmatism.*—This anomaly is of frequent occurrence. I am as yet without satisfactory statistics; but I certainly do not exaggerate when I assert that in forty or fifty eyes, one is, in consequence of astigmatism, disturbed in its function.

Boundaries between normal and abnormal astigmatism do not exist. When it attains the degree of $\frac{1}{40}$, I have called it abnormal, because the disturbance of vision is then of that nature, that cylindrical glasses are desirable for its improvement. But otherwise it is evident, that the limit I have fixed upon is rather arbitrary. With much slighter degrees the acuteness of vision is no longer perfect. Thus I was formerly of opinion, that an astigmatism of about $\frac{1}{100}$, such as exists in both my eyes, under no circumstances interfered with the distinctness of the images, and was therefore not capable of correction; and yet I found that $\frac{1}{80} c$ (the weakest glasses I possess) held with the axis perpendicular before my eye, unmistakably increase the distinctness of the images, while, *vice versâ*, with the axis in a horizontal position, the same glasses produce a pretty considerable disturbance. The improvement which is produced by the addition of $\frac{1}{40} c$, with a vertical axis is now most striking. Hence, we see again, that too high a degree has been considered as normal by Dr. Knapp.

The cases which have occurred to me, presented an astigmatism of from $\dfrac{1}{40}$ to $\dfrac{1}{4\frac{1}{2}}$. In the majority it amounted to more than $\frac{1}{18}$, not unfrequently to more than $\frac{1}{10}$.

Astigmatism is often hereditary. Not unfrequently one of the parents labours under the same defect. But more frequently still it happens, that different children, born of the same parents, exhibit this anomaly, and mostly in the same form; in this case we are equally justified in calling the condition hereditary, as when it occurs in one of the parents.

In the majority of instances both eyes are affected. Often, however, one is completely or almost completely free. Mr. R. had in both eyes Ah between $\frac{1}{6}$ and $\frac{1}{7}$; in his brother, Ah existed $= \frac{1}{9\frac{1}{3}}$ of precisely the same form, only in one eye: his left eye was almost perfectly free from astigmatism. It is remarkable that, with such a difference between the two eyes, the upper part of the face likewise is usually asymmetric. Also, when a high degree of ametropia occurs only on one side, asymmetry of the bones bounding the orbit is a very common phenomenon. This is connected with the peculiarities in the form of the face in myopic, and especially in hypermetropic, individuals,—an important subject, which has already long engaged my attention, but on which I cannot here further dilate.

Thus far I have met with many more cases of abnormal astigmatism in men than in women. I do not, however, feel justified in assuming that this is not partly accidental. This point must remain for future decision.

As to time of life, it is evident that this can have no influence. So long as the power of accommodation remains active, the disturbance of vision from a moderate degree of astigmatism is, however, productive of less inconvenience. Slight cases, therefore, usually first present themselves, when the range of accommodation (about the thirtieth year) is already perceptibly diminished, while in high degrees of astigmatism the disturbance is early remarked, and the ophthalmic surgeon is not unfrequently consulted even before the patient has attained his seventh year. On the other hand, at an advanced period of life, in consequence of the diminution of the pupil, a certain degree of astigmatism produces less disturbance. With all this the astigmatism certainly maintains about its original degree.

The disturbance of vision, connected with this anomaly, is very peculiar. It is neither to be compared with that proceeding from defects of the retina (amblyopia), nor with that from obscuration of the media, nor even with that which is the result of ametropia. In the ordinary forms of amblyopia, the projection into the field of vision is uncertain and not accurately circumscribed; in obscurations the diffuse light scattered over the retina produces a mist before the eye, which diminishes the contrast between light and shade of the objects; in a state of refraction not corresponding to the distance at which the objects are, each point is represented by a circle of diffusion, and by the mutual overlying of these numberless circles, the contours of the objects are, as it were, effaced. In astigmatism, on the other hand, in contrast to amblyopia, the projection in the field of vision is as yet perfectly accurately defined, and is correctly described : thus the astigmatic individual will state, to the minutest particulars, under what partly black, partly grey lines, a figure, for example the

33

compound roman letter W, appears. But the retinal image itself, placed
in an unaltered shape before the eyes, by the projection, deviates in
form and in distribution of light so much from the object, that he is not
in a position to recognise the latter from it, at least when the images
of different adjoining objects cover one another, and the component
lines, in all directions and with different degrees of distinctness, cross
one another.   Clearly also irregular astigmatism here plays a great
part : it causes, that in the meridian wherein the refraction deviates
most from the required condition of accommodation, double images
arise, which may exceedingly magnify the confusion.   It is now easy
to understand how, in the endeavour to guess at the form of objects,
from the alternating images which appear in the agitation of accommodation, psychical fatigue is soon created, with which, under some
circumstances, as the result of the excessive tension of accommodation, phenomena of asthenopia are combined.   It is therefore no
wonder that astigmatic persons should feel so exceedingly pleased at
the correction of their anomaly, and should manifest their pleasure
in a more lively manner than ordinary ametropic individuals.

It has already been shown, that regular congenital astigmatism
generally depends upon asymmetry of the cornea, while the cases in
which the lens plays the principal part, are among the rarest exceptions.

A.—Of *congenital regular astigmatism of the cornea* we have,
from the point of view of refraction in the two principal meridians,
distinguished three forms (compare p. 482) : the myopic, the hypermetropic, and the mixed.   Each of these has its peculiarities, which
will best appear by describing, after a short introduction, one or more
cases of each form.

1. *Myopic astigmatism.*—Of this we have two forms : *a*, simple
myopic astigmatism, Am, when emmetropia in the one principal
meridian is combined with myopia in the other; *b*, compound myopic
astigmatism, M + Am, when myopia exists in both the principal meridians, but in a different degree.   To this latter form belongs,
among others, the case of Airy.

At first I supposed that myopic astigmatism occurs only exceptionally.   The first cases which I saw, all belonged to the hypermetropic form, a few to the mixed.   Subsequently, the proportion
changed, and now I think it may be established, that in eight cases
of astigmatism nearly one belongs to the myopic form.   In general,
however, it is only,

a. Simple myopic astigmatism.—Absolute emmetropia in one of the principal meridians is a condition not easily met with. Strictly speaking, therefore, cases of *simple* myopic astigmatism scarcely occur.

But shall we, where the slightest trace of myopia exists in the second meridian, consider the anomaly to be compound myopic, or when combined with the least trace of hypermetropia, to be compound hypermetropic astigmatism? This would, it appears to me, not be practical. To the idea of simple astigmatism a certain latitude must be allowed. $M = \frac{1}{80}$ in general requires no correction, nor does $H = \frac{1}{80}$ in young persons: a simple cylindrical glass is then quite sufficient. Only it will appear, that in proportion as correction by a simple cylindrical glass leaves a little H or M, as accommodation diminishes, respectively earlier or later than usual, combination with a convex spherical surface will be required for near objects.

CASE I. *Simple myopic astigmatism.*—Mr. O., student in divinity, now twenty-one years of age, consulted me three years since. I diagnosed myopia about $= \frac{1}{16}$, complicated with amblyopia. The degree of myopia was, however, not strictly definable, on account of the diminished acuteness of vision. The latter, in fact, amounted to scarcely $\frac{1}{3}$, so that the patient could distinguish ordinary print only at a short distance, in which the existing myopia was very serviceable to him.

He had large prominent eyes, clear media, only a trace of atrophy of the membranes, on the outside of the optic disc,—moreover, this disc was redder than is normally the case, without being redder than it usually appears in young myopic persons, who read and write much. He thought that his power of vision had latterly diminished; but he had never had easy sight, and had never been able, particularly in the evening, to continue long at a time engaged in close work.

Such a disturbance is very common in myopes. But in them it has usually developed itself at a definite time, and as the result of continued work in a stooping position, while the power of vision had previously been quite sufficient. I have therefore doubted, whether in this case the cause of the amblyopia was to be sought therein, and moreover, derivative means, artificial leeches, cold douches to the eye, &c., were employed in vain. Finding no improvement, the patient ceased his visits.

Some weeks ago he again presented himself. His power of vision, he stated, was so defective that he feared he should not be able to continue his studies. He was anxious, before finally making up his mind, to consult me once more. My former notes were referred to. I immediately suspected that astigmatism, previously overlooked by me, must exist in this case.

2

In favourable light he saw with both eyes, and with each eye separately, No. I at the distance of from $2\frac{1}{2}''$ to $3''$. At a great distance the acuteness of vision was, for the right eye, $= \frac{1}{4}$, for the left eye, $= \frac{1}{5}$. Negative glasses improved the sight, but comparatively little: and yet he preferred a strong glass, about $\frac{1}{10}$, with which the acuteness of vision rose to $\frac{2}{7}$. The existence of astigmatism had thus become probable.

We therefore proceeded to the trial with the point of light (compare p. 454). The right eye saw the point of light as a line /, inclining nearly 30° outwards, and to it, armed with $\frac{1}{30}$, the line appeared still longer and slighter; with $\frac{1}{30}$ and with $\frac{1}{20}$ it was, on the other hand, at the same time broader and complicated with secondary lines. With from $-\frac{1}{40}$ to $-\frac{1}{13}$, the image was nearly round, with $-\frac{1}{8}$ it was spread out in a direction perpendicular to its primary one. It was, however, rather changeable, so that the glass with which the most slender horizontal image was obtained was difficult to define, the more so, as this image was not a pure line, but a rather compound figure extended in a recumbent position. The eye was now armed with $\frac{1}{40}$ and a negative glass was alternately placed before the positive one, on which the opposite directions formed a cross, which, when the negative glass was $\dfrac{1}{6\frac{1}{2}}$, consisted of the slenderest lines.

The direction of both principal meridians was thus ascertained. Through a slit, $1\frac{3}{4}$ mm. wide ═══, held in the direction of the horizontal principal meridian, the acuteness of vision rose to $\frac{1}{3}$; positive and negative glasses held in front of the slit produced no further improvement. The same slit, held before the vertical principal meridian, produced no essential advantage; on the addition of $-\frac{1}{10}$ the acuteness of vision rose to $\frac{1}{3}$. As to reading at a short distance, this was only slightly improved by looking through the horizontal slit, on the contrary it was very considerably improved by looking through the vertical slit.

A glass of $\frac{1}{16}c$, the axis of the surface being held in the direction of the vertical meridian, caused No. I to be easily read at nearly double the distance, $\frac{1}{11}c$, and $\frac{1}{9}c$ at more than double the distance; on the contrary, when the axis of the cylindrical surfaces coincided with the horizontal principal meridian, even No. IX could no longer be deciphered. At a distance $-\frac{1}{10}c$, the axis coinciding with the horizontal principal meridian, was found excellent: with it the acuteness of vision rose, under favourable circumstances, nearly to $\frac{3}{4}$. The patient had never before had an idea what acute vision was, and felt uncommonly happy.

Black lines, inclining 30° outwards, were pretty accurately seen at a distance without glasses, while lines, perpendicular to these, were scarcely recognised as lines. When a glass of $-\frac{1}{10}$ was held before the eye, the greatest sharpness of the latter was obtained, and the first could only with tension of accommodation be tolerably satisfactorily seen.

Time did not admit of the radii of curvature of the cornea being measured.

That asymmetry existed in this coat could, however, be inferred from the form of the reflected image of a square surface inclining 30°.

The atrophy of the membranes, observable on the outside of the optic disc, had increased since the first examination. The retinal vessels, running in the direction of the vertical principal meridian, were in the non-inverted image accurately recognised by an emmetropic eye; in order to see those running in the direction of the horizontal meridian in the non-inverted image, a negative glass of about $-\frac{1}{10}$ was required. In the inverted image it was difficult to establish the difference in distance of the variously directed blood-vessels.

The *left* eye presented a remarkable correspondence with the right. Here, too, Am existed about $=\frac{1}{10}$, and the vertical principal meridian inclined about 30° outwards \. A more accurate description appears therefore to be quite superfluous.

Epicrisis, or critical remarks.*—The case here described is one of the thousands, in which astigmatism has been looked upon as amblyopia, and has been treated as such. If the aimless and energetic treatment was only vexatious to the patient, his joy, when he found his sight at all distances improved by suitable glasses, was indescribably great. He was accustomed always to hold even large print at a very short distance from the eye, partly in order by looking under a greater angle to make amends for his diminished acuteness of vision, partly, as an associated movement, with the convergence and tension of accommodation, to contract his pupil, and thereby to diminish the diffusion-images. On this excessive tension of accommodation required for more accurate definition, depend the phenomena of asthenopia, usually observed in astigmatic persons. Probably the amblyopia remaining after correction of the astigmatism, is likewise a result of the excessive strain connected with the strongly stooping position so injurious to the eye.—It will have been observed that the patient saw better at a distance with tolerably strongly-negative spherical glasses: this, too, appears attributable to the fact, that the tension of accommodation required in the use of these glasses, gave rise to constriction of the pupil, and thus to diminution of the diffusion-images.

I prescribed for the patient provisionally, only glasses of $-\frac{1}{10}c$, with which he saw both distant and near objects satisfactorily. His range of accommodation amounted to nearly $\frac{1}{4}$, and as he had accustomed himself to strain his power of accommodation, it cannot appear strange, that he at first required no other spectacles for reading and writing. However, it is to be expected, that the excessive tension of accommodation will soon cease, and

---

* This term, employed in the original, ought to be introduced into our medical vocabulary; it has the sanction of Galen for its use—ἡ τῶν διὰ τῆς πείρας εὑρισκομένων βοηθημάτων ἐπίκρισις.—S. H.

should continued work then cause some inconvenience, I propose to recommend him the use of bi-cylindrical glasses of

$$\tfrac{1}{36} c \ \Gamma \ - \tfrac{1}{14} c,$$

whereby the astigmatism shall be corrected, and a slight degree of myopia in all meridians shall be produced. Should the acuteness of vision become perfect, of which (now that excessive tension in a stooping position is no longer necessary) there is some prospect, he will not require these latter glasses until a more advanced period of life.

b. Compound myopic astigmatism, M + Am.—Of compound myopic astigmatism I have seen only a few cases. It occurs under the form of myopia, complicated with amblyopia. It is easily recognised according to Airy's method. This accounts for the fact that this form, notwithstanding its rarity, was the first to be discovered. Eyes so affected see near comparatively better than distant objects; and by spherical negative glasses, which correct the myopia in the principal meridian of greatest curvature, the acuteness of vision of distant objects is, particularly in young persons, improved. Perfect acuteness of vision at a distance is, however, attainable only by means of negative spherico-cylindrical glasses, while for near objects, when, as occurred in most of the cases observed by me, the myopia is slight in the principal meridian of weakest curvature, simple negative cylindrical glasses are in general the best.

CASE II. *Compound myopic astigmatism.*—While these sheets are passing through the press, a case occurs to me, remarkable enough to justify its insertion here. Mrs. F., nearsighted from youth, and having in neither eye perfect acuteness of vision, complained some years ago, of occasionally recurring flickerings before the right eye, followed by a very transitory disturbance of vision. About six months since these flickerings returned, but on this occasion the disturbance of vision was permanent. At first there was a considerable scotoma, in which the yellow spot was included, while, moreover, the superior half of the field of vision in general appeared fainter. After numerous slight modifications in form, during the first weeks after it set in, a small, circumscribed scotoma finally remained, in part absolutely, in part relatively, insensible, with a defined boundary, projecting almost immediately above the point of direct vision; in the higher parts also of the field of vision a slight degree of torpor remained. The eye reads, however, but not without trouble, while the line above what is read is in great part invisible.

The ophthalmoscopic investigation is negative. Certainly nothing abnormal is to be seen in the portion of the retina corresponding to the scotoma (bordering inferiorly upon the yellow spot), and whether the smooth, glittering appearance of a part of the optic disc is to be considered as due to atrophy, is at least very doubtful.

The left eye gives M about $= \tfrac{1}{11}$, but at the same time possesses acuteness of vision of only $\frac{1}{3}$. Ophthalmoscopically, no abnormity was found. Suspecting astigmatism, I turned, while the eye was armed with $-\frac{1}{9}, \frac{1}{24} c$ round before the eye, and thereupon, the axis being horizontal, the acuteness of vision immediately rose to $\frac{2}{3}$, to descend, when it was perpendicular, below $\frac{1}{10}$. Trial with the point of light gave, with the addition of a weakly positive glass, an extension in breadth; with a negative glass of $-\frac{1}{7}$ or more, scarcely any extension in length. Much irregular astigmatism exists.

With the aid of the stenopæic slit I found:

$$\text{in v, M} = \tfrac{1}{14\cdot5};$$
$$\text{in h, M} = \tfrac{1}{9},$$

indicating an astigmatism of $(\frac{1}{9} - \frac{1}{14\cdot5})$ about $\frac{1}{24}$.

At a distance, horizontal strokes are seen better than vertical; with $\frac{1}{14}$ the horizontal are perfectly defined, and at the same time the vertical ones have become more distinct, attaining perfect distinctness, however, first with $-\frac{1}{9}$.

Without glasses No. I is recognised at the distance of about 5″. With $\frac{1}{24} c$, the axis being horizontal, whereby in all meridians $M = \frac{1}{9}$, No. I is read at 8″: the greater acuteness is very striking; the patient emphatically distinguishes between simple recognition and acute vision. The right eye is found to be affected by the same form, and by almost the same degree of As as the left.—For both eyes I prescribed,

(1.) $- \frac{1}{15} s \supset - \frac{1}{24} c$, as a double eye-glass for distant objects, whereby $R = \infty$,

(2.) $\frac{1}{24} c$, whereby R is brought to 9″,—very well adapted for seeing minute objects accurately, and

(3.) $- \frac{1}{20} s \supset - \frac{1}{24} c$, whereby R is brought to lie at $4\frac{1}{2}$ feet; these glasses, specially destined to look at the model, which is painted, might, at pleasure, be worn as spectacles.

I shall, moreover, have a glass ground, in which the cylindrical surface shall represent $- \frac{1}{24}$, and the spherical surface shall have two foci (verres à double foyer), acting, namely, in its upper part as $- \frac{1}{20}$, in its lower as $\frac{1}{\infty}$ or as $- \frac{1}{60}$. By this the astigmatism will be removed, and the farthest point, seen through the upper part of the glass, will be brought to $4\frac{1}{2}$ feet, through the inferior, to 15″ or 20″ respectively.

Remarks.—I have already (p. 60) stated, that in almost all the cases of abnormal astigmatism observed by me, without exception, the principal meridian of maximum of curvature approximated to the vertical position. In the case here described we find the confirmation of the rule: that there is no rule without an exception. Here, in fact, just as with Young, the maximum of curvature coincides nearly with the horizontal meridian, the minimum of curvature with the vertical. The patient had not been aware that she saw less acutely than other people. I therefore think it probable that Young also, whose astigmatism was of about the same degree, incorrectly ascribed perfect acuteness of vision to himself; and should many of his accurate observations be adduced as proofs of the contrary, I would state, on the other hand, that my patient drew and painted very respectably. This apparent enigma is easily solved. Myopic persons are accustomed, in order to see more acutely, to squeeze their eyelids close together : the narrow slit thus produced diminishes the circles of diffusion in the vertical dimension. If astigmatism coexist, a narrow slit has a doubly advantageous effect, as it allows only the rays to enter, which fall in meridians of nearly equal radius of curvature. Hence it follows that, while ordinary myopes, from narrowing the slit, derive advantage only in looking at remote objects, situated beyond the distance of distinct vision, astigmatics find their power of vision improved also for near objects. A very slender slit almost entirely removes the disturbance dependent on astigmatism, and the acuteness of vision would thereby become nearly perfect, if the disadvantages of diffraction and diminution of light did not intervene. My patient undoubtedly also made use of narrowing the slit, even in looking at near objects, and the question is whether Young did not also do so. Meanwhile she was loud in her commendation of the advantage obtained from a cylindrical glass: little pictures especially were with it seen much more acutely. And by holding a cylindrical glass before the eye, non-astigmatic persons can easily convince themselves, how rapidly the definition of a picture suffers from that defect.

Narrowing the slit between the eyelids, so universal in myopia, does not belong to astigmatism in general. Especially in hypermetropic astigmatism it is almost always absent. This would appear to have its explanation in the fact, that in this instance, in the horizontal meridian a high degree of hypermetropia exists, which, not being overcome by the accommodation, leaves great diffusion in this direction, and therefore affords no advantage. Could the eyelids admit of a vertical slit, hypermetropic astigmatics would undoubtedly have made use of it.

The scotoma which exists in the right eye of my patient, is in no way connected with the astigmatism.

Respecting the glasses prescribed, little remains to be said : only a word in reference to the glasses à double foyer. In old people, with acquired hypermetropia, I have often applied them with much advantage, for example, positive glasses of $\frac{1}{30}$ in the upper, of $\frac{1}{10}$ to $\frac{1}{8}$ in the lower part. Moreover, in painters, who in the upper part desired and also really needed $R = \infty$, in the lower part $= 24''$ to $12''$. My patient used $-\frac{1}{14}$, in order to see at a distance; and in painting, looked over her spectacles. At the same time narrowing the slit, she had her farthest point at only $9''$. This distance, in one sense too short, made good on the other hand the want of acuteness of vision. I thought, the habit once formed of painting at so short a distance, that the farthest point might be brought to not more than $15''$ or $20''$.—So far I had never yet combined a cylindrical surface with a spherical one, à double foyer. Such a combination cannot, however, in my opinion, produce any inconvenience.

2. *Hypermetropic astigmatism.*—Most cases of abnormal astigmatism belong to the hypermetropic form. In general experience has

shown, that in hypermetropic eyes, even when the astigmatism continues within the limits of the normal, the asymmetry is greater than in myopic and emmetropic eyes; and it is therefore not surprising that precisely those eyes are also most subject to abnormal, and indeed to the highest degrees of astigmatism. We shall certainly not be far from the truth in assuming, that of six hypermetropic eyes, one suffers from abnormal astigmatism, and that the imperfect acuteness of vision so often combined with hypermetropia is, in one-half of the cases, in a great measure attributable to astigmatism.

The majority of cases belong to *simple* hypermetropic astigmatism. While, namely, in the horizontal meridian the hypermetropia is considerable (from $\frac{1}{30}$ to $\frac{1}{8}$ and more), we find in the vertical if not emmetropia, at least such slight degrees of myopia or of hypermetropia, that the limits of simple hypermetropic astigmatism are not surpassed. However, I have also seen numerous cases of compound hypermetropic astigmatism, rising even to $H\frac{1}{7}$ in the principal meridian of strongest curvature with $H\frac{1}{5}$ in that of weakest.—In young persons hypermetropia in the meridian of maximum of curvature appears first on artificial paralysis of the accommodation.

As to the form of the eye, I would remind the reader, that in hypermetropic astigmatism the radius ρ_o of the cornea in the horizontal meridian is often unusually great. Moreover, we can, in extensive movements of the eye, often satisfy ourselves, that the visual axis is short, and that the vertical axis of the globe is less than the horizontal.

The function of the eye characterises the condition as H, with diminished acuteness of sight. With this a great degree of asthenopia is connected. For a short while large print can still be read, but soon fatigue, and sometimes even pain, occurs. One of the patients (with $Ah = \frac{1}{18}$) aged 26, recorded the following :—"My occupation is that of a clerk. The first effort to work was the most painful. Thereupon dazzling soon followed, obliging me to shut my eyes, and to keep them closed for some time. After that my work went on somewhat better, but I found it impossible to work all the forenoon; I was constantly obliged to leave off. At the end my eyes were painful, and I felt best when I walked for a considerable time in the open air, out of the sun. In the evening, by gaslight, my work went on at first pretty well, but soon red dazzling came on. I was then obliged every time to leave off, and with fatigued and painful eyes I returned home." He got $\frac{1}{18}c$ to work with and to wear. Thereupon he communicated to me :—" On using the spectacles I found, even on the first day, an incredible improvement (his acuteness of vision was, in fact brought from $\frac{2}{7}$ to $\frac{3}{4}$). Next day I experienced no painful affection, and I found it easy to work uninterruptedly the whole morning. I saw everything infinitely sharper. In the evening I experienced not the slightest inconvenience from the light.—In the open air, too, when I walk without the spectacles, I am free from pain. Spectacles which I had before tried (ordinary spherical glasses), had been of no use to me."

In hypermetropic astigmatism the vision of distant objects is improved by positive glasses, particularly in the compound form; but even when the accommodation is removed by a mydriatic, it appears to be impossible to determine with precision the degree of H. This circumstance in itself leads us to suspect astigmatism. Horizontal stripes are, moreover, seen at a distance more distinctly than vertical ones. Some have of themselves observed this; some even mention it unasked. In this respect we have here, therefore, precisely the opposite of what we observe in myopic astigmatism : in the latter, vertical lines alone are distinct at a distance. Especially in the simple forms Am and Ah, this contrast is strongly marked. By means of a spherical negative glass we can change Am into Ah; and by a positive, Ah into Am, the direction of distinctly seen stripes being at the same time inverted.

a. Simple hypermetropic astigmatism. — Of this I observed a case.

CASE III. Am *in the right, with* Ah *in the left eye.* — Mr. R. M., burgomaster at O., aged 38, could in earlier years, at intervals, read and write, though only with great exertion. Latterly this has become almost impossible to him. In vain he endeavoured by means of spectacles to remedy this state of things. Very strong light still avails him most. The left eye has, at a distance, acuteness of vision of $\frac{1}{3}$, the right of $\frac{1}{5}$. He expressly states that the left eye at a distance sees double, and that the lines of adjoining letters cover one another. I immediately suspected astigmatism. With $\frac{1}{18}c$, turned round before this eye, the acuteness of vision was, in the horizontal position of the axis, diminished to $\frac{1}{18}$, in the vertical it was brought to perfection $= 1$. The same glass produces no improvement whatever before the right eye: however the glass may be turned, everything at a distance remains indistinct. And yet it was with this eye he could read better. That in the left eye about $\frac{1}{16}$ Ah existed, was ascertained by the above experiment; what was deficient in the right eye was not yet evident. Strokes having been fixed at a distance, he stated that with the left eye he saw the horizontal ones distinctly; but he now at the same time discovered, that with the right eye he saw the vertical ones almost quite acutely, while, on the contrary, he could distinguish little or nothing of the horizontal. I now perceived that in the right eye Am must exist, and with $-\frac{1}{16}c$, the axis being held horizontally, he saw with this eye at a distance almost quite acutely. Hence it followed at the same time, that with $\frac{1}{16}c$, in a vertical position of the axis, he should read admirably, and, in fact, with it No. I was seen at the distance of a foot: the acuteness of vision was perfect. He now stated to me, that objects appeared smaller to the unaided left eye than to the right, and on strict inspection it was not to be mistaken, that the left eye was less prominent.

Thus, by an unusual mode, I had immediately ascertained, tolerably clearly, the condition of both eyes. The systematic investigation, was, however, not neglected. The right eye saw the point of light as a vertical, the left saw it as a horizontal stroke; by $-\frac{1}{16}$ the first was changed into a horizontal, by $\frac{1}{16}$ the second was changed into a vertical stroke: the principal meridians did not perceptibly deviate from the horizontal and vertical planes. Through a slit $1\frac{3}{4}$ mm. wide, held in a vertical direction, the left eye had, at a distance, $S = \frac{1}{3}$, with glasses of $\frac{1}{80}$ something still to be improved; the right only $\frac{1}{3}$, with $-\frac{1}{18}$ rising to $\frac{2}{3}$. Near at hand, on the contrary, the right eye read very easily through the slit held vertically, the left, under similar circumstances, read with difficulty. Through a horizontal slit the right eye had, at a distance, acuteness of vision of $\frac{2}{3}$, which was not to be improved by glasses; while the left eye saw at a distance very imperfectly, and required glasses of from $\frac{1}{18}$ to $\frac{1}{13}$. That through the horizontal slit the left eye can scarcely read at all, the right eye only imperfectly, is in accordance with all the foregoing.

From the above experiments we now deduced:

Right eye, in v, M $= \frac{1}{18}$;

in H, E;

Left eye, in v, H $= \frac{1}{80}$;

in H, H $= \frac{1}{14}$.

In the right eye there was therefore Am $_{.18}$ without complication. In the left, properly Ah $= \frac{1}{14} - \frac{1}{80} = \frac{1}{17}$.

With $\frac{1}{17}c$ on the left, and $-\frac{1}{18}c$ on the right, there was good vision at a distance, and spectacles furnished with these glasses were worn with much satisfaction. The same spectacles were quite insufficient for reading. It appeared that there was only slight accommodation. Consequently it was thought necessary, for near work, to bring the farthest point R to from 18 to 20''. This was accomplished by placing before the right eye a simple cylindrical glass of $\frac{1}{18}c$, before the left a spherico-cylindrical,

$$\frac{1}{20}s \supset \frac{1}{18}c.$$

Remarks.—The above case serves to show how astigmatism may sometimes be discovered by a more direct method than the systematic investigation. Examination with the ophthalmoscope might also have led directly to the same result: on relaxation of accommodation I saw in the left eye only the horizontal, in the right only the vertical vessels well-defined. However, to save time, it is better for those who have not examined many astigmatic patients, to keep to the rules laid down. But in cases where perfect emmetropia exists in one of the meridians, we may attain our object more quickly by the trial with cylindrical glasses; such cases are, however, exceptional.

On a subsequent visit of this patient, I caused him to look through dark violet glasses, towards a square illuminated opening (compare p. 473). What I expected, took place: with the right eye he saw the upper margins blue, with the left the outer margins red; and on holding before his eyes glasses of $- \frac{1}{30}$, the upper margins appeared to the right eye blue, the outer margins red, while for the left eye both were reversed.

It was above remarked, that objects appeared smaller to the left eye than to the right. This does not depend upon astigmatism. Astigmatism caused the vertical dimensions of objects to appear greater in both eyes (compare p. 471), and this, too, was actually the case. On the other hand, that objects were apparently greater to the right eye than to the left, was the result of the longer visual axis in the first eye. In both the cornea had the same form, most probably the same was true of the lens, and the only difference between the two eyes would therefore be the difference in the length of the visual axis. Now where this difference exists, the second nodal point lies in the right eye farther from the retina than in the left, and the retinal images are therefore greater in the first. If no extension of the retina be combined therewith (atrophy of the membranes was not seen with the ophthalmoscope), the greater retinal image is also projected greater.

By this the difference in magnitude, exhibited by the objects in the two eyes, is explained. On correction with glasses, the magnitude of the objects is altered: with positive glasses the nodal point moves forward, with negative, backward. Nearly always we shall find, that where the eyes are unequal, the placing of R at an equal distance for both, produces an inversion in the magnitude of the images: the eye, which required the strongest negative or the weakest positive glasses, now sees objects smallest. If the difference be great, it may cause disturbance, and the latter must often be avoided at the sacrifice of distinctness of vision in one eye. By placing the glasses very close before the eye, and by correct calculation of the curvature of the surfaces of the glasses, whereby their nodal points, at a similar focal distance, acquire another position, we can partly counteract this defect.

In the case under consideration, the difference in magnitude of the objects before both eyes was nearly corrected by the cylindrical glasses, provided they were held close in front of the eye. At least no inconvenience proceeded from it. Only when the glasses were not close to the cornea, did the difference in magnitude of the images become rather confusing. The cause is to be sought in the fact, that the hypermetropia of the left eye was not completely corrected by the glasses, and on this side, with the glasses intended for reading, the farthest point continued more remote from the eye. Certainly a slight degree of latent hypermetropia was also present, and, moreover, I gave $\frac{1}{20} s$ in place of $\frac{1}{18} s$. In reading, the left eye saw less acutely with the glasses than the right.

b. Compound hypermetropic astigmatism has, with a high degree of hypermetropia in the horizontal meridian, usually a relatively slight degree of it in the vertical. In the latter I have rarely found the hypermetropia greater than $\frac{1}{22}$; several times about $\frac{1}{28}$, while in the horizontal meridian the hypermetropia may amount to $\frac{1}{5}$ and more. It thus appears that the compound hypermetropic astigmatism often keeps very close to the simple.

It is remarkable, that in general the disturbance of vision was less than should have been expected from the degree of the astigmatism. Usually we find the disturbance of vision not proportionate to the degree of the astigmatism: the size of the pupil, its position in reference to the axis of the cornea, its constriction in accommodation, the form, too, of the curvature in the different meridians, the complication, finally, with irregular astigmatism, exercise, all combined, a great influence.

CASE IV. *Compound hypermetropic astigmatism.*—Mr. R., aged 18 years, has never seen acutely; he states that he observes a shadow along the margins of objects; at his work he has always sought for strong light, and has nevertheless soon perceived symptoms of asthenopia. Notwithstanding this, he has applied himself pretty closely to study. Some years ago he had consulted an oculist, who had referred the disturbance to congenital amblyopia, and had therefore considered it to be incurable. This opinion found the more acceptance, as his brother (with a normal condition of the right eye) had in the left a disturbance, corresponding to that in the two eyes of our patient. In his parents, and the other children, the acuteness of vision is satisfactory in both eyes.

Having been attacked by a slight conjunctivitis, the patient called upon me. This soon gave way; but it appeared that the acuteness of vision of the left eye was only $\frac{2}{7}$; of the right, for near objects, it was $\frac{2}{3}$, for distant, $\frac{1}{3}$. Ophthalmoscopic examination showed, in the first place, that the optic discs were as red as the fundus oculi in general, — which capillary hyperæmia, in consequence of great strain, with the head in a stooping position, is frequently developed, especially in young people. But at the same time I observed that, while the horizontal retinal vessels, in slight tension of accommodation, were easily seen, the vertical exhibited themselves most distinctly with a lens of $\frac{1}{8}$. This held good for both eyes. Consequently there was no doubt of the existence of astigmatism. On being asked whether he saw horizontal and vertical stripes at a distance equally well, the patient immediately answered, that he had formerly remarked, that he could distinguish the vertical lines on a target accurately, only when he inclined his head quite horizontally.

The radii of curvature of the two corneæ were measured, in the first place, in the horizontal plane (H), exactly in the visual line ρ°, 10° to the nasal side $\rho n'$, 20° to the nasal side $\rho n''$, 10° and 20° to the temporal side, $\rho t'$ and $\rho t''$; and in like manner in the vertical plane (V), first in the visual line ρ°, and subsequently 10° and 20° upwards $\rho s'$, $\rho s''$, and 10° and 20° downwards $\rho i'$ and $\rho i''$. In each place the mean of six observations was taken. The calculated results are as follow:

	In II		In V
Right eye, $\rho n''$ =	9·80	$\rho i''$ =	8·04
$\rho n'$ =	8·76	$\rho i'$ =	7·47
ρ° =	8·32	ρ° =	7·30
$\rho t'$ =	8·24	$\rho s'$ =	7·08
$\rho t''$ =	8·61	$\rho s''$ =	7·82
Left eye, $\rho n''$ =	10·38	$\rho i''$ =	7·59
$\rho n'$ =	8·58	$\rho i'$ =	7·43
ρ° =	8·38	ρ° =	7·38
$\rho t'$ =	8·30	$\rho s'$ =	7·21
$\rho t''$ =	8·57	$\rho s''$ =	7·55

Hence it appears in the first place, that the cornea exhibits a high degree of astigmatism (the difference of the radii of curvature in the visual line gives for the right eye, As = 1 : 6·374, for the left eye, As = 1 : 6·8); secondly, that the eccentricity of the vertical elliptical section, especially in the left eye, is very slight; thirdly, that the form of the curvature deviates considerably from the ellipse; fourthly, that the visual line cuts the cornea in a point, which is situated very much to the inside of, and at the same time very much beneath, the apex of the cornea.

In the right eye, the accommodation was paralysed by sulphate of atropia. Thereupon the acuteness of vision diminished considerably, and improved comparatively little by positive glasses = $\frac{1}{16}$ to $\frac{1}{7}$. The diffusion-images of a point of light showed, that the vertical principal meridian inclined about seven degrees outwards, the horizontal an equal number of degrees outwards and downwards. With $\frac{1}{28}$ to $\frac{1}{24}$ the most slender horizontal line was seen, from which, however, numerous accessory lines proceeded; with $\frac{1}{12}$ the diffusion-image was a horizontal rhomb **<>**, with $\frac{1}{7}$ it was a vertical rhomb, with $\frac{1}{9}$ it was a very irregular square figure, bent in at both sides, which, with $\frac{1}{5}$ changed into a vertical line, thickened in the centre and with ramified extremities, and was slightest with $\frac{1}{5}$, held at $\frac{1}{2}''$ from the eye. Evidently, therefore, there was much irregular astigmatism; the regular appeared to amount to $\frac{1}{4\cdot5} - \frac{1}{28} = 1 : 5\cdot36$. However, we found on examination with the ophthalmoscope, and on trying the cylindrical glasses, a slighter degree, namely about $\frac{1}{7}$. Manifestly no accurate result was to be obtained with the linear diffusion-images. The application of the method of determining the refractive condition in the two principal meridians, with the aid of a slit, I had not yet learned. Moreover, I still possessed only one cylindrical glass, and that of $\frac{1}{8}$. This glass, held at most $1''$ from the eye, improved the sharpness of vision from $\frac{2}{7}$ to $\frac{2}{3}$. The question is, whether with ample choice of glasses no greater acuteness of vision would have been attainable. Probably, in order wholly to exclude asthenopia, this eye would, for proximity, require a spherico-cylindrical glass, while provisionally, a simple cylindrical glass is sufficient for distance: for in the range of accommodation of youth, the then remaining total hypermetropia of $\frac{1}{28}$ is easily enough overcome.

Of the left eye it is noted only, that it likewise is hypermetropic in the two principal meridians, that the acuteness of vision at a distance amounts to $\frac{2}{9}$, with $\frac{1}{24}$ increases to $\frac{2}{7}$, moreover, that glasses of $\frac{1}{8}c$ produce a considerable improvement.

On other phenomena I think it unnecessary to dwell. From what has preceded we are in a position to predict them without fear of being put to shame by the result. A recapitulation and analysis would be only repetition. I prefer recording some points from

CASE v.—relating to the brother of the above patient, Mr. R., Jr.

In the first place, as to the radii of curvature of the two corneæ, we found :—

	In H		In V	
Right eye,	$\rho n'' = 9\cdot10$		$\rho i'' = 8\cdot42$	
	$\rho n' = 8\cdot38$		$\rho i' = 8\cdot10$	
	$\rho^\circ = 8\cdot11$		$\rho^\circ = 8\cdot10$	
	$\rho t' = 8\,10$		$\rho s' = 8\cdot27$	
	$\rho t'' = 8\cdot10$		$\rho s'' = 8\cdot04$	
Left eye,	$\rho n'' = 9\cdot74$		$\rho i''' = 8\cdot06$	
	$\rho n' = 8\cdot78$		$\rho i' = 7\cdot98$	
	$\rho^\circ = 8\cdot44$		$\rho^\circ = 7\cdot69$	
	$\rho t' = 8\cdot61$		$\rho s' = 7\cdot85$	
	$\rho t'' = 8\cdot77$		$\rho s'' = 7\cdot63$	

A glance at these numbers shows, that the left cornea has a much smaller radius of curvature in the centre of the vertical section, than in the centre of the horizontal section, while for the right cornea the radii of curvature are equal in both directions. In accordance herewith, the acuteness of vision in the right eye is perfect, and for the left amounts to only $\frac{1}{10}$, and at the same time the large letters of the same line which are still recognised do not appear to stand regularly in a straight line. Further, the curvature of the cornea is in both eyes very irregular: in the first place the radius 20° above the visual line is still shorter than in that line—an anomaly which I had never before met with, either in sound or in astigmatic eyes, and, secondly, in the horizontal meridian of the right eye, the radius of curvature towards the temporal side appears to remain unaltered throughout a great extent. It is evident, that from the ascertained value, therefore, no ellipses are to be calculated. Further, it deserves attention, that the form of the astigmatism of the left eye quite agrees with that observed in both eyes of the patient's brother. An hypermetropic astigmatism, probably with hypermetropia in both meridians, prevails in this instance. If without glasses a point of light be seen as the most slender horizontal stroke, and with $\frac{1}{8}$ as the most slender vertical stroke, it is to be expected that with artificial mydriasis a weakly positive glass should be required to see the most slender horizontal stroke, and a glass stronger than $\frac{1}{8}$ to see the most slender vertical stroke. The direction, too, of the principal meridians, nay, even the peculiar form of the diffusion-images agrees in both cases, so that neither did the irregular astigmatism present any remarkable difference.

The nearest points at which vertical and horizontal wires were acutely seen, were determined comparatively for the right and left eye of this person : these distances lay, for the right eye, respectively at $9\frac{1}{3}''$ and $6\frac{1}{8}''$, with glasses of $\frac{1}{8}$ at $3\frac{5}{8}''$ and $3\frac{1}{12}''$; for the left eye, with glasses of $\frac{1}{5}$ at 8 and at $3\frac{1}{4}$ inches. The accuracy with which these distances were obtained, left nothing to be desired; but evidently the difference of asymmetry was also reflected in these numbers, and it even appears from them, that in the vertical meridian the two eyes did not differ much from one another. That the right eye, even in the vertical meridian, has some latent hypermetropia, is, with the great distance of the nearest point of distinct vision, scarcely to be doubted.

With a cylindrical glass of $\frac{1}{12}c$ the disturbance of vision of the left eye was almost entirely corrected, and *vice versâ*, a glass of $-\frac{1}{11}c$ (with opposite direction of the axis) produced a condition in the right eye, nearly agreeing with that of the left. The experiments tried in this respect were remarkable. In particular, in alternate production and correction of the astigmatism in each of the two eyes the difference in form of the objects and in distinctness of the strokes of different direction, were as satisfactory to us as they were surprising to the patient. What has been above said respecting the apparent magnitude of the different dimensions of a square, before and after the crroection of the astigmatism, was in this instance also fully confirmed.

I had recently an opportunity of again examining Mr. R., and noted the following:

In the perpendicular image the emmetropic individual sees, with relaxation of his accommodation, the horizontal retinal vessels of the left eye;

with strong tension, or with glasses of $\frac{1}{10}$, he sees the vertical. The optic disc, seen in the inverted image, is extended in breadth, which is particularly striking on comparison with the optic disc of the right eye.

Examination with the stenopæic slit gives for the vertical meridian H $= \frac{1}{40}$, for the horizontal H $= \frac{1}{10}$. With the vertical slit, the acuteness of vision rises at a distance from $\frac{1}{10}$ to $\frac{1}{3}$, and a remote point of light is with it seen as a point. The horizontal slit produces, as such, no improvement, but, with the addition of $\frac{1}{10}$, it causes the acuteness of vision to rise to $\frac{1}{4}$.—The patient prefers holding the slit at from 1″ to 1½″ from the eye. —With $\frac{1}{40}$ s $\subset$ $\frac{1}{18}$ c the acuteness of vision becomes about $\frac{3}{8}$, with $\frac{1}{12}$ c it becomes about $\frac{1}{10}$.

3. *Mixed Astigmatism.*—Amh and Ahm. We have remarked, that most cases of myopic, and especially of hypermetropic, astigmatism, differ little from the simple; the same may be predicated of the mixed, whether we find a high degree of H in the horizontal principal meridian, combined with a slight degree of M in the vertical, or a high degree of M in the latter, with slight hypermetropia in the horizontal. The occurrence of nearly equal degrees of the two forms of ametropia in the opposite principal meridians is an exception. To this the subjoined case most nearly approaches, in which, however, the degree of asymmetry was not considerable.

CASE VI.—*Amh in the left eye.*—Mr. V., aged 59 years, has in the right eye S $= \frac{1}{2}$, in the left S $= \frac{1}{12}$. The *right* eye is nearly emmetropic: improvement of vision at a distance by $\frac{1}{60}$ is doubtful; — $\frac{1}{60}$ acts injuriously. Experiments with the point of light afford no proof of abnormal regular astigmatism, but indicate a highly-developed irregular astigmatism.

From youth, the patient has been unable to use his *left* eye; however, there exists neither obscurity nor organic change in the fundus oculi. Positive and negative spherical glasses produce no improvement. The reflected images of the cornea had suggested the idea of asymmetry. Examination with the ophthalmoscope afforded the proof of it: in the non-inverted image I, as an emmetrope, saw, with some tension of my accommodation, vertical vessels of the retina perfectly acutely; horizontal vessels, on the contrary, appeared, on tension of accommodation, very faint, and on perfect relaxation were not well defined. I hence inferred the existence of myopia in the vertical, and of hypermetropia in the horizontal meridian. On examination with the point of light the principal meridians seemed to deviate little from the vertical and horizontal planes; the most slender vertical line was seen with $\frac{1}{45}$, the most slender horizontal with $- \frac{1}{30}$. The diagnosis was: mixed astigmatism $= \frac{1}{18}$, composed of

$$M \frac{1}{30} + H \frac{1}{45}.$$

The cornea more than fully accounted for this: the radius of curvature in

34

the visual line amounted, in the horizontal plane, to 8·29 mm., in the vertical = 7·69,—indicating an astigmatism of 1 : 11·67. While (at least by the method with the point of light) only Amh $\frac{1}{18}$ was found, the crystalline lens appeared to compensate in part for the astigmatism of the cornea.

Quite in accordance with the ametropia in both principal meridians, the left eye sees at a distance vertical lines a little better than horizontal. With $\frac{1}{45}$ horizontal lines are still more indistinctly visible, while vertical lines are acutely seen. *Vice versâ*, with — $\frac{1}{30}$ horizontal lines are very well seen, vertical lines, on the contrary, are only faintly perceptible. The astigmatic lens of Stokes, brought to the action of $2 \times \frac{1}{32} = \frac{1}{16}$, makes the acuteness of vision at once four times greater, by bringing it from $\frac{1}{10}$ to $\frac{2}{3}$. With $\frac{1}{18} c$, combined with — $\frac{1}{30} s$, it rose above $\frac{1}{2}$, and was therefore still better than in the right eye.

For distance a flat glass was prescribed for the right eye ; for the left a bi-cylindrical glass of $\frac{1}{45} c \sqcap — \frac{1}{30} c$. For close work, I was anxious, the acuteness of vision not being perfect, to bring R to 12″. This was effected by means of a spherico-cylindrical glass of $\frac{1}{20} s \subset \frac{1}{18} c$: with $\frac{1}{20}$, in fact, R in the vertical meridian $(\frac{1}{30} + \frac{1}{20} = \frac{1}{12})$ becomes = 12″, and with $\frac{1}{18} c$ R in the horizontal is made equal to R in the vertical. Hereby the right eye now acquired simply $\frac{1}{12} s$. The images were of nearly equal magnitude, and the vision was with both eyes at the same time very pleasant. Vision with the left eye was more acute than with the right.

Remarks.—This case was, notwithstanding the slight degree of H in the horizontal meridian, referred to mixed astigmatism. I felt justified in this because, with the very slight range of accommodation belonging to the patient's time of life, the hypermetropia could by no means be overcome. The latter must, therefore, necessarily be corrected, and this would have been serviceable also even in a young person, although the latter should, with — $\frac{1}{18} c$, have seen acutely at a distance, and even in reading should have experienced but little inconvenience.

The acuteness of vision of the left eye was, in comparison with the degree of astigmatism, very imperfect. One might have been inclined to connect the important disturbance with the singular circumstance, that the ascertained degree of astigmatism was the resultant of a double asymmetry, namely, of a greater asymmetry of the cornea, and of an opposite and slighter asymmetry of the crystalline lens ; but, were this supposition correct we could not, in my opinion, have expected the considerable improvement from cylindrical lenses, which we have indicated. Raising the acuteness of vision from $\frac{1}{10}$ to above $\frac{1}{2}$ may be considered extraordinary.

The diminished acuteness of vision of the right eye also appears to me somewhat enigmatical. It is indeed true that at 59 years of age it is only exceptionally still perfect ; but it is equally rare to find it fallen to $\frac{1}{2}$, without any perceptible anatomical change. Moreover, it is the rule, that, in astigmatism of the one eye, notwithstanding the most perfect correction, the acuteness of vision of the astigmatic eye continues inferior to that of the other. In this instance the opposite was found. I am therefore strongly inclined to assume, that in the right eye also astigmatism was present in a degree which interfered with the acuteness of vision. No accurate investigation was made on this point; nor were the radii of curvature of the cornea measured.

The spectacles intended for seeing at a distance could afford the patient no great advantage, commensurate with the trouble of wearing them; but neither was there any objection to allow their use, if desired. Spectacles for near objects were much more important. Leaving out of consideration even the advantage of stereoscopic vision, reading with two eyes is much pleasanter, and, if the acuteness of vision of both eyes is imperfect (provided there be no obscuration), also much easier than with one eye: the acuteness of vision is even perceptibly increased by it. In order to distinguish small objects, still stronger spectacles might be allowed: in that case, in the combination of the spherico-cylindrical glass, $\frac{1}{18}$ c remains constant and $\frac{1}{20}$ s needs only to be increased.

B. We have seen that when the cornea, by itself, produces an abnormal degree of congenital astigmatism, the lens may increase, but commonly diminishes the same. In the latter case, the astigmatism of the cornea continues to predominate; in the former the action of the lens is weaker, and is therefore to be considered only as accessory. But in a few cases it occurs, on the other hand, that the existing abnormal degree of astigmatism may be said to be dependent on the crystalline lens; and a very remarkable case of this nature is described by Dr. Knapp,* in which the peculiar form of the crystalline lens was the cause of an astigmatism, in great part regular. Less rarely, an abnormal position is the cause. This condition may, in the first place, be congenital. Numerous cases have been known in which the lens was situated so eccentrically, that the equator passed through the plane of the pupil, and thus a portion of the plane of the pupil remained without a lens. In this case, then, astigmatism exists in a manner to produce great disturbance, but it is of an irregular nature, and cylindrical glasses are incapable, in this instance, of producing any improvement (see Irregular Astigmatism, in § 40). Some cases, however, occur, where the displacement of the crystalline lens is so slight that the latter still occupies the whole plane of the pupil, but at the same time has so oblique a position, as to give rise to a considerable degree of tolerably regular astigmatism. Some years ago, before I was in the habit of investigating the disturbance of function in asymmetry with the requisite accuracy, a case of this nature occurred to me. I shall here merely communicate what was noted at the time.

* *Archiv f. Ophthalmologie*, B. viii. Abth. 2, p. 229.

2

CASE VII.—*Astigmatism, from congenital eccentricity of the crystalline lens.*—Jacob D., aged 20, called on me on the 24th of April, 1860: he had myopia $= \frac{1}{4}$ in both eyes, S $= \frac{1}{2}$ in the left, S $= \frac{1}{4}$ in the right eye. By holding the negative glass obliquely before the right eye, the acuteness of vision could be brought nearly to $\frac{1}{2}$. Long visual axis; on the whole large eyes. In neither, however, was there atrophy of the chorioidea, but in the left was a white irregularly circumscribed spot, narrower than the optic disc, beneath which it was, and concealing the vessels of the retina. The chambers of the eyes were shallow; at the same time there was a very marked iridodenosis, particularly at the inferior portion of the iris; there was good reflecting, but little accommodating, movement of the pupils. The total range of accommodation of the left eye was $\frac{1}{8\frac{2}{3}}$; nevertheless, when the myopia was neutralised by $\frac{1}{3\frac{1}{2}}$, placed at $\frac{1}{2}''$ from the nodal point, the nearest point in the left eye lay, R being $= \infty$, at $17''$.

Through the action of sulphate of atropia, the pupils acquire an apparent diameter of $8\frac{1}{4}$ mm. The iridodenosis at the same time continues. Now it appears, that a certain space exists between the iris (displaced, it is true, very much forwards) and the crystalline lens, and at the same time that this last lies eccentrically. On examination with the ophthalmoscope, we see on the outside, a narrow, scythe-shaped red margin around the equator of the crystalline lens; this bright margin becomes broader when we look a little from within outwards into the eye, but if we pass still more inwards, it rapidly becomes again narrower, and in the right eye even altogether disappears. Evidently, therefore, the outer margin of the lens displaced inwards and upwards lies more forward than the upper and inner margin, particularly in the right eye. The reflected image of the anterior surface of the lens is faint in both eyes, difficult to see, situated very near the reflected image of the cornea, and on movement of the flame moving more than the last. The reflected image formed by the posterior surface of the crystalline lens stands at a tolerably great distance, and considerably higher than the corneal image. With the phacoidoscope* (conf. the method in *Nederl. Lancet*, 3rd Series, Part III., p. 242), looking from the outer side into the left eye under an angle of 30° with the visual line, while the flame stood in the line, which on the other side made an angle of 30° with the visual line, the distance between the reflected corneal image and the posterior lenticular image amounted to $3\frac{1}{4}$ mm., and the line uniting these images made an angle of 35° with the horizontal plane, in which the visual line, the flame, and the eye of the observer were.

On examination with the ophthalmoscope in the inverted image the vessels exhibit in and near the optic disc, with the ordinary movements of the objective lens, in the left eye scarcely any, in the right eye a very considerable parallactic movement (the direction of which, in connexion with the movement of the lens, is not noted).

The corneæ, measured in a plane, carried horizontally through the

---

* The author's instrument for measuring the change of shape of the lens in accommodation (see p. 16).—TRANSLATOR.

visual line, gave, as ρ°, in the visual line, as $\rho n'$ and $\rho n''$, 11° 23'' and 22° 46' on the nasal side, and as $\rho t'$ and $\rho t''$, 11° 23' and 22° 46' on the temporal side of the visual line, the following results (each number being the mean of four measurements) :

Right eye.	Left eye.
$\rho n'' = 8\cdot70$	8·87
$\rho n' = 8\cdot16$	8·16
$\rho^\circ = 8\cdot14$	8·10
$\rho t' = 8\cdot21$	8·17
$\rho t'' = 8\cdot61$	8·50.

Hence it appears, that the corneæ have a great radius, that the ellipsoidal curvature in the horizontal plane is very regular, and has a slight eccentricity, and finally, that the axis of the cornea and the visual line nearly coincide.

Remarks.—I wish only to establish more fully, that the crystalline lens, particularly in the right eye, had an oblique position, causing its axis to deviate very much from that of the cornea, and that at the same time a diminished acuteness of vision existed, admitting of improvement by means of an oblique position of the negative lens of $-\dfrac{1}{3\frac{1}{2}}$, whereby the myopia was corrected. Astigmatism therefore existed. And although we must regret, that neither the direction, nor the degree of the requisite inclination of the axis of the negative lens were noted, and that therefore the direction and degree of the existent astigmatism thereby corrected are unknown, and although we should, moreover, have been glad to know the curvature of the cornea in the vertical plane, in order to exclude the cornea as a cause of the astigmatism, I nevertheless feel justified in ascribing the observed astigmatism to the oblique position of the crystalline lens. The existence of this category of astigmatism is thus proved, and this may for the present suffice.—The different results of measurement, which I have communicated, may subsequently, when it shall be thought desirable for the comparison of more of such cases with one another, be employed in calculation.

It also deserves mention, that three elder brothers and one sister of the patient have normal eyes, but that a younger brother, and perhaps also the mother, suffer from the same defect.

II.—ACQUIRED REGULAR ASTIGMATISM.

A. *Depending on the Cornea.*—In all the foregoing, acquired astigmatism has scarcely been mentioned. I must acknowledge that, until a short time ago, I thought it of little importance. Very seldom does it depend on an oblique position of the crystalline lens caused by partial luxation ; and if disturbances of the cornea be its cause, irregular astigmatism is almost without exception to be expected. I therefore supposed, *à priori*, that cylindrical glasses would in this case but little or not at all remedy the disturbance of vision. The result has, however, in many instances proved the contrary. In a case of a central speck upon the cornea, I performed iridectomy, and obtained a well-formed pupil, only in the centre admitting some diffuse, but otherwise regularly refracted, light through the cornea. Nevertheless, the acuteness of vision was very imperfect : while the eye had $\frac{1}{30}$ hypermetropia, No. VI could not even with glasses of $\frac{1}{10}$, be read. The letters had a strange form; in an oblique direction they exhibited an irregular prolongation. On ophthalmoscopic investigation, the movement of the objective lens appeared to produce a considerable parallax. I tried the combination of a convex with a cylindrical glass, and the acuteness of vision was nearly doubled. Ordinary print could now be read.—The matter is, *à posteriori*, evident enough. The existing astigmatism may be resolved into a regular and irregular astigmatism, and after correction of the regular, the irregular causes less disturbance. *I have found that in many cases in which, on account of opacity of the cornea, iridectomy, or iriddesis is performed, great advantage may be obtained by a cylindrical glass.* Let it be tried only, whether a cylindrical glass of, for example, $\frac{1}{30}$ c, turned round before the eye, will not produce alternately increased and diminished acuteness of vision; and when the required direction is thus ascertained, it remains only to find out in these cases, to what strength of cylindrical glasses the preference is given. By the more indirect methods above described, this object is, in general, less easily attained. *After the extraction of cataract, too, the cornea often acquires a form, which gives great value to the combination with a cylindrical glass.*

Cylindrical glasses are also often very useful in acquired modifications in the form of the cornea, without the necessity of performing any operation upon the iris.

CASE VII.—M. Kr., a girl aged 14, has, some years ago, lost the left eye, in consequence of perforating ulcers of the cornea, with subsequent atrophy. On the lower and inner part of the right eye, too, remains a cicatrix from destruction of tissue and prolapse of the iris. The pupil is thereby drawn downwards and inwards, but it is otherwise unaltered, and only little diffused light enters the eye. Nevertheless, the acuteness of vision leaves much to be desired, and is scarcely improved by the total cutting off of the diffused light. Moreover, there exists a tolerably great degree of myopia, with which, therefore, amblyopia seems to be combined. Supposing that the form of the cornea might be the cause of the diminished acuteness of vision, I made an examination, and found, in fact, that a point of light was seen with — $\frac{1}{3}$ as an obliquely vertical, with — $\frac{1}{8}$, removed somewhat further from the eye, as an obliquely horizontal line. By the use of the slit, held in one of the two directions, the acuteness of vision was very considerably improved. With — $\frac{1}{30}$ c minute work could now be performed close to the eye, which without cylindrical glasses was altogether impossible.

I shall communicate, somewhat more in detail, a case which is certainly an extremely rare one.

CASE VIII.—*Acquired regular astigmatism of the cornea.*—J. F., brigadier in the army, aged 31, complains that for the last two years his sight has become worse and worse. Perfect acuteness of vision he never had. The corneæ exhibit, particularly on focal illumination, a slight general opacity, stated to have remained as the result of purulent inflammation which set in three days after birth. In the right eye, moreover, the boundary between the cornea and the sclerotic is, in consequence of peripheral spots, not to be determined; in the centre of the anterior surface of the lens there is also a small, sharply-defined, not elevated white speck. Neither had formerly prevented his entering the service. Now, however, the acuteness of vision had fallen in the right eye to $\frac{1}{10}$, in the left to $\frac{1}{3}$, and the patient was no longer in a condition properly to discharge his duties.

The existing opacity of the cornea did not fully explain the disturbance of vision. Moreover, without any fresh inflammatory attack, the power of vision had become more and more disturbed. It appeared to me that the curvature of the corneæ was abnormal,—a supposition which was fully confirmed by ophthalmometric investigation. The results of the latter were as follow:—

	In H.	In V.
Right eye,	$\rho n'' = 9{\cdot}64$	$\rho i'' = 9{\cdot}69$
	$\rho^\circ = 8{\cdot}72$	$\rho^\circ = 7{\cdot}13$
	$\rho t'' = 7{\cdot}77$	$\rho s'' = 7{\cdot}38$
Left eye,	$\rho n'' = 10{\cdot}97$	$\rho i'' = 7{\cdot}59$
	$\rho^\circ = 8{\cdot}40$	$\rho^\circ = 7{\cdot}25$
	$\rho t'' = 8{\cdot}45$	$\rho s'' = 7{\cdot}17$

Evidently the radius of curvature is much longer in the horizontal plane than in the vertical. Therefore, although in the form of the curvature much irregularity was observable, and the experiment with the point of light afforded no result, improvement was in this instance to be expected from cylindrical glasses: and in fact with a glass of $\frac{1}{8}$ c, the only one which I had at the time at my disposal, the acuteness of vision was raised to $\frac{1}{4}$. With a more extensive choice of glasses still further improvement would doubtless have been obtained.

I regret that an opportunity did not later present itself of examining the patient more particularly by different methods.

Remarks.—The cause of the abnormal curvature of the cornea existing in this case was not very clearly ascertained. We may, however, with tolerable probability assume, that the ophthalmia neonatorum had left behind it some change of form, and that this, combined with unequal resistance, whether in consequence of modified intra-ocular pressure, or under the influence of attendant, almost imperceptible, changes of nutrition, had gradually increased. Manifestly the curvature was very irregular. In both eyes the curvature was particularly great in the horizontal plane towards the temporal side, and in the vertical plane at the upper portion, in part it was still greater at 20° from the visual line than in the line of vision itself, although the latter, as direct determination showed, deviated in the horizontal plane only $3\frac{1}{2}$° from the centre. But, notwithstanding this irregularity, the great difference of curvature for the vertical and horizontal meridian was most striking ; and therefore also much advantage was to be expected from cylindrical glasses.

In connexion with this subject, it is remarkable that the cornea, if it originally possessed an average curvature, had both in the horizontal meridian acquired a longer, and in the vertical a shorter radius.

I have said that the case is rare. Usually, in fact, in *acquired* alterations of form of the cornea, whether on account of conical curvature, or of absolute irregularity or inequality of the surface, examination with the ophthalmometer is unattended with any satisfactory result, and it can only empirically be determined, whether cylindrical glasses are of any use or not.

B. *Acquired regular astigmatism, seated in the lens.*—Either the acquired or the congenital displacement of the lens (of which I have spoken at p. 531) may be the cause of regular astigmatism. Often the lens is thereby so much displaced, that it no longer corresponds to the entire plane of the pupil, with which a high degree of irregular astigmatiºm is then combined. But if the lens assumes an oblique direction in the plane of the pupil, regular astigmatism must be the consequence, and the use of cylindrical glasses will then produce improvement. A not unimportant example of this is afforded by—

CASE IX.—J. S., aged 42 was, four years ago, successfully operated on for cataract in the left eye. Rather more than a year later, he received a blow in the right eye from a bent branch. Up to this time he had had acute vision at a distance with this eye. Now everything appeared to him misty. On examination, I found iridodenosis in a high degree, quivering movements of the lens (established on every strong movement, both in the reflected images and in the lens itself, by lateral focal illumination), and, moreover, a slight degree of myopia. When a glass of $-\frac{1}{36}$ was held before the eye, the patient declared that he saw as well as formerly. I could not satisfy myself as to the existence of an oblique position of the lens. I therefore regarded his condition as myopia, in consequence of laceration of the zonula Zinnii, and saw in the myopia a reason for Helmholtz's explanation of the mechanism of accommodation. To the quivering movements of the lens a quivering of the objects, after each strong movement of the eye, corresponded. These quite agreed with those which occurred on little shaking movements of the neutralising positive glass before his lensless eye, and were thus explained.

A few months ago the patient applied to me again. The acuteness of vision in the right eye was then diminished. Even with the aid of his spectacles, he could no longer see acutely at a distance. I supposed that the somewhat luxated lens was passing into a state of opacity. This was found not to be the case: the lens had continued quite transparent. But I had at once perceived that, since the first examination, the pupil had deviated to the nasal ˙side, so that on this side only a slender margin of iris remained. This slender margin lies deeper than the outer margin, and has a convex curve forwards: the pupillary margin is directed backwards; thence the curve is formed, and the marginal portion deviates again in such a manner backwards, that it is most probably somewhat prolapsed through the lacerated zonula.

To this relation of the iris an oblique position of the lens corresponds. On the temporal side, the latter is almost in contact with the iris; on the nasal side it must therefore lie much deeper. After instillation of sulphate of atropia a considerable dilatation of the pupil occurs upwards, downwards, and to the temporal side, so that the lens comes to lie more in the centre. Looking in an oblique direction into the eye, we can, however, nowhere succeed in seeing the equator of the lens. The centre of the vortices also appears to correspond nearly to the centre of the cornea.

With the oblique position therefore there is no, or only slight, lateral displacement of the lens.

The acuteness of vision is only about $= \frac{3}{8}$. This diminution is ascribed to the oblique position of the lens, and consequently to astigmatism. Numerous experiments were performed, which also established this point. I shall mention only some of them. With $- \frac{1}{12}$ the patient sees, at a distance, vertical, with $- \frac{1}{20}$ horizontal lines most accurately. Even with $- \frac{1}{36}$ the horizontal lines are tolerably well defined, but the vertical exhibit a shadow, which nearly disappears when the nasal portion of the pupil is covered.—The point of light under no circumstances appears as a line of light, but is, on the contrary, always double. With $- \frac{1}{24}$, each of the double images is smallest. With $- \frac{1}{20}$ they lie above one another, with $- \frac{1}{12}$, close to one another.

The astigmatism is, on account of these experiments, estimated at $\frac{1}{12} - \frac{1}{20} = \frac{1}{30}$.

Remarks.—In the observation of this case no cylindrical glasses availed me. It may, however, be inferred, that with a spherico-cylindrical glass of $- \frac{1}{20} s \supset - \frac{1}{30} c$ (the axis of the cylinder having a vertical direction) R in all meridians should be about $= \infty$. Such a glass might be useful as a spyglass. For near objects it would not answer, because the range of accommodation, which at the time of the former examination was still tolerably considerable, was now reduced almost to nothing. For reading,

R must therefore be brought to about 12″: this would be effected by placing $\frac{1}{30} c$, with the axis directed horizontally, before the eye.

The cause of the astigmatism in this instance lay clearly exclusively in the lens, the measurements of the cornea even revealing an unusual symmetry.

In H.	In V.
$\rho n'' = 8\cdot64$	$\rho i'' = 8\cdot30$
$\rho n = 7\cdot94$	$\rho i' = 7\cdot98$
$\rho^\circ = 7\cdot74$	$\rho^\circ = 7\cdot74$
$\rho t' = 7\cdot74$	$\rho s' = 7.76$
$\rho t'' = 8\cdot09$	$\rho s'' = 8\cdot09$

The visual line deviated 5° inwards from the apex of the cornea.

It is remarkable, that the astigmatism dependent on an oblique position of the lens gave rise to diplopia, which in ordinary cases depending on asymmetry of the cornea, is not so expressly indicated. The diplopia appeared most distinctly in looking at a point of light. We have to suppose that the sectors of the lens formed four images clearly distinguishable, which, in looking with the naked eye, had already decussated. With $- \frac{1}{20}$ they were situated over one another, with $- \frac{1}{12}$ those adjoining one another were brought to a focus. In the first case the acuteness of vision was improved, when the inner or outer half, in the latter when the superior or inferior half of the pupil was covered.

In former years it often occurred to me to observe, particularly in myopes, that of a point of light two or three images were seen, which with too weak and with too strong glasses, stood in opposite directions in one line. In these cases no other stripes were acutely seen, than those corresponding to one of the two directions. Evidently, as agrees also with the above observations, the manifold images must cover one another in the stripe, if the latter is to be acutely seen. Whether in these cases the astigmatism depended on a congenital oblique position of the lens, I did not at the time investigate. I hope to find opportunity to do so.

On many remarkable points, peculiar to this case, I will not dilate. Only with respect to the myopia I would observe, that this seems to have arisen as the result of laceration of the zonula Zinnii, notwithstanding that the falling backward, as such, of the crystalline lens, must have given rise to the opposite, that is to hypermetropia. On the first examination, when no oblique position of the crystalline lens had as yet occurred, I had not been able to discover any atrophy of the chorioidea; and the patient stated that with the aid of a weakly negative glass, just as before, he could again see quite acutely at a distance. Now, however, a narrow atrophic meniscus had become visible at the outside of the optic disc, which in any case is strongly in favour of the view, that a slight degree of myopia had originally been present.

NOTE.

HISTORY OF OUR KNOWLEDGE OF REGULAR ASTIGMATISM.

In Mackenzie's justly-celebrated book (A Practical Treatise on the Diseases of the Eye. London, 1854), and still more completely in the excellent French edition by Warlomont and Testelin (Traité pratique des Maladies de l'œil, par Mackenzie. Paris, 1856), we really find almost everything comprised, which science, up to the dates of the publication of those works, possessed upon the subject under consideration. From them I have for the most part become acquainted with its literature, and whenever I had no opportunity of consulting in the original the works mentioned in them, my friend Mr. Hulke, of London, with great readiness and in the most obliging manner, consulted them for me, and sent me accurate extracts from them.

It is remarkable that we find the subject treated of almost exclusively in English literature. In the first place we meet with two men, of whom England may well boast: Thomas Young, who discovered normal astigmatism, and the Royal Astronomer Airy, who first recognised and described the asymmetry of his own eye as a defect.

Respecting Young's observation, I have above (compare p. 456), already stated what is necessary, in connexion with other investigations relating to the subject of normal astigmatism.

Airy's case (Transactions of the Cambridge Philosophical Society, 1827, vol. ii. p. 267), on the contrary, described in a manner worthy of the great master, must here occupy us more fully. It relates to a high degree of compound myopic astigmatism. Thus, according to his method, Airy could determine the farthest point of distinct vision in the two principal meridians, and at the same time the direction of the latter: in the vertical (with an inclination of 35°) R was $= 3\cdot5''$, in the horizontal, R $= 6''$. Hence he calculated the glass required for correction, and also stated the reasons, why a negative spherico-cylindrical glass is to be preferred to a negative bi-cylindrical one.

Many years later he again described his state (Id., 1849, vol. viii. p. 361). At this time, the farthest point lay in the vertical meridian at $4\cdot7''$, in the horizontal at $8\cdot9''$. His myopia had therefore decreased in both meridians, and at the same time the astigmatism appeared to have undergone some diminution,—from $\dfrac{1}{8\frac{1}{4}}$ to $\dfrac{1}{10}$. But Airy himself supposes, that the farthest point in the vertical meridian might lie somewhat nearer than $4\cdot7''$, and he is inclined to infer that his astigmatism had continued unaltered. With a man like Airy we may assume, that he observed for his farthest point with unalterd accommodation; otherwise we should venture the supposition that, in his earliest observations, in consequence of accommodation on the approach of the point of light, the myopia in the vertical meridian had turned out too great, whereby the recession of the farthest point with the increase of years (which certainly with the existing degree of myopia is extremely rare), should only apparently have taken place.

Airy's observation seems at first to have attracted attention only at Cambridge : to Stokes (*The Report of the British Association for the Advancement of Science for* 1849, p. 10), namely, we are indebted for the astigmatic lens for determining the degree of astigmatism, and Dr. Goode (*Monthly Journal of Medical Science*, Edinb. 1848, p. 711,—and *Transactions of the Camb. Philosoph. Society*, vol. viii. p. 493), who studied at Cambridge, first communicated some fresh cases of this anomaly. Just like Airy, he had astigmatism in one of his eyes, to which his attention was directed by the observations of the Astronomer Royal on the subject. From the complicated changes of form, which, according to his accurate description, a point of light underwent at different distances from his eye, it may be inferred that the asymmetry was combined with a high degree of irregular astigmatism. As to the regular, the distances of distinctness in the two principal meridians lay about at 6·13 and 25 English inches. Chamblant, the optician at Paris, prepared for him a plano-cylindrical lens, the cylindrical surface of which was ground with a radius of 9″ concave. Goode states that, with the aid of this glass he saw both near and distant objects acutely.

In a second case a point of light appeared as a horizontal line at 37 centimètres (about 14½ English inches), without at a greater distance being replaced by a vertical one. Horizontal stripes were not seen distinctly at 37 cent. or upwards ; vertical stripes at no distance whatever. A plano-cylindrical glass, with 2½″ radius of the convex cylindrical surface, was too strong, with 3″ radius it was too weak. A bi-cylindrical concavo-convex glass, with intersected axes, the concave surface having 7½″, the convex 4½″ radius of curvature, would probably have answered the purpose.

In a third case a point of light appeared at 35 centim. as a transverse line, and at a greater distance was indistinct. At a similar distance horizontal stripes were acutely seen, and a little further off a vertical stripe. A plano-cylindrical *concave* lens of 16″ radius produced a considerable improvement.

Goode found three other gentlemen in the University of Cambridge, whose astigmatism in one eye was improved by a plano-cylindrical lens of 12″ radius.

These cases, much as we value the communication of them, show that Airy's method was insufficient, accurately to determine the farthest point in the two principal meridians, and in general the degree of astigmatism. The seat, too, of the latter was unknown to Goode. Even in the highest degrees of astigmatism he could not satisfy himself as to the asymmetry of the cornea, and he was therefore inclined to seek the cause in the crystalline lens.

A case of abnormal astigmatism was almost at the same time communicated by Hamilton in the same journal (*Monthly Journal*, 1847, p. 891). In this instance, torpor of the retina existed as a complication, as it appears, without limitation of the field of vision. As to the astigmatism, it was characterised by distinctness of horizontal, and indistinctness of vertical lines. If I understand the case aright, vertical lines were acutely seen at a shorter, horizontal lines at a greater, distance, and a plano-concave cylindrical lens, placed before the eye with a vertical position of the axis, produced an improvement. Dr. Thompson found the vertical diameter of the cornea somewhat greater than the horizontal, and he thought, moreover, that the horizontal meridian was somewhat more highly curved.

Further, the cases are known which are appended by Hays to the American edition of Lawrence's work (Lawrence *On Diseases of the Eye*, edited by J. Hays, Philadelphia, 1854, p. 669). The first is that of a clergyman, whose description affords an excellent picture of simple myopic astigmatism. With the naked eye he saw vertical, with a concave glass horizontal lines distinctly. That he did not perceive both lines equally acutely, escaped him, until, by the use of negative glasses, the distinctness was inverted. After an able analysis of his case, the patient came to the conclusion, that he should need a spheroidal or cylindrical glass for correction, but he did not venture to decide whether it should be convex or concave. Hays' note states merely that M'Allister, the optician, ground for him a plano-cylindrical (positive or negative?) glass, and that vision was remarkably improved by it.

" We have," continues Hays, " within the past year seen two cases in which this defect of vision existed.

" The subject of the first was a lady, sixteen years of age, who consulted me in consequence of her vision being so defective as to materially interfere with her education. I accompanied her to Mr. M'Allister's, and found that, with the assistance of a double concave lens of high power, she could read sufficiently well with her left eye ; but none of the ordinary glasses, either concave or convex, would enable her to distinguish ordinary-sized letters with her right eye. I then instituted some experiments to ascertain, if possible, the cause of this defective vision. Having drawn two bold dark lines of equal length, crossing each other at their centres, at right angles, and shown them to the patient, she was able to see them sufficiently well to state that the perpendicular line appeared to her longer than the horizontal. Mr. M'Allister furnished me with some mathematical diagrams, which, being shown to the patient, she stated that circles appeared to be ovals, the circles appearing elongated perpendicularly. Various other trials were made, all, however, tending to show that objects seemed to her to be elongated in their perpendicular, and shortened in their transverse diameters. Mr. M'Allister, having fortunately some lenses, plane on one side, and with a concave and cylindrical surface on the other, I soon found one which corrected the distortion. I had prepared for her spectacles with a double concave lens of the proper number for her left eye, with a plano-concave cylindrical lens for the right eye, with which she can read ordinary print with either eye, and still better when using both eyes.

" The second case occurred in a gentleman, about fifty-five years of age, who consulted me for an inflamed eye, about which he was very anxious, as he stated it was his best eye, the other having been always so defective as to be nearly useless. On examining into the nature of this defect, I found that it was similar to that in the preceding case, except that objects were elongated in their horizontal diameter."

Besides the above cases, only one more has been recorded, which was observed on the Continent of Europe. It was described by Pastor Schnyder, of Menzburg (Switzerland, canton of Lucerne), who discovered this anomaly in his own person (*Ann. d'Oculistique*, t. xxi. p. 222. Bruxelles, 1849—taken from the *Verhandlungen der Schweizerischen Naturforschenden Gesellschaft* —to which I have not an opportunity of referring). He was nearsighted for vertical, farsighted for horizontal lines. For correction he used bi-convex cylindrical glasses, combined with bi-concave spherical. I find no record of what the focal distance of the glasses was. Mr. Schnyder had no other means of discovering the defect than the fact that horizontal and vertical wires were not accurately distinguished at the same distance. In order to determine what glasses were required, he seems to have tried which he needed, in order to see acutely horizontal and vertical wires, placed at the same distance.

I might here close the history of our knowledge of astigmatism. At least, no other facts have come under my cognizance. It, however, occurs to me that something further should be stated as to what has been assumed or suspected by different writers respecting the seat of the anomaly.

As might be expected from Airy,—in the absence of satisfactory reasons, he has wisely refrained from expressing any opinion as to the seat of the asymmetry. He appears also to have used no effort, to attain to certainty respecting this point. Goode, on the contrary states, that in a case of highly-developed astigmatism, he in vain endeavoured to satisfy himself, from the form of a reflected image, of the existence of peculiar asymmetry of the cornea, and he justly adds that he was therefore inclined to look for the seat of the defect in the crystalline lens.

In the case described by Hamilton, Dr. Thompson examined the cornea, whose vertical measurement he found somewhat greater than the horizontal, " being shaped somewhat irregularly, and the diameter projecting slightly upwards and inwards." Hamilton adds, " Dr. Thompson thought he perceived a somewhat more marked curvature of the cornea in the transverse diameter." According to what method the examination was made, is not stated. The result, however, renders it probable that the cornea was concerned in the asymmetry.

Wharton Jones (Manual of Ophthalmic Medicine and Surgery. 2nd Edition, London, 1855, p. 352), and Wilde (Dublin Journal of Medical Science, 1st Series, vol. xxviii. p. 105) go still further. Without more accurate investigation, they assume, that the foundation of astigmatism is really to be sought in the cornea. Both put it prominently forward as an established fact, that the cornea, in its vertical meridian, has a shorter radius of curvature than in the horizontal, and they explain Airy's case (they themselves observed no cases) by a peculiar development of that difference. What W. Jones (Cyclopædia of Practical Surgery, Art. *Cornea*, p. 832) describes as "a case of cylindrical deformation of the cornea, produced by injury," does not apply here. Whence they derive the proof of the fact put forward by them, is a puzzle to me. So far as I know, previously to the date of the communications of Jones and Wilde, the radius of curvature of only one cornea was determined in the vertical and in the horizontal meridian,—viz., by Senff (conf. Volkmann, Art. *Sehen*, p. 271, in Wagner's *Handwörterbuch der Physiologie*, 1846). In this instance the radius was found scarcely shorter in the vertical meridian. How little importance, moreover, was to be attached to one observation, appears from the investigation of Knapp, who found in the majority of his measurements the radius longer in the vertical meridian. It was, therefore, not until after the numerous measurements made by us, that we ventured to assert, that the horizontal meridian usually has the longest radius.—A little work, however, which I found quoted in more than one place, I have been unable to consult: I mean Gerson (*De forma corneæ*, Göttingen, 1810). Mackenzie (*l. c.* p. 926) borrowed from it the fact, that Fischer could not at the same time distinctly see horizontal and vertical lines. Here, therefore, astigmatism is in question. This circumstance, taken in connexion with the title of the work, leads us to suppose, that Gerson sought the seat of the defect in the cornea. Might we perhaps find in it reasons for the assertion of Wharton Jones and Wilde? It seems to me that it is not to be supposed that the form of the cornea was satisfactorily determined by Gerson,—and still less, that subsequent writers would not have mentioned it. Wharton Jones gave his explanation only as a supposition. Wilde, on the contrary, says expressly, " It is well known that the cornea is not a correct surface of revolution, but that the curvature of its horizontal plane is less than that of its vertical. When this exceeds the normal extent, it gives rise to irregular refraction, causing a circle to appear an oval," &c., &c. Wilde was so convinced of the correctness of this opinion, that he did not hesitate to replace the name of cylindrical eye, chosen by Wharton Jones, by that of ' cylindrical cornea.'

That, with some exceptions, Wharton Jones and Wilde approached the truth, has appeared from our investigation. But do they deserve credit for this? In my opinion, Young's observation on his own eye should rather have led them to look for the seat of the defect in the crystalline lens, and so long as the asymmetry of the cornea was not satisfactorily ascertained by measurement, it appeared more philosophical to keep to that view. Their assertion was therefore a very bold one. We see that in science also the quotation is sometimes applicable, that " *audaces fortuna juvat.*"

---

§ 40. Irregular Astigmatism.

Irregular astigmatism may, as well as the regular, be divided into *normal* and *abnormal*. The normal form is connected with the structure of the lens; the cornea does not participate in producing it. The abnormal degrees, on the contrary, which considerably disturb the power of vision, may depend upon irregularities of the cornea as well as upon those of the lens.

We commence with *normal irregular astigmatism*. The principal phenomenon attending this irregularity is known under the name of *polyopia monocularis*. With some attention any one can observe this polyopia in himself. Eyes in which, the lens being present, it should be entirely wanting, are undoubtedly rare exceptions. The following experiments will be sufficient to satisfy us of its existence and of its importance.

1°. Let a small *black* spot, on a *grey* or *white* ground (as .), be gradually brought nearer to the eye than the distance of distinct vision : most people will then observe that the black spot passes into a circle of greyish spots, which, when the spot is removed from the eye, again approach one another, and, at the distance of distinct vision, coalesce to form a black spot. It is desirable in this and in the following experiment to keep our eye, without alteration, accommodated for the farthest point, in order that the magnitude of the pupil may continue the same ; we must therefore, if not myopic, arm the eye with a positive glass, say of $\frac{1}{8} - \frac{1}{10}$, in order thus, while the eye continues relaxed, to be able to bring the point to either side of the distance of distinct vision. If we subsequently carry the spot beyond the distance of distinct vision, and for the greater correctness of comparison we may for the greater distance, take a proportionately larger point (as **.**), several spots usually again appear ; but in this case a central darker spot remains, around which the other paler spots are more or less regularly grouped. This central spot was absent when the black spot was nearer than the distance of distinct vision : on this account with equal deviation of accommodation we distinguish better (the diameter of the pupil being assumed to be unchanged), when the eye is accommodated for a too near, than for a too distant, object.

2°. We may repeat this experiment with a *white* spot on a *black* ground. As white spots, we may make use of small granules of whitelead, got by scraping an ordinary visiting card, and spread upon black velvet. Among these granules we find a great variety of sizes. If we take one of the largest, of about $\frac{1}{8}$ mm. in diameter, the experiment will yield nearly the same results as were obtained with the black spot. It will then, however, more distinctly appear, that each spot is radiatingly elongated, and exhibits dispersion,— with the blue turned towards the centre, when the spot is nearer than the distance of distinct vision, with the red towards the centre, if the point lies beyond it.

3°. Let the experiment be repeated with one of the smallest granules. The radiatingly elongated spots have now given way to slender rays, which, when the granule lies nearer than the distance of distinctness, do not run together in the middle, and which, on the contrary, have a white spot in the centre, when the object is beyond the distance of distinct vision.

4°. Let the observer look at a little point of light, for example, at a small opening turned towards the light, but still better (in order to avoid diffraction), at a small image of light formed by reflexion. The phenomena are then observed, in proportion to the magnitude, precisely as they have been described under 2° and 3°.

By these experiments we have now learned that polyopia, in looking at a small object, is the same phenomenon as that of the rays, under which at a distance a bright star or light appears, for which the eye is not accommodated. To each principal ray corresponds one of the marginal spots, under which the black dot appears. Therefore, too, those have the most distinct polyopia, who in a point of light perceive a comparatively small number of distinctly separated rays.

5°. Let a small point of light, a little reflected image or an opening of $\frac{1}{8}$ mm. (0·00492 of an English inch) in a metal plate, turned towards the sky, be gradually brought near the eye. Having arrived nearer than the distance of distinct vision, the point of light divides into a certain number of bright rays, and even, when it has reached the anterior focus, the circle of diffusion in the retina being as large as the pupil, the rays are still visible: they are the lines of light of the well-known entoptic image (compare Fig. 103, p. 200), which occurs in most eyes under this form. The transition of the bright rays into the lines of light of the entoptic image is very easily observed. While the light in the entoptic luminous circle, attaining on the retina the magnitude of the pupil, has been more uniformly divided, the few very bright rays, of which the image of a star almost exclusively consists, are therein only faintly represented by the said lines of light. The number and direction, however, remain precisely the same.

From these experiments it appears, that polyopia uniocularis, rays of stars, and radiating lines of light in the entoptic spectrum are dependent on the same cause, rest upon the same peculiarity in the structure of the eye. If, therefore, we have ascertained the source of one of these phenomena, we know that of all.

Now we have already, in treating of the entoptic phenomena, seen that the lines of light of the entoptic spectrum (compare Fig. 103) are to be sought in the crystalline lens: on moving in fact, the eye behind the point of light, no parallax is perceptible, and their cause therefore lies nearly in the plane of the pupil, and consequently in

35

the lens.   Hence it follows, that both the rays emerging from points of light and the polyopia, have their origin in the lens.   This is more decisively proved by the circumstance, that all these phenomena are wanting when the lens is absent from the eye (aphakia).   Moreover we can now further show that the cornea has no essential part therein.   In the first place, in examining the reflected images of the cornea, if such irregularities were here present, as are required for the explanation of the phenomena in question, they must have been apparent.   And, in the second place, I have excluded the action of the cornea by plunging my eye into water in a little bowl, bounded by a convex glass replacing the cornea, and the phenomena have then continued under the usual form.

If the cause be thus situated in the lens, the question suggests itself, how these phenomena are to be explained by it.   In the first place we observe, that the form of the rays, under similar circumstances perfectly constant for each eye, immediately reminds us of the peculiar structure of the lens, namely of the radiating figure from which its fibres proceed.   Those of the anterior surface we can observe in any one in the living eye, by lateral focal illumination (Helmholtz), especially by employing a lens, and better still with the aid of the phacoidoscope (compare p. 16).   The lines of the posterior surface differ in form and in direction.   Meanwhile the crystalline lens is by those lines divided into irregular sectors.   Now the explanation of the polyopia is this, that each sector forms a separate image.   The proof of this I have given twelve years ago, by moving a rather small opening (about ½ mm., or 0·01968 of an English inch, in diameter) before the pupil, while the multiple image of a point of light falls upon the retina.   We thus see a simple image when the opening corresponds to a given sector, and when by shifting the opening we come to the boundary between two sectors, two faint images appear, of which, on further displacement, that first seen disappears, while the one which has supervened remains alone and brighter. On more rapidly moving the opening it appears as if the little image of light jumps, which really happens in the transition from one sector to another.—In proportion as we accommodate with more precision, the multiple images approach one another, and finally coalesce into one image.   However, even with the most perfect accommodation, they do not exactly cover each other.   In the first place, regular astigmatism, and in so far the cornea also, here plays a part.   This regular astigmatism manifests itself precisely by the fact, that the images placed opposite to each other more speedily reach each other in one direction than in the opposite. The result of this is, that a point of light always appears somewhat angular, and even a black spot undergoes a peculiar change of form on a slight play of accommodation, without at the same time ceasing to be black. But even when we completely correct the regular astigmatism by means of a suitable cylindrical glass, all the multiple images do not meet precisely in one place: in one direction or another a single one projects beyond the rest into the centre, and accurate consideration of a point of light shows that all have not even their focus exactly in the same axis.

In this, therefore, lies, in the first place, *an element of irregular astigmatism*. A *second element* we find in the image of each sector in itself. It is very difficult by experiments to get a correct idea of the image of each sector. The impression of light on each point is, in fact, not proportional to the strength of the light, and consequently we obtain a different result with respect to the distribution of light, in proportion to the brightness of the light with which we experiment. On repeating the experiments above stated we had abundant opportunity to satisfy ourselves of this. While, for example, a bright fixed star (Sirius I have often taken as the object), with slightly hypermetropic arrangement of my right eye, gives seven or eight extremely fine bright rays, partly ramifying towards the periphery, and terminating at a short distance from the centre, a less bright luminous point appears rather as a circle of spots, with comparatively very strong illumination in the periphery, about agreeing with the circle of spots under which, with a similar arrangement, we see a black spot. The rule, however, remains with each illumination, and also in experimenting with a spot of a certain extent, that each image is elongated in the direction of the rays of the whole circle of diffusion, so that we can in it distinguish an outer and an inner margin, which last is turned towards the centre of the circle of diffusion. We can now further satisfy ourselves:—

1°. That the image of each sector is astigmatic. Through an opening of about 0·5 mm., held before a given sector, a fixed star, which under the greatest magnifying power remains a point, forms, with the most perfect accommodation, an image on the retina, which, were it accessible to our investigation, would certainly be very perceptible. The light of a lantern, seen at a great distance through a single sector, is nearly as great as if we had approached it by half

2

the distance. By using monochromatic light, the astigmatism of each sector remains unmistakeable.

2°. That the image has an aberration, agreeing with the spherical aberration. In the circle of diffusion, formed by a spherical lens from a monochromatic point of light, the light is not uniformly distributed. Before the focus of the rays (as both construction and direct experiment readily show) the illumination is strongest at the outside, behind the intersection; in the centre of the circle of diffusion. Now the same is true of the light, refracted by one of the sectors. Therefore a point of light, and even a little luminous spot, seen through the whole lens, is more strongly illuminated in the centre or at the circumference, accordingly as the eye is accommodated for a shorter or longer distance than that at which the spot is. We have already remarked that, consequently, the magnitude of the circles of diffusion being equal, the acuteness of vision suffers more when the retina lies behind than when it lies in front of the focus.

We have thus indicated *two causes of normal irregular astigmatism*, namely, the imperfect coincidence, even after accommodation, of the images of the different sectors, and the astigmatism proper to the image of each sector in itself.

In the image of each sector we can, moreover, easily recognise the chromatic aberration. In front of the intersection each image is red at the outer, and blue at the inner margin; behind the intersection the outer margin appears blue, and the central light is reddish. Now, if we examine the multiple images of a thin line, the lateral images have also coloured edges, and only the central image is uncoloured. It is very instructive, as Helmholtz has done, to combine a line with a point, placed near the extremity of the line. We now see, with imperfect accommodation, especially with adjustment for a greater distance, different lines close to one another, and we can satisfy ourselves that these, in each direction of the line, correspond to the multiple images of the point of light to which they are directed. It is now evident, that the edges of the central line will be colourless, because the radiating elongation of the sector-image, whence it arises, lies in the direction of the line, and the colours thus fall over one another. We obtain the sharpest, brightest, and most achromatic line, by giving the line such a direction, that two opposite radiating sector-images cover one another on the line. On the contrary, the lateral images of the line have coloured edges, and are at the same time fainter and broader: their section is equal to the longitudinal section of the elongated image, to which they correspond.—The phenomena here described may also be observable at the boundaries of brightly illuminated surfaces, with imperfect accommodation, as the transition from the bright to the dark takes place through two or three degrees. Even with perfect accommodation, some can satisfy themselves by the fact, that they see the bright moon as images covering one another. I was particularly struck with the distinctness and well-defined boundary, over the whole surface of the round images covering one another, of an opening, through which the nearly homogeneous light of the flame of alcohol containing salt was seen. But more especially when the accommodation is not perfect, we see in that experiment a number of circles, for the most part covering one another, and by covering a portion of the pupil we can never make one of these circles *partly* disappear—cut a segment off it: the circle only grows faint, to disappear suddenly and completely, when the whole sector of the lens belonging to that circle is entirely covered. It needs scarcely to be remarked that, on covering the pupil, the figure, as a whole, disappears on the same side, when the eye is accommodated for a nearer object, but on the opposite side, when, on the contrary, it is accommodated for a more remote point.

In the foregoing the cause of the peculiar distribution of light of the circles of diffusion was found in the crystalline lens, and was in general terms brought into connexion with the radiating figure, from which the fibres of the lens proceed. The perfect explanation is, however, not thus attained. The multiple images of a point were seen so early as by de la Hire.[*] Thomas Young[†] examined the circles of diffusion of a point of light at different distances, even delineates them, and said respecting their cause: " The radiating lines are probably occasioned by some slight inequalities in the surface of the lens, which is very superficially furrowed in the direction of its fibres." Listing[‡] discovered that, in many persons, in the entoptic spectrum of rays of light, which, proceeding from the anterior focus, run parallel in the vitreous humour, some bright lines, mostly in the form of an irregular star, occur with some off-shoots, which he looks upon as the image of an umbilical body with suture-like and elevated ramifications, derived from the separation, in the fœtal state, of this part of the capsule from the inner surface of the cornea.

[*] *Mémoires de l'académie de Paris*, 1694, p. 400.
[†] *Philosophical Transactions* for 1801, i. p. 43.
[‡] *Beitrag zur physiologischen Optik.* Göttingen, 1845.

In examining the entoptic phenomena I found* that multiple images, lines radiating from points of light and the entoptic star of Listing pass imperceptibly into one another, and therefore have one and the same origin; but respecting the proper cause in the structure of the lens I could form no satisfactory idea, and even now I have not been sufficiently successful in my attempts, to make known their result. Further investigation on this point appears to me to be necessary.

The astigmatism, of which we have thus far spoken, may be considered to be normal. The acuteness of the power of vision suffers very little under it, and least of all when we look with both eyes together, and when these have about the same refraction. We never find the astigmatism of both eyes exactly equal. The images of the same point, formed on the two retinas, therefore, deviate a little from one another. Both, however, coalesce in idea, and the correctness of the judgment respecting the form of a point or of a very small object, sometimes gains considerably thereby. Thus the acuteness of vision, apart from the stereoscopic effect, is greater with two eyes than with one : if vision takes place with only one eye, the form of the retinal image is, at least in the vicinity of the yellow spot, projected with greater accuracy; in vision with two eyes, on the contrary, the object is more correctly estimated.

If the acuteness of the power of vision, in monochromatic light, suffers little by ordinary astigmatism, the achromatism of the eye, with imperfect accommodation, may even gain thereby, as different coloured images fall over one another, and are thus partially neutralised. This also is especially the case in using both eyes.

II. *Abnormal irregular astigmatism.*—This has its seat either in the cornea or in the lens. As to the cornea, the *kerato-conus* or *cornea conica* first comes under observation. High degrees strike the eye at once. Slight degrees, on the contrary, are often enough overlooked. The disturbance of the power of vision frequently suggests the idea of amblyopia, combined with myopia. Three cases have already occurred to me which were long treated as amblyopia. That in this instance an anomaly of refraction, and indeed astigmatism, is the cause of the diminished sharpness of sight, is evident. A complete theoretical development would, even did we know precisely the surface of curvature, which is to be ascertained only by examination with the ophthalmometer, be very difficult. In high degrees, the mere inspection of the

---

* *Nederlandsch Lancet*, 1846-1847, D. ii. p. 432.

curvature and profile at once satisfy the observer, that the radius of curvature in the centre of the cornea is much shorter, so that the rays falling thereon from each cone of light must much sooner unite. Especially in reference to these rays the eye is myopic. There must, however, be not only a difference in focal distance, but the foci are also imperfect even for small portions of the refracting surface, and moreover, certainly do not all lie in the same axis. The high degree of astigmatism connected with this state, therefore, needs not to be further proved.—It would be very troublesome if, in order to recognise slight degrees, we should be obliged to have recourse to the ophthalmometer, in order to determine the radius of curvature in different parts of the cornea.   Fortunately, we have a more practical auxiliary. The already long-existing disturbance of vision leads us to resort to the ophthalmoscope, chiefly with the idea of finding the cause in the fundus oculi, and unexpectedly we discover the anomaly of the refracting surface.   This has happened to me more than once. Sometimes the degree was still so slight, that even after the discovery of the true cause, the observer, on taking a profile view, could not satisfy himself as to the state of things, so that full certainty as to the existence of the anomaly was attainable only with the ophthalmometer.   How the ophthalmoscope exhibited it is very simple.   In the inverted image, where there is a tolerably wide pupil, we overlook, at the same time, a rather large portion of the fundus oculi; the image, therefore, of one part or other, for example of the optic disc, remains in the field of vision both on moving the head of the observer, and on shifting the lens held before the observed eye.   At the same time, however, the rays, which, proceeding from the optic disc, strike the eye of the observer, pass each time through other parts of the cornea: now if its curvature is irregular, the result is, that the form of the disc each time alters, that it shortens in this direction, extends in that direction, and, moreover, is never seen acutely in its integrity.   In somewhat higher degrees, too, the side of the conical projection opposite to the incidence of the light is darker,—as if shaded.

That it is important to recognise these slight degrees of conical cornea, and not to treat them as amblyopia, is evident.

Where the form is favourable and the position advantageous, stenopæic spectacles may produce considerable improvement.   If this assistance be not sufficient (the field of vision too small, the spectacles an annoyance), an improvement by operation may be attempted. The chief object of the operation is easily stated: we desire to place the pupil before that part of the cornea, whose curvature is most uniform and approaches most nearly to the spherical, in order that a sharper image may be formed in the visual line, and especially that direct vision may be improved. *A priori* it will be evident, that this object will be more easily attained by a small pupil, not only because the circles of diffusion are thus rendered smaller, but particularly because we may expect the less difference in the radius of curvature, the smaller the portion of the cornea is, which participates in the formation of the image. Bowman* has made the pupil slit-like by double iriddesis.† Von Graefe‡ confined himself to iridectomy. Both obtained favourable results with respect to the acuteness of vision. Von Graefe proposed besides to procure diminution of the pressure in the eye, which result of iridectomy had in his hands obtained such brilliant and useful application in glaucoma: he hoped thus to oppose the further development of the conicity, if not to lessen the existing degree of it. Bowman, on his part, has actually seen diminution of the conicity take place after iriddesis. The results of the latter operation upon the power of vision are still more favourable, so that at present iriddesis, by which we also obtain a small pupil, seems to deserve the preference. Theoretically, however, the slit-like pupil, obtained by double ireddesis, appears to me, narrow as it may be, not the most favourable: when the direction of the slit is horizontal, the diffusion for vertical lines will still be considerable, and though for horizontal lines the eye will have little diffusion, it will be highly myopic. It certainly seems better, by simple iriddesis, to exclude the apex of the cone. By means of stenopæic spectacles (with artificial mydriasis) the most suitable place and form of the pupil can be discovered, and perhaps also the seat of most favourable curvature may be sought with the ophthalmometer; and when by this or any other mode we have ascertained where and in what form the pupil must act most advantageously, the further task of operative surgery is, to apply the means so as to realise what is found to be desirable.§

* *Ophthalmic Hospital Reports*, etc., No. ix. 1859, p. 154.

† Compare, upon this operation, also Critchett, *Ophthalmic Hospital Reports*, etc., No. ix. 1859, p. 145.

‡ *Archiv f. Ophthalmologie*, B. iv. H. ii. p. 271.

§ In this respect, very ingenious proposals have been made by Bowman, the object of which is to bring the pupil by means of a second iriddesis on the same side, proceeding from the margin of the pupil obtained by the first

To be classed with conical cornea, though usually producing less disturbance, are *partial bulgings* or flattenings of this membrane, which, in consequence of suppuration or of softening, not unfrequently occur. These are often accompanied with so much opacity as to render the displacement of the pupil by iriddesis or iridectomy desirable. But the astigmatism is not thereby removed, since the clear part of the cornea has lost its regular curvature. Von Graefe has remarked, that after iridectomy the form of the cornea* gradually improved—and I have repeatedly found this confirmed. Moreover, it appears, that in these cases improvement is often to be obtained by cylindrical glasses, the asymmetry being partly reducible to regular astigmatism.

To the very ordinary causes of altered, and consequently irregular arching of the cornea, belongs the *extraction of cataract*. Especially when prolapsus iridis or threatening prolapsus has existed, whereby the pupil has lost its central position, or where, with forward projection of the flap, the wound-surfaces do not perfectly correspond, we seldom obtain a completely normal arching of the cornea. If the deviation is slight, the power of vision may still be quite sufficient; but on accurate investigation it now appears that the acuteness is defective, and the astigmatism is in this instance also partly capable of correction by giving an oblique position to the convex glass, or by combination with a cylindrical one.

A common cause of irregular astigmatism we find further in *spots on the cornea*. That slight spots cause much more disturbance by scattering diffused light in the eye, than by reflecting and cutting off a part of the light, has been shown many years ago, and hereupon the indication for stenopæic spectacles was subsequently founded. Even in my first communication I had referred to the irregular refraction of light, connected with spots. How much effect this has, the ophthalmoscope afterwards taught me. Through a rather transparent spot we distinguish the fundus oculi with tolerable accuracy; but, while, in the mode described above, the rays are brought consecutively through different parts of the spot to the eye of the observer, he is surprised

iriddesis, still nearer to the edge of the cornea. He has also proposed to try, by means of a glass with corresponding curvature, still further to improve the astigmatism for this place, at least for the stationary eye.

* In the acute process of softening or suppuration it is a matter of recognised importance, to keep the form of the cornea as perfect as possible. To attain this object, repeated experience shows that timely support by means of a bandage causing pressure, cannot be sufficiently recommended.

at the extremely irregular displacement, shrinking and distortion of the forms, connected with a peculiar glancing,—very characteristic for any one who has once seen it. Spots, whose existence was not perceived on superficial inspection, sometimes, on examination with the ophthalmoscope, produced in a remarkable degree the phenomena just mentioned. Thus by ophthalmoscopic investigation we are led to examine the cornea with focal illumination, and then we find, in a scarcely perceptible opacity, the cause of the astigmatism, and at the same time of the diminished acuteness of vision, which had at first suggested the presence of other causes.—Under these circumstances the surface of the cornea is often not perfectly smooth, as readily appears from the irregular images of a flame reflected on the opaque part. This occurs chiefly when superficial ulceration of the cornea has existed. But this inequality is not necessary to produce astigmatism, and therefore local change of the coefficient of refraction, with condensation of the corneal tissue, seems equally capable of taking part in its production.—If we have not examined the astigmatism with the ophthalmoscope, we shall often think we find a disproportion between the degree of opacity and the disturbance of the acuteness of vision, which must be explained partly by irregular astigmatism.

Finally, in some *acute affections of the cornea*, particularly *with transparent ulcers*, a high degree of irregular astigmatism coexists.

So much with respect to the cornea. As to the crystalline lens, irregular astigmatism may by it in two ways attain a high degree, namely, by a change in the lens itself, and by displacement of the lens. With reference to the change of the lens itself, my friend Bowman recently wrote to me as follows: "I have often thought that some defects of vision may depend on physical alterations of the lens, sometimes independent of cataract, sometimes attending the earlier stages of cataract; making the changes of shape of the lens under the same action of the ciliary muscle more or less incomplete." To these remarks I give my full adhesion. Even independently of the changeability by accommodation irregularities are developed in the lens, which when the eye is still in a state of rest manifest themselves as irregular astigmatism. Usually, as Giraud-Teulon observed, this astigmatism increases at a more advanced time of life, especially when opacity of the lens is superadded. Even Mackenzie says: "Uniocular diplopia is sometimes a precursor of cataract," and Ruete very correctly explains, how radiating opacity of the lens may give rise to diplopia. We hear the latter complained of mostly, when one eye no longer takes much part in vision, which is very easily explicable on the principles already laid down (p. 550).

Besides, it very seldom occurs, that multiple images producing any disturbance remain, when by the assistance of suitable spectacles the accommodation has been made as perfect as possible. In youth the phenomena of irregular astigmatism may, both without and with tension of accommodation, be almost wholly absent.—The irregular astigmatism which depends on displacement of the lens, produces much more disturbance, especially when the lens has only partially remained in the plane of the pupil, and the rays, therefore, in part, refracted solely by the cornea, penetrate to the retina. This may take place in incomplete luxation, whether spontaneous, or produced by external injury; but it appears to occur more frequently as the result of congenital ectopia of the lens. Of this I have seen remarkable cases, three of which belonged to the same family. In such instances the power of vision is very imperfect. Just like highly hypermetropic individuals, the patients see near objects comparatively better, though still very defectively. Even when the lens occupies half of the plane of the pupil, they comport themselves as hypermetropes. This led me to infer that convex glasses would be beneficial to them, and it appeared that in this I was not mistaken. The glasses required were similar to those indicated in aphakia. On accurate examination with the ophthalmoscope and with focal illumination this result cannot appear strange. If the lens even in the normal eye is less homogeneous near the equator than near the axis, this is especially true of the abnormally situated lens. The reflection is, moreover, very strong, particularly when the lens lies obliquely. At the side of the lens the fundus oculi is seen perfectly clear; through the crystalline lens it usually appears less clear and acute. This we observe especially in examining the inverted image, as we can then see the optic disc in two closely adjoining pictures, one larger and brighter by the side of the crystalline lens, the other smaller and less brilliant, formed by the co-operation of the crystalline lens. Thus, also, the image, formed by the medium of a glass lens on the retina, is clearer, more perfect, and at the same time larger than that produced through the edge of the natural lens ; and, on the other hand, the disturbance from the rays, which form no sharp image on the retina, must in the latter case be greater than in the first. A stenopæic apparatus, by which either the rays entering the eye through the crystalline lens,

or those passing in beside it, are cut off, very much improves the
acuteness of vision.   In a still youthful lad, labouring under congenital ectopia of the lens, cataract was developed; in proportion as the
lens became more opaque, the sight improved.   I had absolutely no
inducement to operate on this cataract, even after it had become
ripe, although the diffuse light still continued somewhat inconvenient.

The literature and history of our knowledge of irregular astigmatism have
been sufficiently dwelt upon in the foregoing. I shall here add only that the
literature of normal irregular astigmatism, with a brief statement of its
contents, is given by Helmholtz (*l. c.*, p. 146), and that the cases of normal
irregular astigmatism which have occurred, are communicated in Stellwag
von Carion's monograph (*Denkschriften der k. k. Akad.* v. 2, p. 172. *Ueber
doppelte Brechung und davon abhängige Polarisation des Lichtes im menschlichen Auge* (on Double Refraction and Polarisation of Light dependent
thereon in the Human Eye), pp. 19 *et seq.*, Wien, 1853) as diplopia (polyopia) monophthalmica.   The theory of Stellwag von Carion, which is evident
from the title of his work, is refuted by Gut (*Ueber Diplopia monophthalmica*, Zurich, 1854).

CHAPTER IX

DIFFERENCE OF REFRACTION IN THE TWO EYES.

§ 41. Occurrence, Phenomena, Results.

Like the organs of animal life in general, the eyes present a great symmetry between the right and the left side. The statement so often made, that the right and the left eye usually differ considerably is an error, or, more strictly speaking, an exaggeration. In all respects, similarity is rather to be met with. This extends, not only to the magnitude of the eyeball, the diameter of the cornea, the colour of the iris, the size of the pupil, and other external properties, even some congenital morbid deviations, such as microphthalmos, cataracta congenita, iridemia, and acquired changes of form, such as cornea conica, often occur in both eyes in about the same way. The same is found to obtain with respect to the refractive condition of both eyes. Even the degrees of progressive myopia in most cases differ little in the two eyes. We have already seen that the majority of eyes are nearly emmetropic, and this generally holds good, in fact, for both. This emmetropia is the result of the convexity of the cornea, of the position and of the focal distance of the crystalline lens, and of the length of the visual axis, each of which may in itself differ considerably in the normal emmetropic eye, and then mutually compensate each other. But the similarity in the same individual usually goes so far that, as numerous measurements have shown me, the radius of curvature of the cornea coincides almost perfectly for both eyes; whence we may infer that for two eyes of the same individual the crystalline lens and the length of the visual axis approach more nearly to each other than they do for emmetropic eyes in general. A certain harmony also unmistakeably exists in general in the course of the subconjunctival blood-vessels, in many peculiarities of the optic disc and its blood-vessels, in the entoptic figure of the lens, and in the position of the yellow spot (angle a). Even in the asymmetry of the cornea there exists symmetry between the right and the left side.

All this is the rule. Exceptionally it occurs that both eyes differ much originally from each other, particularly with respect to their refractive condition.   Thus, as we have already remarked (p. 252), this asymmetry of the eyes is usually combined with asymmetry of other parts, especially of the orbit, and of the bones composing it, so that the difference of the eyes is reflected both in the form of the forehead and of the face.   Since my former observations on this subject, I have taken much pains in endeavouring to discover fixed rules on this point.   In this, however, I have not succeeded.   I can only in general maintain, that at the side where the strongest refraction, or rather the longest visual axis occurs, the orbit (and with it the eye) is situated closer to the median line, while its surrounding edges are placed more forward.   If the left and right half differ in this respect from one another, there exists also in general a difference in the refractive condition, and *vice versâ*. Hence there is evidently a connexion between the two.   But that the connexion is not absolute is not strange, for just as with differing form and position of the orbits the two eyes may be emmetropic, it must be possible that equality of the eyes should coexist with difference of the orbits of the same individual.   Though *homo dexter* and *homo sinister* may be dissimilar, they may both be emmetropic or equally ametropic.

The differences occurring in refraction may be divided into *congenital* and *acquired*.   We shall speak first of the *congenital*, which are the more important.   Among these must be reckoned the difference in myopia, though in youth this is often but slight.   The predisposition was original and the further development was included in it: where both eyes become highly myopic, that high degree of myopia was not present also in youth.

All imaginable combinations of refraction occur in fact.   With emmetropia of the one eye, the other may be either myopic or hypermetropic; hypermetropia or myopia may occur in very different degrees in the two eyes; lastly, the one eye may be hypermetropic and the other myopic.   It is remarkable that, when astigmatism occurs only on one side, there is in general in other respects harmony of refraction on both sides; that is, with H of the one eye, we find hypermetropic astigmatism of the other; with M of the one, myopic astigmatism of the other; with emmetropia, the astigmatism is mixed.—When with difference in refraction of the two eyes, the corneæ have nearly equal radii, this is to be considered as accidental: in general, under these circumstances, the difference is as great as is usually the case in eyes of different individuals.   The same may be admitted also respecting the crystalline lens, since the length of the visual axis for each eye is connected with the nature and with the degree of the ametropia.

As to the use of the eyes, with difference of refraction, this is possible in three ways: 1°. binocular vision, 2°. vision with each of the two eyes alternately, 3°. constant exclusion of the one eye.

1. *Simultaneous vision with two eyes,* even when the eyes were similar, was formerly doubted. It was asserted, that, although both eyes are properly directed, only one eye sees at the same time, and that in this the eyes relieve one another. This assertion has long since been refuted. But it certainly is true, that we usually abstract from the one eye more easily than from the other. If any one causes the sight to be directed to a remote object, it appears, on subsequent closing of the left eye, almost always, that the right eye has been used. If a distant object be covered with the extended finger, this covering will by most people be effected for the right eye. Now where there is difference in refraction that eye is used, with which, at the required distance, vision is most acute and easiest. But if the ordinary observation of an object be in question, there may be binocular vision even with unequal eyes, within the limits of easy convergence. This occurs in many cases, even where there is considerable difference in refraction. Experience, in fact, shows that in spite of the unequal magnitude and unequal acuteness, the images of the two retinas assist one another in observation: not only are the solidity and the distance more correctly estimated, but even acuteness of vision and the facility of reading, writing, &c., may gain thereby. This, indeed, cannot surprise us. In the first place, even for normal and equal eyes, there are no absolutely identical or corresponding points, and it is certain that such are much less still to be expected, when, from original inequality of the two eyes, the condition for connecting these points by practice more and more perfectly in a symmetrical position, has been wanting (compare p. 165). In the second place, as will more particularly be seen, the feeble tints of diffuse images forthwith disappear, when the acute image of the second eye is combined with them. In speaking of irregular astigmatism, I have already alluded to a remarkable co-operation of two unequal images (compare p. 550). How unequal in magnitude and acuteness the two retinal pictures of a near object, viewed laterally by both eyes, often are in equal eyes! In truth, the second eye is rarely disturbing to vision, unless, in consequence of an opacity, it

admits much diffused light to the retina; and that even then this disturbance is by no means the rule, is proved both by the rarity of the deviation of an eye affected by cataract, and by the possibility of the development of cataract in one eye being totally unobserved.

To satisfy ourselves, whether both eyes take part in vision, we cover them alternately, having fixed an object, by putting the hand before them. Whichever eye we cover, that which has remained uncovered must continue to fix without movement, and if the covered eye had deviated behind the hand, it must, on removing the latter, immediately again occupy its former place. If the result of this examination leaves any doubt, we place a weak prismatic glass with the angle inwards before the one eye, whereupon, if vision is binocular, double images arise, which are overcome by a distinct movement inwards.

When there is a difference in refraction, we can determine the farthest and nearest point of each eye separately. If the acuteness of vision is sufficient in both, we usually find the ranges of accommodation also equal. And if these are greater than the difference in refraction, they fall partly on one another: the nearest point of the least refracting eye lies at a shorter distance than the farthest point of the most refracting eye. But still we should be very much deceived, if we supposed, that in binocular vision the distance for which accommodation takes place could be equal. Buffon held this opinion, but we have called it an error. Even a slight difference in refraction we are not able to adjust by accommodation, if this has an equal range in both eyes, so inseparably is the tension of accommodation in one eye connected with that in the other. Of this we can easily satisfy ourselves. Let any one who has equal eyes, hold only a weak negative or positive glass before the one eye, look at any object, and then close alternately the one and the other eye. Experiments of this nature are really important. We perceive in the first place, that we continue to accommodate acutely with the one eye, and indeed by preference with the eye, which, with less tension of the relative accommodation, forms the sharpest and largest images. I myself, for example, read the finest diamond type for hours together, without fatigue, in the evening, without spectacles, but if I bring a glass of $\frac{1}{24}$ before one eye, I nevertheless, by preference use this eye for looking at near objects. Now it further appears, that with the unaided eye we have in this case a diffusion-image. By no tension whatever can we succeed in getting a sharply-defined image for both eyes together. Finally, we observe, if we now again open the assisted eye, that the feeble parts of the diffuse-image almost entirely disappear, while the darker parts coincide with those of the acute image. With glasses of $\frac{1}{48}$ I experience no disturbance whatever; with those of $\frac{1}{24}$ there is something misty, which disappears on covering the eye which is not properly adjusted; but in spite of that mistiness, both the solidity and the distance of objects are more correctly estimated, and with the stereoscope a stereoscopic image is obtained. Undoubtedly the advantages of binocular vision extend much farther, if the difference in refraction existed originally, the reasons of which have already been given. Besides, just as in the experiments with artificial difference by means of glasses, the one eye in this case also accommodates sharply, at the expense of the other, rather than by average tension of accommodation to obtain half acute images in both eyes. This, however, does not prevent the acuteness of vision, when it is imperfect in both eyes, being rendered greater by the assistance of the less correctly accommodated eye: this I have observed especially in disturbance, the result of astigmatism. But even when in consequence of too great difference in refraction, the second eye no longer assists, it at least produces no disturbance. I recently made the acquaintance of an optician of great merit, who told me, that he was emmetropic in one eye, while in the other, he had M = 1 : 5·5. The eyes were properly directed for any distance. In ordinary vision he experienced no disturbance and used his emmetropic eye. With the emmetropic eye a small light at a distance appeared to him to be, in fact, very small; with the myopic eye it presented a large diffused image. But if he now opened the emmetropic eye, the diffused image diminished to one-half. He asked me for the explanation of this fact. I found it partly in the diminution of the pupil of the myopic eye, on opening the other, partly in the circumstance that the most external and fainter portion of the diffusion-image actually became invisible; the outermost part was fainter, because the eye was accommodated for a *nearer point*.

Not unfrequently it has occurred to me, that the patient has thought that with one eye he could scarcely distinguish anything, notwithstanding that the acuteness of vision was still tolerably good. I have found this in high degrees both of myopia and of hypermetropia. That the power of vision of a strongly hypermetropic eye, which requires glasses of $\frac{1}{8}$, or even of $\frac{1}{6}$, in order to have defined images on the retina, has been overlooked, cannot surprise us; but it is singular that clever and well-informed men have so often continued ignorant that they still see satisfactorily with their strongly myopic eye, when they only bring the object near enough. In these cases the unused eye has often deviated somewhat, and indeed almost without exception in the outward direction. This direction I have even met with, when the deviated eye was strongly hypermetropic, provided that myopia, or at least emmetropia, existed in the other used eye. Under these circumstances the direction of the eye may for certain distances have still continued correct. In general, I must observe that deviation is never produced by difference in refraction. At most the latter may be the cause, why the deviation was not prevented, and it is, in fact, no longer prevented, so soon as the difference in refraction is so great that the one eye loses all importance for binocular vision : this eye is then equivalent to a blind eye, and just like the latter, therefore deviates outwards. But if the eye has still any co-operation in binocular vision, vision is improved by it, and certainly the deviation never arises in order to prevent binocular vision, as has been asserted.

2. *The eyes are alternately used.*—In difference in refraction it not unfrequently occurs, that the one eye is employed for near, and the other for distant, vision. I allude to those cases in which a certain deviation exists, and where, consequently, binocular vision, properly speaking, does not occur : evidently this alternation exists as a rule, so long as binocular vision is maintained, in which, as we have seen, the one eye is always acutely accommodated, and therefore, in the whole region of accommodation, each eye in part takes the office on itself. Now, in these cases, it may appear as if the range of accommodation is extraordinarily great. Thus one of my friends boasted, that at a distance he saw with perfect acuteness, and that in vision for near objects he was inferior to none. On examination this was at once explained. His right eye was emmetropic, and his left presented myopia $= \frac{1}{5\cdot5}$. He was himself not aware of this. After his twenty-eighth year this last eye began to deviate outwards, and was thus excluded from binocular vision ; but he continues to use it, when he wishes to distinguish very small objects. Thus a deviated myopic eye is most certainly preserved from ambly-

opia, while, on the contrary, that which has deviated inwards becomes amblyopic throughout the greater part of its field of vision. That it is of importance, if possible, to preserve it from amblyopia, need scarcely be observed.

3. *One eye may, in observation, continue wholly excluded.*—Under this head two kinds of cases are to be distinguished: those in which a morbid condition of the eye (*e. g.*, detachment of the retina) has set in, and has given rise to the exclusion with deviation, and those where the deviation was primary, influenced by the tension of the muscles, and the disturbance of vision is the result of want of use. With respect to the first we may be silent. As to the last, we must distinguish between the deviation inwards and that outwards. In the deviation outwards the field of vision is enlarged, and extends over objects, which are not seen by the other eye. In the deviation inwards the field of vision is diminished, and that of the deviated eye falls more over the other. This may produce confusion, and therefore we mentally neglect the impressions received on the corresponding part of the deviated eye, which consequently, so far as the common binocular field of vision extends, becomes amblyopic. In the deviation outwards only a small portion of the field of vision is common; and, moreover, abstraction is less required, because the usually strongly myopic eye receives very diffuse images. Therefore, in these cases the power of vision is generally tolerably satisfactorily maintained, even though the eye is not used.

A word still as to the *acquired* differences in refraction. They are limited chiefly to aphakia and to loss of accommodation in one eye. The mode in which vision takes place in aphakia of one eye has been investigated by von Graefe, particularly with reference to the question, whether it is desirable to operate for cataract in one eye, while the other is sound? His answer is, that, taking everything together, " the operation for cataract in one eye, with important advantages, is attended with no essential injury, and is therefore always indicated, if we can, with tolerable certainty, reckon upon a favourable result." In this opinion I can cordially concur. Particularly in active young persons, in whom at the same time the danger of the operation is slight, the advantages of a wider field of vision, diminishing the risk of wounds upon the second eye, the removal of the deformity and the greater self-confidence inspired by the possession of two eyes, throw a considerable weight into the scale. Moreover, I can confirm the observation of von Graefe, that in young persons the existence of combined vision can often be established, whereby the

2

estimation of distance and of solidity is improved, and that where combined vision is wanting, the lensless eye at least extremely rarely causes any disturbance. On a single occasion double vision produced disturbance where there was deviation outwards. Besides, that strabismus should occur as a result of the operation, I cannot admit. At most, it is comprehensible that it should increase where it had already existed, and produced, immediately after the operation, double images, near to one another, which it was difficult to unite again by muscular action.

Finally, where the power of accommodation is lost or diminished in the one eye, the distance of distinct vision does not proceed equally on both sides. On looking to a distance both eyes may, for example, be properly accommodated; this proper accommodation disappears in proportion as the object approaches. The inequality which has usually suddenly set in, probably still more its changeable degree, gives rise to complaints of dazzling. The large pupil is doubly injurious, as it makes the circles of diffusion larger and increases the strength of the light in the eye which does not see acutely. In speaking of the anomalies of accommodation we shall revert to this point.

§ 42. Treatment and Optical Remedies in Difference of Refraction in the Two Eyes.

In the establishment of the indication, the principal thing is to determine, whether binocular vision exists, or not.

Where *binocular vision* is present, at any distance, the point is to maintain this, and if possible, to render it capable of extension over a greater region. In the choice of glasses we start from the more acutely-seeing eye, to which the other must remain subordinate. Where there is little difference in acuteness of vision, it may also be considered which eye needs the weaker glass for correction, that is indeed also in general the eye which has the more acute vision. For this eye now, according to its refraction and accommodation, quite independently of the other, all the rules hold good, that guide us in the choice of glasses (compare §§ 18, 23, and 32). The question then remains, what glass the other eye requires?

At first view we might suppose, that for this latter we should have simply to choose the glass that brings the farthest point to the same distance, at which it lies for the first eye. This is in fact the opinion of laymen: "My eyes differ, consequently I need different glasses,"—such is the ordinary reasoning. It is so evident, so palpable, and apparently so logical, that we cannot be surprised at it, the less so, as the so-called "opticians" support it, and are quite prepared to put two different glasses in the same frame. It is, however, far from being the case, that we should keep to this rule. Even from habit a great difficulty arises. One person has, in spite of hypermetropia in one eye, in his youth always seen and read without spectacles, and has never experienced any difficulty in binocular vision. Another reads admirably and suffers no fatigue, although his eyes are in different degrees myopic. If we now give such people convex or concave glasses similar for both eyes, they will be satisfied, for the relation between the two eyes, to which they are accustomed, remains almost unchanged. If, on the other hand, we give them different glasses, whereby the range of accommodation in both eyes becomes more equal, we shall often enough find the proverb confirmed "le mieux est l'ennemi du bien." The cause of this is principally that when the distance of distinctness is made equal, the images of the two eyes are not equal, but different, particularly in magnitude. Within certain limits a difference in magnitude, such as, with equal eyes, can be produced by a combination of a positive and negative glass for the one eye, is, as is shown by the experiment, attended with no essential difficulty, especially not in looking at objects situated in the same plane, as in reading, writing, &c. If we consecutively close each eye, it is found that the letters appear with one eye larger, with the other smaller, while both eyes combine them in a medium magnitude. It is well known that this is equally the case when we look at two uniform figures, with a slight difference in magnitude, through the stereoscope. It is the result of the varying and imperfect correspondence of the symmetrical points which must result from the ordinary use of the eyes, in which letters and other forms are so often met with at somewhat unequal distances from the two eyes. But if the difference in magnitude exceeds a certain degree, double vision becomes evident, with larger letters corresponding to one, smaller to the other eye, which cannot be brought to cover one another, and which the person is, therefore, inclined, by deviation of one of the visual lines, to separate still further. The same thing occurs when the same distance of distinct vision has been produced in cases of great differences in refraction by difference of glasses.* This has led me to adopt the rule

---

* We might turn highly periscopic glasses (whose nodal points lie outside the body of the glass) for the one eye with the convex, for the other

to give similar glasses for both eyes, when the binocular vision of eyes of different refraction is acute and easy at any distance without glasses, and shifting of this distance is necessary, and I find this to answer very well. But may we never deviate from this rule? Undoubtedly. In the first place we may do so when the difference in refraction is slight, amounting to not more than $\frac{1}{48}$ or $\frac{1}{36}$. I have met, particularly, with myopes, who have for distant vision given the preference to such corresponding difference in glasses. Moreover, where there is a greater difference in refraction, we may, by a moderate difference in glasses, partly correct this; for example, with $M = \frac{1}{12}$ in one eye, and $M = \frac{1}{8}$ in the other eye, we may give a glass of $-\frac{1}{12}$ for the first (if there is no contra-indication to neutralisation), and at the same time one of $-\frac{1}{10}$ for the other eye; but the difference in glasses can rarely exceed $\frac{1}{40}$ or $\frac{1}{30}$. Lastly, there may often be an advantage in producing by different glasses, in imperfect acuteness of vision, nearly accurate images on the two retinas, by whose co-operation then the power of distinguishing is sometimes really increased. This refers especially to hypermetropes: these, even, are also the cases in which the patients, under the existing difference in refraction, were not satisfied with their power of vision at any distance whatever. But under all circumstances the combination of the different glasses ought to be tried, to ascertain if it is really suitable. *A priori* we can give no certain opinion, as the existing difference of the eyes has become habitual, and may have had an influence on the corresponding points.

When an eye takes part in combined vision, its function is maintained, even when it constantly receives very imperfect diffused images. Particularly the field of vision continues in its integrity, and if the acuteness of sight may somewhat diminish, it returns, when more is required from this eye, for example, when disturbance occurs in the other and on systematic practice. This last I consider in every case desirable, especially in high degrees of ordinary hypermetropia, likewise in aphakia; it is accomplished, the eye ordinarily used being closed, simply with a convex glass. Thus remaining unenfeebled, this eye is then always ready to afford assistance so soon as the other may come to fail, and at the same time it can still better

with the concave surface towards the eye, or by a peculiar combination of a concave and a convex glass, different for each eye, we might endeavour to bring the resulting nodal points on both sides to an equal distance from the retina, and thus to make the images equally large; but the method is very delicate, and I can scarcely imagine that it will ever be adopted in practice.

aid in binocular vision. A highly myopic eye can practise without a glass. This, however, has usually deviated outwards, and it then belongs to another category, namely, to those cases in which

Binocular vision is absent.—It is chiefly under this head that the remarkable examples fall, in which a defect in refraction is looked upon by the patient as total uselessness. I will communicate a couple of them.

1. Mr. R., aged 58, an architect, has from his youth been much occupied with architectural drawing. In this he has always made use of his left eye. Since an attack in the eyes, from which he suffered, he has seen less acutely with that eye. " It is my only eye," he says, "and I am much perplexed." I establish the existence of $M = 1 : 11\cdot5$, $S = 0\cdot6$, diffuse light being warded off, and of synechia, with opacity of the anterior surface of the crystalline lens, the result of iritis. On glancing with the ophthalmoscope also into the right, somewhat outwardly deviated eye, I find it free from synechia and see with $\frac{1}{10}$ (compare my method at p. 337) the fundus oculi scarcely diffused in the non-inverted image : the eye was therefore hypermetropic. On asking him how he saw with that eye, I received for an answer that at a distance everything was confused, and that he could distinguish nothing near with it. His amazement, when he looked at a distance through a glass of $\frac{1}{10}$, is still vividly before me. " I actually see better with this eye," he exclaimed, "than I ever did with the right, even with the aid of my concave glass." Objects appeared to him at the same time much larger, and if he looked at those with which he was acquainted, he thought the distance shorter than it really was. With $\frac{1}{6}$ he read without difficulty ; with $\frac{1}{3}$ he distinguished the smallest type. His hypermetropia amounted to not more than $\frac{1}{8}$; S being at the same time $= 0\cdot7$.

Two points here deserve our attention. In the first place, that in apparent disuse the eye had continued so good : I am, however, convinced that in looking at distant objects the patient not unfrequently made use also of this eye. In the second place, that with the comparatively slight degree of H, he did not know the value of the eye. This is certainly to be ascribed to the fact, that the other eye was myopic, and that in youth, its degree of myopia being somewhat less, it saw near objects almost without exertion, and at the same time distinguished at a distance better than the hypermetropic eye did. In this way there was no occasion to put the accommodation much upon the stretch. If both eyes had been in the same degree hypermetropic, Mr. R. would undoubtedly have read with them.

II. Mrs. L., aged 40, has a number of general ailments, and to them she ascribes it, that during the last six months her sight has fallen off very much. " With the right eye she has never seen." It is rather strongly deviated outwards. The left eye has $M = 1 : 5$, $S = 10 : 70$; the diminished acuteness of vision is dependent on chorioiditis disseminata and motes in the vitreous humour. A glance into the right eye with the ophthalmoscope shows me with $\frac{1}{10}$ at a distance the inverted image of the fundus oculi, bearing a rather considerable circular atrophy. It therefore appears that the myopia has here a much higher degree; and while I now approximate No. 1 to 2″, she reads it without any difficulty, to her own amazement: "She had never tried this." In this eye M was $= 1 : 2\cdot5$, S $= 10 : 40$, and with a glass of $-\frac{1}{5}$ she could still read satisfactorily with this eye. While the left eye was under treatment, I advised her to practise the right eye cautiously, partly without a glass, partly with $-\frac{1}{5}$. Thus S within some months increased to $9 : 20$, and the eye was, and continued, much more useful than the left.

In general, the optical treatment in difference in refraction, is much easier where there is deviation of one eye than when there is binocular vision. In this case, we keep the better eye for ordinary use, and keep up the other by regular practice, with exclusion of the better. In rare cases, with deviation outwards, the one eye is used exclusively for distant, the other for near, objects. This task they must continue to fulfil, and we keep up each, so far as is necessary, according to the general rules. This is, therefore, still simpler. Lastly, almost always with deviation inwards, and not unfrequently also with deviation outwards, the one eye is wholly out of use: perhaps it was even originally less sharpsighted, and now it is quite amblyopic. If it no longer fixes on closing the other eye, there is nothing to hope for. Practice is then in vain.—The question, when it is expedient, in deviation, to perform tenotomy, cannot be here investigated at length. On this subject, I may refer to the well-known essay of von Graefe. A couple of remarks may here be made. As the result of my investigation, I have assumed that difference of refraction never produces strabismus, but only does not prevent its occurrence. Consequently, from the difference in refraction, a decided contra-indication to tenotomy is never to be deduced. We must say only, that binocular vision can acquire no particular value. But is not tenotomy performed for appearance' sake, even when one eye has lost its sight?—A second remark is, that in the highest degrees of myopia an eye deviated outwards acquires, through simple tenotomy, a better position in looking at distant objects, but seldom learns to converge.

In aphakia of the one eye, with normal acuteness of vision of the other, especially with deviation of that eye, some practice with a convex glass is to be recommended, in order to prevent retrogression of the acuteness of vision. Some minutes daily are sufficient.

To the indication, in loss of accommodation of one eye, I shall revert, in speaking of the anomalies of accommodation, at the consideration of which we have now arrived.

II.—ANOMALIES OF ACCOMMODATION.

INTRODUCTION.

WE commenced the second chapter of this work by demonstrating that the anomalies of refraction and those of accommodation form two different categories. We laid stress upon the fact that, as the first are anomalies of the form, the latter disturbances in the function of muscles, they must be rigidly distinguished from one another. But with this difference in nature, the connexion between the two is not to be overlooked. Thus we had, in speaking of the emmetropic eye, to treat of presbyopia, which, although the normal condition at a more advanced time of life, is, with respect to its essential nature, related to the anomalies of accommodation. Thus, in aphakia, the refraction is abnormal, but, at the same time, the accommodation is removed. Thus we saw further how hypermetropia, and sometimes also myopia, leads to spasm of accommodation, and how, in the two forms, the connexion between accommodation and convergence is peculiarly modified. If we add that the symptoms differ, accordingly as the anomaly of accommodation occurs in emmetropic or ametropic eyes, and that the differential diagnosis between the two categories is not always free from difficulty, it will certainly be admitted that it is practically useful to append, in the same work, to the detailed treatise on the anomalies of refraction, a short description of the disturbances of accommodation.

Accommodation depends upon muscular action. We are here therefore to expect the anomalies which are proper to muscles in general: paralysis and spasm. In connexion with the former, the action of mydriatics; in connexion with the latter, that of myotics, is to be studied. Each investigation must be based upon a knowledge of the nerves, which are implicated in either condition, and we have to treat thereof in connexion with the movements of the iris, which are associated with those of accommodation.

We therefore treat, in three chapters, of :—

I. The influence of the nerves upon accommodation, and upon the movements of the iris.

II. Paralysis and debility.

III. Spasm.

CHAPTER X.

INFLUENCE OF THE NERVES UPON ACCOMMODATION AND UPON THE MOVEMENTS OF THE IRIS.

§ 43. The Movements of the Iris.

THE mechanism of accommodation has already come under our consideration (§ 4). Here we may therefore confine ourselves to the movements of the iris.

The movements of the iris are of two kinds : reflex and voluntary. Reflex action is exhibited as constriction of the pupil, in consequence of the stimulus of incident light upon the retina. Fontana* has shown that the light falling upon the iris produces no remarkable contraction. We have confirmed this result by causing the image of a small distant light to fall, by means of a convex lens, upon the iris, whereby during slight perception of light, a doubtful contraction occurred, which gave way to a strong contraction so soon as the light, entering through the pupil, excited a vivid perception.† That this contraction takes place by reflex action of the optic nerve upon the oculo-motor nerve in the brain was proved by Mayo,‡ by striking experiments upon pigeons. Nevertheless, the experiments of Harless§ and of Budge‖ have shown, that even after death, so long as irritability remains, the pupil still contracts upon the continued action of light. Of the correctness of this observation we have satisfied ourselves. In a dog, killed by loss of blood, the one eye was closed, the other was opened and turned to the light : after the lapse of an hour the pupil of the opened eye was perceptibly smaller than that of the closed eye. The latter now remained also exposed to the light, and on the following day the diameter of both

---

* *Dei Moti dell'Iride*. Lucca, 1765. Compare also *Programma*, etc., cui inest Diss. E. H. Weberi, *Summam doctrinæ de motu iridis continens*, 1821.

† Compare de Ruiter, *De actione Atropæ Belladonnæ in iridem*. Trajecti ad Rhenum, 1853, and in *Nederl. Lancet*, III. p. 433. From these investigations, made under my direction and with my assistance, upon the iris and belladonna, I have borrowed, when I use the plural " we," and quote the dissertation.

‡ Mayo, *Anatomical and Physiological Commentaries*, No. II. 4to. London, 1823.   § *Die Muskelirritabilität*, München, 1850.

‖ *Comptes rendus*, T. xxxv. p. 561.

eyes was equal. The upper jaw, alone with the eyes, was taken out of some frogs, one eye was exposed to the light, while the other was covered with a closely-folded piece of black paper : after the lapse of half-an-hour, the pupil turned to the light was narrow, the other was wide. But the latter also contracted almost immediately after the removal of the paper.*

When light falls upon one side, the pupil contracts on both sides : the contraction on the same side we call direct, that on the opposite side, we call consensual.† We may accurately study these two, as well as the accommodative (Listing), by ourselves, after the entoptic method (compare p. 197). A small opening in an opaque plate, held at about 6″ from the eye, and turned towards the light, gives, in the vitreous humour a bundle of nearly parallel rays, of the size of the pupil, and is therefore seen as a round, illuminated disc, whose diameter increases and diminishes with that of the pupil. If both eyes had been closed, and if one be now opened, the pupil is seen almost immediately to contract, and then slowly and vibratingly to dilate again : the little light entering the eye through the opening is sufficient to excite strong contraction. The consensual contraction, on the contrary, according to Listing,‡ does not begin until $\frac{2}{3}$ second after the opening of the other eye, lasts about $\frac{1}{3}$ second, after which the pupil again dilates slowly and vibratingly for some seconds. The consensual dilatation, he observed to commence about $\frac{1}{2}$ second after the closing of the other eye, and with diminishing rapidity to continue for one or two seconds. This last continues in my eyes considerably longer.§ The whole course of consensual contraction and dilatation (opening of the left eye, contraction of the right, closing of the left, dilatation of the right), which, with Listing, lasts $\frac{2}{3} + \frac{1}{3} + \frac{1}{2} + 1$ to $2 = 2\cdot1$ to $3\cdot1$ seconds, with me occurs ten times in the minute, and therefore lasts six seconds. The dif-

* Further investigations on this subject have been instituted by Kuyper (*l. c.*), H. Müller (*Würzb. Abhandlungen*, x. p. L.), and especially by Brown-Sequard (*Journal de physiologie de l'homme et des animaux*, 1859, T. ii. pp. 281 et 451).

† When, in the absence of the direct, consensual contraction is present in one eye, we are justified in inferring the existence of blindness in that eye. If both are present, or both are wanting, no certain conclusion is to be drawn as to the power of vision. Compare, with respect to this last, Mackenzie, *The Physiology of Vision*, London, 1841, p. 198.

‡ *Beitrag zur physiologischen Optik*, Göttingen, 1845.

§ Conf. *Nederlandsch Lancet*, 2ᵉ Serie, 1846, D. ii. p. 442.

ference has reference especially to the duration of the consensual dilatation, whose maximum it is difficult exactly to determine. —In these experiments the closing must, for more than one reason, be effected only by holding a screen before the eye.

The accommodative movement is, as well as the accommodation itself, to be considered voluntary. It is true, we contract our pupil, without being conscious of the contraction of muscular fibres, but this holds good for every voluntary movement. When a person raises the tone of his voice, he is not conscious that by muscular contraction he makes his chordæ vocales more tense; he attains his object without being aware of the means by which he does so. The same is applicable to accommodation for near objects, and to the contraction of the pupil accompanying it. The fact that this last is only an associated movement, does not deprive it of its voluntary character, for there is perhaps no single muscle which can contract entirely by itself.

E. H. Weber* has discussed the question, whether the contraction of the pupil is associated with the convergence of the visual lines, or with the accommodation. From his experiments of seeing acutely the same object, alternately through concave and through convex glasses, he came to the conclusion that the pupil neither contracts nor dilates without change of convergence. Cramer† repeated these experiments, but without taking sufficient care that vision took place through the axes of the glasses, so that, on removing the latter, some change of convergence was readily produced. Nevertheless, in my experiments with Dr. de Ruiter, I came to the same conclusion as Cramer, namely, that tension of accommodation, even without increase of convergence, is attended with contraction of the pupil. Now, on repeating the experiments, also without the use of glasses, and being able, the fixation of the same point remaining unchanged, to put my accommodation alternately more and less upon the stretch, I find that, especially in looking at a remote object, each stronger tension is combined with contraction of the pupil. These experiments, in which the contraction of the pupil presents so completely the voluntary character, are still more unassailable than those with glasses, in which the change of the intensity of light is not altogether avoidable.—That increased convergence of the visual lines without change of accommodation also makes the pupil to contract, is easily proved by simple experiments with prismatic glasses.

* *l. c.* p. 12.
† *Het accommodatie-vermogen der oogen.* Haarlem, 1853, p. 115.

Listing observed that the accommodative contraction of the pupil takes place almost contemporaneously with the will, just as is the case in movements of ordinary muscles. It is, however, easy to show that, even if contraction and extension commence almost simultaneously with the will, they by no means take place with the rapidity which is peculiar to voluntary muscles. By alternating the accommodation for a remote and a near object, I cannot voluntarily strongly contract and dilate the pupil more than thirty times in the minute.

§ 44. The Ciliary System and its Function.

We have already shown that accommodation is dependent on muscular action in the eye. In this organ there are no other muscles than those of the iris and the ciliary muscle, which have been described at p. 23. Now, accommodation is produced by the ciliary muscle, probably even exclusively by this muscle (compare p. 26). But the movements of the iris are associated with the accommodation; they are governed by the same nerves as the latter; even a direct relation cannot be considered impossible, so long as the mechanism of accommodation has not been clearly elucidated; if we add that the disturbances of accommodation are most distinctly revealed in deviation of the movements of the iris, it will certainly be allowable to treat in common of the nerves of the iris and of the ciliary muscle.

The parts enumerated derive their nerves from the ciliary, also called the ophthalmic, ganglion. This ganglion gives off from 10 to 16 minute branches, the ciliary nerves, which perforate the sclerotic, not far from the optic nerve, and proceeding straight forwards between the sclerotic and the chorioidea, reach the ciliary muscle and the iris, and give some filaments to the cornea. One or two ciliary branches come directly from the naso-ciliary nerve, perforate, as well as the others, the sclerotic, and, according to Bernard's statement,[*] finally pass into the conjunctiva and the iris, but not into the cornea: their origin indicates that they act chiefly as nerves of sensation.—Into the ciliary ganglion three so-called roots enter: the short root from the oculo-motor nerve, the long root (often existing double[†]) from the naso-ciliary nerve; and, lastly, a branch, derived from the sympathetic nerve

[*] Bernard, *Leçons sur la physiologie et la pathologie du système nerveux*, Paris, 1858, T. ii. p. 86.

[†] Conf. Hyrtl. *Berichtigungen über das Ciliarsystem des menschlichen Auges*, in *Med. Jahrb. Oesterr.* B. xxviii. s. 1.

in the neck. In the ciliary ganglion numerous ganglionic cells are met with. What the connexion is between the three kinds of nerve-fibres enumerated and these ganglionic cells, has not been ascertained, nor whether fresh nerve-fibres here have their origin, joining the ciliary nerves. All the ciliary nerves, the commencement of whose course we have already described, divide in the first instance near at hand and farther up the outer surface of the ciliary muscle into two, and afterwards into more numerous branches, which form a rich plexus (*orbiculus ciliaris* of W. Krause), whence many little fasciculi penetrate into the ciliary muscle. I examined them in 1853, with Dr. de Ruiter, in white rabbits, and as the result of that investigation, the following was noted:* " Many branches proceed, after having formed a plexus on the ciliary muscle, to the periphery of the iris, and there again form, near the margin of the latter, a plexus of tolerably large branches, whence smaller branches take their origin and establish a third plexus of the iris, in that part where the muscular fibres are observed to run a circular course. The nerve-tubes belong for the most part to the slighter kind, become by ramification still slighter, have a very long isolated course through the iris, which is particularly true of the thicker nerve-tubes, and in their progress form many loops, from whose extremities new fibres again arise by division, which again form loops, not, however, to be considered as terminal loops, as we can often observe further ramifications of the tubes, which, after having lost the medullary sheaths, in many places terminate in an invisible manner." This result has been confirmed by subsequent investigators. I have now, in reference to the nerve-fibres, nothing essential to add. In the meantime, in the peripheral distribution of different nerves, especially in those of the involuntary muscles, ganglionic cells are found, and this is true also of the ciliary nerves. Not only have they been demonstrated by H. Müller and Schweigger (compare p. 381), and recently also by Saemisch,† in the chorioidea, where, too, the muscular fibres are not wholly wanting, but also particularly by H. Müller,‡ in the orbiculus ciliaris, where C. Krause § already mentions them. Müller saw, in the ramifications of the first and second order of the ciliary nerves in the ciliary muscle, some beautiful and distinct cells, some-

---

* *Nederlandsch Lancet*, D. iii. p. 436.

   † *Beiträge zur normalen und pathologischen Anatomie des Auges*, Leipzig, 1862. Pl. II. Figs. 2 and 3.   ‡ *Würzb. Abhandl.* x'. p. 108.

   § C. Krause, *Handbuch der Anatomie*, 2e Aufl. B. i. p. 526.

times with two or three efferent branches, whose transition into nerve-fibres with medullary sheaths was not, however, with certainty recognised. He thinks, nevertheless, that they may be regarded as ganglionic cells. This discovery was confirmed by W. Krause* in all its parts. Moreover, Müller (*l. c.*) found even in the finest nerve-bundles of the ciliary muscle, where the primitive fibres also ramify, little thickenings of the fibres, in which a small round or oval body was to be seen, presenting the appearance of a bipolar ganglionic cell. While Müller remains in doubt as to the nature of these corpuscles, W. Krause (*l. c.*), who found them constantly present in twelve subjects, thinks they must be regarded as genuine ganglionic cells, although he agrees that they are not connected with the axes of the fibres. It is not improbable that, in connexion with the ciliary nerves, still more of these groups of ganglionic cells will be found in the eye.

After this brief anatomical exposition, we may now proceed to the consideration of the function of the ciliary system. Except the above-mentioned one or two ciliary nerves of separate origin, all the branches destined for the iris and for the ciliary muscle proceed from the ciliary ganglion. In this ganglion consequently the function is comprised. The question is therefore, properly, what influence each of the three nerves exercises on the ganglion, and what conditions of the internal muscles of the eye correspond to the conditions of the ganglion. On this subject, however, nothing can with certainty be said, and we can at present investigate only the influence of the roots of the ganglion, as this manifests itself indirectly upon the muscles.

The action of the oculo-motor nerve upon the sphincter of the pupil is established beyond doubt. Not only is the pupil dilated and immovable in paralysis of this nerve, but on irritating the nerve in the base of the brain in animals, we see it strongly contract. If Volkmann and E. Weber had, in opposition to previous investigations, seen dilatation produced by irritation, Budge† showed that this was to be ascribed to simultaneous irritation of the sympathetic branch running in the neighbourhood, and retaining its irritability longer, and Nuhn,‡ who in a decapitated criminal had likewise seen dilatation, recognised, after experiments on different animals, the same source of error as Budge had indicated. In the beheaded man also, contraction

---

* *Anatomische Untersuchungen*, Hannover, 1861, p. 91.

† *Archiv f. physiol. Heilkunde*, 1853, B. xi. p. 780.

‡ *Zeitschrift f. rationelle Medicin*, N. F. 1853, B. iii.

of the pupil on irritation of the nerve in question was subsequently seen.* Most decisive, however, are the cases of complete paralysis, because they show that this nerve is the condition *sine quâ non*, both for reflex and accommodative movement of the pupil, and for the accommodation itself : no trace thereof remains, when its paralysis is complete. If other nerves also have influence upon the sphincter of the pupil and the ciliary muscle, they have it only by the intervention of the oculo-motor nerve. Nor are these positive facts shaken by the negative results of the investigations of Bernard,[†] who saw no change take place in the diameter of the pupil, either upon dividing the oculomotor nerve, or upon irritating its peripheral portion, in rabbits.— No other disturbances than those above-mentioned take place on irritating the oculo-motor nerve. The only fact which exhibits the influence of the intervening ganglion, is the comparative slowness of the contraction of the pupil.—Whether the oculo-motor nerve sends also some sensory filaments to the internal eye, cannot be ascertained.

The influence of the sympathetic nerve upon the pupil was discovered even before 1727, by Petit :[‡] after dividing the nervus vagus he found the pupil smaller. That Petit had correctly ascribed this phenomenon to the division of the sympathetic nerve, which, in many animals, is in the neck united with the nervus vagus, was proved by Dupuy,[§] who observed the same phenomenon after extirpation of the first ganglion. The accuracy of the fact was still further demonstrated by the careful experiments of Reid.[||] Budge and Waller[¶] have the merit of having shown, that the filaments of the sympathetic nerve acting on the pupil arise from the spinal cord, and pass into the anterior roots of the two inferior cervical, and the six· superior dorsal, nerves. In frogs and rabbits the contraction consequent on division of the nerve is slight (and in the last it is certainly not greater

---

* By Budge and Waller (*Archiv f. physiol. Heilk.* B. xi. p. 775), and by Duval, Rochart and Petit (*Gazette médicale de Paris*, 1852, p. 457).

† *Leçons sur la physiologie et la pathologie du système nerveux*, Paris, 1858, t. ii. pp. 207 and 209.

‡ Mémoire dans lequel il est démontré, que les nerfs intercostaux fournissent des rameaux qui se portent des esprits dans les yeux, in *Histoire de l'Académie royale des sciences*, Année 1727.

§ *Journal de médecine, de chirurgie*, etc. 1816, T. xxxvii. p. 340.

|| *Edinburgh Medical and Surgical Journal*, August, 1839 ; and *Physiological and Pathological Researches*, Edinburgh, 1841, p. 291.

¶ *Comptes rendus*, 1852, tomes xxxiv., xxxv., in different places.

when the first ganglion also is extirpated), in dogs it is very considerable; but the dilatation on irritation of the sympathetic nerve of the
neck, which, though it does not directly follow, rapidly attains its
maximum, is still the most striking phenomenon.—The difference of
the two pupils after division of the nerve is greatest while the eyes
are exposed only to faint light: where there is a strong action of the
sphincter muscle, the resistance even of the undiminished action of
the radiating fibres, at least in rabbits, is almost annihilated. The
difference in magnitude is, however, permanent; at least we have
seen it continue in dogs and rabbits longer than six months; Budge
has observed it even for a year.—Budge and Waller showed, that
after division of the nervus vagus and of the sympathetic in the
neck, in connexion with the difference in origin, of the former the
inferior part, of the latter the superior, pass into degeneration (fatty
metamorphosis). We have confirmed this in many cases, but in the
first ganglion itself, and in the efferent fasciculi, whose number seems
far to exceed that of the afferent, no change was met with. Irritation
of the ganglion then also still produces dilatation of the pupil after the
lapse of many weeks. If the first ganglion itself is extirpated, the
efferent bundles too pass into a state of degeneration, but then also
the ciliary nerves continue unchanged even into the iris, where we examined them many weeks after extirpation of the ganglion, which is
most probably due to the influence of the ciliary ganglion. Thus,
too, it is intelligible, that the extirpation of the first ganglion is not
followed by more contraction, than the division of the nerve below
the ganglion.

The foregoing shows that the action of the sympathetic root consists in a persistent exaltation of the tone of the radiating fibres.
Thus the dilatator pupillæ is with constant force the antagonist of the
sphincter muscle. The action of the sphincter changes, as we have
seen, both with the incidence of light and with accommodation; but
if the sphincter is paralysed, the pupil is immovable. Meanwhile we
may assume that, just as for the vaso-motor nerves, the tonic action
in the dilatator muscle may, under certain still unknown circumstances (irritation of the fifth pair?) somewhat fall and rise.—It has,
indeed, hypothetically been assumed that the sympathetic nerve
acts also upon the accommodation. Though it might appear somewhat rash absolutely to deny an influence, for which the analogy of
the iris may be appealed to, yet we find that it is supported by
no fact whatever. We are acquainted with no muscle capable of

2

acting antagonistically to the ciliary muscle; nor have we any reason to admit the existence of *active* accommodation for distance (compare p. 20). On the other hand, the action of the sympathetic branch on the tone of the blood-vessels is fully established. It is known that division of the sympathetic nerve in the neck is followed by considerable dilatation of the vessels of the head, most distinctly observable in the ears of rabbits, while irritation of that nerve is attended with contraction of the same vessels (Bernard). With Dr. van der Beke Callenfels,* I showed that the vessels of the pia mater are governed by the same nerve; and I subsequently satisfied myself, with Dr. Kuyper,† that the vessels of the iris also contract on irritation of the sympathetic nerve, even when they are distended under the influence of the instillation of digitaline or in consequence of discharge of the aqueous humour, or, as I recently found in conjunction with Mr. Hamer, when after the action of the Calabar bean, the same irritation scarcely makes the pupil dilate. This last confirms my opinion, that this contraction of the vessels cannot be the mechanical result of dilatation of the pupil, but that it occurs independently. Formerly, indeed, I was inclined to attribute the dilatation of the pupil attendant on irritation of the sympathetic nerve to the contraction of the vessels, as I supposed that the diminution of blood in the iris would at the same time lessen the contraction of the sphincter muscle. The phenomenon is, however, equally evident, when the circulation of the blood has already ceased, and the dilatation is moreover, too considerable, to be explained by the contraction of the vessels. We must, therefore, take refuge in contraction of the radiating fibres of the iris, which, as they are in some animals highly developed, can with certainty be demonstrated.

The *influence of the nervus trigeminus* upon the iris and upon the accommodation is still doubtful. By exclusion we may assume that this nerve gives sensation to the iris; for neither the oculo-motor nor the sympathetic possesses sensitive filaments by which the great sensibility of the iris might be explained. Moreover, sensation ceases when the nervus trigeminus is divided. The difficulty lies in the determination of the influence of the nervus trigeminus upon the motion of the iris. It has been found experimentally that irritation of the trunk of the fifth pair, as well as of its ophthalmic division

* *Nederlandsch Lancet*, 1855, D. iv. p. 689.

† *Onderzoekingen over de kunstmatige verwijding van den oogappel*, Diss. naug. 1859.

(the nervus ophthalmicus Willisii) causes the pupil to contract. Now we are acquainted with no other contractions of the pupil than those produced by the reflex action of light, and by accommodation, and these both wholly disappear on paralysis of the oculomotor nerve. The existence of a direct influence of the fifth pair upon the sphincter of the pupil (through motor-filaments) is therefore improbable. We are consequently led to assume that stimulation of the nervus trigeminus acts, both in its trunk and in its branches, upon the ciliary ganglion, so as there either to increase the action of the fibres of the oculo-motor, or to diminish that of the sympathetic nerve. The influence still takes place, if the sympathetic and oculo-motor nerves have previously been divided. This is, however, by no means strange, since the ciliary ganglion and the internal nervous system of the eye continue permanently normal after the sections alluded to, as is proved, with respect to the latter, by the unaltered action of atropia and of the Calabar bean dropped into the eye.

The mechanism, whereby the nervus trigeminus acts upon the ciliary ganglion is, however, rather obscure. Since this influence, as we have seen, continues after division of the oculo-motor and sympathetic nerves, it must be capable of taking place without reflexion in the central organs. Indeed, we can, from the fact that on stimulation of a nerve the change of the electrical condition is continued in both directions, very well comprehend the direct influence of a stimulus, without assuming in the nervus trigeminus the existence of fibres, whose ordinary function should be centrifugal conduction towards the ciliary ganglion. But if such exist (in the nervus lachrymalis centrifugally conducting fibres are undoubtedly present), the contraction of the pupil which occurs in an irritated state of the peripheral sensitive filaments of the eye, might be explained by reflex action, upon those centrifugally conducting fibres, in the Gasserian ganglion. At any rate, in an irritated condition of the cornea, to which the ciliary nerves are distributed, reflex action even in the ciliary ganglion may be assumed from analogy, as, with reference to the secretion of saliva, reflex action through the submaxillary ganglion has been demonstrated by Bernard.

The principal experiments on which the above view of the action of the nervus trigeminus upon the iris is based, are the following :—

a. After division of the n. trigeminus at the base of the skull, the pupil contracts in rabbits (in dogs ?) ; but this contraction often does not occur before the lapse of some minutes, and in a few days or hours for the most part disappears again (Longet, Budge). The same is true of frogs (Budge): also on division of the half of the medulla oblongata (Joh. Mueller).

b. On merely compressing the nervus ophthalmicus Willisii, Budge and Waller observed contraction of the pupil. Bernard observed the same after division of this nerve. The mobility of the pupil on the incidence of light is not impaired in this experiment, and if no inflammation of the eye ensues, the diameters of the two pupils are soon again nearly equal.

c. If the oculo-motor nerve be previously divided (Budge), or torn out (Bernard), contraction of the pupil nevertheless ensues, on division of the n. trigeminus.

d. Bernard (*l. c.* T. II. p. 90) tore the oculo-motor nerve at one side, whereupon the pupil became dilated, acquired, however, the same dilatation on both sides upon the instillation of extract of belladonna, and subsequently, upon dividing the n. trigeminus on the same side on which the oculo-motor nerve was torn, he saw the pupil contract.

e. In a young rabbit he divided the optic nerve, and all the motor nerves of the eye; even then stimulation of the fifth pair produced contraction of the pupil.

f. In another animal the first ganglion of the sympathetic nerve was removed, whereupon the pupil became small, with long vertical diameter; the nervus trigeminus having been then divided, the pupil became round, while the contraction increased.

In all that I had seen and read respecting the influence of division of the n. trigeminus, the doubt had occurred to me, whether this section did not act upon the pupil principally in consequence of the filaments of the sympathetic nerve being at the same time divided, which filaments, according to Budge, reach the ciliary, through the Gasserian ganglion. I therefore determined, in concert with Dr. P. O. Brondgeest, my assistant in the physiological laboratory, to make some experiments upon the subject. In rabbits the sympathetic nerve was exposed on one side of the neck, and was very gently stimulated for a moment (with the aid of the galvanic apparatus of du Bois-Reymond) in order to ascertain that the exposed nerve acted on the pupil; thereupon the skin was again closed with *serres fines*, and the trigeminus was divided on the same side, in the manner indicated by Bernard. If anæsthesia of the eye was obtained without further general disturbance, the sympathetic nerve was, after a shorter or longer interval, again stimulated, in order to see whether it had maintained its influence upon the pupil. The experiment succeeded in eleven rabbits. The following results were obtained, upon the bearing of which I need not further dwell.

1°. Division either of the Gasserian ganglion, or of the n. ophthalmicus Willisii produces constant contraction of the pupil, with longer vertical diameter. Even with imperfect anæsthesia of the surrounding parts of the eye, the contraction is still present, provided the cornea be insensible.

2°. The contraction diminishes within a few hours, but does not disappear, if irritation of the eye occurs, and if the blood-vessels of the iris are highly distended. The pupil then sometimes becomes angular.

3°. The contraction gives way to some dilatation when, even with complete anæsthesia, the eye being properly protected, the state of irritation is absent. Dr. Snellen (*De invloed der zenuwen op de ontsteking*, Utrecht, 1857) showed that the inflammation which is known to occur after division of the nervus trigeminus is the result of external injuries, which are not avoided owing to the existing anæsthesia, and that it can be prevented by systematic protection from all external injury.

4°. From comparative experiments on both sides, it appeared that the contraction is much greater on division of the n. trigeminus than on that of the sympathetic nerve in the neck, or on extirpation of the first ganglion.

5°. The tension of the eyeball remains at first the same, sometimes becomes even rather greater, while the pupil is very narrow, and the iris lies near the cornea. The tension, however, in a short time, regularly diminishes, and indeed in the highest degree, when the eye by proper protection remains free from irritation. This diminished tension is in accordance with my theory of glaucoma, as being originally neurosis of the nerves of secretion.

6°. After division and acquired anæsthesia, stimulation of the sympathetic nerve produced, in seven out of eleven cases, dilatation of the pupil, though in a much slighter degree than when the n. trigeminus is not divided. In four instances the dilatation of the pupil on stimulation of the sympathetic nerve was entirely absent. In all these cases the cornea was completely insensible. In three of the seven cases, in which dilatation followed stimulation of the sympathetic nerve, there was sensibility of the lower, and in one there was, in addition, sensibility of the upper, eyelid; in the three other cases there was no sensibility.

7°. In all cases, too, where the pupil continued immovable, the vessels of the ear contracted on stimulation of the sympathetic nerve, showing that the nerve was sensitive. Before the division of the trigeminus it was seen, that on stimulation simultaneous dilatation of the pupil and contraction of the vessels of the ear occurred.

8°. After division Calabar produces contraction, atropia, dilatation of the pupil,—the latter not in a high degree.

9°. Dissection showed that in general, the nervus ophthalmicus Willisii had been divided in front of the ganglion; sometimes also the second, and partly the third branch. In other cases the Gasserian ganglion itself was touched. It did not account satisfactorily for the cases in which little or no dilatation of the pupil occurred on stimulation of the sympathetic nerve.

CHAPTER XI.

PARALYSIS AND DEBILITY OF ACCOMMODATION.

§ 45. MYDRIATICS AND THEIR ACTION.

A COMPARATIVE examination of a number of substances and of preparations has shown, that the most useful mydriatics are to be found among the Solaneæ, and that of these the Atropa Belladonna is, for various reasons, to be preferred to all others, even to the Datura Stramonium and the Hyoscyamus niger.* Above all, where strong action is not required, atropia (soluble in 450 parts of water), and where a stronger effect is indicated, the very soluble sulphate of atropia, which were first introduced into practice in England, are to be recommended. For the full effect, a drop of a solution of one part of sulphate of atropia in 120 parts of water (we express this strength by 1 : 120), is quite sufficient.† The internal exhibition of the remedy also, with which it is necessary to be cautious, produces mydriasis.

The principal phenomena consequent on the instillation of sulphate of atropia, are : 1°, increasing dilatation, followed by insensibility of the pupil; 2°, diminution, and soon total loss of accommodation.

The dilatation of the pupil, considerable in man (especially in youth), the dog, and the cat, is less so in the rabbit, slight in birds, in whom it was formerly overlooked, very perceptible in frogs, and not at all, or scarcely so, in fishes. After the instillation of 1 : 120 the dilatation begins in man within fifteen minutes, and in the course of

---

* Compare Kuyper, *Onderzoekingen over de kunstmatige verwijding van den oogappel.* Diss. inaug. Utrecht, 1849.

† If the instillation is followed in the course of an hour and a-half by pain and injection of the vessels, the preparation is not suitable, and there then arises, on its repeated employment, a peculiar inflammation, described by me as atropinism. Even when suitable, it produces in some persons, after having been used for many months, a similar inflammation, and it must then be altogether laid aside. In such cases other mydriatics are then seldom borne. Chemical reagents were not decisive in distinguishing the inapplicable sulphate of atropia. Compare Kuyper, *l. c.*

from twenty to twenty-five minutes attains its maximum, with absolute immobility. The younger the individual, and the thinner the cornea is, the more rapidly does the action occur. In frogs and in birds the dilatation disappears within one or two hours, and gives place to a brief contraction. The course of the dilatation in man, after the instillation of 1 : 120, is represented by the line *d d* of Fig. 166, with the return to the normal diameter in 167. On the absciss *a a'* (Fig. 166) the minutes are indicated after the instillation, which

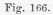

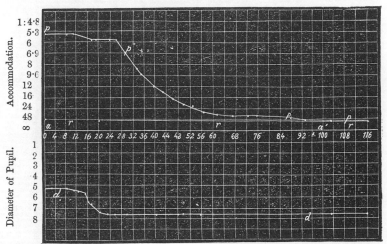

took place at 0, the lengths of the ordinates downwards perpendicular to *a a'*, are the transverse diameters of the pupil, to be read off in mm. before the line. The pupil was always accurately measured at short intervals, with the ophthalmometer, with perfectly equal illumination of the eye, the other being closed. Fig. 167, whose absciss marks in days the total duration of the change of the pupil, in like manner gives the diameters in the curve under *a a'*. The *diminution of the accommodation* commences somewhat later than the dilatation of the pupil. The accommodation gradually returns after some days, together with the mobility of the pupil. Fig. 166 indicates by the curve *p p*, the course of the absolute nearest point; by the curve *r r*, that of the farthest point. It will be seen that the latter undergoes scarcely any change; the nearest point, on the contrary, removes from the eye. This removal commences in from twelve to eighteen

minutes after the instillation, is in twenty-six minutes, when the dilatation is already nearly complete, still little remarkable; then rapidly,

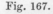

Fig. 167.

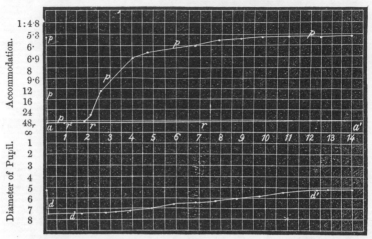

and subsequently slowly, proceeds, and attains its maximum in one
hundred and three minutes after the instillation, when p and r coincide and the accommodation is therefore wholly removed. When,
after forty-two hours, the pupil is somewhat smaller, a slight degree
of mobility has also returned, and, at the same time, some accommodation is to be observed, which now rather rapidly increases until
the fourth day, but is not perfect until after the lapse of eleven days.
The observation was made on the eye of my assistant, Mr. Hamer,
who has practised himself in very accurately determining his absolute
nearest point at the maximum of convergence, while one eye is closed
(compare p. 117).—Besides the results to be deduced from the
figures, we have still to remark :—

1°. After the return of the accommodation with the third and
following days, the relative range of accommodation has a position
similar to what it occupies in myopes : with moderate convergence,
only a very small fraction of the existing accommodation can be obtained. Thus, Mr. Hamer, on the sixth day found, that, while with
convergence to 9″ of his eye which had not been subjected to instillation, about the half of the total accommodation came into play, the
eye which had undergone the operation attained only a fifth of what

it was now again capable of at the maximum of convergence.   2°.
The farthest point has here, with a slight degree of M, continued
nearly unaltered.   Usually, it removes somewhat further from the
eye.   If there exists permanent tension of accommodation, such as
is proper to H, and not unfrequently occurs in some amblyopes, astigmatics and in young myopes, this gives way under the influence
of atropia, and r then removes to a much greater extent.   3°.   With
tension of accommodation, objects appear to become smaller (micropia) : in this case we imagine the object nearer, and as the visual
angle has not become greater, we suppose the object to be smaller.*

4°. To the eye which has undergone instillation, objects appear
much more strongly illuminated, especially when both eyes are at
the same time open, under which circumstances, in consequence of
consensual reflexion, the pupil of the eye not subjected to instillation
is narrower than usual.   The comparison is effected by looking at a
bright object upon a darker ground, a prismatic glass, with the
angle outwards, being brought before one of the eyes.

The loss of accommodation, after the action of atropia, is the
more troublesome, because the pupil is so extremely wide, which,
even in slight variation of accommodation, produces great circles
of diffusion; therefore for each distance different glasses are necessary for acute vision, affording scarcely any range.   The *disturbance*,
moreover, differs according to the *refraction of the eye*.   Emmetropes see well at a distance, but can distinguish nothing near without convex glasses.   Myopes complain less, because, although
their distant vision is much more diffuse, they can still often read,
their farthest point remaining unaltered.   In hypermetropes, even the
slightest action of the mydriatic produces such disturbance, that
without convex glasses nothing is distinguished.—If the mydriatic
have been dropped into only one eye, the disturbance is the greater,
because the defined image of the eye not operated on is so feebly
illuminated, compared with the diffuse image of the other: the
mydriatic eye is then by preference closed.   In atropia-mydriasis of
both eyes there is no difficulty in using convex glasses.

With respect to the action of *weaker solutions* of sulphate of
atropia, Dr. Kuyper has made some investigations.   His researches
have yielded the following results :—

a. The solution of 1 : 1800 produces good dilatation within 30

---

* I observed this phenomenon first in myself, and gave the above explanation of it in *Ned. Lancet*, 1851, D. vi. p. 607.

minutes; this attains its maximum, with complete immobility of the pupil, and generally with almost total annihilation of the power of accommodation, at the end of from 45 to 60 minutes. So early as on the following day, some mobility has returned. On the third day, no inconvenient disturbance remains, although two, three, or more days later, a difference in the diameters of the pupils is still perceptible.

b. The solution of 1 : 2400 produces dilatation after from 25 to 33 minutes; this attains almost the maximum (diameter = $8\frac{1}{4}$ mm.), after the lapse of from 45 to 50 minutes, without complete loss of mobility and accommodation; after 55 minutes, sometimes no mobility is perceptible: after 70 minutes, the power of accommodation is very much diminished, but by no means removed. Even in a few hours later, the dilatation again diminishes. The following day it is still distinctly perceptible; on the third day it is slight; it is not until the fourth day that it has wholly disappeared.

c. The solution of 1 : 9600 produces dilatation after 60 minutes, which slowly increases; after the lapse of 90 minutes, the pupil is perfectly dilated, but is not immovable; the power of accommodation is but little diminished. The following day the pupil is very movable, and is much smaller. On the third day there is no trace of mydriasis.

d. The solution of 1 : 14,400 causes commencing dilatation, after from 35 to 40 minutes; in from two to four hours the diameter of the pupil is 2 mm. greater; after the lapse of seven hours, contraction has again taken place, and on the following day no trace of mydriasis is perceptible.

The *mode of action* of mydriatics I have investigated with Dr. de Ruiter. Independently of our researches, von Graefe, as he stated to me by letter, had arrived at the same results. Our experiments have established beyond doubt the passage of atropia into the aqueous humour.

a. The action exhibits itself the more rapidly, the thinner the cornea, and the younger the animal is. Removal of the outermost layers of the cornea hastens the action (von Graefe). When some dilatation ensues upon inunction above the eye, a trace of the matter rubbed in may always have reached the organ. On strong action in the wounded skin (in dogs) some dilatation (the result of general action) rapidly sets in also on the other side. *b.* The application, confined to the cornea, in the eyes of frogs, after excision of the heart, after decapitation, after removal of the brain and spinal cord, and even after complete isolation of the eyes, produces distinct dilatation within a few minutes.   The same took place in a chopped-off calf's head, and in recently killed rabbits.   c. A trace of an extremely dilute solution, introduced by means of a capillary tube into the anterior chamber of the eye, produced dilatation in rabbits.   d. After repeated instillation in a rabbit, the whole eye was washed out with a broad jet of water : the aqueous humour then discharged, introduced into the eye of a dog, and long kept in contact with it (von Graefe also injected it into the chamber), produced considerable dilatation of the pupil.   This is incontestably the *experimentum crucis*.   The quantity which penetrated is, however, extremely small, for the solution of 1 : 120,000 kept equally long in contact with the cornea, acted still more strongly.   On internal administration and consequent mydriasis, the evacuated aqueous humour was inefficacious.

Lastly, the question is, through the intervention of *what nerves* the absorbed atropia acts.   In the first place, we cannot admit that the matter acts directly upon the muscular fibre-cells : the similar nature of these contractile elements in the sphincter and the dilator should then lead us to expect a similar influence upon both, and strong dilatation of the pupil could not take place.   We therefore infer that the atropia acts on the nerve fibres, or on the ganglionic cells.   *a. The sphincter muscle becomes paralytic :* reflex and accommodative movements are abolished ; and, moreover, paralysis of accommodation (of the m. ciliaris) ensues, which, however, remains much longer incomplete than that of the sphincter of the pupil.   Hence it follows, that the elements of the oculo-motor nerve are paralysed,—the more deeply-seated (of the ciliary muscle) being the last to be affected (an additional argument for the direct action of the atropia on the nerve-elements).   *b. The dilator muscle becomes strongly contracted*.   The proof consists in the fact that, as Ruete* was the first to show, in complete paralysis of the oculo-motor nerve, the size of the pupil is still considerably increased by atropia ; additional dilatation also occurs under atropia after removal of the nerve in question in animals.   To explain this we assume a stimulating action on the sympathetic nerve, which we can scarcely imagine to be persistent unless it takes place by the intervention of ganglionic

* *Klinische Beiträge z. Pathologie und Physiologie der Augen und Ohren.* Braunschweig, 1843, p. 250.

cells.   Of these it is known that they are specific in their action, and of
a condition of persistent stimulation by a given substance we have an
example in the action of strychnia brought into direct contact with the
grey substance of the spinal cord.*   After a powerful effect of atropia,
I saw still further dilatation of the pupil arise on stimulation of the
sympathetic nerve in the neck in rabbits, a proof that this nerve at
least is not paralysed.   If division of the sympathetic nerve have
previously taken place, the pupil on the same side is not so fully
dilated by atropia as that upon the other.   Biffi† and Cramer‡ saw
also in this phenomenon a proof of the stimulating action upon the
sympathetic nerve.   We cannot admit it to be such : the difference
between *normal* and increased action of the sympathetic nerve, as
opposed to paralysis of the oculo-motor nerve, may be sufficient to
explain the difference observed.

The influence of atropia on the n. trigeminus is probably nar-
cotising.   However, both in cases of paralysis in man, and after
the division of this nerve in the rabbit, the action of atropia is as
usual : if the pupil was, as in Dr. Snellen's case, originally wider
than in the other eye, it remained wider also after instillation in
both eyes ; if it was narrower, as in experiments on rabbits, it
remained narrower also upon instillation.

Respecting the influence upon the vaso-motor nerves of the iris,
nothing can with certainty be stated.

The ancients (Conf. Plinius, *Hist. Naturalis*, liber xxv. cap. 13) were
acquainted with the mydriatic action of some plants, and employed it in the
depression of cataract.   Such an action was ascribed especially to Anagallis,
which, however, has not been confirmed.   Of the influence of belladonna on
the pupil we find mention first made by van Swieten (*Comment. in Boerhavii
Aphorismos*, t. iii.) ; moreover, by Reimarus (conf. Dariès. *Diss. de Atropa
Belladonna*. Lipsiæ, 1776), Mellin, Ray and others ; and Loder (conf. Schi-
ferli, *Ueber den grauen Staar*, p. 85) employed the infusion in the extraction of cataract.   Karl Himly (*Gött. Gelehrte Anzeige*, 1800), who discovered
the mydriatic action of hyoscyamus, has, however, the merit of being the first
to make mydriatics in an extended sense available in ophthalmic surgery.
Almost at the same time Darwin (*Zoonomia*, iii. 132, London, 1801) sug-

---

* That Harley did not obtain this effect, is probably to be attributed to
the employment of too strong a solution (conf. Kölliker, *Verhandl. der
Gesellsch*.   Würzburg, B. ix. p. xvii.).

† *Intorno all'influenza che hanno sull'occhio i due nervi grandi sympathico
e vago*.   Pavia, 1846, p. 12.

‡ *Het accommodatie-vermogen*, 1853, p. 127.

gested the advantage to be derived therefrom in some forms of ophthalmia.—
The influence of mydriatics on the accommodation was not investigated until
a later period, and then, indeed, with wonderful accuracy, by Dr. Wells
(*Philosophical Transactions*, 1811, p. 378). In his experiments upon Dr.
Cutting, it appeared that the accommodation was wholly lost, and even
that the farthest point somewhat receded. In a couple of myopes, too,
diminution of accommodation with unaltered farthest point was established.
In connexion with the observation which we here find, that, on the passing
off of the effect, the diminution of the pupil and the increase of the range of
vision did not keep regular pace with each other (the occurrence of dilatation
before the loss of accommodation was unobserved), Brewster came to the
conclusion that, after the application of belladonna, another organ than
the iris must also be paralysed.—Numerous other investigations were communicated from many quarters, but contributed nothing essential beyond
what is comprised in the foregoing section. Only it still deserves to be
mentioned that, according to von Graefe, diminished tension of the fluids of
the eye might also be admitted as a result of the use of atropia, of the correctness of which view Dr. Schneller (*Archiv f. Ophthalmologie*, B. II.,
Abth. 2., p. 95.) thought he found a proof in the dilatation of the vessels of
the retina observed by him. I suggested a doubt whether, supposing that
the observation is correct, it indicates diminished tension (conf. Kuyper, *l. c.*).
The paralysis of the accommodation certainly could not explain this, for, even
if with accommodation temporary increased tension may arise, the relation
between absorption and secretion, just as we observe in consequence of
pressure with the finger on the eye, would immediately remove it by the
absorption of a little fluid. The tension of the eye depends upon the action
of the secretory nerves, and these lie in the path of the n. trigeminus, the
division of which, as numerous experiments have shown me, considerably
lessens the tension of the eye. We should thus, *à priori*, think it possible
that atropia, by paralysing these nerves, should diminish the tension, but I
have never been able with certainty to satisfy myself of it.

§ 46. MORBID PARALYSIS OF ACCOMMODATION.

Paralysis of accommodation as disease is by no means an
unusual occurrence. Emmetropic and ametropic eyes are alike
liable to it. It occurs too at every age, but in old persons, who
have already lost their accommodation by senile changes, it is of
little importance. As we know, that the accommodation is effected
exclusively by the internal muscles of the eye, we can seek paralysis
also only in the fibres of the short root of the ciliary ganglion.
Now, in fact, it often occurs that only these fibres are paralysed,
and in this case we have paralysis of accommodation alone: except
that paralysis of the sphincter pupillæ, which derives its motor fibres

from the same root, is usually combined therewith. But in about an equal number of cases there exists at the same time paralysis of other fibres of the oculo-motor nerve, and not unfrequently the paralysis extends even to all the branches of this nerve. It is remarkable, that while paralysis of accommodation very often occurs separately, paralysis in the domain of the oculo-motor nerve is comparatively rarely met with, without paralysis of accommodation. I may add, that so far as my experience goes, uncomplicated paralysis of accommodation occurs much more frequently in women, often too in children ; paralysis of the oculo-motor nerve on the contrary, including paralysis of the accommodation, is much more frequently found in men, and ordinarily not until after the twenty-fifth year. In either case, the paralysis is rarely complete : generally speaking, it is only paresis, inasmuch as a certain, though usually only a slight degree of accommodation, has remained.

Uncomplicated paralysis of accommodation has only one objective symptom : dilatation and immobility of the pupil. The dilatation is not considerable ; for even with complete paralysis, a wider pupil than the normal in the dark is not to be expected. Nevertheless, in complete paralysis not a trace of either accommodative or of reflex movement is to be seen. But I may add, that these cases are extremely rare. Further, the connexion between paralysis of the pupil and of accommodation cannot be called absolute : once I found satisfactory accommodation still coexistent with absolute immobility of the pupil. In one instance too, paralysis of accommodation disappeared without a return of the mobility of the pupil,—and, on the other hand, with perfect or almost perfect loss of accommodation, the motion of the pupil may be but little disturbed.

From all this it is evident, that the *subjective* phenomena are the most important. Now, upon these the refraction of the eye has a considerable influence.

Myopes, whose farthest point is not more than 14″ from the eye, find no difficulty in reading, for this point remains unchanged, and although their nearest point then coincides with it, they see, with unalterable refraction, perfectly acutely at the distance of 14″ or less. The disturbance is confined to this, that on the one hand, objects at a greater distance appear, on account of the greater circles of diffusion of the larger pupil, more diffuse than usual,—on the other, that within the distance of their combined nearest and farthest point, they cease to see acutely. Both disadvantages are in great part removed when the paralysis of accommodation is incomplete, and we then hear few complaints from myopes. It is only when they wear neutralising spectacles, and use them at their work, that they are on a footing with

Emmetropes.—These, on the occurrence of paralysis of accommodation, immediately resort to the oculist. They can no longer read nor write, and they are aware that an important disturbance exists : even when, as is usual, only one eye is affected, a certain dimness is, on account of the acute origin of the paralysis, forthwith observed, causing each eye to be separately tried, and thus the lesion is discovered. If we find that vision at a distance is acute, and with either concave or convex glasses becomes diffuse, while for near objects convex glasses are necessary, the diagnosis is made, which finds only a still further confirmation in the torpidity of the dilated pupil.

The paralysis of accommodation is productive of yet greater disturbance in *Hypermetropes :* not only for near, but also for distant objects, with respect to which an involuntary accommodation formerly easily overcame their hypermetropia, is their vision diffuse. It is evident, that such a condition suggests the idea of amblyopia, and I have already (p. 286) communicated a case in which the patient's father, himself a medical man, feared the worst. By attending to the direction, in any disturbance of vision, systematically to define with glasses the refraction, and the acuteness of sight in distant vision (compare § 9), we shall be sure to avoid error : amblyopia is thereby forthwith excluded, and while the glasses required for distant vision are insufficient for seeing near objects, the paralysis of accommodation is recognised.

The phenomena are less characteristic when no complete paralysis, but only paresis is present. The myope then often experiences no actual disturbance; the emmetrope complains of fatigue only on tension for near objects, resembling the asthenopia of the hypermetrope (compare Chap. V., p. 287) ; but the hypermetrope very rapidly experiences considerable asthenopia for near objects, and even difficulty in seeing acutely at a distance. In general with paresis of accommodation, asthenopia very quickly occurs; in the first place, because the wider pupil requires more accurate accommodation to distinguish satisfactorily ; in the second place, because, just as in atropia-paresis, the relative range of accommodation is very unfavourably situated : while with the maximum convergence, the closest point is found

38

comparatively little farther from the eye, with medium convergence, only a slight tension of accommodation appears to be possible.— Sometimes in paresis of accommodation micropia is also complained of ;* the explanation of which is given above (p. 586).

The foregoing refers more particularly to the uncomplicated paralysis of accommodation. Often, however, this is, as we have seen, only *a part of a more general morbid condition*, and most frequently of *paralysis of the oculo-motor nerve*. If this is complete the upper eyelid hangs, and the outer angle of the slit even stands considerably lower than that of the other side (compare Fig. 168, taken from a photograph)—a proof that the (now paralysed) elevator of the upper eyelid is also the elevator of the conjoined lower lid. A very slight upward movement of the eyelid remains, in consequence of the fact that, on endeavouring to raise it, the musculus orbicularis palpebrarum, which is governed by the facial nerve, can relax itself still more : the latter muscle remains in any case capable of strong contraction. If we raise the paralysed eyelid, we find the cornea deviated outwards (Fig. 169), and on looking to the opposite side it

Fig. 168. Fig. 169.

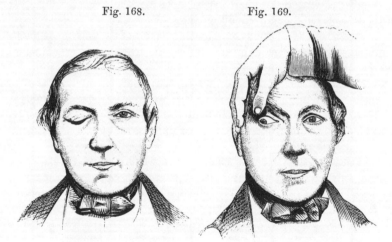

scarcely reaches the middle of the slit (paralysis musculi recti interni). On endeavouring to look upwards, the paralysed eye remains unaltered in its place (paralysis mm. recti superioris et obliqui inferioris). On endeavouring to look downwards, the m. obliquus superior,

* Demours in particular (*Traité des maladies des yeux*, T. i. p. 444) has remarked this. Compare also Duval, *Ann. d'Oculist*, T. xxiii. p. 154.

which is governed by the n. trochlearis, alone acts, and this, especially when the eye is turned outwards, produces a slight inward rotation around the visual axis rather than a downward movement of this axis.* With these phenomena a misapprehension of the position, and an apparent movement of the objects, on every attempt at movement of the eye, are combined—the first dependent on an incorrect estimation of the position of the eye, the second on the loss of adequate correspondence between the attempt at movement voluntarily made and the real movement of the field of vision on the retina. The complaint of vertigo is thus explained.—In other cases only a part of the muscles, influenced by the third pair, is implicated in the paralysis; sometimes the m. levator palpebræ superioris, which does not readily remain wholly free, and also very easily shows the disturbance, alone is affected, sometimes the m. rectus internus; very seldom the m. obliquus inferior is implicated, notwithstanding that it is precisely the branch destined for this muscle, which gives off the short root of the ciliary ganglion, of which wholly uncomplicated paralysis very often occurs.—Not unfrequently, too, in both eyes, different muscles governed by the third pair are at the same time or consecutively, more or less paralysed, whether with the accommodation or not.—Further, we observe that the fourth and sixth pairs are also affected (I have even seen a case in which only the musculus rectus externus and the

---

* The rotation mentioned here, was observed and analysed by me in a case described in the *Nederlandsch Lancet*, 1850, D. vi. p. 425. Compare also Ruete, *Klinische Beiträge*, p. 242. It demands some explanation here. In the movements of the visual axis directly upwards and downwards, as well as in those to both sides in a horizontal plane, the vertical meridians of the primary position remain perfectly vertical, as appears from the coincidence of the secondary images of a vertical coloured ribbon with the images of other vertical lines, so that in the last case the eye rotates round a vertical, in the first, round a horizontal, axis. To make this possible, the m. rectus superior and the m. obliquus inferior must in the movement upwards assist each other in the rotation around the horizontal axis, and in the rotation around the visual axis they must neutralise one another; the same is true of the m. rectus inferior and the m. obliquus superior in looking downward. This explains the effect, observed in paralysis of the oculo-motor nerve, of the m. obliquus superior, governed by the n. trochlearis, on an effort to look downward, the musculus rectus inferior being paralysed. Compare Ruete, *Das Ophthalmotrop*, 1846, p. 9, and F. C. Donders, Beitrag zur Lehre von den Bewegungen des menschlichen Auges in *Holländische Beiträge zu den anatomischen und physiologischen Wissenschaften*, 1846, B. i. pp. 105, *et seq.*

2

accommodation were paralysed) ; and occasionally, too, paræsthesia exists in some branches of the fifth pair.—Lastly, the paralysis of accommodation is wholly subordinate to that of different parts of the body, and then depends upon disturbance of the central organs. Under all these combinations, however, the disturbance connected with paralysis of accommodation continues of the same kind.

. On what morbid alteration the paralysis of accommodation depends, is often obscure. Experience shows that in sudden changes of temperature, particularly on exposure to storms or draughts of air, paralysis of the motor nerves of the eye, sometimes of a single nerve or of particular branches, not unfrequently occurs. When the days are extremely warm, and the evenings cool, a larger number of cases of this paralysis is in general met with. Such cases are called rheumatic, and are referred by some to an inflammatory affection of the nerve-sheath. The paralysis in these cases occurs suddenly ; often it is observed on awaking in the morning. We may hope that after some weeks or months it will again give way, but at the end of six months such hope must be abandoned. If the other eye also subsequently becomes affected, as I have often seen it, the idea of constitutional predisposition is naturally suggested ; but for this view there is frequently no ground.—Only, syphilis is recognised as a constitutional cause, and, if mercurials are used, it may produce paralysis even many years after infection. Under such circumstances the paralysis is rarely limited to the accommodation. The seat is especially considered to be central, when both sides are affected ; by periostitis, by peculiar tumours of the nerves, perhaps also by inflammation of the nerves, syphilis may produce paralysis. Usually, however, nothing of these morbid changes is apparent during life. The prognosis is in such instances less favourable.—Moreover, we find cases recorded in which injury, abscesses in the orbit, tumours in the cranial cavity, and different morbid changes in the brain were in operation, and credulous people have admitted hysteria and hypochondriasis into the list of causes.

On the subject of treatment we may be brief. The so-called rheumatic paralysis often gives way spontaneously, most frequently after two or three months. It is pretty generally the custom, under such circumstances, to apply an ointment with Veratria around the eye, and to give secale cornutum internally, and in this respect I myself follow the example of others ; but it is very hard to satisfy one's self by comparative observation that this plan is attended with any benefit.

The myosis, which is the result of the employment of Calabar, even in paralysis of the oculo-motor nerve, may in every case produce symptomatic improvement. How far this remedy is otherwise indicated, further experience must decide (compare the close of § 48 on Myosis and Myotics). On the supposition of the existence of constitutional syphilis, an antisyphilitic treatment is often tried, and the preference is generally given to a short course of inunction, which, however, as every other treatment, is frequently unattended with any marked result.—Where the nervous system is more generally implicated, regimen and treatment are directed to that condition, without special attention to the paralysis of accommodation.

Respecting the use of spectacles in paralysis of accommodation, it is almost sufficient to observe, that there is scarcely ever any objection to bringing the point of distinct vision to the distance which the existing acuteness of vision and the nature of the work to be performed render desirable. Sometimes, however, especially when the paralysis is incomplete, we give weaker glasses, so that the tension required ensures practice of accommodation. But if asthenopia then occurs, we do not withhold stronger glasses. Whether in paralysis of accommodation of one eye the assistance of a convex glass is to be afforded, must be judged from what has been said as to the use of glasses in difference of refraction of the two eyes (compare § 42). We should bear in mind, that in the stationary refraction of the one eye, the same glass can in this case be useful only for a given distance.

The principal objective phenomenon of paralysis of accommodation—the wide, immovable pupil—was the first to attract attention, and was designated by the ancients under the term *mydriasis*. But a dilated pupil being a symptom of amaurosis, the disturbance of vision in simple paralysis of accommodation was also looked upon as a slight degree of amblyopia, or was ascribed to the excess of incident light. Even in our own day this error is not unusual. It was in fact incredibly long, before ophthalmologists in general had a sufficiently correct idea of accommodation properly to comprehend its deviations. And this in spite of the excellent example of Dr. Wells (*Philosophical Transactions*, vol. ci., p. 378, London, 1811), who, in 1811, correctly recognised and understood a case of paralysis of accommodation, and terminated his description with the following pregnant words :—" From these circumstances it was plain that this gentleman, at the same time that his pupils had become dilated, and his upper eyelids paralytic, had acquired the sight of an old man, by losing suddenly the command of the muscles, by which the eye is enabled to see near objects distinctly ; it being known to those who are conversant with the facts relating to human vision, that the eye, in its relaxed state, is fitted for distant objects, and that the seeing of near objects accurately is dependent upon muscular exertion." Now, as Ruete states, we find mention made by some writers, as E. Home, Sichel, and Canstatt, in cases of paralysis of the oculo-motor nerve, of diminished accommodation for near objects; but still we miss the accurate determination, and, in general, any correct idea of the state of the case. James Hunter (*Edinburgh Medical and Surgical Journal*, Jan. 1840, p. 124) even thinks that a case of mydriasis occurring suddenly in a child, in which near objects could be distinguished only with the aid of convex spectacles ($\frac{1}{5}$), must be ascribed to spasm. With reference to this case, Himly (*l. c.*, B. 2, p. 481) proposes the question, whether paralysis should not rather produce presbyopia, and, in fact, he describes paresis of accommodation under the name of suddenly-occurring presbyopia. In like manner, what was described by von Walther (*Journal* von Graefe *und* Walther, B. iii. p. 22), as amaurosis ciliaris; by Sichel (*Ann. d'oculist.*, 1853) as amblyopie presbytique, might also be nothing else than paresis of accommodation. Meanwhile Ruete (*l. c.* 1843, p. 246) treated in detail of the influence of paralysis of the third pair upon the accommodation; but, as in the three cases which he happened to meet with, scarcely any disturbance existed, he thought that no very great influence upon the accommodation is to be attributed to this nerve.

Thus ignorance or doubt remained. I know not who was the first to suggest clearer and correct ideas. But it seems as if these were included in the discovery of the principle of accommodation, and on that discovery, as it were, spontaneously came to light in different quarters, although Cramer, who discovered that principle himself, was still deceived as to the nervous influence in accommodation. A more accurate observation of the cases which presented themselves certainly proceeded from the introduction of the determination of the range of accommodation.

Mydriasis, as a symptom of blindness, almost always depending on a cerebral cause, does not belong to my subject. With respect to mydriasis, independent of paresis of accommodation, I might probably also be silent. I believe, in fact, that in the great majority of cases, either the paresis of accommodation was overlooked, or the existence of mydriasis was lightly assumed. Certainly it has not been sufficiently kept in view, that young children usually have large pupils, and thus all sorts of causes have been called upon, but especially the presence of worms, to explain a phenomenon which, in childhood, needed no explanation. Accurate determinations of the size of the pupil, the light being the same, may in each case be required: in my own investigations, in which the measurement was effected with the ophthalmometer, I was struck with the great similarity of the pupil in the same individuals at different times, the illumination and the accommodation only being equal. Moreover, cases are communicated in which, with a general tendency to spasm, with anæsthesia, also with irritation of the fifth pair, there was a particularly wide pupil, but respecting the accommodation nothing is here noted. A remarkable case, with irregular, almost whimsical, sometimes periodically recurrent, mydriasis, for a time alternating in the two eyes, with accompanying paresis of accommodation, is recorded by von Graefe (*Archiv f. Ophthalmologie*, B. iii., H. 2, p. 359). In this instance the power of vision was permanently disturbed, and probably a cerebral affection was at the bottom of it. Von Graefe says he has also observed mydriasis to be a precursor of mania.—That an irritated condition of the sympathetic nerve in the neck (irritation of the abdominal portion in animals does not produce mydriasis) might lead to uncomplicated mydriasis, without any influence on the accommodation, is, *à priori*, very probable; but the cases in which the occurrence thereof should be proved are almost wholly wanting in literature, and in nature I have so far not met with them.

§ 47. Paresis of Accommodation after Diphtheria faucium and weakening of Accommodation.

For some years past a malignant disease, known by the name of *diphtheria faucium*, or *angina diphtheritica* (better *diphtherina*), has prevailed in certain countries of Europe. In the commencement of 1860 it began to manifest itself in several places in the Netherlands, where it is still prevalent, and even in the course of the past year carried many to the grave.* In France and elsewhere, different forms of paralysis had been observed, as sequelæ of this diphtheria. Among these mention had been made of disturbance of vision, but without just appreciation of its nature.† Soon after the occurrence of the disease, cases presented themselves to me, to the connexion of which with the angina in question I was led by a particular circumstance. It immediately appeared to me, that what was considered as disturbance in the function of the retina, was a simple paresis of accommodation; and I subsequently had opportunities of satisfying myself of the correctness of this view in a great number of patients.

* See the Reports in the *Nederlandsch Tijdschrift voor Geneeskunde*, 1863.

† Mention had already been incidentally made of paralysis after diphtheria, by Bretonneau, Trousseau and Blache, and a detailed description of a case observed by him, with a brief report of six others, was given by Faure (*L'Union Méd.*, Nos. 15 and 16, 1857). Although general paralytic symptoms are the most prominent, mention is made also of paralysis of the palate and of "weakness of sight," once too of strabismus. Cases are given also by Richard and by Mayer (conf. Eisenmann, *Canstatt's Jahresbericht*, 1858), in which mention is made of disturbance of vision.—Since my own investigations, confirmatory observations have reached me from various quarters.

The following is a history of the course of my observations on this subject :—*

1. Miss D., aged 26, applied to me on the 22nd of May, 1860, complaining of disturbance of vision. On examination, it was found that this disturbance depended on diminution of the power of accommodation. Remote objects were seen quite acutely, and were rendered diffuse both by convex and concave glasses: emmetropia, therefore, existed. The distance P of the *nearest point* (at 26 years of age, with normal range of accommodation of the emmetropic eye = from $4\frac{1}{2}$ to 5 Parisian inches) was reduced for the right eye to about 24″, for the left to 12″. With glasses of $\frac{1}{24}$, R was for the right eye = 12″; for the left R was = 8″. The pupils were wider than usual, particularly the right one; the reflex movement was tolerably good, the accommodative movement, particularly in the right eye, was very limited.

Rather more than five weeks previously the patient, then lodging at Bennekom, had suffered from inflammation of the throat. Having returned to Utrecht, she for the first time remarked, about fourteen days before, that she could no longer see near objects acutely. She could read only a few lines, and that not unless at a comparatively great distance; thereupon everything ran together; the letters were unrecognisable; the lines appeared to be strokes; the eyes were as if fatigued.

These symptoms resemble those of *asthenopia*. But there was no manifest hypermetropia; and with atropia-paralysis scarcely Hm $\frac{1}{60}$ appeared, which is usual with emmetropic eyes. We had, therefore, not to do with ordinary asthenopia. Indeed, both the history of the case and the present symptoms were opposed to the affection being of that nature. As to the first,—the disturbance had occurred suddenly, at least within a few days, without any particular fatigue having been remarked before, even on continued work. In *asthenopia from hypermetropia*, on the contrary, the troublesome symptoms come on either very slowly, at first apparently periodically, or after particularly weakening causes. And as to the symptoms : the nearest point was too far from the eye ; reading, &c., was, even on the first attempt, too difficult ; rest of the eye was attended with too little temporary improvement. Moreover, the peculiar feeling of pressure in the forehead, which brings the hand involuntarily to that part, was wanting ; while, on the other hand, the wide and, in accommodation, too slightly movable pupils, pointed directly to paresis.

The cause of this paresis was meanwhile obscure. In children,

* The particulars have been given in detail by me in the *Archiv für die Holländische Beiträge zur Natur. und Heilkunde*, published by F. C. Donders and W. Berlin. B. 10, 1861.

according to my experience, loss or diminution of the accommodation, without paresis of the muscles of the eye, in both eyes alike, does not occur so rarely, and usually gets well within two or three months : the cause then remains quite unknown, and recovery ensues without anything particular having been done. In adults this is quite different : paralysis of accommodation *in both eyes together* is in such persons a very unusual occurrence, certainly still rarer without further paralysis of the muscles of the eye and eyelids. I was therefore unable to give any certain prognosis from experience. The prognosis, however, could not be favourable, inasmuch as the simultaneous occurrence of the affection on both sides led me to suspect the existence of a central cause, to which dulness in the head, slight attacks of vertigo, and sometimes even violent headache, gave still further support. Derivation by the intestinal canal, pediluvia, stimulating frictions in the frontal region, were prescribed, and rest was recommended. Subsequently glasses of $\frac{1}{16}$ were permitted for near objects, by which all difficulty for close vision was removed.

In examining this patient, *a peculiar lesion of speech* did not escape me. I suspected that it must have depended on a congenital defect. Through motives of delicacy I was unwilling to ask the patient directly about it ; nor did she allude to it.

II. About a fortnight after, a youth named R., aged 15, of fair complexion, pale, and rather slight, was brought to me. His complaints were in all respects the same as those of Miss D. The power of vision was, however, still more limited : at a distance he saw acutely ; as for near objects, on the contrary, he could absolutely not read ordinary type. The closest point of distinct vision could not be directly determined ; with glasses of $\frac{1}{8}$ it lay at 7″. The pupils were large, reflex motion was slight, accommodative movement was scarcely perceptible.

It struck me that in this boy there was a lesion of speech similar to that in the case of Miss D. He, too, had suffered from sore throat. Moreover, he came from Ede, a village in the immediate neighbourhood of Bennekom. Still more : I heard that in the same Bennekom several other people, who had likewise suffered from inflammation of the throat, presented both disturbance of vision and difficulty of speech. This fact appeared to me to be truly important.

In R., I now, in the first place, investigated everything which had reference to the modification of the voice and speech. The disturbance had in this boy remained directly after the inflammation of the throat ; in Miss D. it had not, as I subsequently ascertained, been developed until some time after the sore throat had given way.

The mucous membrane of the mouth and throat was normal, rather pale than red; the tonsils were scarcely swollen. *The uvula, however, was extremely long and was absolutely immovable.*—If we look at the palate in the normal state, the tongue being a little depressed and the nose closed, so that respiration must take place through the widely-opened mouth, the palate becomes retracted, and the uvula is at the same time usually short-ened and elongated alternately. On an effort at swallowing, which mechanism succeeds best in this position when the lower jaw is steadily fixed, the soft palate ascends still more, the arches contract, and the first time at least the uvula is simultaneously retracted. About the same is observed on every effort to speak: it is best to make the patient utter the sound *a* (as in art), which is very possible with wide-opened mouth and depressed tongue. Still greater are the contraction of the arches and the elevation of the palate, with retraction of the uvula in the commencement of the vomiting movement, which occurs on tickling the pharynx with a fine feather. Now, in all these experiments the uvula of our patient remained equally long and immovable, the ascent of the palate was very limited, and the pharyngo-staphyline arches approached each other but slightly. Evidently, therefore, the azygos uvulæ was paralysed, and the other muscles of the palate were more or less affected by paralysis.

With respect to speech, a double abnormity presented itself, namely, *speaking through the nose*, and the accompaniment of many sounds with a *rattling or snoring accessory sound*. The rattling sound was evidently dependent on a quivering of the uvula which had come into contact with the root of the tongue, and it was strongly heard with particular consonants, as well as with the vowel *a* (as in able).

The speaking through the nose was in itself a proof that, in consequence of the paresis of the soft palate, the nasal cavity was not closed. The nasal sound was most strongly heard in the pronunciation of *o*; but with all vowels it existed more or less, and it was also audible with all the soft con-sonants. (I use here the terms employed by Dr. R. Lepsius. *Standard Alphabet*, etc. London, 1855.) Moreover, the communication with the nose in the pronunciation of each vowel was shown by the movement imparted to the down of fine feathers, when this was kept under the nostrils upon a sheet of paper held against the upper lip. Also, in the compression of the alæ nasi, the slight descent of the tone in each sound, as well as the increase of the nasal sound was distinctly established. Lastly, the impeded or retarded movement of the palate appeared from the impossibility of giving a soft pro-nunciation to the explosive consonants. These consonants are uttered by closing the opened, or opening the closed, mouth. On closing between the lips, *p* is uttered; on closing between the anterior part of the tongue and the anterior part of the hard palate, *t* is pronounced; on closure between the more posterior parts of the tongue and palate, *k* is expressed. If at the same time we make the voice ring, *p*, *t*, and *k* give way to the soft con-sonants *b*, *d*, and *g* (as in game). Now, to produce these sounds, the nose must be shut off from the throat. If this separation be wanting, we produce, instead of *b*, *d*, and *g*, the resonants *m*, *n*, and *ng*. This appeared to be actually the case in our boy: a soft explosive consonant at the end of the word gave way to the corresponding resonant. English words, whose explosive sounds are expressed also at the ends of the words with a ringing voice, best illustrate this,—for example, *rub, head,* and *egg.* Now, if R. tried to pronounce these words well, he invariably said *rum, hen,* and *eng ;* or, *rump, hent,* and *enk.* Even after having heard how much these sounds differed from the required, *rup, het,* and *ek* were sometimes elicited. But it was only necessary to impress upon him that the final consonant should be expressed with a ringing voice, and then it again became each time, *rum, hen,* and *eng.* If the soft explosive consonants were not at the end of the words, their sound was characteristically heard, but yet it began with the resonant; band was pronounced *m*band, door as *n*door, give as *ng*give. On the contrary, scarcely any deviation was perceptible in the pronunciation of the hard non-ringing explosive consonants, *p, t,* and *k.**

---

* I formerly paid much attention to the subject of articulation, and was therefore in a position to observe accurately the phenomena connected with that function. They often give the first indication to the oculist. I may therefore be allowed here briefly to explain them. When after a vowel, pronounced through the nose, the soft explosive consonant is to follow, the nose must be completely separated from the throat, at the same moment as the cavity of the mouth between the lips (with *b*), or between the tongue and palate (with *d* and *g*) is closed. If the separation does not take place at the same time, we hear the resonants *m, n* and *ng,* in place of the explosive consonants *b, d,* and *g.* For the mechanism is precisely the same for both, except that in the resonants there is a continuity between the cavity of the nose and that of the throat, which is wanting in the explosive consonants. Now if there be paresis of the palate, in the articulation of the vowels the nose is not completely closed, and it is evident, that on the effort immediately after to produce a soft ringing explosive consonant, the complete closing follows either not at all, or at least too late. Instead of *rub, head,* and *egg,* we therefore hear in our patient, *rum, hen,* and *eng.* On increased exertion they become *rump, hent, enk* (properly *engk*—for the *n* before *k* is always *ng*) : the hard explosive consonant is added. The mechanism of this last, in fact, presents no difficulty. After the sound of the voice has ceased, the closing of the mouth needs only to be interrupted by some impulse of air, to make the hard explosive consonants heard. The nose indeed remains open, but the sound of an explosive consonant is with a non-ringing voice much stronger than that of a resonant, and therefore we hear the first distinctly, the latter not so. Hence it will be understood that our patient had no difficulty in producing *rup, het,* and *ek.* For this the voice needed only to be brought to silence immediately after the vowel, then the resonant was not heard, and the interruption of the closing of the mouth caused the hard explosive consonant to be heard. If it be asked, lastly, why the soft explosive consonants could be produced better at the beginning of a word than at the end, the answer is simply that in that case the closing of the cavity of the mouth and the removal of the continuity of the cavities of the throat and nose needed not to take place precisely at the same moment. In pronouncing *band, door,* &c., the cavity of the mouth was first closed and, before the voice

The semiparalytic condition of the palate led me to suppose, that swallowing also would not take place regularly. When questioned on the subject, the patient stated, too, that he could swallow solid food only with great effort, and that in drinking he was obliged to proceed slowly and cautiously. Fluids passed very readily into the nose, and that usually gave rise to regurgitation into the larynx, and, consequently, to cough.

So much, as yet, with respect to the boy R.

Soon after I had an opportunity of again seeing Miss D. *The agreement of the phenomena relating to the palate, speech, and deglutition*, with everything noted above respecting R., was striking. The rattling accessory sound was, however, less, and she complained more of the secretion of viscid mucus in the throat, which there was much difficulty in removing.

The two cases here described kept up my interest. There could, it seemed to me, be no doubt as to the connexion between the paralytic symptoms and the preceding inflammation\ of the throat. Further investigation appeared, however, desirable, and I therefore repaired to Bennekom, where the physicians, Dr. Thomas and Mr. Ketting, with the greatest readiness, gave me all the information I requested; they also afforded me the opportunity of examining some other patients, in whom secondary paralytic symptoms had manifested themselves. The first four cases had proved fatal in the acute stage of the disease.

III. I saw in the first place (on the 10th of June) a girl aged 17, who had been attacked on the 7th of April, and after the separation of considerable gangrenous spots, appeared within a fortnight to have recovered. I heard that immediately after the inflammation of the throat, a slight lesion of speech seemed to exist, but that it nevertheless had not become considerable until a fortnight later, that then for the first time the rattling sound was heard, and the nasal tone of the voice had become really distinct. Moreover, that about a week after the termination of the disease, difficulty in reading was for the first time observed. This symptom also soon increased; the patient had always, however, been able to read some lines. During the month of May the symptoms connected with speech and sight remained almost unchanged. In the commencement of

---

was heard, a powerful effort was made to close the palate by the way to the nose. If this in great part succeeded, a sound was heard, which held the medium between the explosive consonant and the resonant, or, rather, because the closing still went on during the sound of the voice, it was as if the explosive sound was preceded by a resonant: *m*band, *n*door, &c. It needs no proof that, if the continuity had remained equally free, at the beginning of the words also, in place of the explosive consonant, only the resonant would have been heard.

June evident improvement took place. At the time of my visit, on the 10th of June, the movements of the palate were normal ; a rattling accessory sound of the voice was no longer audible. Yet the nasal tone was usually still perceptible in the pronunciation of the vowels ; *rub*, *head*, and *egg* were still heard as *rump*, *hent*, and *engk* ; sometimes *rub* was well pronounced ; *head*, never ; *be* sounded almost always as *pe* ; if the nose was held close externally, she could say *be*, *de*, and *ge* better.—The power of accommodation was still far from having attained its normal range. Myopia existed about $= \frac{1}{40}$. The nearest point still lay, however, at 6″. The range of accommodation, therefore, amounted to $\frac{1}{6} - \frac{1}{40} =$ rather more than $\frac{1}{7}$; it ought, at the patient's age, to have amounted to more than $\frac{1}{4}$, and was consequently reduced by about one-half. There still also existed difficulty in continuing reading and fine work. On the whole, the symptoms were similar to those of ordinary asthenopia,—they were only so far different that reading was much easier when the book was held somewhat further off. Reflex and accommodative movements of the pupil were little disturbed.—After my visit the improvement steadily progressed. On the 7th of September I received from Mr. Ketting the following report :—G. v. N. again sees perfectly well ; the pronunciation of *rub*, *head*, and *egg*, cannot yet, however, be called quite perfect. Strengthening regimen and treatment.

Respecting Miss D., (the patient of I.), I learned here that she came under treatment on the 15th of April, that the symptoms were in every respect moderate : there was little pain in the throat, there was but slight fœtor, nor was there much swelling ;—that, nevertheless, diphtheritic spots had appeared in the throat, that in this case also mineral acids were employed, whereupon separation had ensued, and the patient rapidly recovered. In the beginning of the month of May she returned to Utrecht. It has above (p. 599) been stated at length how, some time subsequently, loss of the power of accommodation and lesion of speech and deglutition had appeared. In this, however, improvement gradually occurred. I saw her on the first of September. The rattling sound had quite disappeared ; the uvula was easily moved ; deglutition was normally performed. The vowels had still a weakly nasal sound ; the tone changed a little on closing the nose externally. *Rub* and *head* were still often heard as *rumb* and *hend* ; *egg* was better pronounced.—The accommodative power had returned : on accurate optometric investigation the nearest point was found for both eyes at 5″, for the right eye at 5·1″, for the left, at 5·3″. Nor was close work attended with any inconvenience whatever ; the pupils were normal. The headache, dulness, &c., had quite disappeared.

iv. Moreover I saw a boy, aged 9, who had been attacked on the 16th of April with violent symptoms and with great swelling of the external glands of the neck. At the end of three weeks he had recovered, but was still feeble. About a fortnight later the lesion of speech was observed ; little complaint was made as to vision. Meanwhile he was and continued weak, and about a month after his illness it was observed that he began to run badly. On the 9th of June I find him a pale, emaciated boy, with sunken eyes, somewhat hanging under jaw, unhealthy complexion, and a painful expression of countenance. His gait is tottering ; in running he often falls on his knees, and then finds difficulty in rising up again. For the last three days, too, he could not turn in bed ; he had to be raised in order to be placed upon his side. At the same time he complains of pain in the forehead, sometimes also in the neck. All this does not prevent his being very cheerful and gay, running and playing about, nor when among his companions does he think of illness. Nevertheless he finds chewing, and particularly swallowing, especially of solid food, very difficult ; therefore he always wishes to drink with his meals, the morsel invariably goes wrong, the water comes out through his nose, and cough, and sometimes nausea and vomiting, ensue. In fine, he gets but little food into his stomach. His voice is strongly nasal, the rattling accessory sound is almost constantly heard,—in a word the lesion is the same as that above described at length, and the limited movement of the palate testifies of a semiparalytic condition.—His power of accommodation is less interfered with than was the case with the other patients. He sees well at a distance, and his nearest point lies at 6″. It ought to lie at 4″ or 3·5″.

Stress was laid upon the necessity for nourishing diet and tonic treatment. General improvement gradually took place. On the 7th of September I received the following favourable report :—" P. v. L. is again at school ; he pronounces *rub*, *head*, and *egg* like an Englishman, no longer totters or falls in running ; all his movements are easy and free ; his appetite is better than it ever was before ; he sees acutely up to 6″ ; there is no nausea whatever."

Of the case, communicated under II., the result was unfortunate. The course of the disease had been violent, and was combined with swelling in both the throat and the salivary glands. The convalescence, nevertheless, appeared to be progressing favourably. Soon, however, the lesion of speech became developed, and shortly afterwards, that of the power of accommodation supervened. In other respects the patient now seemed to be perfectly well. But after I had seen him at Utrecht (compare p. 601) weakness of the limbs set in ; the arms became so powerless that he could neither strip nor dress himself. The emaciation increased, and difficulty of breathing not unfrequently occurred. A first attack of violent dyspnœa subsided favourably. Some weeks later a second followed. In spite of all the stimulating remedies employed, the breathing became rapidly rattling, and the patient died with symptoms of so-called paralysis of the lungs. A post-mortem examination could not be obtained.

Besides those here communicated, I saw a few cases, in which also disturbance of vision had existed, but where the power of accommodation appeared to have already completely returned. It is remarkable that in the epidemic in the village visited by me, all those who had recovered, as it seemed without exception, exhibited paralytic symptoms. Subsequently in other places the mortality was less, and paralysis much more rarely ensued. Nevertheless the number of those who applied to me was upwards of thirty, and in the majority of these the paresis was confined to the palate and to the accommodation. One case I had seen even before those related above. It was that of Miss V., of Weesp, aged twenty, who called upon me for the second time on the 17th of June. Referring to my note-book I read literally:—" Diminution of range of accommodation ; symptoms resembling those of hebetudo ; hypermetropia $= \frac{1}{10}$; she has also had aphonia, has been very hoarse, the cavities of the nose and throat communicate permanently—these symptoms were developed after inflammation of the throat, with great external swelling, without pain, but with fever and distress." In this case, too, I had made experiments as to the pronunciation of different sounds, and as the patient now stated, had found that she had difficulty in pronouncing d, b, and g (in game) at the end of words. But at that time I had not recognised the connexion either between the paralysis of the internal muscles of the eye and of the palate, or between these two and the preceding angina,—and therefore I had retained no distinct recollection of the case. Now she had completely recovered, with respect both to sight and speech. The hypermetropia, too, had given way. Such patients apply, it appears, to the oculist. The knowledge of their cases is, therefore, important to him. About the same time Dr. Fles informed me that he had been called at Utrecht in consultation respecting a boy who, after angina (as it appeared on subsequent investigation, diphtherina) was attacked with paralysis of the palate and of the muscles of accommodation, together with incomplete ptosis and strabismus divergens, all indicating paralysis of the oculo-motor nerve; at the same time, want of power of the limbs, and of the cervical and masticating muscles, had occurred. Only the debility of the muscles of the limbs remained ; the other symptoms of paresis had again disappeared.

Among the cases which afterwards occurred to me there were many in which the angina ran its course without important symptoms, several in which the angina was not recognised as diphtheria, and yet the subsequent paresis of accommodation left, I am convinced, no doubt upon the subject. In this we have a hint to the physician, to make an accurate inspection in every case of angina, even when the symptoms appear to be of slight importance. And let the oculist, on his part, never neglect, in paresis of accommodation, to inquire whether angina has preceded the attack or not. It is important for him to ascertain this, both in a prognostic and in a thera-

peutic point of view.   As to the former, it is favourable; for in all
the cases which occurred to me, recovery ensued, in one instance, not
until ten months after the attack of angina, general debility, too,
remaining all that time.   We must not, however, conceal the fact,
that besides the case given above, a second, as we were informed, ended
fatally two or three months after the attack.

The proximate cause of this paresis after diphtheria has not been
satisfactorily explained.   Besides the contagious character, which in
this first epidemic might appear most distinctly, and was also quite
clear to me, the subsequent paralytic symptoms also show especially,
that the so-called angina is a general disease, and we may suppose that the altered blood-crasis has excited a secondary morbid
process in the central organ, which becomes the cause of the paralytic symptoms : pathological anatomy must decide the question.
Besides, the supposition of Bretonneau deserves consideration, who
looks upon the paralysis as a secondary symptom of the morbid
poisoning, to be compared with the secondary phenomena of syphilis.
It is certainly remarkable, that since strong cauterisation of the
white spots in the throat has been generally adopted, the ratio of
mortality has become more favourable, and the consecutive paresis
has been of rarer occurrence—as if the absorption of the matters
formed in the local process was in truth injurious.

I closed my original essay with the following words :—" As to the
treatment of the paralysis after angina diphtheritica, little can as yet
be said.   In every typical deviation, which we encounter for the first
time, *reason* is our guide.   It appeared here to recommend tonics—
of which, in general, our age has need.   Has experience also as yet
expressed any opinion?   I would not venture to assert it.   It has,
however, been found, that with nourishing diet (to ensure which,
under the existing difficulty of chewing and swallowing, double care
must be taken), combined with tonic medicines, complete recovery
has, in the great majority of cases, been the result."   Now I may
add that these inferences have been fully confirmed by later cases.
Under the use of sulphate of quina combined (the digestive organs
being in a normal state) with small doses of sulphuric acid, sometimes also of preparations of iron, and with due attention to nutri-
tious diet, the lesion almost invariably gave way within a couple of
months.

The phenomena of paresis after diphtheria have been ascribed to
general debility.   This explanation appears to me to be unsatisfactory :

the very circumstance, that, besides the soft palate, frequently only the accommodation and the sphincter iridis have suffered, must lead us to suspect the existence of a special process. It is true that after considerable loss of blood, and after exhausting diseases, the accommodation is often seriously affected, that then in the slightest degrees of hypermetropia, and even in emmetropia, symptoms of asthenopia are not unfrequent; but in such cases the whole muscular system also exhibits a proportionate condition of debility. After diphtheria, on the contrary, we often observe the want of proportion in this respect. If individuals are sometimes weak, there are others who feel perfectly well, have resumed their work and run for hours, while the paresis of accommodation continues. They complain of nothing else than lesion of vision, and for it apply to the oculist. Further information we can expect only from anatomical investigation, the opportunity for which, fortunately, rarely presents itself.

CHAPTER XII.

SPASM OF ACCOMMODATION.

§ 48. MYOTICS AND MYOSIS.

THE year just elapsed has put us in possession of a myotic, which immediately proved itself an able opponent of the best mydriatics. It is the *ordeal bean* of old Calabar, obtained from the *Physostigma venenosum* (Balfour), belonging to the Leguminosæ. This remedy has at once superseded all myotics, before tried or recommended as such. The preparations so far known, and sent to me are—a dark brown alcoholic extract, two sorts of paper, brown and violet (prepared according to Streatfeild's method), and two solutions of the extract in glycerine, a weaker c and a stronger c'. On the last we read—" 1 Minim equal to 4 grains of Bean."

Among the principal phenomena observed after the application of these agents to the conjunctiva, *contraction of the pupil and spasm of accommodation* are the most prominent.

The first effect, immediately after the application, is a brief irritation; upon this, after the lapse of four minutes, slight spasms supervene in the lower eyelid. The contraction of the pupil, and almost simultaneously, the spasm of accommodation now follow.

The *contraction*, after a sufficient dose ($\frac{1}{4}$ drop of c', diluted or not with water), commences after from five to ten minutes, attains its maximum after from thirty to forty minutes, at which it remains only a short time, diminishes slowly after three hours, and disappears entirely in from two to four days, occasionally being replaced even by some dilatation. The whole process is, therefore, more rapid than that of the effect of atropia, probably in consequence of a greater power of imbibition. The subjoined Figures 170 and 171 (compare those of the action of atropia at pp. 585 and 586) indicate the course of the contraction in Mr. Hamer. Fig. 170 extends over two hours; Fig. 171 over three days. The action was moderately strong, and was almost painless. The pupil I measured with the ophthalmometer, always with equal illumination, and I directed the whole investigation.

Fig. 170.

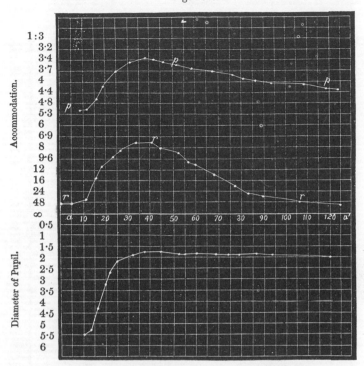

With respect to the contraction and the phenomena connected with it the following are to be noted :—

  a. The diameter of the pupil becomes still less (from 1½ to 2 mm.) than, in the normal condition, with the strongest light which can be borne and with the most powerful accommodation (von Graefe).

  b. The influence of the light does not, however, cease: one can easily observe in himself particularly the consensual contraction, employing the entoptic method, by closing and opening the other eye (compare p. 197), as von Graefe also did.   The movements are slow ; the consensual contraction lasts three, the consensual dilatation lasts four, seconds (compare p. 573).   Moreover, the pupil at the same time often appears to be somewhat angular.   It is in the middle like a crape, and has a tolerably sharply circumscribed, more strongly illuminated diffuse border (Fig. 172 A), which on consensual contraction is broader (B), and has a dark-green tint, while the

2

middle of the surface appears yellow.   (In the entoptic observation

Fig. 171.

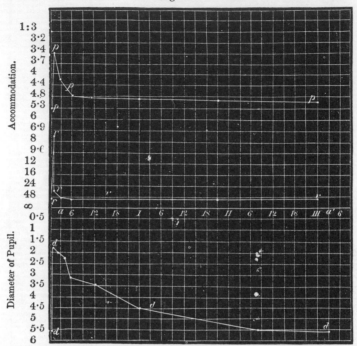

the figure is seen inverted, but it is here (Fig. 172) inverted, and therefore gives the true form of the pupil for the left eye).

c. Especially in the commencement of the contraction involuntary spasmodic vibrations occur in the diameter of the pupil.

d. The illumination of objects is feeble, with an unusual brownish tint (Bowman). The effect is similar to that of solar eclipses, in which, notwithstanding sunshine with its usual strongly contrasting shadows, the light is unusually feeble. If the instillation has been performed on only one eye, the great difference in illumination is best seen on doubling the image by a prism (compare p. 133).

e. The circles of diffusion of a point of light, situated beyond the distance of distinct vision, become less the smaller the pupil is, and vision therefore becomes much less diffuse beyond the limits of accommodation.

f. After the disappearance of the myosis the pupil sometimes becomes somewhat larger than before.

Fig. 172.

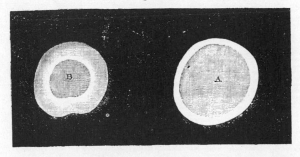

The *spasm of accommodation* appears from the altered position both of the farthest (Figs. 170 and 171 *r r*) and of the nearest (*p p*) point of distinct vision, drawn above the absciss *a a'*. The said curves exhibit the whole course of both. We have, moreover, to note the following :—

a. In the determination of the farthest point clonic spasms of accommodation alternately arise, so that objects appear with the same glass (at a distance) alternately distinct and diffused. Now the points of the curve *r r* correspond to the moments of relaxation. In an hour after the employment of the myotic, the accommodation is again completely under control. The curve *r r* shows further, that with a moderate dose, pain being virtually absent, the farthest point has still approached the eye from 56″ to 7″·3, that is to nearly two-thirds of the absolute range of accommodation, originally present.

b. The determination of the nearest point was effected with the aid of the most perfect optometrical instruments. The course of the points, as shown by these, is very satisfactory. In an earlier experiment of Mr. Hamer the action, after the application of a piece of Calabar paper too strongly impregnated, was much more violent, the painful spasms lasted more than six hours, and the pain increased so much on endeavouring to accommodate, that the idea of determining the nearest point was given up.

c. The figures show that, with *diminution* of the action, the range of accommodation is absolutely increased, most considerably after about 100 minutes (Fig. 170), and that this increase diminishes only slowly (Fig. 171). In a previous investigation an increased range of accommodation was found also at the commencement of the action, the influence on the nearest point being in the first period greater than on the farthest. In the observation represented by Fig. 170, rather the opposite took place.

d. The great effect upon the accommodation with slight impulse of the will is very important. This is still strongly felt when the farthest point has again returned nearly to its original position : 105 minutes after the application, the point of distinct vision lay, with convergence to 10″, for the right eye naturally at 10″; for the left, on the contrary, at 4‴·5, thus nearly attaining the absolute nearest point ; after the lapse of three hours and a-half, the said point lay, with similar convergence, at 5″·6 ; after nearly seven hours, at 6″·2 ; after rather more than eleven hours at 8″·3 ;—and so long as the range of accommodation remained greater in the left eye, some difference in accommodation continued perceptible also with equal convergence of the two eyes. (It was determined, what negative glass the eye which had undergone instillation must have before it, in order, in looking at 10″ and with rapid alternation pushing the hand before each of the eyes, to obtain equal sharpness of letters and of optometer-wires.) The relative accommodation has, therefore, approached to that of hypermetropes : much accommodation with slight convergence,—the reverse of what is met with under the influence of atropia.

e. In the condition described under *d*, the determination of the nearest point with horizontal and vertical lines presents more difference than usual (Bowman). This apparently exalted astigmatism is certainly in part dependent on the greater difference in refraction with difference of convergence (compare p. 451).

f. So long as with a given tension accommodation takes place for a shorter distance than usual, objects appear larger (macropia), just as in the opposite case (compare p. 587) they appear smaller (micropia).

g. The increased refraction on relaxation usually lasts in any perceptible degree only an hour. With a very large dose, which produces persistent and violent pain, it may last many hours. With a small dose considerable contraction of the pupil, without any very perceptible influence on the accommodation, might be obtained.

Finally, it remains to be stated : that, according to von Graefe, 1° the acuteness of vision sometimes diminishes, particularly in the period of development of the spasm, probably in consequence of insufficient stability of accommodation, in any case, independently of the want of light from constriction of the pupil; 2° that, also in defect of the iris, the influence on refraction and accommodation remains the same.

The action of Calabar is not equally great *in all animals*. In this respect it presents much analogy to Belladonna, inasmuch as in man, and moreover in the dog and cat, a high degree of myosis is obtained, even with small doses, while in the rabbit, as in birds, and especially in amphibious animals and fishes, a slighter effect is observed. With a stronger dose too, than we can employ in man, still stronger myosis is obtained in these (von Graefe). Immobility of the pupil we could not obtain.

With respect to the *mode of action*, similar experiments lead to a like conclusion as in the case of mydriatics. As to transition into the aqueous humour, however, von Graefe could not directly satisfy himself from the myotic action on instillation into the eye of another animal.—After repeated strong application, however, it succeeds, if the discharged fluid is long kept in contact with the eye into which it is dropped.

We have also been specially engaged in the investigation of the question, *by the intervention of what nerves* the Calabar acts.

It is quite evident that spasm of the m. sphincter pupillæ ensues. Indeed the high degree of contraction renders paralysis of the dilator muscle alone insufficient to explain it; and the increased refraction, in which a more powerful action of the muscles of accommodation is included, puts altogether beyond doubt a spasmodic contraction of the sphincter pupillæ, as being governed by the same nerve as the ciliary muscle, and associated with it in its action: moreover, according to our experiments upon rabbits, after division, both of the sympathetic nerve and of the trigeminus, the contraction of the pupil under the influence of Calabar still increases considerably. The nerve alluded to is the oculo-motor nerve, and, more especially, the short root, which this nerve sends to the ciliary ganglion. It is opposed to our idea of the similar nature of all nerve-fibres, that a particular substance, as Calabar, should have on some fibres a paralysing, on others a stimulating, and still more a tonic stimulating, influence. Consequently, in this case also, we prefer to assume (compare p. 590) an action upon specific nerve-cells present in the eye itself. With a stimulated condition of this internal ciliary system, however, as we have seen, increased action, both voluntary and reflex, is not excluded, —quite analogous to the effect of strychnia upon voluntary muscles.

It is not so easy to show, how far the Calabar exercises upon the
dilator muscle also the opposite influence of atropia. In the first
place, it certainly does not give rise to complete paralysis of this
muscle; for after long and repeated application of Calabar, stimulation of the sympathetic nerve in rabbits and in dogs always
still produced some dilatation of the pupil. We performed,
among others, the following experiment:—the nervus trigeminus
was divided on the left side,—insensibility of the eye and contraction of the pupil ensued; the cervical sympathetic nerve of
the same side was three times stimulated,—each time there was
dilatation of the pupil; it was then divided,—the pupil appeared still
more contracted than before the stimulation; in both eyes Calabar ($\frac{1}{3}$
drop of c') was long kept in contact,—after eight minutes there was
incipient, at the end of fifteen minutes there was the strongest contraction, greater on the left side; after the lapse of eighteen minutes
there were spasms of the extremities, difficulty of breathing, impend-
ing suffocation; artificial respiration was kept up,—four minutes later
death ensued with slight spasms of the limbs; the sympathetic was
again irritated,—dilatation of the pupil still invariably followed.
Thus, after slow death, in consequence of poisoning by the instillation of Calabar, the sympathetic nerve in the eye is still excitable.
Consonant to this is the fact, that on division of the cervical sympathetic nerve, before or after the employment of Calabar on both
sides, the pupil appears smaller on the side on which the nerve is
divided.—We supposed that the action of Calabar, in cases of
paralysis of the oculo-motor nerve, would elucidate the question still
farther. In different quarters it was observed that this paralysis did
not prevent the myotic action. In a first case, in which, in the ordinary investigation, the pupil appeared absolutely immovable, some
mobility was still seen, under strong incident light, in observation
with the ophthalmometer: the paralysis was therefore not complete,
and we consequently desisted from an investigation which promised
no certain result. In a second case, in a lady aged 32, there was
absolute paralysis of the whole right oculo-motor nerve, which had
set in gradually six weeks previously, after repeated complaints of
headache for four years, often combined with erysipelas of the right
half of the face; in this instance the strongest incident light on one
or both eyes gave no appearance of contraction on this side. The
Calabar employed (the extract), however, produced contraction,
as strong as usual, as the subjoined figure (173) shows, and at
the same time somewhat increased refraction. Now, we were disap-

pointed in so far as this *considerable* contraction teaches nothing respecting the influence of the sympathetic nerve; for evidently

Fig. 173.

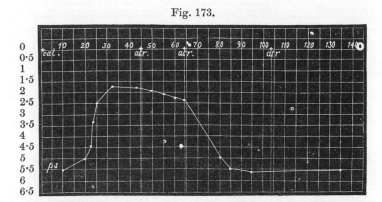

spasm of the sphincter muscle is at the same time in operation. But such local spasm, where there is complete paralysis of the trunk of the oculo-motor nerve, is still an important phenomenon : in the first place, because it confirms the fact that the Calabar acts by direct contact ; and in the second place, because this action cannot well be imagined to occur otherwise than by the intervention of a ganglionic-cell-containing centre in the eye.—Meanwhile it is, on other grounds, more than probable, that Calabar, if it does not paralyse, at least lowers the action of the sympathetic nerve. When, in fact, by a moderate action of Calabar, the accommodation is brought at most by half into tonic tension, the pupil is already narrower than with intense light and strong accommodation; and this half takes place without the sphincter, which continues sensitive for reflex and accommodative impulses, attaining the maximum of its action : consequently, without diminished action of the dilator, such strong contraction is not explicable. The circumstance, too, that the contraction of the pupil continues for a few days in so much a higher degree than the spasm of accommodation, is in favour of a diminished action of the radial fibres, and consequently of a lowering influence of the Calabar upon the sympathetic nerve.

There was no evidence of a special action on the trigeminus and on the vaso-motor nerves of the iris ; we observed only that on the side on which the trigeminus was divided, the action of Calabar was not less distinct than on the other side.

The struggle between atropia and Calabar, when applied simultaneously, or soon after one another, is remarkable. When applied together, some contraction of the pupil and spasm of accommodation first occur, as the effect of Calabar. The spasm of accommodation still continues, when the action of the atropia on the iris gains the upper hand, and the pupil consequently becomes wider. Von Graefe in particular has investigated how, when employed consecutively to the action of atropia, that of Calabar may become intercalated. He showed that in weak action of atropia, and in the period of diminution of its strong action, Calabar is capable of temporarily constricting the pupil and increasing the refraction, and that after the giving way of these phenomena, the more tedious atropia-process again follows its regular course. We were particularly desirous to ascertain whether, with absolute atropia-paralysis of the sphincter and of the muscles of accommodation, a powerful employment of Calabar still has influence; and this, in fact, we most distinctly found to be the case, observing, moreover, that this influence was still greater upon the refraction and accommodation, than upon the

Fig. 174.

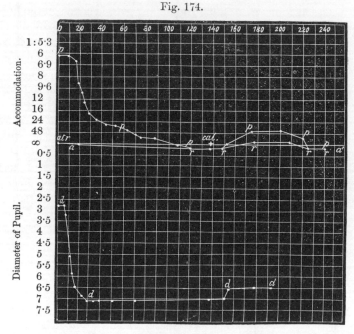

diameter of the pupil. Fig. 174, an observation on the eye of Mr.

Müller, surgeon in the navy, furnishes an example of this : according to the cross, on the absciss $a\,a'$, 137 minutes after the application of atropia, while p and r coincided and the mydriasis had attained its maximum, Calabar was dropped in,—and ten minutes later the refraction ascends $(r\,r)$, accommodation is again present $(p\,p)$, and at the same time the diameter of the pupil is a little diminished.   In a second, likewise very practised observer (Mr. van Leent, surgeon in the navy), the effect of Calabar was on the first day, and particularly on the second day, after the renewed application of atropia, much stronger still.   Notwithstanding that the pupil contracted only slightly, he could each time, after some rest, read for a few moments No. 1½ of Snellen's test-types at 12″; and the nearest point was, in fact, determined at about from 14″ to 16″, while, on relaxation, his usual slight hypermetropia had given way to emmetropia. After the cessation of the action of the Calabar, that of the atropia was in these three accurately investigated cases, after fourteen days or longer, still recognisable from the wider pupil, —in itself a proof that the mydriatic had been strongly applied. Hence it appears, that the paralysis, produced by a specific agent, may be overcome by the effect of another specific agent, even in such a way that voluntary action again becomes possible.

The subjoined Figure 175 indicates the influence of atropia on the

Fig. 175.

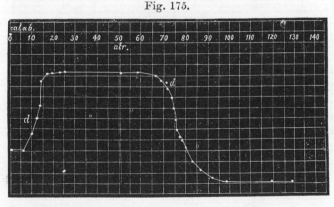

pupil, fifty minutes after the employment of Calabar : the complete dilatation of the pupil is produced evidently somewhat more slowly. Rather more than three hours later Calabar is again dropped in in the same person (Dr. Land).   The existing hypermetropia of $\frac{1}{60}$ entirely gives way, for a short time spasmodic myopia occurs, and with convergence undoubtedly accommodation, which, however, just as in the previous cases, is not perfectly under control, and after a few moments becomes fatigued. The pupil at the same time becomes somewhat narrower = 6·75. On the following day H is again = $\frac{1}{60}$; the pupil is somewhat movable. After seven days the pupil = 6·35; it is not until the seventeenth day that both pupils are equal, = 4·37— thus less than at the commencement.

On the discovery of the physiological action of Calabar, it followed as a matter of course that this agent should be tried in various anomalies. In the first place, it is found to be useful to lessen the inconvenience of atropia-mydriasis; and according to v. Graefe the atropia process may be shortened by a systematic employment of the Calabar. How far it may lead to cure, or at least afford permanent benefit in paralysis of accommodation and in mydriasis, in which its use had already been suggested by Robertson, experience only can decide. But it is certainly important, that in ordinary paralysis of accommodation, whether self-existing, or connected with further paralysis of the oculo-motor nerve (in cerebral mydriasis the effect of Calabar is found to be entirely absent), the pupil is contracted and the refraction is increased by Calabar: in a case of unilateral paresis of accommodation which occurred to me, and which very much interfered with binocular vision, the inconvenience was completely removed by a glycerine solution diluted with eight parts of water, used once daily. Thus, too, the myosis connected with the weak action of Calabar, may often be useful in many cases where a stenopæic apparatus improves the sight (compare pp. 128 et. seq.), as in diffusion of light (opacities of the cornea, &c.), in irregular astigmatism (keratoconus, luxation of the lens, &c.); (compare pp. 553 et. seq.), further in aphakia, especially when the plane of the pupil is not clear. The improvement of the acuteness of vision in ordinary ametropia is indeed remarkable: precisely with very weak action of Calabar myopes distinguish much more accurately at a distance, and hypermetropes, under the double advantage of smaller circles of diffusion and of easier tension of accommodation, lose for a time their asthenopia.—The great question, which practice has to answer is, whether Calabar is permanently as harmless* for accommodation as atropia is, and whether the conjunctiva will permanently bear its repeated application. Until these points are decided, the future of Calabar in therapeutics cannot be foretold.

I have now to add only, that v. Graefe has advantageously applied the contraction of the pupil in glaucoma, in order to facilitate the performance of iridectomy, and that in his opinion the alternating action of Calabar may probably contribute to tear synechiæ.

The want of an efficient myotic was long felt in ophthalmic surgery. But the longer it was unsupplied, the feebler must the hope of finding such have become. It is true that all myotic action could not be denied to the agents which were formerly placed in this category: Semen Santonicum (Himly), Daphne Mezereum (Hahnemann), Nicotiana Tabacum (Heise), Aconitum Napellus, Secale Cornutum, &c.; but their stimulating action was in itself sufficient to forbid their employment in practice. The same conclusion was arrived at by myself with Dr. Kuyper (*l. c.*) in a systematic investigation with respect to nicotin, conia, extract of aconite, and digitaline; and Ad. Weber (*Verhandlungen der von 3 bis 6 September*, 1859, *in Heidelberg versammelten Augenärzte*, Berlin, 1860) had to pay the penalty of an attack of keratitis for an imprudent application of digitaline to his own eye. Fresh tobacco leaves appeared to be somewhat better borne. Finally, a subcutaneous injection of morphia, in which von Graefe (*Deutsche Klinik*, 20 April, 1861) discovered a tolerably powerful agent, not only for contracting the pupil, but also for increasing the refraction, was also certainly inapplicable to this special object.—In the Calabar the wished-for agent appears to have been bestowed upon us. The general effect of this ordeal Bean had already been studied by Dr. Daniell (1846), and more fully by Christison (1855); van Hasselt had also (1856) found myosis to be a principal symptom in its general action, when Thomas Fraser (*Diss. inaug.*, defended at Edinburgh on the 31st July, 1862) discovered that its local application contracts the pupil, and Dr. Argyll Robertson (*Edinburgh Medico-Chirurgical Society*, 4th February, 1863), pointed out its influence on accommodation, and introduced the Calabar as a new remedy into ophthalmological practice. Upon this followed investigations by Harley (conf. *Med. Times and Gazette*, 20th June, 1863), especially with respect to its general action, with some additional remarks by Hulke; moreover by Bowman and by Soelberg Wells (*Medical Times and Gazette*, 16th May, 1863); lastly, by von Graefe (*Deutsche Klinik*, 1863, No. 29, and *Archiv f. Ophthalmologie*, B. ix.), Hamer (*Geneeskundig Tijdschrift*, July, 1863), Rosenthal (*Archiv f. Anatomie und Physiologie*, Jahrgang, 1863), and Schelske (*Klinische Monatsblätter f. Augenheilkunde*, 1863, p. 380); and, in concert with Mr. Hamer, I have continued them. Our object was, rather by the accuracy than by the number of our experiments, in following up the previous valuable investigations, somewhat to increase our knowledge of this remarkable agent. The principal results of our researches are comprised in the foregoing pages.

§ 49. Spasm of Accommodation.—Myosis.—Painful Accommodation.

We have to distinguish different forms of spasm of accommodation. That which most frequently occurs is nothing else than an
exalted tone of the muscles concerned in the latter function. In
healthy emmetropic eyes this tone is, keeping in view the extremely
slight diminution of refraction in atropia-paralysis, undoubtedly very
trifling. On the other hand, we have in hypermetropia found a permanent tension, which wholly or partially conceals the abnormal condition : it can exist only in virtue of the accommodation, and must therefore be destroyed by the paralysing influence of the atropia. The increased tension is here the natural result of the persistent effort to overcome the existing anomaly of refraction. In amblyopes and astigmatics
where the same sometimes occurs, it is explicable by the constant endeavour, in accommodating for the nearest point, to see the smaller
objects under a greater angle. It is less evident, how myopes also
acquire a tonic spasm of their accommodation. That this not unfrequently occurs, especially when the eyes are in a state of irritation,
we have already observed. Dr. Fles now informs me, and I readily
believe it, that he met with this condition in many cases in young
persons, especially in boys, who had been prepared for an examination at one of the military schools. Partly irritation of the eye,
reflected on the accommodating system, partly excessive tension
of accommodation during the constant work, particularly with defective light, may be the cause of it. It is invariably the paralysis by
atropia which reveals its existence. In young children under these
circumstances, I have seen slight degrees of myopia give way even to
hypermetropia, so extremely sensitive is their play of accommodation.

The tonic spasm of which we have here been speaking, seldom
acquires much pathological importance. In myopia we must attend
only to the accompanying symptoms of irritation; in hypermetropia
we must recognise it, in order to direct the optical treatment
accordingly.

We must here once more remind the reader, that von Graefe, where
there was an attempt to relax the accommodation, thinks that he has
sometimes established the existence of an involuntarily exalted, and
therefore spasmodic, action (compare p. 351), and that some very
slightly myopic persons, who endeavoured without a negative glass to

see the fundus oculi in the non-inverted image, have complained to me of something similar.

Of the acute occurrence of myopia, in which the idea of spasm of accommodation naturally suggests itself, we find some examples related by the earlier writers, which Ruete* has collected. I am, however, not convinced that, in these instances, anything else than amblyopia had occurred. When in consequence of the latter, smaller objects, as for example letters, could be distinguished only when near, the existence of near-sightedness was often inferred. Generally speaking, among the earlier observations, the determination of the farthest point of distinct vision, whereby nevertheless alone the presence of myopia could with certainty be proved, is omitted. Acute spasm of accommodation, such as, for example, is produced by Calabar, is undoubtedly very rare. I myself have never met with a clear case of it, and this may excuse my scepticism. My task is confined to quoting those few cases which afford satisfactory evidence. Von Graefe † communicates two of them.

The first is that of an engineer, in whom the right cornea had been injured by the finger-nail of a child. When the irritation consequent thereon had, after some days, wholly subsided, the patient saw indistinctly with this eye, and small objects were multiplied. The pupil was of normal diameter, with slow and slight reflex-, and without accommodative movement. At the precise distance of distinct vision the polyopia had disappeared. Accommodation was almost entirely lost, and the eye was, at the same time myopic: with the naked eye the patient was accommodated for $3\frac{1}{4}''$, with $-\frac{1}{6}$ for $8''$, with $\frac{1}{10}$ for $2\frac{1}{3}''$. The left eye had the usual range of accommodation, and was about emmetropic: with $\frac{1}{10}$ vision ranged from $3''$ to $9\frac{1}{2}''$.—The patient had often previously satisfied himself that both eyes were equal. Cure ensued, and indeed very rapidly, after Heurteloupian abstractions of blood: after the first the eye accommodated from $3\frac{1}{2}''$ to $5\frac{1}{4}''$; after the second, from $4''$ to $8\frac{1}{2}''$; after the third the accommodation was nearly equal to that of the other eye, whose nearest point lay at about $4\frac{3}{4}''$.

Perhaps this affection is to be considered, as von Graefe says, as a reflex neurosis, in like manner as injuries of sensory nerves sometimes excite tonic spasms in ordinary voluntary muscles.

The second case is that of a girl aged 18, with painful spasm of the

---

* Ruete, *Pathologie und Physiologie der Augen und Ohren*, p. 262.
† *Archiv f. Ophthalmologie*, B. ii. H. 2, p. 304.

orbicular muscle [of the right side], which on tension of the eyelids, and also sometimes spontaneously, became more violent. Pressure on the supra-orbital nerve had no effect, a slight pressure on the facial nerve increased the pain and the spasm, strong pressure lessened both. A brief improvement, after the application of leeches, was followed by aggravation of the symptoms, with disturbance of vision. The refraction appeared to be increased, and the accommodation to be very limited, namely from $2\frac{3}{4}''$ to $3\frac{1}{4}''$. The right pupil was somewhat narrower than the left, with slight reflex-, and without any accommodative movement. The left eye was normal. The endermic employment of sulphate of atropia behind the ear was at first followed by no improvement; but, on the contrary, the same condition in all respects was developed also in the left eye. When, on the third day, belladonna-symptoms arose, the spasm and pain diminished, and on increase of the intoxication they entirely ceased, and the patient could accommodate with the right eye from $5\frac{1}{2}''$ to $14\frac{1}{4}''$, with the left from $5\frac{1}{2}''$ to $17''$. However the symptoms returned when the employment of atropia was suspended. The result of the case is not communicated.

Von Graefe sees in this case a combination of spasm of the muscles of accommodation (oculomotor nerve), with neurosis of the facial nerve, in which it is important that, although we cannot admit the existence of any connexion between the nerves mentioned, the affection increased and diminished *pari passu* in both.

A third case was described by Liebreich.*

Miss F., aged 21, complained of dazzling before the left eye; fatigue on exertion and nearsightedness had set in a year before after constant work, often continued at night. On examination it was found that with parallel visual lines, sight was acute at a distance with $-\frac{1}{40}$, but that with commencing convergence, such strong accommodation supervened, that she then needed even stronger negative glasses to see acutely in the point of convergence, until finally, at the distance of $6''$ both eyes could distinguish sharply without glasses. As the existence of spasm of accommodation was hence inferred, atropia was repeatedly dropped in, in consequence of which the myopia gave way to hypermetropia $= \frac{1}{24}$. Meanwhile it appeared further, that the convergence was difficult, the possible divergence particularly great, while other symptoms indicated insufficiency of the mm. recti interni. The spasm of accommodation might be connected herewith; but still it was determined first to suppress this with atropia in both eyes, and the employment of the remedy was continued for fourteen days. When the accommodation had subsequently returned, the patient seemed to have recovered: the spasm had altogether given way, and even with glasses of $\frac{1}{25}$, which were prescribed for her, distant and near objects were acutely seen, and work was continued without fatigue.

---

* *Archiv f. Ophthalmologie*, B. viii. H. 2, p. 259.

It was evident that in this case the insufficiency of the mm. recti interni had not been the immediate cause of the asthenopia. But might not the spasm of accommodation, with the long-continued excessive tension, have been produced by the effort to overcome that insufficiency? It is extremely remarkable how accurately the spasm observed in this case agrees with that excited by Calabar: by it too the refraction is increased, and convergence gives a relatively too strong tension of accommodation. The diameter of the pupil is not given.

The cases here communicated may suffice to illustrate the different forms of spasm of accommodation.

We have still to speak briefly of pain with tension of accommodation, which is probably combined also with spasm. At p. 289 I have already communicated a case of this nature. I may be allowed here shortly to relate two others.

Mrs. O., aged 29, called upon me in October, 1859, complaining of violent pain in the eye on any effort to see near objects, which had already existed in a greater or less degree for more than ten years. She had a flat face and shallow anterior chamber of the eye. The pupils were small, but movable. The nearest point lay at 11″, the farthest at ∞ ; upon artificial mydriasis, H appeared $= \frac{1}{16}$. The acuteness of vision was normal. I gave her glasses of $\frac{1}{16}$, believing that after the return of the accommodation she would be able to work with them at a distance.—Some time after she called upon me again. Her state had continued the same, and the spectacles had been of no use to her. Other glasses were tried, but with no better result. A derivative treatment was also adopted quite in vain. I determined then to have atropia dropped in for some time, in order to counteract all tension of accommodation, and I permitted her to wear light blue glasses of $\frac{1}{16}$, and to use $\frac{1}{7}$ for near objects. Repeatedly, after one month, two months, &c., it was tried whether the mydriatic could be omitted. The results of these trials were unfavorable. But at the end of six months, she observed with joy, that leaving off the use of atropia, with the return of accommodation, reading without glasses, she was free from pain. She now, moreover, occupied herself at close work with glasses of $\frac{1}{16}$.—When after a year-and-half, a relapse occurred, the employment of atropia for three months was again sufficient to overcome the painful spasm.

In this case, the pain is much more prominent than spasmodic contraction. But what suggests the idea of the latter, is the whole latency of the hypermetropia, with comparatively slight range of accommodation. At the time of the relapse the patient was at Dresden, and she consulted me by letter. I should have been glad then to have examined her anew, particularly in order to satisfy myself still further respecting the relative range of accommodation.

40

A second case of this nature was that of a friend of mine, who had held an important office in the East Indies, in which he had to work hard and to make observations with optical instruments. During his observations, he for the first time felt pain, which made him cautious. His state was considered to be hyperæmia of the retina. On reading and in calculating his observations the pain increased. Examination now showed, that after the use of atropia, hypermetropia $= \frac{1}{24}$ existed. At first weak, afterwards strong convex glasses were given, quite in vain. Derivants, leeches, and Heurteloup's artificial leeches were tried, with equal want of success. Reading for a few minutes produced a degree of pain, which compelled him to desist. This state had already lasted for a-year and a-half, and his return to his native country was spoken of. But it occurred to those about him, that they might first consult me by letter, for which purpose both the patient and his oculist, formerly a pupil of mine, sent me a very detailed report, dated the 15th February, 1861. My advice was :—for a time to employ sulphate of atropia (1 : 120) at least twice a-week, and meanwhile during the paralysis of accommodation thus obtained, to make vision at different distances possible by means of different convex glasses. Some months later I received the report, that " the atropia treatment had instantly afforded the best results. Hope revives in me," thus wrote the patient, " that we shall overcome the malady. In the morning I can already work tolerably steadily. In the evening, reading or writing inconveniences me less, but I do not yet venture upon it, in order not to retard the progress of my recovery. Your suspicion that my hypermetropia might be more than $\frac{1}{24}$ is not confirmed ; every time we get the same result. I now use $\frac{1}{24}$ for distance, $\frac{1}{16}$ when sitting at table, and $\frac{1}{11}$ when at work. These numbers are, however, ' nominal '—(N.B. They are the numbers of Paetz and Flohr, compare p. 142), and are too great :

$$\frac{1}{24} \text{ is, properly speaking, } \frac{1}{22} ;$$

$$\frac{1}{16} \qquad ,, \qquad ,, \qquad \frac{1}{14} ;$$

$$\frac{1}{11} \qquad ,, \qquad ,, \qquad \frac{1}{9 \cdot 5}.$$

This last is still too weak when I have just dropped in atropia ; then I have $\frac{1}{9 \cdot 5}$ and $\frac{1}{22}$ as equivalent to $\frac{1}{7}$." Thus my friend wrote to me (and, as is evident, he was master of the subject), on the 31st of August, 1861. The hopeful expectation he expressed was fully justified by the result. When, after a first disappointment, the use of atropia was, a few months later, for the second time suspended, the pain on tension of accommodation did not return, and, so far as I am aware, no disturbance whatever has since recurred in making observations, reading, writing, or calculating.

This case scarcely needs any comment. It shows that in slight degrees of H a condition may be developed by continued tension, in which the least accommodation for near objects becomes very painful. Spectacles are then of no use, because with the convergence involuntary accommodation is combined, and this again excites the pain. The above-quoted observation of Liebreich has suggested to me the possibility, that in these cases, just as in Liebreich's, tension of accommodation too strong in proportion to the convergence sets in. Spasm of accommodation would then really exist.

NOTE.

From time to time cases occur of extremely contracted pupil, myosis, without established modification of accommodation. Usually it exists in both eyes, and, as Mackenzie says, the small, black, round pupil is at the same time " slow in its motions, scarcely dilating in the dark, and with belladonna." In the highest degrees not only does the acuteness of vision suffer from want of sufficient light, but the field of vision is also limited by the thickness of the margin of the iris,—in any case it is peripherally very dark.

Even Plenck (*De morbis oculorum*, 1777, p. 120) distinguished two forms : myosis *spastica* and myosis *paralytica*. Theoretically, in fact, both spasm of the sphincter, and paralysis of the dilator may give rise to myosis. Now it is to be expected, that with spasm of the sphincter, the accommodation should often be affected, which is less to be anticipated with paralysis of the dilator. A case probably of paralytic nature has been recorded by Dr. Felix v. Willebrand (*Archiv für Ophthalmologie*, B. I. i. p. 319), in which the cause of the myosis was sought in pressure on, and paralysis of the sympathetic nerve by masses of swollen lymphatic glands in the neck, with the diminution of which, under the use of mercurial ointment with iodide of potassium, and of warm alkaline baths, the myosis and the disturbance of vision depending on it gave way. To this class, too, a case of myosis appears to belong, communicated by Dr. Gairdner to the Medico-Chirurgical Society of Edinburgh (see 'Monthly Journal of Medicine,' vol. xx. p. 71, 1855), in which an aneurism of the subclavian artery may be supposed to have compressed and paralysed the sympathetic nerve in the neck. The want of an antagonist might in such cases lead to secondary shortening of the sphincter.—The narrow pupil met with in inflammatory states of the cornea, and in connexion with intolerance of light, must certainly be considered rather as the result of *spasm* of the sphincter muscle. The same is probably true of myosis observed in violent neuralgia of the ophthalmic nerve (Ruete, *Lehrbuch der Ophthalmologie*, 1853, B. i. p. 328), particularly of that which occurs with a violent attack of prosopalgia, only on the affected side, of which my colleague Prof. Loncq has related two cases to me. It will be important, in the occurrence of such cases, to ascertain with precision how far the accommodation is implicated.

Those cases are still more obscure which are observed to be attended with permanent headache, especially in weak cachectic subjects, with tabes dorsalis (conf. Romberg, *Nervenkrankheiten*, B. i. Abth. 3, p. 684), and with different cerebral affections. More than one instance has occurred to me, where I could discover nothing with respect to the cause.—I think I have remarked, that continued close work, at an advanced time of life, gives rise to permanent contraction of the pupil, and slight degrees of myosis may find their explanation in this fact.

2

INDEX.

Printed by J. W. Roche, 5, Kirby Street, Hatton Garden.